Sturdevant's
Art and Science of
OPERATIVE DENTISTRY

Sixth Edition

Harald O. Heymann, DDS, MEd
Professor
Department of Operative Dentistry
The University of North Carolina
School of Dentistry
Chapel Hill, NC

Edward J. Swift, Jr., DMD, MS
Professor and Chair
Department of Operative Dentistry
The University of North Carolina
School of Dentistry
Chapel Hill, NC

André V. Ritter, DDS, MS
Professor and Graduate Program Director
Department of Operative Dentistry
The University of North Carolina
School of Dentistry
Chapel Hill, NC

ELSEVIER

ELSEVIER
MOSBY

3251 Riverport Lane
St. Louis, Missouri 63043

Sturdevant's Art and Science of Operative Dentistry   ISBN: 978-0-3230-8333-1

Notices

Knowledge and best practice in this field are constantly changing. As new research and experience broaden
our understanding, changes in research methods, professional practices, or medical treatment may become
necessary.

Practitioners and researchers must always rely on their own experience and knowledge in evaluating and
using any information, methods, compounds, or experiments described herein. In using such information
or methods they should be mindful of their own safety and the safety of others, including parties for
whom they have a professional responsibility.

With respect to any drug or pharmaceutical products identified, readers are advised to check the most
current information provided (i) on procedures featured or (ii) by the manufacturer of each product to be
administered, to verify the recommended dose or formula, the method and duration of administration,
and contraindications. It is the responsibility of practitioners, relying on their own experience and
knowledge of their patients, to make diagnoses, to determine dosages and the best treatment for each
individual patient, and to take all appropriate safety precautions.

To the fullest extent of the law, neither the Publisher nor the authors, contributors, or editors, assume
any liability for any injury and/or damage to persons or property as a matter of products liability,
negligence or otherwise, or from any use or operation of any methods, products, instructions, or ideas
contained in the material herein.

Library of Congress Cataloging-in-Publication Data or Control Number
Sturdevant's art and science of operative dentistry.—6th ed. / [edited by] Harald O. Heymann,
Edward J. Swift Jr., Andre V. Ritter.
       p. ; cm.
   Art and science of operative dentistry
   Includes bibliographical references.
   ISBN 978-0-323-08333-1 (hardcover : alk. paper)
   I. Heymann, Harald.   II. Swift, Edward J.   III. Ritter, Andre V.   IV. Sturdevant, Clifford M.
V. Title: Art and science of operative dentistry.
   [DNLM: 1. Dentistry, Operative. WU 300]
   617—dc23

                                                                    2011053083

ISBN: 978-0-3230-8333-1

Vice President and Publisher: Linda Duncan
Executive Editor: John Dolan
Senior Content Developmental Specialist: Courtney Sprehe
Publishing Services Manager: Catherine Jackson
Project Manager: Sara Alsup
Design Direction: Teresa McBryan
Designer: Jessica Williams

Printed in Canada

Last digit is the print number: 9   8   7   6   5   4   3   2   1

Contributors

Stephen C. Bayne, MS, PhD
Professor and Chair
Department of Cariology, Restorative Sciences,
   and Endodontics
School of Dentistry
University of Michigan
Ann Arbor, MI

Lee W. Boushell, DMD, MS
Assistant Professor
Department of Operative Dentistry
The University of North Carolina
School of Dentistry
Chapel Hill, NC

James J. Crawford, MA, PhD
Professor Emeritus
The University of North Carolina
School of Dentistry and Medicine
Chapel Hill, NC

Terrence E. Donovan, DDS
Professor
Department of Operative Dentistry
The University of North Carolina
School of Dentistry
Chapel Hill, NC

R. Scott Eidson, DDS
Clinical Associate Professor
Department of Operative Dentistry
The University of North Carolina
School of Dentistry
Chapel Hill, NC

Harald O. Heymann, DDS, MEd
Professor
Department of Operative Dentistry
The University of North Carolina
School of Dentistry
Chapel Hill, NC

Ralph H. Leonard, Jr., DDS, MPH
Director
Dental Faculty Practice
Clinical Professor
Department of Diagnostic Sciences and General
   Dentistry
The University of North Carolina
School of Dentistry
Chapel Hill, NC

Jorge Perdigão, DMD, MS, PhD
Professor
Division of Operative Dentistry
Department of Restorative Sciences
School of Dentistry
University of Minnesota
Minneapolis, MN

André V. Ritter, DDS, MS
Professor and Graduate Program Director
Department of Operative Dentistry
The University of North Carolina
School of Dentistry
Chapel Hill, NC

Theodore M. Roberson, DDS
Professor Emeritus
Department of Operative Dentistry
The University of North Carolina
School of Dentistry
Chapel Hill, NC

Daniel A. Shugars, DDS, PhD, MPH
Research Professor
Department of Operative Dentistry
The University of North Carolina
School of Dentistry
Chapel Hill, NC

Gregory E. Smith, DDS, MSD
Professor Emeritus
Department of Restorative Sciences
University of Florida
College of Dentistry
Gainesville, FL

John R. Sturdevant, DDS
Associate Professor
Department of Operative Dentistry
The University of North Carolina
School of Dentistry
Chapel Hill, NC

Edward J. Swift, Jr., DMD, MS
Professor and Chair
Department of Operative Dentistry
The University of North Carolina
School of Dentistry
Chapel Hill, NC

Jeffrey Y. Thompson, PhD
Professor
Section of Prosthodontics
Director
Biosciences Research Center
College of Dental Medicine
Nova Southeastern University
Ft. Lauderdale, FL

Ricardo Walter, DDS, MS
Assistant Professor of Restorative Dentistry
Department of Preventive and Restorative
   Sciences
The Robert Schattner Center
School of Dental Medicine
University of Pennsylvania
Philadelphia, PA

Aldridge D. Wilder, Jr., DDS
Assistant Dean
Professor
Department of Operative Dentistry
The University of North Carolina School of
   Dentistry
Chapel Hill, NC

Foreword

Not long ago I picked up and read Charles Pappas' lively 1983 account of "The Life and Times of G.V. Black."* I rapidly marveled at the scintillating accomplishments of a man whose only dental training comprised a few weeks as an apprentice to a Mount Sterling, Illinois, dentist. Often referred to as the father of Operative Dentistry, Greene Vardiman Black was born in 1836, and opened his first dental practice in 1857, in Winchester, Illinois. Coincident with starting his practice, G.V. Black imposed on himself a rigorous self-education routine, focused primarily on the basic sciences that were emerging and/or developing so impressively during most of the 1800s. Utilizing a few precious hours each evening, after his children had been sent to bed, Black began intensive studies of chemistry, microbiology, and pathology. At that time most of the books and scientific essays available to Black were authored by Europeans, some writing in English, but many in Latin, German, and French. Consequently, Black studied these foreign languages until he was sufficiently proficient to absorb the science he needed in order to advance in his chosen professional and early academic life.

Beginning in the mid-1860s, Black began to apply what he drew from his basic science studies, and started to publish increasingly learned articles about various facets of Dentistry. With his dental experience growing, and his academic capabilities ever more obvious, Black was invited in 1866 to become a founding trustee of the Missouri Dental College, where he subsequently taught from 1870 to 1881. In 1877 Black was awarded an honorary DDS by the Missouri Dental College, and in 1884 he received an honorary MD degree from the Chicago Medical College (later to become Northwestern University Medical School). In 1883 Black had begun to teach at the Chicago College of Dental Surgery as Professor of Dental Pathology and Bacteriology. In 1897, G.V. Black became Dean and Professor of Operative Dentistry, Dental Pathology and Bacteriology at the Northwestern University Dental School, a position he held for 17 years. Black died on August 31, 1915.

Black himself published six books, of which his magnum opus was *Operative Dentistry: Volumes I and II* (1908). Quickly receiving wide acclaim, that work was revised and republished seven times over the period of a half-century. What would G. V. Black say if today he were handed, and asked for comments on, the sixth edition of *Sturdevant's Art and Science of Operative Dentistry*? My guess is that Black would, first of all, express quiet satisfaction that as a science Operative Dentistry has made so much progress that some of the key, enduring principles he enunciated were no longer relevant, having been overtaken by modern science and technology. An example would be Black's famous principle of extension for prevention, a dictum no longer followed because of the improvements in oral hygiene, fluoride therapy, remineralization formulations, and fissure sealants, that together have greatly reduced the incidence and severity of recurrent caries.

I think that Black would also be pleased that the authors collaborating on *Sturdevant's* sixth edition have retained the impressively comprehensive nature of this textbook. With his own background in microbiology and pathology, Black would have seen as very relevant the extensive coverage devoted to anatomy, histology, physiology, microbiology and cariology within the Operative Dentistry framework. For example, and as is more apparent than ever, modern cariology has become a fast moving field with changing ideas on etiology, detection, measurement, risk assessment, prevention, and treatment of caries. *Sturdevant's* editors and co-authors fully immerse themselves in such topics, and skillfully blend and present the established understandings with the new, emerging scientific developments.

Black was also a student of chemistry and materials science. He carefully studied the chemistry of dental cements, and he shared his findings via many scientific publications. Black conducted numerous studies on amalgams, their composition and properties. These experiments were also written up and published. Because of the central place amalgams held in dental practice a century ago, I think Black would be astounded by the enormous role adhesive resins and various composite restorative materials play today in contemporary Operative Dentistry. The transition from amalgam to non-metallic restorations is far from complete, yet the adhesive dentistry revolution has been accompanied by modifications of G. V. Black's venerable six principles of cavity preparation, as originally codified in 1908. Black would surely think of this as a definitive and welcome sign of dentistry's scientific progress, a goal for which he always advocated.

Black would likely be impressed by the functional and greatly improved esthetic results achievable with the modern composite restorative materials. Yet it is probably safe to assume that Black the scientist would urge even more research to develop still better dental materials with which to treat patients, and thereby improve the public's health. That is the type of challenge the sixth edition of *Sturdevant's* Operative Dentistry has embraced, and represents the type of vision and spirit that guided the major revisions contained within this book.

G.V. Black was a consummate operative dentist, a life-long scientist, and a widely respected teacher. He was aware of the importance of scientific papers and well-illustrated textbooks as critical learning materials for the dental student, and the conscientious practitioner alike. Black would likely, therefore, appreciate and applaud the well organized structure and the up-to-date content of *Sturdevant's* sixth edition. (The first edition appeared in 1968.) It is also likely that after a stellar academic career, G.V. Black would lightly tug on his beard and smile in admiration as his eyes fell on the electronic

*Pappas, C.N. *The Life and Times of G.V. Black*. Quintessence Publishing Co., Chicago, 1983.

renderings and colorful digital images that grace *Sturdevant's* sixth edition. Furthermore, the always inquisitive Professor Black would surely want to access the website that accompanies this book, and view for himself the supplemental book chapters, videos, and weblinks that round out a truly comprehensive Operative Dentistry learning system. For the dental students who may immerse themselves in this book, and for practitioners who will wish to use it as the standard reference to the subject, the skillful employment of digital tools and technology will be welcome, and will make this superb master work more comprehensive, more accessible, and surely more valued.

John W. Stamm, DDS, MScD, DDPH
Alumni Distinguished Professor and Dean Emeritus
School of Dentistry
The University of North Carolina at Chapel Hill
Chapel Hill, NC
June 30, 2011

Preface

Sturdevant's Art and Science of Operative Dentistry is considered to be the most comprehensive operative dentistry text on the market. Drawing from both theory and practice, and supported by extensive clinical and laboratory research, it presents a clearly detailed, heavily illustrated step-by-step approach to conservative restorative and preventive dentistry. Based upon the principle that dental caries is a disease, the book provides both a thorough understanding of caries and an authoritative approach to its treatment and prevention. Throughout the book, emphasis is placed on the importance of treating the underlying causes of the patient problem(s), not just restoring the damage that has occurred. It is organized in a sequential format; the early chapters present the necessary general information while the later chapters are specifically related to the practice of operative dentistry, including conservative esthetic procedures.

The sixth edition of *Sturdevant's Art and Science of Operative Dentistry* has been **significantly revised** in order to streamline the text and improve readability. The order of chapters has been reorganized, redundant and outdated information has been deleted, and several chapters have been moved to the new companion website. In addition, the book is now in **full color**. The line art for the book has been completely redrawn in full color to better show techniques and detail, and new, full color photos have been added where appropriate. Conservative esthetic procedures, which are covered at length, especially benefit from the addition of color.

The sixth edition is much more than just a printed book, however. The new **companion website** features the entire text online, plus six chapters that are exclusively online. In addition, videos demonstrate key procedures addressed in the text. See the inside front cover for a complete listing of the chapters and videos available.

New to this Edition

- **Streamlined for improved readability**
- **Full color**
- **Companion website**

Chapter Synopses

CHAPTER 1: CLINICAL SIGNIFICANCE OF DENTAL ANATOMY, HISTOLOGY, PHYSIOLOGY, AND OCCLUSION

This chapter provides a thorough understanding of the histology, physiology, and occlusal interactions of the dentition and supporting tissues.

CHAPTER 2: DENTAL CARIES: ETIOLOGY, CLINICAL CHARACTERISTICS, RISK ASSESSMENT, AND MANAGEMENT

This chapter presents basic definitions and information on: dental caries, clinical characteristics of the caries lesions, caries risk assessment, and caries management in the medical model, all in the context of clinical operative dentistry.

CHAPTER 3: PATIENT ASSESSMENT, EXAMINATION AND DIAGNOSIS, AND TREATMENT PLANNING

This chapter provides an overview of the process through which a clinician completes a patient assessment, clinical examination, diagnosis, and treatment plan to operative dentistry procedures.

CHAPTER 4: FUNDAMENTAL CONCEPTS OF ENAMEL AND DENTIN ADHESION

The chapter presents the basic concepts of adhesion, along with detailed descriptions of the factors affecting enamel and dentin adhesion, and the different approaches for resin bonding to tooth structure.

CHAPTER 5: FUNDAMENTALS OF TOOTH PREPARATION AND PULP PROTECTION

This chapter emphasizes procedural organization for tooth preparation and associated nomenclature, including the historical classification of carious lesions.

CHAPTER 6: INSTRUMENTS AND EQUIPMENT FOR TOOTH PREPARATION

This chapter reviews hand instruments for cutting, powered cutting equipment, and rotary cutting instruments. It also looks at cutting mechanisms, as well as the hazards of cutting instruments, and the precautions that should be taken when using them.

CHAPTER 7: PRELIMINARY CONSIDERATIONS FOR OPERATIVE DENTISTRY

This chapter addresses routine, chairside, pre-operative procedures (before actual tooth preparation). Primarily, these procedures include patient and operator positions and isolation of the operating field.

CHAPTER 8: INTRODUCTION TO COMPOSITE RESTORATIONS

This chapter provides a general introduction to composite restorations (the predominant direct esthetic restorative material), and describes the properties and clinical uses of composite materials. There is also information about various types of composites, including macrofill, microfill, hybrid, nanofill, nanohybrid, flowable, and packable types as well as other direct tooth-colored restorative materials such as glass ionomers and resin-modified glass ionomers. A brief historical perspective of other tooth-colored materials that may still be encountered clinically is provided.

CHAPTER 9: CLASS III, IV, AND V DIRECT COMPOSITE AND GLASS IONOMER RESTORATIONS

This chapter presents the specific rationales and techniques for use of direct composite resin in Class III, IV, and V direct composite restorations. It also presents information about any differences in these classes of restorations when a glass ionomer material is used for the restoration.

CHAPTER 10: CLASS I, II, AND VI DIRECT COMPOSITE RESTORATIONS AND OTHER TOOTH-COLORED RESTORATIONS

This chapter presents techniques for restoring the occlusal (including the occlusal thirds of facial and lingual surfaces) and proximal surfaces of posterior teeth with direct composite resin and other directly placed tooth-colored materials. The least invasive treatments are presented first, followed by progressively more involved methods of treatment. Consequently, first the rationale and technique for pit-and-fissure sealants, preventive resin or conservative composite restorations, and Class VI composite restorations are presented. Next, Class I and II composite restorations are presented, followed by composite foundations.

CHAPTER 11: INDIRECT TOOTH-COLORED RESTORATIONS

This chapter reviews the indications, contraindications, advantages, disadvantages, and clinical techniques for Class I and II indirect tooth-colored restorations, restorations which are made on a replica of the prepared tooth in a dental laboratory or by using computer-aided design/computer-assisted manufacturing (CAD/CAM) either at chairside or in the dental laboratory.

CHAPTER 12: ADDITIONAL CONSERVATIVE ESTHETIC PROCEDURES

This chapter presents conservative esthetic procedures in the context of their clinical applications. Fundamental principles in conservative esthetic dentistry are reviewed in detail. A complete review of esthetic procedures is included, ranging from conservative treatments, such as vital bleaching, to more extensive procedures involving etched porcelain veneers. Detailed step-by-step procedures are systematically presented, and exquisitely illustrated.

CHAPTER 13: INTRODUCTION TO AMALGAM RESTORATIONS

This chapter presents the fundamental concepts of amalgam restoration, including the types of amalgam restorations, properties, clinical procedures, controversial issues, and safety.

CHAPTER 14: CLASS I, II, AND VI AMALGAM RESTORATIONS

This chapter presents the techniques and procedures for Class I, II, and VI amalgam restorations. Class I restorations restore defects on the occlusal surface of posterior teeth, the occlusal two thirds of the facial and lingual surface of molars, and the lingual surfaces of maxillary anterior teeth. Class II restorations restore defects that affect one or both of the proximal surfaces of the posterior teeth. Class VI restorations restore rare defects affecting the cusp tips of posterior teeth or the incisal edges of anterior teeth.

Chapter 1

Clinical Significance of Dental Anatomy, Histology, Physiology, and Occlusion

Lee W. Boushell, John R. Sturdevant

A thorough understanding of the histology, physiology, and occlusal interactions of the dentition and supporting tissues is essential for the restorative dentist. Knowledge of the structures of teeth (enamel, dentin, cementum, and pulp) and their relationships to each other and to the supporting structures is necessary, especially when treating dental caries. The protective function of the tooth form is revealed by its impact on masticatory muscle activity, the supporting tissues (osseous and mucosal), and the pulp. Proper tooth form contributes to healthy supporting tissues. The form of a tooth and its contour and contact relationships with adjacent and opposing teeth are major determinants of muscle function in mastication, esthetics, speech, and protection. The relationships of form to function are especially noteworthy when considering the shape of the dental arch, proximal contacts, occlusal contacts, and mandibular movement.

Teeth and Supporting Tissues

Dentitions

Humans have primary and permanent dentitions. The primary dentition consists of 10 maxillary and 10 mandibular teeth. Primary teeth exfoliate and are replaced by the permanent dentition, which consists of 16 maxillary and 16 mandibular teeth.

Classes of Human Teeth: Form and Function

Human teeth are divided into classes on the basis of form and function. The primary and permanent dentitions include the incisor, canine, and molar classes. The fourth class, the premolar, is found only in the permanent dentition (Fig. 1-1). Tooth form predicts the function of teeth; class traits are the characteristics that place teeth into functional categories.

Because the diet of humans consists of animal and plant foods, the human dentition is called *omnivorous.*

Incisors

The incisors are located near the entrance of the oral cavity and function as cutting or shearing instruments for food (see Fig. 1-1). From a proximal view, the crowns of these teeth have a relatively triangular shape, with a narrow incisal surface and a broad cervical base. During mastication, incisors are used to shear (cut through) food. Incisors are essential for the proper esthetics of the smile, facial soft tissue contours (e.g., lip support), and speech (phonetics).

Canines

Canines possess the longest roots of all teeth and are located at the corners of the dental arch. They function in the seizing, piercing, tearing, and cutting of food. From a proximal view, the crown also has a triangular shape, with a thick incisal ridge. The anatomic form of the crown and the length of the root make these teeth strong, stable abutment teeth for a fixed or removable prosthesis. Canines not only serve as important guides in occlusion because of their anchorage and position in the dental arches but also play a crucial role (along with the incisors) in the esthetics of the smile and lip support (see Fig. 1-1).

Premolars

Premolars serve a dual role: (1) they are similar to canines in the tearing of food, and (2) they are similar to molars in the grinding of food. Although the first premolars are angular, with their facial cusps resembling the canines, the lingual cusps of the maxillary premolars. The occlusal surfaces present a series of curves in the form of concavities and convexities

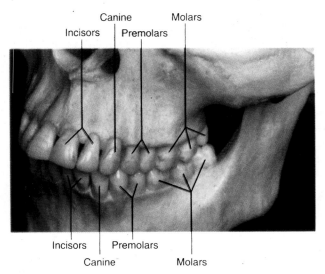

Fig. 1-1 Maxillary and mandibular teeth in maximum intercuspal position. The classes of teeth are incisors, canines, premolars, and molars. Cusps of mandibular teeth are one-half cusp anterior of corresponding cusps of teeth in the maxillary arch. *(From Logan BM, Reynolds P, Hutchings RT: McMinn's color atlas of head and neck anatomy, ed 4, Edinburgh, Mosby, 2010.)*

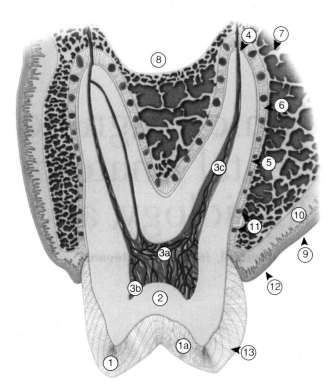

Fig. 1-3 Cross-section of the maxillary molar and its supporting structures. *1*, enamel; *1a*, gnarled enamel; *2*, dentin; *3a*, pulp chamber; *3b*, pulp horn; *3c*, pulp canal; *4*, apical foramen; *5*, cementum; *6*, periodontal fibers in periodontal ligament; *7*, alveolar bone; *8*, maxillary sinus; *9*, mucosa; *10*, submucosa; *11*, blood vessels; *12*, gingiva; *13*, striae of Retzius.

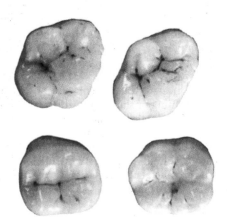

Fig. 1-2 Occlusal surfaces of maxillary and mandibular first and second molars after several years of use, showing rounded curved surfaces and minimal wear.

that should be maintained throughout life for correct occlusal contacts and function. Although less visible than incisors and canines, premolars still can play an important role in esthetics.

Molars

Molars are large, multi-cusped, strongly anchored teeth located nearest the temporomandibular joint (TMJ), which serves as the fulcrum during function. These teeth have a major role in the crushing, grinding, and chewing of food to the smallest dimensions suitable for swallowing. They are well suited for this task because they have broad occlusal surfaces and multi-rooted anchorage (Fig. 1-2 and 1-3). Premolars and molars are important in maintaining the vertical dimension of the face (see Fig. 1-1).

Structures of Teeth

Teeth are composed of enamel, the pulp–dentin complex, and cementum (see Fig. 1-3). Each of these structures is discussed individually.

Enamel

Enamel formation, *amelogenesis*, is accomplished by cells called *ameloblasts*. These cells originate from the embryonic germ layer known as *ectoderm*. Enamel covers the anatomic crown of the tooth and varies in thickness in different areas (see Fig. 1-3). It is thicker at the incisal and occlusal areas of a tooth and becomes progressively thinner until it terminates at the cementoenamel junction (CEJ). The thickness also varies from one class of tooth to another, averaging 2 mm at the incisal ridges of incisors, 2.3 to 2.5 mm at the cusps of premolars, and 2.5 to 3 mm at the cusps of molars. The cusps of posterior teeth begin as separate ossification centers, which form lobes that coalesce. Enamel usually decreases in thickness toward the junction of these developmental features and can approach zero where the junction is fissured (noncoalesced).

Chemically, enamel is a highly mineralized crystalline structure. Hydroxyapatite, in the form of a crystalline lattice, is the largest mineral constituent (90%–92% by volume). Other minerals and trace elements are present in smaller amounts. The remaining constituents of tooth enamel include organic matrix proteins (1%–2%) and water (4%–12%) volume.

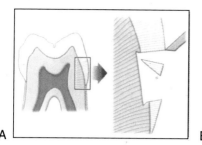
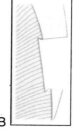

Fig. 1-4 **A,** Enamel rods unsupported by dentin are fractured away readily by pressure from hand instrument. **B,** Cervical preparation showing enamel rods supported by dentin.

Structurally, enamel is composed of millions of enamel rods or prisms, which are the largest structural components, rod sheaths, and a cementing inter-rod substance in some areas. The inter-rod substance, or sheath, may be the increased spacing between crystallites oriented differently to where the "tail" portion of one rod meets the "head" portion of another. This spacing apparently is partially organic material. The rods vary in number from approximately 5 million for a mandibular incisor to about 12 million for a maxillary molar. The rods are densely packed and intertwined in a wavy course, and each extends from the DEJ to the external surface of the tooth. In general, the rods are aligned perpendicularly to the DEJ and the tooth surface in the primary and permanent dentitions except in the cervical region of permanent teeth, where they are oriented outward in a slightly apical direction. In the primary dentition, the enamel rods in the cervical and central parts of the crown are nearly perpendicular to the long axis of the tooth and are similar in their direction to permanent teeth in the occlusal two thirds of the crown. Enamel rod diameter near the dentinal borders is about 4 μm and about 8 μm near the surface. This difference accommodates the larger outer surface of the enamel crown compared with the dentinal surface at the DEJ.

Enamel is the hardest substance of the human body. Hardness can vary over the external tooth surface according to the location; also, it decreases inwardly, with hardness lowest at the DEJ. The density of enamel also decreases from the surface to the DEJ. Enamel is a rigid structure that is both strong and brittle (high elastic modulus, high compressive strength, and low tensile strength) and requires a dentin support to withstand masticatory forces. Dentin is a more flexible substance that is strong and resilient (low elastic modulus, high compressive strength, and high tensile strength), which essentially increases the fracture toughness of the more superficial enamel. Enamel rods that lack dentin support because of caries or improper preparation design are easily fractured away from neighboring rods. For optimal strength in tooth preparation, all enamel rods should be supported by dentin (Fig. 1-4).

Human enamel is composed of rods that, in transverse section, have a rounded head or body section and a tail section, forming a repetitive series of interlocking prisms. The rounded head portion of each prism (5 μm wide) lies between the narrow tail portions (5 μm long) of two adjacent prisms (Fig. 1-5). Generally, the rounded head portion is oriented in the incisal or occlusal direction; the tail section is oriented cervically.

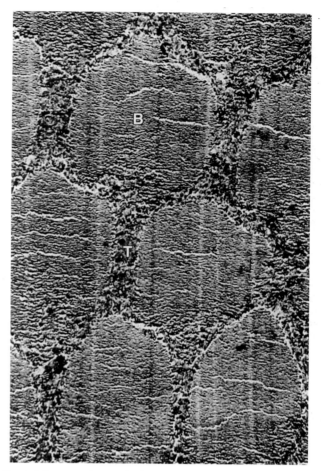

Fig. 1-5 Electron micrograph of cross-section of rods in mature human enamel. Crystal orientation is different in "bodies" (*B*) than in "tails" (*T*). Approximate level of magnification 5000×. *(From Meckel AH, Griebstein WJ, Neal RJ: Structure of mature human dental enamel as observed by electron microscopy, Arch Oral Biol 10(5):775–783, 1965.)*

The structural components of the enamel prism are millions of small, elongated apatite crystallites that vary in size and shape. The crystallites are tightly packed in a distinct pattern of orientation that gives strength and structural identity to the enamel prisms. The long axis of the apatite crystallites within the central region of the head (body) is aligned almost parallel to the rod long axis, and the crystallites incline with increasing angles (65 degrees) to the prism axis in the tail region. The susceptibility of these crystallites to acid, from either an etching procedure or caries, may be correlated with their orientation. Although the dissolution process occurs more in the head regions of the rod, the tail regions and the periphery of the head regions are relatively resistant to acid attack. The crystallites are irregular in shape, with an average length of 160 nm and an average width of 20 to 40 nm. Each apatite crystallite is composed of thousands of unit cells that have a highly ordered arrangement of atoms. A crystallite may be 300 unit cells long, 40 cells wide, and 20 cells thick in a hexagonal configuration (Fig. 1-6). An organic matrix or prism sheath also surrounds individual crystals and appears to be an organically rich interspace rather than a structural entity.

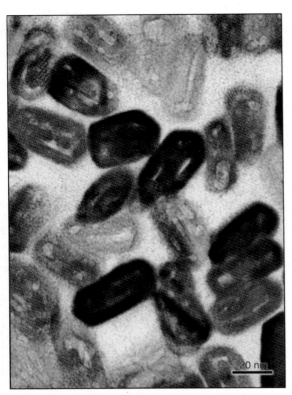

Fig. 1-6 Electron micrograph of mature, hexagon-shaped enamel crystallites. *(From Nanci A:* Ten Cate's oral histology: development, structure, and function, *ed 7, St Louis, 2008, Mosby.)*

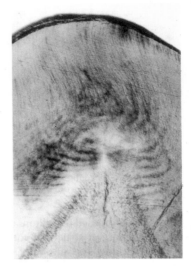

Fig. 1-7 Gnarled enamel. *(From Berkovitz BKB, Holland GR, Moxham BJ:* Oral anatomy, histology and embryology, *ed 4, Edinburgh, 2009, Mosby.)*

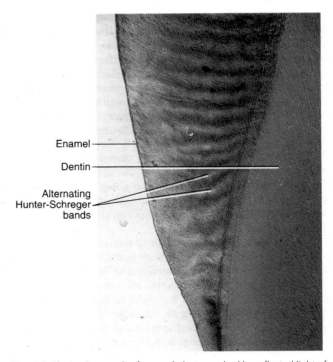

Enamel — Dentin — Alternating Hunter-Schreger bands

Fig. 1-8 Photomicrograph of enamel photographed by reflected light of Hunter-Schreger bands. *(From Avery JK and Chiego DJ:* Essentials of oral histology and embryology: A clinical approach, *ed 3, St Louis, 2006, Mosby.)*

Enamel rods follow a wavy, spiraling course, producing an alternating arrangement for each group or layer of rods as they change direction in progressing from the dentin toward the enamel surface, where they end a few micrometers short of the tooth surface. Enamel rods rarely run a straight radial course, as there is an alternating clockwise and counterclockwise deviation of the rods from the radial course at all levels of the crown. They initially follow a curving path through one third of the enamel next to the DEJ. After that, the rods usually follow a more direct path through the remaining two thirds of the enamel to the enamel surface. Groups of enamel rods may entwine with adjacent groups of rods, and they follow a curving irregular path toward the tooth surface. These constitute gnarled enamel, which occurs near the cervical regions and the incisal and occlusal areas (Fig. 1-7). Gnarled enamel is not subject to fracture as much as is regular enamel. This type of enamel formation does not yield readily to the pressure of bladed, hand-cutting instruments in tooth preparation.

The changes in direction of enamel prisms that minimize fracture in the axial direction produce an optical appearance called *Hunter-Schreger bands* (Fig. 1-8). These bands appear to be composed of alternate light and dark zones of varying widths that have slightly different permeability and organic content. These bands are found in different areas of each class of teeth. Because the enamel rod orientation varies in each tooth, Hunter-Schreger bands also have a variation in the number present in each tooth. In anterior teeth, they are located near the incisal surfaces. They increase in numbers and areas of teeth, from canines to premolars. In molars, the bands

occur from near the cervical region to the cusp tips. The orientation of the enamel rod heads and tails and the gnarling of enamel rods provide strength by resisting, distributing, and dissipating impact forces.

Enamel tufts are hypomineralized structures of the enamel rods and the inter-rod substance that project between adjacent groups of enamel rods from the DEJ (Fig. 1-9). These projections arise in dentin, extend into enamel in the direction of the long axis of the crown, and may play a role in the spread of dental caries. Enamel lamellae are thin, leaf-like faults

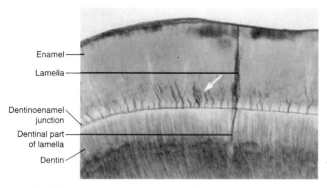

Fig. 1-9 Microscopic view through lamella that goes from enamel surface into dentin. Note the enamel tufts (*arrow*). *(From Bath Balogh M, Fehrenbach MJ: Illustrated dental embryology, histology, and anatomy, ed 3, Saunders, 2011, St Louis. Courtesy James McIntosh, PhD, Assistant Professor Emeritus, Department of Biomedical Sciences, Baylor College of Dentistry, Dallas, TX.)*

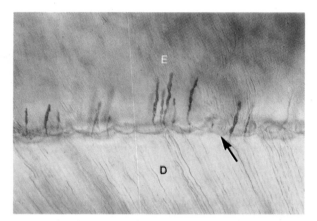

Fig. 1-10 Microscopic view of scalloped dentinoenamel junction (DEJ) (*arrow*). *E*, enamel; *D*, dentin. *(From Bath Balogh M, Fehrenbach MJ: Illustrated dental embryology, histology, and anatomy, ed 3, Saunders, 2011, St Louis. Courtesy James McIntosh, PhD, Assistant Professor Emeritus, Department of Biomedical Sciences, Baylor College of Dentistry, Dallas, TX.)*

between enamel rod groups that extend from the enamel surface toward the DEJ, sometimes extending into dentin (see Fig. 1-9). They contain mostly organic material, which is a weak area predisposing a tooth to the entry of bacteria and dental caries. Enamel rods are formed linearly by successive apposition of enamel in discrete increments. The resulting variations in structure and mineralization are called *incremental striae of Retzius* and can be considered growth rings (see Fig. 1-3). In horizontal sections of a tooth, the striae of Retzius appear as concentric circles. In vertical sections, the lines traverse the cuspal and incisal areas in a symmetric arc pattern, descending obliquely to the cervical region and terminating at the DEJ. When these circles are incomplete at the enamel surface, a series of alternating grooves, called *imbrication lines of Pickerill*, are formed. The elevations between the grooves are called *perikymata*; these are continuous around a tooth and usually lie parallel to the CEJ and each other.

A structureless outer layer of enamel about 30 μm thick is found most commonly toward the cervical area and less often on cusp tips. No prism outlines are visible, and all of the apatite crystals are parallel to one another and perpendicular to the striae of Retzius. This layer, referred to as *prismless enamel*, may be more heavily mineralized. Microscopically, the enamel surface initially has circular depressions indicating where the enamel rods end. These concavities vary in depth and shape, and they may contribute to the adherence of plaque material, with a resultant caries attack, especially in young individuals. The dimpled surface anatomy of the enamel, however, gradually wears smooth with age.

The interface of enamel and dentin (dentinoenamel junction, or DEJ) is scalloped or wavy in outline, with the crest of the waves penetrating toward enamel (Fig. 1-10). The rounded projections of enamel fit into the shallow depressions of dentin. This interdigitation may contribute to the firm attachment between dentin and enamel. The DEJ is also a hypermineralized zone approximately 30 μm thick.

The occlusal surfaces of premolars and molars have grooves and fossae that form at the junction of the developmental lobes of enamel. These allow movement of food to the facial and lingual surfaces during mastication. A functional cusp that opposes a groove (fossa) occludes on enamel and inclines on each side of the groove and not in the depth of the groove.

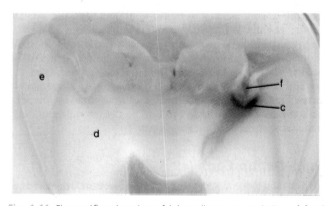

Fig. 1-11 Fissure (*f*) at junction of lobes allows accumulation of food and bacteria predisposing the tooth to dental caries (*c*). Enamel (*e*); dentin (*d*).

This arrangement leaves a V-shaped escape path between the cusp and its opposing groove for the movement of food during chewing. Failure of the enamel of the developmental lobes to coalesce results in a deep invagination of the enamel surface and is termed *fissure*. Non-coalesced enamel at the deepest point of a fossa is termed *pit*. These fissures and pits act as food and bacterial traps that predispose the tooth to dental caries (Fig. 1-11).

Once damaged, enamel is incapable of repairing itself because the ameloblast cell degenerates after the formation of the enamel rod. The final act of the ameloblast is secretion of a membrane covering the end of the enamel rod. This layer is referred to as *Nasmyth's membrane*, or *primary enamel cuticle*. This membrane covers the newly erupted tooth and is worn away by mastication and cleaning. The membrane is replaced by an organic deposit called the *pellicle*, which is a precipitate of salivary proteins. Microorganisms may attach to the pellicle to form bacterial plaque, which, if acidogenic in nature, can be a potential precursor to dental disease.

Although enamel is a hard, dense structure, it is permeable to certain ions and molecules. The route of passage may be

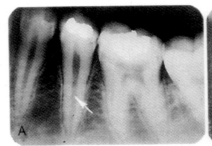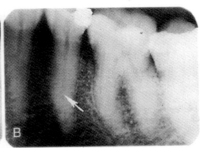

Fig. 1-12 Pulp cavity size. **A,** Premolar radiograph of young person. **B,** Premolar radiograph of older person. Note the difference in the size of the pulp cavity (*arrows*).

through structural units that are hypomineralized and rich in organic content, such as rod sheaths, enamel cracks, and other defects. Water plays an important role as a transporting medium through small intercrystalline spaces. Enamel permeability decreases with age because of changes in the enamel matrix, a decrease referred to as *enamel maturation.*

Enamel is soluble when exposed to an acid medium, but the dissolution is not uniform. Solubility of enamel increases from the enamel surface to the DEJ. When fluoride ions are present during enamel formation or are topically applied to the enamel surface, the solubility of surface enamel is decreased. Fluoride concentration decreases toward the DEJ. Fluoride can affect the chemical and physical properties of the apatite mineral and influence the hardness, chemical reactivity, and stability of enamel, while preserving the apatite structures. Trace amounts of fluoride stabilize enamel by lowering acid solubility, decreasing the rate of demineralization, and enhancing the rate of remineralization.

Pulp–Dentin Complex

Dentin and pulp tissues are specialized connective tissues of mesodermal origin, formed from the dental papilla of the tooth bud. Many investigators consider these two tissues as a single tissue, which forms the pulp–dentin complex, with mineralized dentin constituting the mature end product of cell differentiation and maturation.

The dental pulp occupies the pulp cavity in the tooth and is a unique, specialized organ of the human body that serves four functions: (1) formative or developmental, (2) nutritive, (3) sensory or protective, and (4) defensive or reparative. The formative function is the production of primary and secondary dentin by odontoblasts. The nutritive function supplies nutrients and moisture to dentin through the blood vascular supply to the odontoblasts and their processes. The sensory function provides nerve fibers within the pulp to mediate the sensation of pain. Dentin receptors are unique because various stimuli elicit only pain as a response. The pulp usually does not differentiate between heat, touch, pressure, or chemicals. Motor fibers initiate reflexes in the muscles of the blood vessel walls for the control of circulation in the pulp.

Finally, the defensive function of the pulp is related primarily to its response to irritation by mechanical, thermal, chemical, or bacterial stimuli. The deposition of reparative dentin acts as a protective barrier against caries and various other irritating factors. In cases of severe irritation, the pulp responds by an inflammatory reaction similar to that for any other soft tissue injury. The inflammation may become irreversible, however, and can result in the death of the pulp because the confined, rigid structure of the dentin limits the inflammatory response and the ability of the pulp to recover.

The pulp is circumscribed by the dentin and is lined peripherally by a cellular layer of odontoblasts adjacent to dentin. Anatomically, the pulp is divided into (1) coronal pulp located in the pulp chamber in the crown portion of the tooth, including the pulp horns that are directed toward the incisal ridges and cusp tips, and (2) radicular pulp located in the pulp canals in the root portion of the tooth. The radicular pulp is continuous with the periapical tissues by connecting through the apical foramen or foramina of the root. Accessory canals may extend from the pulp canals laterally through the root dentin to the periodontal tissues. The shape of each pulp conforms generally to the shape of each tooth (see Fig. 1-3).

The pulp contains nerves, arterioles, venules, capillaries, lymph channels, connective tissue cells, intercellular substance, odontoblasts, fibroblasts, macrophages, collagen, and fine fibers.[1] The pulp is circumscribed peripherally by a specialized odontogenic area composed of the odontoblasts, the cell-free zone, and the cell-rich zone.

Knowledge of the contour and size of the pulp cavity is essential during tooth preparation. In general, the pulp cavity is a miniature contour of the external surface of the tooth. Pulp cavity size varies with tooth size among individuals and even within a single person. With advancing age, the pulp cavity usually decreases in size. Radiographs are an invaluable aid in determining the size of the pulp cavity and any existing pathologic condition (Fig. 1-12). A primary objective during operative procedures must be the preservation of the health of the pulp.

Dentin formation, *dentinogenesis,* is accomplished by cells called *odontoblasts.* Odontoblasts are considered part of pulp and dentin tissues because their cell bodies are in the pulp cavity, but their long, slender cytoplasmic cell processes (Tomes fibers) extend well (100–200 μm) into the tubules in the mineralized dentin (Fig. 1-13).

Because of these odontoblastic cell processes, dentin is considered a living tissue, with the capability of reacting to physiologic and pathologic stimuli. Odontoblastic processes occasionally cross the DEJ into enamel; these are termed *enamel spindles* when their ends are thickened (Fig. 1-14). They may serve as pain receptors, explaining the enamel sensitivity experienced by some patients during tooth preparation.

Dentin forms the largest portion of the tooth structure, extending almost the full length of the tooth. Externally, dentin is covered by enamel on the anatomic crown and cementum on the anatomic root. Internally, dentin forms the

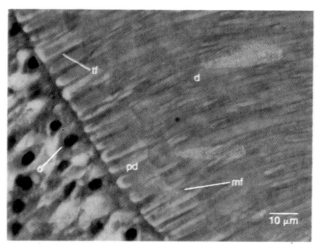

Fig. 1-13 Odontoblasts (*o*) have cell processes (Tomes fibers, [*tf*]) that extend through the predentin (*pd*) into dentin (*d*). *mf*, mineralization front.

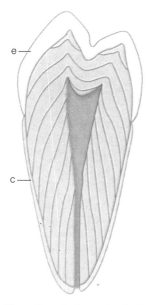

Fig. 1-15 Pattern of formation of primary dentin. This figure also shows enamel (*e*) covering the anatomic crown of the tooth and cementum (*c*) covering the anatomic root.

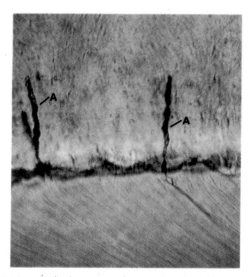

Fig. 1-14 Longitudinal section of enamel. Odontoblastic processes extend into enamel as enamel spindles (*A*). *(From Berkovitz BKB, Holland GR, Moxham BJ: Oral anatomy, histology and embryology, ed 4, Edinburgh, 2009, Mosby. Courtesy of Dr. R. Sprinz.)*

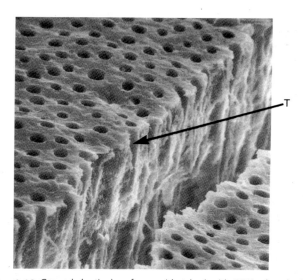

Fig. 1-16 Ground dentinal surface, acid-etched with 37% phosphoric acid. The artificial crack shows part of the dentinal tubules (*T*). The tubule apertures are opened and widened by acid application. *(From Brännström M: Dentin and pulp in restorative dentistry, London, 1982, Wolfe Medical.)*

walls of the pulp cavity (pulp chamber and pulp canals) (Fig. 1-15). Dentin formation begins immediately before enamel formation. Odontoblasts generate an extracellular collagen matrix as they begin to move away from the adjacent amelo-blasts. Mineralization of the collagen matrix, facilitated by modification of the collagen matrix by various noncollage-nous proteins, gradually follows its secretion. The most recently formed layer of dentin is always on the pulpal surface. This unmineralized zone of dentin is immediately next to the cell bodies of odontoblasts and is called *predentin*. Dentin formation begins at areas subjacent to the cusp tip or incisal ridge and gradually spreads to the apex of the root (see Fig. 1-15). In contrast to enamel formation, dentin formation continues after tooth eruption and throughout the life of the pulp. The dentin forming the initial shape of the tooth is called

primary dentin and is usually completed 3 years after tooth eruption (in the case of permanent teeth).

The dentinal tubules are small canals that extend through the entire width of dentin, from the pulp to the DEJ (Figs. 1-16 and 1-17). Each tubule contains the cytoplasmic cell process (Tomes fiber) of an odontoblast and is lined with a layer of peri-tubular dentin, which is much more mineralized than the surrounding intertubular dentin (see Fig. 1-17).

The surface area of dentin is much larger at the DEJ or den-tinocemental junction than it is on the pulp cavity side. Because odontoblasts form dentin while progressing inward toward the pulp, the tubules are forced closer together. The number of

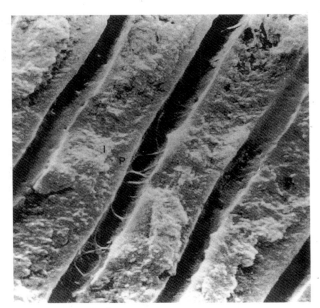

Fig. 1-17 Dentinal tubules in cross-section, 1.2 mm from pulp. Peritubular dentin (*P*) is more mineralized than intertubular dentin (*I*). *(From Brännström M: Dentin and pulp in restorative dentistry, London, 1982, Wolfe Medical.)*

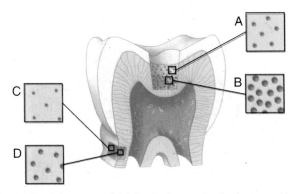

Fig. 1-18 Tubules in superficial dentin close to the dentinoenamel junction (DEJ) (*A*) are smaller and more sparsely distributed compared with deep dentin (*B*). The tubules in superficial root dentin (*C*) and deep root dentin (*D*) are smaller and less numerous than those in comparable depths of coronal dentin.

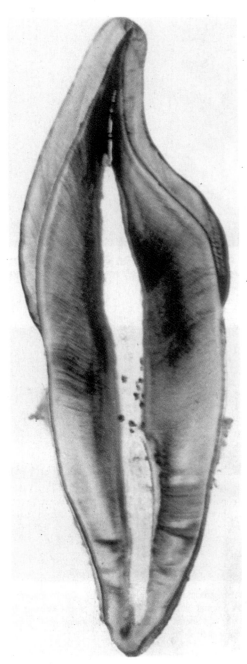

Fig. 1-19 Ground section of human incisor. Course of dentinal tubules is in a slight S-curve in the crown, but straight at the incisal tip and in the root. *(From Young B, Lowe JS, Stevens A, Heath JW: Wheater's functional histology: A text and colour atlas, ed 5, Edinburgh, 2006, Churchill Livingstone.)*

tubules increases from 15,000 to 20,000/mm^2 at the DEJ to 45,000 to 65,000/mm^2 at the pulp.[2] The lumen of the tubules also varies from the DEJ to the pulp surface. In coronal dentin, the average diameter of tubules at the DEJ is 0.5 to 0.9 μm, but this increases to 2 to 3 μm near the pulp (Fig. 1-18).

The course of the dentinal tubules is a slight S-curve in the tooth crown, but the tubules are straighter in the incisal ridges, cusps, and root areas (Fig. 1-19). The ends of the tubules are perpendicular to the DEJ. Along the tubule walls are small lateral openings called *canaliculi*. As the odontoblastic process proceeds from the cell in the pulp to the DEJ, lateral secondary branches extend into the canaliculi and can communicate with the lateral extensions of adjacent odontoblastic processes. Near the DEJ, the tubules divide into several terminal branches, forming an intercommunicating and anastomosing network (Fig. 1-20).

After the primary dentin is formed, dentin deposition continues at a reduced rate even without obvious external stimuli, although the rate and amount of this physiologic secondary dentin vary considerably among individuals. In secondary dentin, the tubules take a slightly different directional pattern in contrast to primary dentin (Fig. 1-21). Secondary dentin forms on all internal aspects of the pulp cavity, but in the pulp chamber, in multi-rooted teeth, it tends to be thicker on the roof and floor than on the side walls.[3]

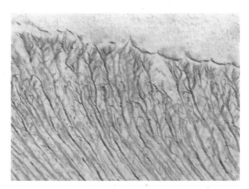

Fig. 1-20 Ground section showing dentinal tubules and their lateral branching close to the dentinoenamel junction (DEJ). *(From Berkovitz BKB, Holland GR, and Moxham BJ: Oral anatomy, histology, and embryology, ed 4, Edinburgh, 2010, Mosby.)*

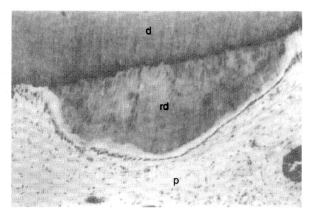

Fig. 1-22 Reparative dentin (*rd*) in response to a carious lesion (*d*, dentin, *p*, pulp). *(From Trowbridge HO: Pulp biology: Progress during the past 25 years,* Aust Endo J *29(1):5–12, 2003.)*

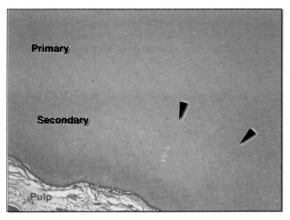

Fig. 1-21 Ground section of dentin with pulpal surface at right. Dentinal tubules curve sharply (*arrows*) as they move from primary to secondary dentin. Dentinal tubules are more irregular in shape in secondary dentin. *(From Nanci A: Ten Cate's oral histology: Development, structure, and function, ed 7, Mosby, 2008, St Louis.)*

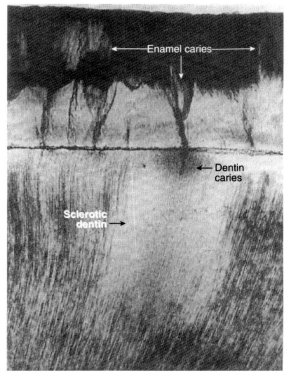

Fig. 1-23 Sclerotic dentin occurring under enamel caries with early penetration of dentin caries along the enamel lamella. *(From Schour I: H. J. Noyes oral histology and embryology,* Philadelphia, 1960, Lea & Febiger.)

When moderate stimuli are applied to dentin, such as caries, attrition, and some operative procedures, the affected odontoblasts may die. Replacement odontoblasts (termed *secondary odontoblasts*) of pulpal origin then begin to form reparative dentin (*tertiary dentin*). The reparative dentin usually appears as a localized dentin deposit on the wall of the pulp cavity immediately subjacent to the area on the tooth that has received the injury (a dentin deposit underneath the affected tubules) (Fig. 1-22). Being highly atubular, the reparative dentin is structurally different from the primary and secondary dentin.

Sclerotic dentin results from aging or mild irritation (e.g., slowly advancing caries) and causes a change in the composition of the primary dentin. The peritubular dentin becomes wider, gradually filling the tubules with calcified material, progressing pulpally from the DEJ (Fig. 1-23). These areas are harder, denser, less sensitive, and more protective of the pulp against subsequent irritations. Sclerosis resulting from aging is called *physiologic dentin sclerosis*; sclerosis resulting from a mild irritation is called *reactive dentin sclerosis*. Reactive dentin sclerosis often can be seen radiographically in the form of a more radiopaque (lighter) area in the S-shape of the tubules.

Human dentin is composed of approximately 50% inorganic material and 30% organic material by volume. The organic phase is approximately 90% type I collagen and 10% noncollagenous proteins. Dentin is less mineralized than enamel but more mineralized than cementum or bone. The mineral content of dentin increases with age. This mineral phase is composed primarily of hydroxyapatite crystallites, which are arranged in a less systematic manner than are enamel crystallites. Dentinal crystallites are smaller than enamel crystallites, having a length of 20 to 100 nm and a width of about 3 nm, which is similar to the size seen in bone and cementum.[3] Dentin is significantly softer than enamel but harder than bone or cementum. The hardness of dentin averages one-fifth that of enamel, and its hardness near the DEJ is about three times greater than near the pulp. Dentin becomes harder with age, primarily as a result of increases in mineral content. Although dentin is a hard, mineralized tissue, it is flexible, with a modulus of elasticity of approximately 18 gigapascals (GPa).[4] This flexibility helps support the more brittle, nonresilient enamel. Often small "craze lines" are seen in enamel, indicating minute fractures of that structure. The craze lines usually are not clinically significant unless associated with cracks in the underlying dentin. Dentin is not as prone to fracture as is the enamel rod structure. The ultimate tensile strength of dentin is approximately 98 megapascals (MPa), whereas the ultimate tensile strength of enamel is approximately 10 MPa. The compressive strength of dentin and enamel are approximately 297 and 384 MPa, respectively.[4]

During tooth preparation, dentin usually is distinguished from enamel by (1) color and opacity, (2) reflectance, (3) hardness, and (4) sound. Dentin is normally yellow-white and slightly darker than enamel. In older patients, dentin is darker, and it can become brown or black when it has been exposed to oral fluids, old restorative materials, or slowly advancing caries. Dentin surfaces are more opaque and dull, being less reflective to light than similar enamel surfaces, which appear shiny. Dentin is softer than enamel and provides greater yield to the pressure of a sharp explorer tine, which tends to catch and hold in dentin.

Sensitivity is encountered whenever odontoblasts and their processes are stimulated during operative procedures, even though the pain receptor mechanism appears to be within the dentinal tubules near the pulp. Physical, thermal, chemical, bacterial, and traumatic stimuli are transmitted through the dentinal tubules, although the precise mechanism of the transmissive elements of sensation has not been conclusively established. The most accepted theory of pain transmission is the hydrodynamic theory, which accounts for pain transmission through rapid movements of fluid within the dentinal tubules.[5] Because many tubules contain mechanoreceptor nerve endings near the pulp, small fluid movements in the tubules arising from cutting, drying, pressure changes, osmotic shifts, or changes in temperature account for most pain transmission (Fig. 1-24).

Dentinal tubules are filled with dentinal fluid, a transudate of plasma. When enamel or cementum is removed during tooth preparation, the external seal of dentin is lost, allowing tubular fluid to move toward the cut surface. Pulpal fluid has a slight positive pressure that forces fluid outward toward any breach in the external seal. Permeability studies of dentin indicate that tubules are functionally much smaller than would be indicated by their measured microscopic dimensions as a result of numerous constrictions along their paths (see Fig. 1-17).[6] Dentin permeability is not uniform throughout the tooth. Coronal dentin is much more permeable than root dentin. There also are differences within coronal dentin (Fig. 1-25).[7] Dentin permeability primarily depends on the remaining dentin thickness (i.e., length of the tubules) and the diameter of the tubules. Because the tubules are shorter, more numerous, and larger in diameter closer to the pulp, deep dentin is a less effective pulpal barrier compared with superficial dentin (Fig. 1-26).

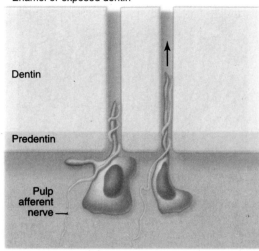

Enamel or exposed dentin

Dentin

Predentin

Pulp afferent nerve —

Fig. 1-24 Stimuli that induce fluid movements in dentinal tubules distort odontoblasts and afferent nerves, leading to a sensation of pain. Many operative procedures such as cutting or air-drying induce such fluid movement (*arrow*).

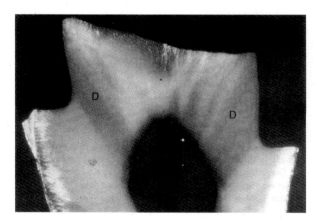

Fig. 1-25 Ground section of MOD (mesio-occluso-distal) tooth preparation on the third molar. Dark blue dye was placed in the pulp chamber under pressure after tooth preparation. Dark areas of dye penetration (*D*) show that the dentinal tubules of axial walls are much more permeable than those of the pulpal floor of preparation.

Cementum

Cementum is a thin layer of hard dental tissue covering the anatomic roots of teeth and is formed by cells known as *cementoblasts*, which develop from undifferentiated mesenchymal cells in the connective tissue of the dental follicle. Cementum is slightly softer than dentin and consists of about 45% to 50% inorganic material (hydroxyapatite) by weight and 50% to 55% organic matter and water by weight. The organic portion is composed primarily of collagen and protein polysaccharides. Sharpey's fibers are portions of the principal collagenous fibers of the periodontal ligament embedded in cementum and alveolar bone to attach the tooth to the alveolus (Fig. 1-27). Cementum is avascular.

Cementum is light yellow and slightly lighter in color than dentin. It is formed continuously throughout life because as the superficial layer of cementum ages, a new layer of

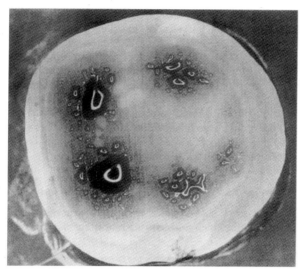

Fig. 1-26 Horizontal section in the occlusal third of molar crown. Dark blue dye was placed in the pulp chamber under pressure. Deep dentin areas (over pulp horns) are much more permeable than superficial dentin. *(From Pashley DH, Andringa HJ, Derkson GD, Derkson ME, Kalathoor SR: Regional. variability in the permeability of human dentin, Arch Oral Biol 32:519–523, 1987, with permission from Pergamon, Oxford, UK.)*

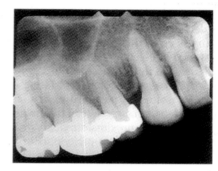

Fig. 1-28 Radiograph showing root resorption on lateral incisor after orthodontic tooth movement.

The cementodentinal junction is a relatively smooth area in the permanent tooth, and attachment of cementum to dentin is firm, but this is not understood completely yet. Cementum joins enamel to form the CEJ. In about 10% of teeth, enamel and cementum do not meet, and this can result in a sensitive area. Abrasion, erosion, caries, scaling, and restoration finishing and polishing procedures can denude dentin of its cementum covering, which can cause the dentin to be sensitive to various stimuli (e.g., heat, cold, sweet substances, sour substances). Cementum is capable of repairing itself to a limited degree and is not resorbed under normal conditions. Some resorption of the apical portion of the root can occur, however, if orthodontic pressures are excessive and movement is too fast (Fig. 1-28).

Physiology of Tooth Form
Function

Teeth serve four main functions: (1) mastication, (2) esthetics, (3) speech, and (4) protection of supporting tissues. Normal tooth form and proper alignment ensure efficiency in the incising and reduction of food with the various tooth classes—incisors, canines, premolars, and molars—performing specific functions in the masticatory process and in the coordination of the various muscles of mastication. In esthetics, the form and alignment of the anterior teeth are important to a person's physical appearance. The form and alignment of anterior and posterior teeth assist in the articulation of certain sounds that can have a significant effect on speech. Finally, the form and alignment of the teeth assist in sustaining them in the dental arches by assisting in the development and protection of gingival tissue and alveolar bone that support them.

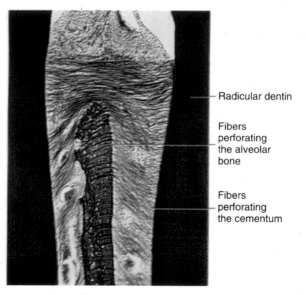

Radicular dentin

Fibers perforating the alveolar bone

Fibers perforating the cementum

Fig. 1-27 Principal fibers of periodontal ligament continue to course into surface layer of cementum as Sharpey's fibers. *(From Avery JK, Chiego DJ: Essentials of oral histology and embryology: A clinical approach, ed 3, St Louis, 2006, Mosby.)*

Contours

Facial and lingual surfaces possess a degree of convexity that affords protection and stimulation of supporting tissues during mastication. The convexity generally is located at the cervical third of the crown on the facial surfaces of all teeth and the lingual surfaces of incisors and canines. The lingual surfaces of posterior teeth usually have their height of contour in the middle third of the crown. Normal tooth contours act in deflecting food only to the extent that the passing food stimulates (by gentle massage) and does not irritate supporting tissues. If these curvatures are too great, tissues usually receive inadequate stimulation by the passage of food. Too little contour may result in trauma to the attachment apparatus.

cementum is deposited to keep the attachment intact. Two kinds of cementum are formed: acellular and cellular. The acellular layer of cementum is living tissue that does not incorporate cells into its structure and usually predominates on the coronal half of the root; cellular cementum occurs more frequently on the apical half. Cementum on the root end surrounds the apical foramen and may extend slightly onto the inner wall of the pulp canal. Cementum thickness can increase on the root end to compensate for attritional wear of the occlusal or incisal surface and passive eruption of the tooth.

These tooth contours must be considered in the performance of operative dental procedures. Improper location and degree of facial or lingual convexities can result in serious complications, as illustrated in Figure 1-29, in which the proper facial contour is disregarded in the placement of a cervical restoration on a mandibular molar. Over-contouring is the worst offender, usually resulting in increased plaque retention that leads to a chronic inflammatory state of the gingiva.

The proper form of the proximal surfaces of teeth is just as important to the maintenance of periodontal tissue as is the proper form of facial and lingual surfaces. The proximal height of contour serves to provide (1) contacts with the proximal surfaces of adjacent teeth, thus preventing food impaction, and (2) adequate embrasure space apical to the contacts for gingival tissue, supporting bone, blood vessels, and nerves that serve the supporting structures (Fig. 1-30).

Proximal Contact Area

When teeth erupt to make proximal contact with previously erupted teeth, initially a contact point is present. The contact point increases in size to become a proximal contact area as the two adjacent tooth surfaces abrade each other during physiologic tooth movement (Figs. 1-31 and 1-32).

The proximal contact area is located in the incisal third of the approximating surfaces of maxillary and mandibular central incisors (Fig. 1-32). It is positioned slightly facial to the center of the proximal surface faciolingually (see Fig. 1-31). Proceeding posteriorly from the incisor region through all the remaining teeth, the contact area is located near the junction of the incisal (or occlusal) and middle thirds or in the middle third. Proximal contact areas typically are larger in the molar region, which helps prevent food impaction during mastication. Adjacent surfaces near the proximal contacts (embrasures) usually have remarkable symmetry.

Embrasures

Embrasures are V-shaped spaces that originate at the proximal contact areas between adjacent teeth and are named for the

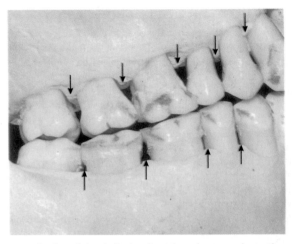

Fig. 1-30 Portion of the skull, showing triangular spaces beneath proximal contact areas. These spaces are occupied by soft tissue and bone for the support of teeth. (*Adapted from Bath-Balogh M, Fehrenbach MJ: Illustrated dental embryology, histology, and anatomy, ed 3, St. Louis, 2011, Saunders.*)

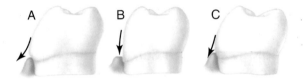

Fig. 1-29 Contours. Arrows show pathways of food passing over facial surface of mandibular molar during mastication. **A,** Over-contour deflects food from gingiva and results in under-stimulation of supporting tissues. **B,** Under-contour of tooth may result in irritation of soft tissue. **C,** Correct contour permits adequate stimulation for supporting tissue, resulting in healthy condition.

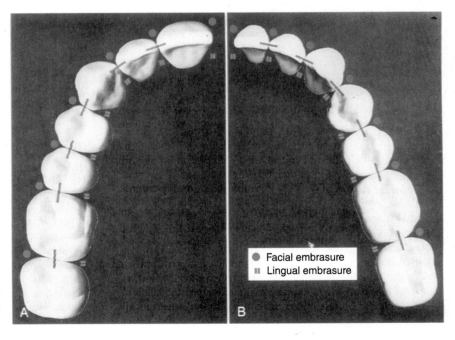

Fig. 1-31 Proximal contact points that have progressed to proximal contact areas. **A,** Maxillary teeth. **B,** Mandibular teeth. Facial and lingual embrasures are indicated.

● Facial embrasure
|| Lingual embrasure

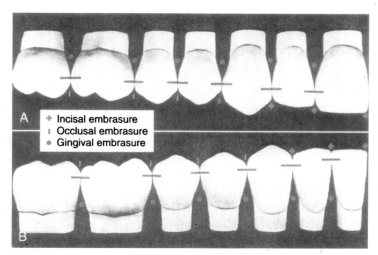

Fig. 1-32 Proximal contact areas. Black lines show positions of contacts incisogingivally and occlusogingivally. Incisal, occlusal, and gingival embrasures are indicated. **A,** Maxillary teeth. **B,** Mandibular teeth.

direction toward which they radiate. These embrasures are (1) facial, (2) lingual, (3) incisal or occlusal, and (4) gingival (see Figs. 1-31 and 1-32).

Initially, the interdental papilla fills the gingival embrasure. When the form and function of teeth are ideal and optimal oral health is maintained, the interdental papilla may continue in this position throughout life. When the gingival embrasure is filled by the papilla, trapping of food in this region is prevented. In a faciolingual vertical section, the papilla has a triangular shape between anterior teeth, whereas in posterior teeth, the papilla may be shaped like a mountain range, with facial and lingual peaks and the col ("valley") lying beneath the contact area (Fig. 1-33). This col, a central faciolingual concave area beneath the contact, is more vulnerable to periodontal disease from incorrect contact and embrasure form because it is covered by nonkeratinized epithelium. The physiologic significance of properly formed and located proximal contacts and associated embrasures cannot be overemphasized; they promote normal healthy interdental papillae filling the interproximal spaces (Fig. 1-34). Improper contacts can result in food impaction between teeth, potentially increasing the risk of periodontal disease, caries, and tooth movement. In addition, retention of food is objectionable because of its physical presence and the halitosis that results from food decomposition. Proximal contacts and interdigitation of teeth through occlusal contacts stabilize and maintain the integrity of the dental arches.

The correct relationships of embrasures, cusps to sulci, marginal ridges, and grooves of adjacent and opposing teeth provide for the escape of food from the occlusal surfaces during mastication (Fig. 1-35). When an embrasure is decreased in size or absent, additional stress is created on teeth and the supporting structures during mastication. Embrasures that are too large provide little protection to the supporting structures as food is forced into the interproximal space by an opposing cusp. A prime example is the failure to restore the distal cusp of a mandibular first molar when placing a restoration (Fig. 1-36). Lingual embrasures are usually larger than facial embrasures and this allows more food to be displaced lingually because the tongue can return the food to the occlusal surface more easily than if the food is displaced facially into the buccal vestibule (see Fig. 1-31). The

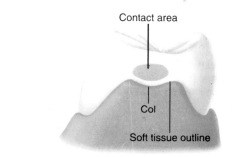

Fig. 1-33 Relationship of ideal interdental papilla to molar contact area.

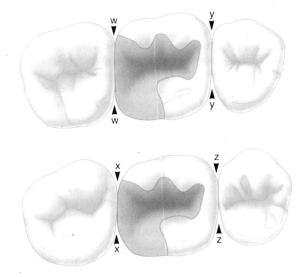

Fig. 1-34 Embrasure form. *w,* Improper embrasure form caused by overcontouring of restoration resulting in unhealthy gingiva from lack of stimulation. *x,* Good embrasure form. *y,* Frictional wear of contact area has resulted in decrease of embrasure dimension. *z,* When the embrasure form is good, supporting tissues receive adequate stimulation from foods during mastication.

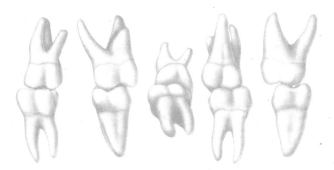

Fig. 1-35 Maxillary and mandibular first molars in maximum intercuspal contact. Note the grooves for escape of food.

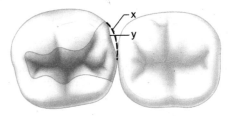

Fig. 1-36 Embrasure form. *x*, Portion of tooth that offers protection to underlying supporting tissue during mastication. *y*, Restoration fails to establish adequate contour for good embrasure form.

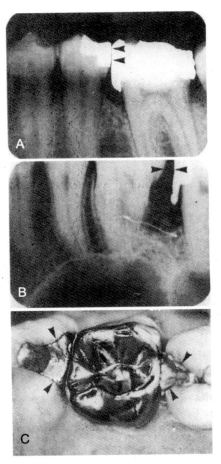

Fig. 1-37 Poor anatomic restorative form. **A,** Radiograph of flat contact and amalgam gingival excess. **B,** Radiograph of restoration with amalgam gingival excess and absence of contact resulting in trauma to supporting tissue. **C,** Poor occlusal margins.

marginal ridges of adjacent posterior teeth should be at the same height to have proper contact and embrasure forms. When this relationship is absent, it causes an increase in the problems associated with weak proximal contacts and faulty embrasure forms.

Preservation of the curvatures of opposing cusps and surfaces in function maintains masticatory efficiency throughout life (see Fig. 1-2). Correct anatomic form renders teeth more self-cleansing because of the smoothly rounded contours that are more exposed to the cleansing action of foods and fluids and the frictional movement of the tongue, lips, and cheeks. Failure to understand and adhere to correct anatomic form can contribute to the breakdown of the restored system (Fig. 1-37).

Maxilla and Mandible

The human maxilla is formed by two bones, the maxilla proper and the premaxilla. These two bones form the bulk of the upper jaw and the major portion of the hard palate and help form the floor of the orbit and the sides and base of the nasal cavity. They contain 10 maxillary primary teeth initially and later contain 16 maxillary permanent teeth in the alveolar process (see Figs. 1-1 and 1-3, *label 7*).

The mandible, or the lower jaw, is horseshoe-shaped and relates to the skull on either side via the TMJs. The mandible is composed of a body of two horizontal portions joined at the midline symphysis mandibulae and the rami, the vertical parts. The coronoid process and the condyle make up the superior border of each ramus. The mandible initially contains 10 mandibular primary teeth and later 16 mandibular permanent teeth in the alveolar process. Maxillary and mandibular bones comprise approximately 38% to 43% inorganic material and 34% organic material by volume. The inorganic material is hydroxyapatite, and the organic material is

primarily type I collagen, which is surrounded by a ground substance of glycoproteins and proteoglycans.

Oral Mucosa

The oral mucosa is the mucous membrane that covers all oral structures except the clinical crowns of teeth. It is composed of two layers: (1) the stratified squamous epithelium and (2) the supporting connective tissue, called *lamina propria*. (See the lamina propria of the gingiva in Fig. 1-38, *label 8*.) The epithelium may be keratinized, parakeratinized, or nonkeratinized, depending on its location. The lamina propria varies in thickness and supports the epithelium. It may be attached to the periosteum of alveolar bone, or it may be interposed over the submucosa, which may vary in different regions of the mouth (e.g., the floor of the mouth, the soft palate). The submucosa, consisting of connective tissues varying in density and thickness, attaches the mucous membrane to the underlying bony structures. The submucosa contains glands, blood vessels, nerves, and adipose tissue.

The oral mucosa is classified into three major functional types: (1) masticatory mucosa, (2) lining or reflective mucosa, and (3) specialized mucosa. The masticatory mucosa comprises the free and attached gingiva (see Fig. 1-38, *labels 6*

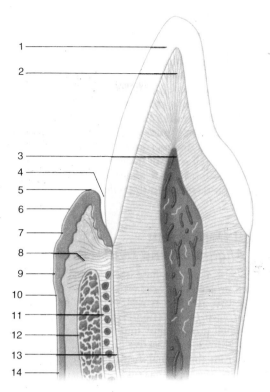

Fig. 1-38 Vertical section of a maxillary incisor illustrating supporting structures: *1,* enamel; *2,* dentin; *3,* pulp; *4,* gingival sulcus; *5,* free gingival margin; *6,* free gingiva; *7,* free gingival groove; *8,* lamina propria of gingiva; *9,* attached gingiva; *10,* mucogingival junction; *11,* periodontal ligament; *12,* alveolar bone; *13,* cementum; *14,* alveolar mucosa.

gingival unit, consisting of free and attached gingiva and the alveolar mucosa, and (2) the attachment apparatus, consisting of cementum, the periodontal ligament, and the alveolar process (see Fig. 1-38).

Gingival Unit

As mentioned previously, the free gingiva and the attached gingiva together form the masticatory mucosa. The free gingiva is the gingiva from the marginal crest to the level of the base of the gingival sulcus (see Fig. 1-38, *labels 4 and 6*). The gingival sulcus is the space between the tooth and the free gingiva. The outer wall of the sulcus (inner wall of the free gingiva) is lined with a thin, nonkeratinized epithelium. The outer aspect of the free gingiva in each gingival embrasure is called *gingival* or *interdental papilla.* The free gingival groove is a shallow groove that runs parallel to the marginal crest of the free gingiva and usually indicates the level of the base of the gingival sulcus (see Fig. 1-38, *label 7*).

The attached gingiva, a dense connective tissue with keratinized, stratified, squamous epithelium, extends from the depth of the gingival sulcus to the mucogingival junction. A dense network of collagenous fibers connects the attached gingiva firmly to cementum and the periosteum of the alveolar process (bone).

The alveolar mucosa is a thin, soft tissue that is loosely attached to the underlying alveolar bone (see Fig. 1-38, *labels 12 and 14*). It is covered by a thin, nonkeratinized epithelial layer. The underlying submucosa contains loosely arranged collagen fibers, elastic tissue, fat, and muscle tissue. The alveolar mucosa is delineated from the attached gingiva by the mucogingival junction and continues apically to the vestibular fornix and the inside of the cheek.

Clinically, the level of the gingival attachment and gingival sulcus is an important factor in restorative dentistry. Soft tissue health must be maintained by teeth having the correct form and position to prevent recession of the gingiva and possible abrasion and erosion of the root surfaces. The margin of a tooth preparation should not be positioned subgingivally (at levels between the marginal crest of the free gingiva and the base of the sulcus) unless dictated by caries, previous restoration, esthetics, or other preparation requirements.

Attachment Apparatus

The tooth root is attached to the alveolus (bony socket) by the periodontal ligament (see Fig. 1-38, *label 11*), which is a complex connective tissue containing numerous cells, blood vessels, nerves, and an extracellular substance consisting of fibers and ground substance. Most of the fibers are collagen, and the ground substance is composed of a variety of proteins and polysaccharides. The periodontal ligament serves the following functions: (1) attachment and support, (2) sensory, (3) nutritive, and (4) homeostatic. Bundles of collagen fibers, known as *principal fibers of the ligament,* serve to attach cementum to alveolar bone and act as a cushion to suspend and support the tooth. Coordination of masticatory muscle function is achieved, through an efficient proprioceptive mechanism, by the sensory nerves located in the periodontal ligament. Blood vessels supply the attachment apparatus with nutritive substances. Specialized cells of the ligament function

and 9) and the mucosa of the hard palate. The epithelium of these tissues is keratinized, and the lamina propria is a dense, thick, firm connective tissue containing collagenous fibers. The hard palate has a distinct submucosa except for a few narrow specific zones. The dense lamina propria of the attached gingiva is connected to the cementum and periosteum of the bony alveolar process (see Fig. 1-38, *label 8*).

The lining or reflective mucosa covers the inside of the lips, cheek, and vestibule, the lateral surfaces of the alveolar process (except the mucosa of the hard palate), the floor of the mouth, the soft palate, and the ventral surface of the tongue. The lining mucosa is a thin, movable tissue with a relatively thick, nonkeratinized epithelium and a thin lamina propria. The submucosa comprises mostly thin, loose connective tissue with muscle and collagenous and elastic fibers, with different areas varying from one another in their structures. The junction of the lining mucosa and the masticatory mucosa is the mucogingival junction, located at the apical border of the attached gingiva facially and lingually in the mandibular arch and facially in the maxillary arch (see Fig. 1-38, *label 10*). The specialized mucosa covers the dorsum of the tongue and the taste buds. The epithelium is nonkeratinized except for the covering of the dermal filiform papillae.

Periodontium

The periodontium consists of the oral hard and soft tissues that invest and support teeth. It can be divided into (1) the to resorb and replace cementum, the periodontal ligament, and alveolar bone.

The alveolar process—a part of the maxilla and the mandible—forms, supports, and lines the sockets into which the roots of teeth fit. Anatomically, no distinct boundary exists between the body of the maxilla or the mandible and the alveolar process. The alveolar process comprises thin, compact bone with many small openings through which blood vessels, lymphatics, and nerves pass. The inner wall of the bony socket consists of the thin lamella of bone that surrounds the root of the tooth. It is termed *alveolar bone proper*. The second part of the bone is called *supporting alveolar bone*, which surrounds the alveolar bone proper and supports the socket. Supporting bone is composed of two parts: (1) the cortical plate, consisting of compact bone and forming the inner (lingual) and outer (facial) plates of the alveolar process, and (2) the spongy base that fills the area between the plates and the alveolar bone proper.

Occlusion

Occlusion literally means "closing"; in dentistry, the term means the contact of teeth in opposing dental arches when the jaws are closed (static occlusal relationships) and during various jaw movements (dynamic occlusal relationships). The sizes of the jaws and the arrangement of teeth within the jaws are subject to a wide range of variation in humans. The locations of contacts between opposing teeth (occlusal contacts) vary as a result of differences in the sizes and shapes of teeth and jaws and the relative position of the jaws. A wide variety of occlusal schemes can be found in healthy individuals. Consequently, definition of an ideal occlusal scheme is fraught with difficulty.[8] Repeated attempts have been made to describe an ideal occlusal scheme, but these descriptions are so restrictive that few individuals can be found to fit the criteria. Failing to find a single adequate definition of an ideal occlusal scheme has resulted in the conclusion that "in the final analysis, optimal function and the absence of disease is the principal characteristic of a good occlusion."[8] The dental relationships described in this section conform to the concepts of normal, or usual, occlusal schemes and include common variations of tooth-and-jaw relationships. The masticatory system is highly adaptable and can function successfully over a wide range of differences in jaw size and tooth alignment. Despite this great adaptability, however, some patients are highly sensitive to changes in tooth contacts, which may be brought about by orthodontic and restorative dental procedures.

Occlusal contact patterns vary with the position of the mandible. Static occlusion is defined further by the use of reference positions that include fully closed, terminal hinge (TH) closure, retruded, protruded, and right and left lateral extremes. The number and location of occlusal contacts between opposing teeth have important effects on the amount and direction of muscle force applied during mastication and other parafunctional activities such as mandibular clenching, tooth grinding, or a combination of both (bruxism). In extreme cases, these forces can cause damage to teeth or their supporting tissues. Forceful tooth contact occurs routinely near the limits or borders of mandibular movement, showing the relevance of these reference positions.[9]

Tooth contact during mandibular movement is termed *dynamic occlusal relationship*. Gliding or sliding contacts occur during mastication and other mandibular movements. Gliding contacts may be advantageous or disadvantageous, depending on the teeth involved, the position of the contacts, and the resultant masticatory muscle response. The design of the restored tooth surface can have important effects on the number and location of occlusal contacts, and both static and dynamic relationships must be taken into consideration. The following sections discuss common arrangements and variations of teeth and the masticatory system. Mastication and the contacting relationships of anterior and posterior teeth are described with reference to the potential restorative needs of the teeth.

General Description
Tooth Alignment and Dental Arches

In Fig. 1-39, *A*, the cusps have been drawn as blunt, rounded, or pointed projections of the crowns of teeth. Posterior teeth have one, two, or three cusps near the facial and lingual surfaces of each tooth. The cusps are separated by distinct developmental grooves and sometimes have additional supplemental grooves on the cusp inclines. The facial cusps are separated from the lingual cusps by a deep groove, termed *central groove*. If a tooth has multiple facial cusps or multiple lingual cusps, the cusps are separated by facial or lingual developmental grooves. The depressions between the cusps are termed *fossae* (singular, is *fossa*). The cusps in both arches are aligned in a smooth curve. Usually, the maxillary arch is larger than the mandibular arch, which results in the maxillary cusps overlapping the mandibular cusps when the arches are in maximal occlusal contact (see Fig. 1-39, *B*). In Fig. 1-39, *A*, two curved lines have been drawn over the teeth to aid in the visualization of the arch form. These curved lines identify the alignment of similarly functioning cusps or fossae. On the left side of the arches, an imaginary arc connecting the row of facial cusps in the mandibular arch have been drawn and labeled *facial occlusal line*. Above that, an imaginary line connecting the maxillary central fossae is labeled *central fossa occlusal line*. The mandibular facial occlusal line and the maxillary central fossa occlusal line coincide exactly when the mandibular arch is fully closed into the maxillary arch. On the right side of the dental arches, the maxillary lingual occlusal line and mandibular central fossa occlusal line have been drawn and labeled. These lines also coincide when the mandible is fully closed.

In Fig. 1-39, *B*, the dental arches are fully interdigitated, with maxillary teeth overlapping mandibular teeth. The overlap of the maxillary cusps can be observed directly when the jaws are closed. *Maximum intercuspation (MI)* refers to the position of the mandible when teeth are brought into full interdigitation with the maximal number of teeth contacting. Synonyms for MI include *intercuspal contact*, *maximum closure*, and *maximum habitual intercuspation (MHI)*.

In Fig. 1-39, *C* (proximal view), the mandibular facial occlusal line and the maxillary central fossa occlusal line coincide exactly. The maxillary lingual occlusal line and the mandibular central fossa occlusal line identified in Fig. 1-39, *A*, also are coincidental. Cusps that contact opposing teeth along the central fossa occlusal line are termed *supporting cusps* (functional, centric, holding, or stamp cusps); the cusps

A. Dental arch cusp and fossa alignment

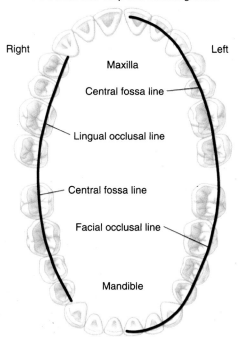

Right   Left

Maxilla

Central fossa line

Lingual occlusal line

Central fossa line

Facial occlusal line

Mandible

1. The maxillary lingual occlusal line and the mandibular central fossa line are coincident.
2. The mandibular facial occlusal line and the maxillary central fossa line are coincident.

B. Maximum intercuspation (MI): the teeth in opposing arches are in maximal contact

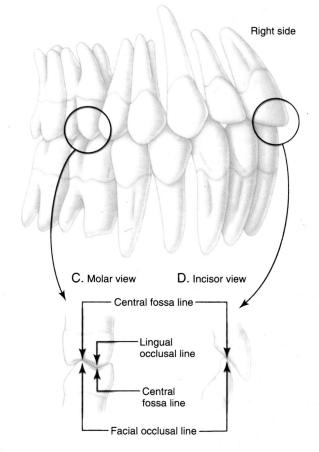

Right side

C. Molar view   D. Incisor view

Central fossa line

Lingual occlusal line

Central fossa line

Facial occlusal line

E. Facial view of anterior-posterior variations

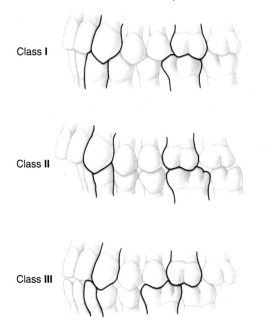

Class I

Class II

Class III

F. Molar Classes I, II, and III relationships

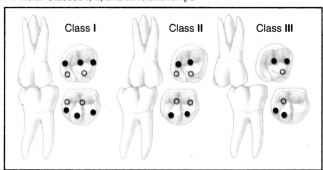

Class I   Class II   Class III

G. Skeletal Classes I, II, and III relationships

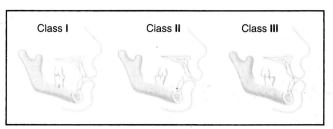

Class I   Class II   Class III

Fig. 1-39 Dental arch relationships.

that overlap opposing teeth are termed *nonsupporting cusps* (nonfunctional, noncentric, or nonholding cusps). The mandibular facial occlusal line identifies the mandibular supporting cusps, whereas the maxillary facial cusps are nonsupporting cusps. These terms are usually applied only to posterior teeth to distinguish the functions of the two rows of cusps. In some circumstances, the functional role of the cusps can be reversed, as illustrated in Fig. 1-40, *C-2*. Posterior teeth are well suited to crushing food because of the mutual cusp–fossa contacts (Fig. 1-41, *D*).

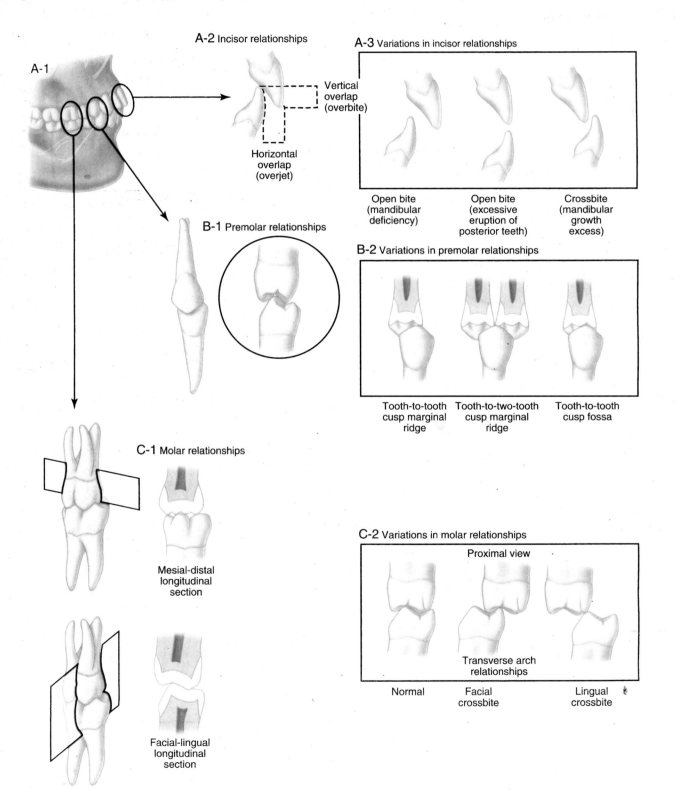

A-1

A-2 Incisor relationships

Vertical overlap (overbite)

Horizontal overlap (overjet)

A-3 Variations in incisor relationships

Open bite (mandibular deficiency)   Open bite (excessive eruption of posterior teeth)   Crossbite (mandibular growth excess)

B-1 Premolar relationships

B-2 Variations in premolar relationships

Tooth-to-tooth cusp marginal ridge   Tooth-to-two-tooth cusp marginal ridge   Tooth-to-tooth cusp fossa

C-1 Molar relationships

Mesial-distal longitudinal section

Facial-lingual longitudinal section

C-2 Variations in molar relationships

Proximal view

Transverse arch relationships

Normal   Facial crossbite   Lingual crossbite

Fig. 1-40 Tooth relationships.

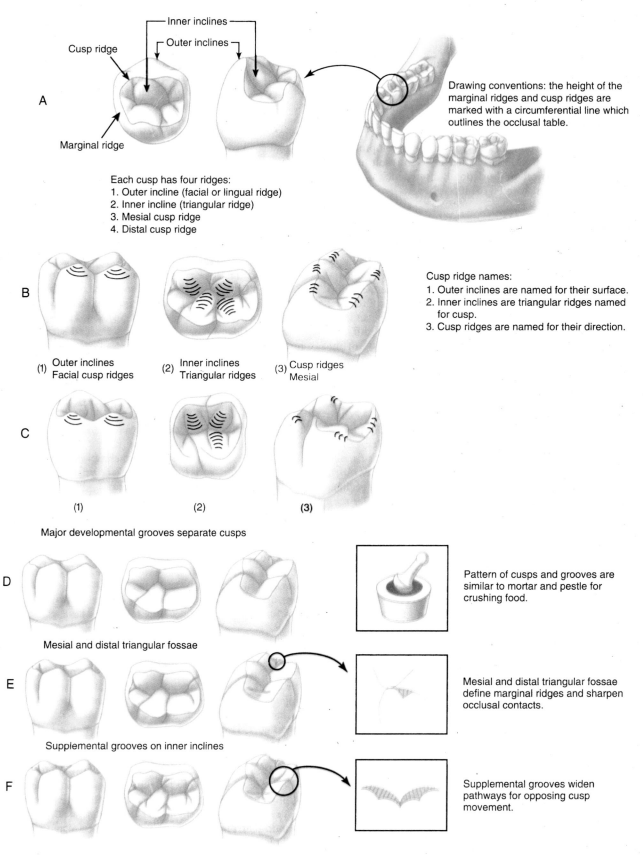

A

Inner inclines

Outer inclines

Cusp ridge

Marginal ridge

Drawing conventions: the height of the marginal ridges and cusp ridges are marked with a circumferential line which outlines the occlusal table.

Each cusp has four ridges:
1. Outer incline (facial or lingual ridge)
2. Inner incline (triangular ridge)
3. Mesial cusp ridge
4. Distal cusp ridge

B

(1) Outer inclines
Facial cusp ridges

(2) Inner inclines
Triangular ridges

(3) Cusp ridges
Mesial

Cusp ridge names:
1. Outer inclines are named for their surface.
2. Inner inclines are triangular ridges named for cusp.
3. Cusp ridges are named for their direction.

C

(1)　　　(2)　　　**(3)**

Major developmental grooves separate cusps

D

Pattern of cusps and grooves are similar to mortar and pestle for crushing food.

Mesial and distal triangular fossae

E

Mesial and distal triangular fossae define marginal ridges and sharpen occlusal contacts.

Supplemental grooves on inner inclines

F

Supplemental grooves widen pathways for opposing cusp movement.

Fig. 1-41 Common features of all posterior teeth.

In Fig. 1-39, *D*, anterior teeth are seen to have a different relationship in MI, but they also show the characteristic maxillary overlap. Incisors are best suited to shearing food because of their overlap and the sliding contact on the lingual surface of maxillary teeth. In MI, mandibular incisors and canines contact the respective lingual surfaces of their maxillary opponents. The amount of horizontal (overjet) and vertical (overbite) overlap (see Fig. 1-40, *A-2*) can considerably influence mandibular movement and the cusp design of restorations of posterior teeth. Variations in the growth and development of the jaws and in the positions of anterior teeth result in open bite, in which vertical or horizontal discrepancies prevent teeth from contacting (see Fig. 1-40, *A-3*).

Anteroposterior Interarch Relationships

In Fig. 1-39, *E*, the cusp interdigitation pattern of the first molar teeth is used to classify anteroposterior arch relationships using a system developed by Angle.[10] During the eruption of teeth, the tooth cusps and fossae guide the teeth into maximal contact. Three interdigitated relationships of the first molars are commonly observed. See Fig. 1-39, *F*, for an illustration of the occlusal contacts that result from different molar positions. The location of the mesiofacial cusp of the maxillary first molar in relation to the mandibular first molar is used as an indicator in Angle's classification. The most common molar relationship finds the maxillary mesiofacial cusp located in the mesiofacial developmental groove of the mandibular first molar. This relationship is termed *Angle* Class I. Slight posterior positioning of the mandibular first molar results in the mesiofacial cusp of the maxillary molar settling into the facial embrasure between the mandibular first molar and the mandibular second premolar. This is termed *Angle* Class II and occurs in approximately 15% of the U.S. population. Anterior positioning of the mandibular first molar relative to the maxillary first molar is termed *Angle* Class III and is the least common. In Class III relationships, the mesiofacial cusp of the maxillary first molar fits into the distofacial groove of the mandibular first molar; this occurs in approximately 3% of the U.S. population. Significant differences in these percentages occur in people in other countries and in different racial and ethnic groups.

Although Angle's classification is based on the relationship of the cusps, Figure 1-39, *G*, illustrates that the location of tooth roots in alveolar bone determines the relative positions of the crowns and cusps of teeth. When the mandible is proportionally similar in size to the maxilla, a Class I molar relationship is formed; when the mandible is proportionally smaller than the maxilla, a Class II relationship is formed; and when the mandible is relatively greater than the maxilla, a Class III relationship is formed.

Interarch Tooth Relationships

Fig. 1-40 illustrates the occlusal contact relationships of individual teeth in more detail. In Fig. 1-40, *A-2*, incisor overlap is illustrated. The overlap is characterized in two dimensions: (1) horizontal overlap (overjet) and (2) vertical overlap (overbite). Differences in the sizes of the mandible and the maxilla can result in clinically significant variations in incisor relationships, including open bite as a result of mandibular deficiency or excessive eruption of posterior teeth, and crossbite as a result of mandibular growth excess (see Fig. 1-40, *A-3*). These variations have significant clinical effects on the contacting relationships of posterior teeth during various jaw movements because anterior teeth do not provide gliding contact.

Fig. 1-40, *B-1*, illustrates a normal Class I occlusion, in which each mandibular premolar is located one half of a tooth width anterior to its maxillary antagonist. This relationship results in the mandibular facial cusp contacting the maxillary premolar mesial marginal ridge and the maxillary premolar lingual cusp contacting the mandibular distal marginal ridge. Because only one antagonist is contacted, this is termed *tooth-to-tooth relationship*. The most stable relationship results from the contact of the supporting cusp tips against the two marginal ridges, termed *tooth-to-two-tooth contact*. Variations in the mesiodistal root position of teeth produce different relationships (see Fig. 1-40, *B-2*). When the mandible is slightly distal to the maxilla (termed Class *II tendency*), each supporting cusp tip occludes in a stable relationship with the opposing mesial or distal fossa; this relationship is a cusp–fossa contact.

Fig. 1-40, *C*, illustrates Class I molar relationships in more detail. Fig. 1-40, *C-1*, shows the mandibular facial cusp tips contacting the maxillary marginal ridges and the central fossa triangular ridges. A faciolingual longitudinal section reveals how the supporting cusps contact the opposing fossae and shows the effect of the developmental grooves on reducing the height of the nonsupporting cusps opposite the supporting cusp tips. During lateral movements, the supporting cusp can move through the facial and lingual developmental groove spaces. Faciolingual position variations are possible in molar relationships because of differences in the growth of the width of the maxilla or the mandible.

Fig. 1-40, *C-2*, illustrates the normal molar contact position, facial crossbite, and lingual crossbite relationships. Facial crossbite in posterior teeth is characterized by the contact of the maxillary facial cusps in the opposing mandibular central fossae and the mandibular lingual cusps in the opposing maxillary central fossae. Facial crossbite (also termed *buccal crossbite*) results in the reversal of roles of the cusps of the involved teeth. In this reversal example, the mandibular lingual cusps and maxillary facial cusps become supporting cusps, and the maxillary lingual cusps and mandibular facial cusps become nonsupporting cusps. Lingual crossbite results in a poor molar relationship that provides little functional contact.

Posterior Cusp Characteristics

Four cusp ridges can be identified as common features of all the cusps. The outer incline of a cusp faces the facial (or the lingual) surface of the tooth and is named for its respective surface. In the example using a mandibular second premolar (see Fig. 1-41, *A*), the facial cusp ridge of the facial cusp is indicated by the line that points to the outer incline of the cusp. The inner inclines of the posterior cusps face the central fossa or the central groove of the tooth. The inner incline cusp ridges are widest at the base and become narrower as they approach the cusp tip. For this reason, they are termed *triangular ridges*. The triangular ridge of the facial cusp of the mandibular premolar is indicated by the arrow to the inner incline. Triangular ridges are usually set off from the other cusp ridges by one or more supplemental grooves. In Figure 1-41, *B-1* and *C-1*, the outer inclines of the facial cusps of the mandibular and maxillary first molars are highlighted. In

Figure 1-41, *B-2* and *C-2*, the triangular ridges of the facial and lingual cusps are highlighted.

The mesial and distal cusp ridges extend from the cusp tip mesially and distally and are named for their directions. The mesial and distal cusp ridges extend downward from the cusp tips, forming the characteristic facial and lingual profiles of the cusps as viewed from the facial or lingual aspect. At the base of the cusp, the mesial or distal cusp ridge abuts to another cusp ridge, forming a developmental groove, or the cusp ridge turns toward the center line of the tooth and fuses with the marginal ridge. Marginal ridges are elevated, the rounded ridges being located on the mesial and distal edges of the tooth's occlusal surface (see Fig. 1-41, *A*). The occlusal table of posterior teeth is the area contained within the mesial and distal cusp ridges and the marginal ridges of the tooth. The occlusal table limits are indicated in the drawings by a circumferential line connecting the highest points of curvature of these cusp ridges and marginal ridges.

Some cusps are modified to produce the characteristic form of individual posterior teeth. Mandibular first molars have longer triangular ridges on the distofacial cusps, causing a deviation of the central groove (see Fig. 1-41, *B-2*). The mesiolingual cusp of a maxillary molar is much larger than the mesiofacial cusp. The distal cusp ridge of the maxillary first molar mesiolingual cusp curves facially to fuse with the triangular ridge of the distofacial cusp (see Fig. 1-41, *C-2*). This junction forms the oblique ridge, which is characteristic of maxillary molars. The transverse groove crosses the oblique ridge where the distal cusp ridge of the mesiolingual cusp meets the triangular ridge of the distofacial cusp.

Supporting Cusps

In Figure 1-42, the lingual occlusal line of maxillary teeth and the facial occlusal line of mandibular teeth mark the locations of the supporting cusps. These cusps contact opposing teeth in their corresponding faciolingual center on a marginal ridge or a fossa. Supporting cusp–central fossa contact has been compared to a mortar and pestle because the supporting cusp cuts, crushes, and grinds fibrous food against the ridges forming the concavity of the fossa (see Fig. 1-41, *D*). The natural tooth form has multiple ridges and grooves ideally suited to aid in the reduction of the food bolus during chewing. During chewing, the highest forces and the longest duration of contact occur at MI. Supporting cusps also serve to prevent drifting and passive eruption of teeth—hence the term *holding cusps*. Supporting cusps (see Fig. 1-42) can be identified by five characteristic features:[11]

1. They contact the opposing tooth in MI.
2. They support the vertical dimension of the face.
3. They are nearer the faciolingual center of the tooth than nonsupporting cusps.
4. Their outer incline has the potential for contact.
5. They have broader, more rounded cusp ridges than nonsupporting cusps.

Because the maxillary arch is larger than the mandibular arch, the supporting cusps are located on the maxillary lingual occlusal line (see Fig. 1-42, *D*), whereas the mandibular supporting cusps are located on the mandibular facial occlusal line (see Figs. 1-42, *A* and *B*). The supporting cusps of both arches are more robust and better suited to crushing food than are the nonsupporting cusps. The lingual tilt of posterior teeth increases the relative height of the supporting cusps with respect to the nonsupporting cusps (see Fig. 1-42, *C*), and the central fossa contacts of the supporting cusps are obscured by the overlapping nonsupporting cusps (see Figs. 1-42, *E* and *F*). Removal of the nonsupporting cusps allows the supporting cusp–central fossa contacts to be studied (see Figs. 1-42, *G* and *H*). During fabrication of restorations, it is important that supporting cusps are not contacting opposing teeth in a manner that results in the lateral deflection of teeth. Rather, the restoration should provide contacts on plateaus or smoothly concave fossae so that masticatory forces are directed approximately parallel to the long axes of teeth.

Nonsupporting Cusps

Figure 1-43 illustrates that the nonsupporting cusps form a lingual occlusal line in the mandibular arch (see Fig. 1-43, *D*) and a facial occlusal line in the maxillary arch (see Fig. 1-43, *B*). The nonsupporting cusps overlap the opposing tooth without contacting the tooth. The nonsupporting cusps are located in the anteroposterior plane in facial (lingual) embrasures or in the developmental groove of opposing teeth, creating an alternating arrangement when teeth are in MI (see Figs. 1-43, *E* and *F*). The maxillary premolar nonsupporting cusps also play an essential role in esthetics. In the occlusal view, the nonsupporting cusps are farther from the faciolingual center of the tooth than are the supporting cusps. The nonsupporting cusps have sharper cusp ridges that may serve to shear food as they pass close to the supporting cusp ridges during chewing strokes. The overlap of the cusps helps keep the soft tissue of the tongue and cheeks out from the occlusal tables, preventing self-injury during chewing.

Mechanics of Mandibular Motion
Mandible and Temporomandibular Joints

The mandible articulates with a depression in each temporal bone called the *glenoid fossa*. The joints are termed *temporomandibular joints (TMJs)* because they are named for the two bones forming the articulation. The TMJs allow the mandible to move in all three planes (Fig. 1-44, *A*).

A TMJ is similar to a ball-and-socket joint, but it differs from a true mechanical ball-and-socket joint in some important features. The ball part, the mandibular condyle (see Fig. 1-44, *B*), is smaller than the socket, or glenoid fossa. The space resulting from the size difference is filled by a tough, pliable, and movable stabilizer termed the *articular disc*. The disc separates the TMJ into two articulating surfaces lubricated by synovial fluid in the superior and inferior joint spaces. Rotational opening of the mandible occurs as the condyles rotate under the discs (see Fig. 1-44, *C*). Rotational movement occurs between the inferior surface of the discs and the condyle. During wide opening or protrusion of the mandible, the condyles move anteriorly in addition to the rotational opening (see Figs. 1-44, *D* and *E*).

The disks move anteriorly with the condyles during opening and produce a sliding movement in the superior joint space between the superior surface of the discs and the articular eminences (see Fig. 1-44, *B*). The TMJs allow free movement of the condyles in the anteroposterior direction but resist

Synonyms for
supporting
cusps include:
1. Centric cusps
2. Holding cusps
3. Stamp cusps

A. Mandibular arch

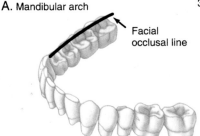

Facial
occlusal line

The mandibular arch is smaller than
the maxillary arch so the supporting
cusps are located on the facial occlusal
line. The mandibular lingual cusps that
overlap the maxillary teeth are
nonsupporting cusps.

B. Mandibular right quadrant

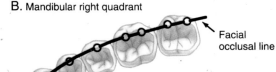

Facial
occlusal line

Mandibular supporting cusps are located
on the facial occlusal line.

C. Proximal view of molar
teeth in oclusion

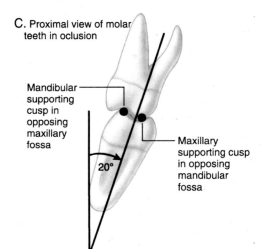

Mandibular
supporting
cusp in
opposing
maxillary
fossa

Maxillary
supporting cusp
in opposing
mandibular
fossa

20°

D. Maxillary right quadrant

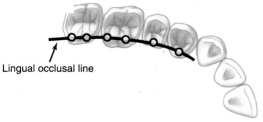

Lingual occlusal line

Supporting cusps are located on the
lingual occlusal line in maxillary arch.

E. Lingual view of left dental arches in
occlusion

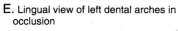

F. Facial view of left dental arches in
occlusion

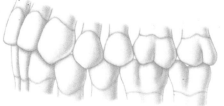

Supporting cusp features:
1. Contact opposing tooth in MI
2. Support vertical dimension
3. Nearer faciolingual center of
tooth than nonsupporting
cusps
4. Outer incline has potential for
contact
5. More rounded than
nonsupporting cusps

G. Mandibular nonsupporting cusps
removed

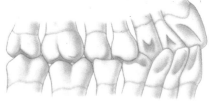

Maxillary supporting cusps occluding in
opposing fossae and on marginal ridges

H. Maxillary nonsupporting cusps removed

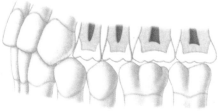

Mandibular supporting cusps occluding in
opposing fossae and on marginal ridges

Fig. 1-42 Supporting cusps.

A. Maxillary arch

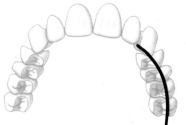

The maxillary arch is larger than the mandibular arch causing the maxillary facial line (nonsupporting cusps) to overlap the mandibular teeth.

Synonyms for nonsupporting cusps include:
1. Noncentric cusps
2. Nonholding cusps

B. Maxillary left quadrant

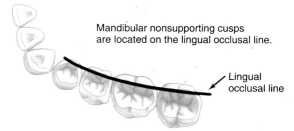

Facial occlusal line

Maxillary nonsupporting cusps are located on the facial occlusal line.

C. Molar teeth in occlusion

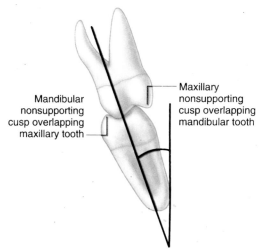

Mandibular nonsupporting cusp overlapping maxillary tooth

Maxillary nonsupporting cusp overlapping mandibular tooth

D. Mandibular left quadrant

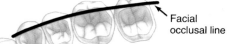

Mandibular nonsupporting cusps are located on the lingual occlusal line.

Lingual occlusal line

Nonsupporting cusp features:
1. Do not contact opposing tooth in MI
2. Keep soft tissue of tongue or cheek off occlusal table
3. Farther from faciolingual center of tooth than supporting cusps
4. Outer incline has no potential for contact
5. Have sharper cusp ridges than supporting cusps

E. Views of left dental arches in occlusion showing interdigitation of nonsupporting cusps

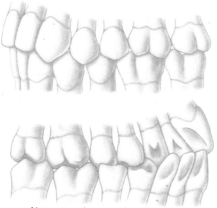

Nonsupporting cusp location:
1. Opposing embrasure
2. Opposing developmental groove

F. Views of left dental arches in occlusion showing facial and lingual occlusal lines

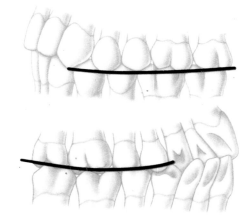

Fig. 1-43 Nonsupporting cusps.

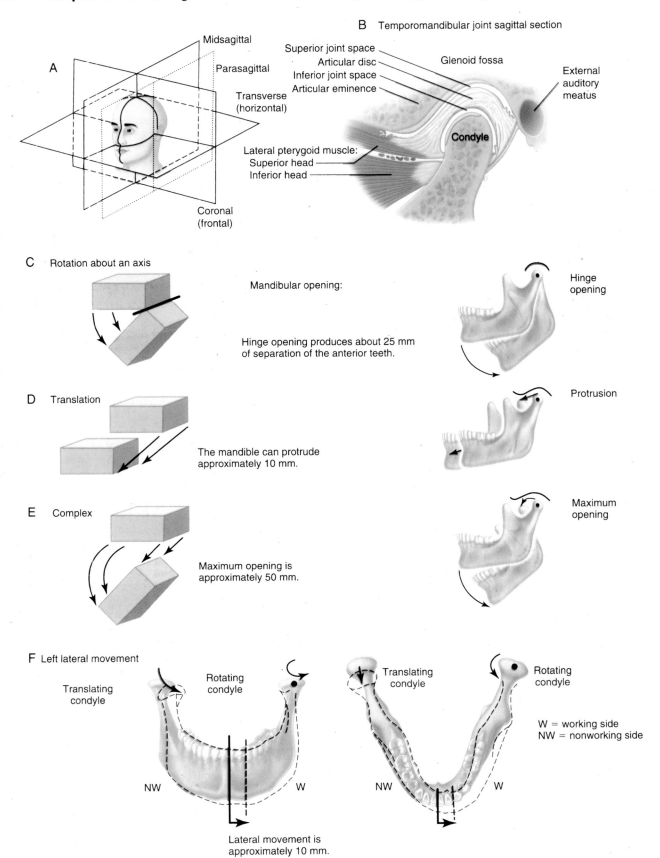

A

Midsagittal

Parasagittal

Transverse
(horizontal)

Coronal
(frontal)

B Temporomandibular joint sagittal section

Superior joint space
Articular disc
Inferior joint space
Articular eminence
Glenoid fossa
External auditory meatus
Condyle

Lateral pterygoid muscle:
Superior head
Inferior head

C Rotation about an axis

Mandibular opening:

Hinge opening produces about 25 mm of separation of the anterior teeth.

Hinge opening

D Translation

The mandible can protrude approximately 10 mm.

Protrusion

E Complex

Maximum opening is approximately 50 mm.

Maximum opening

F Left lateral movement

Translating condyle

Rotating condyle

Translating condyle

Rotating condyle

W = working side
NW = nonworking side

NW

W

NW

W

Lateral movement is approximately 10 mm.

Fig. 1-44 Types and directions of mandibular movements.

lateral displacement. The discs are attached firmly to the medial and lateral poles of the condyles in normal, healthy TMJs (see Fig. 1-45, *B*). The disk–condyle arrangement of the TMJ allows simultaneous sliding and rotational movement in the same joint. Therefore, the TMJ may be described as a *ginglymoarthroidal* joint.

Because the mandible is a semi-rigid, U-shaped bone with joints on both ends, movement of one joint produces a reciprocal movement in the other joint. The disk–condyle complex is free to move anteroposteriorly, providing sliding movement between the disk and the glenoid fossa. One condyle may move anteriorly, while the other remains in the fossa. Anterior movement of only one condyle produces reciprocal lateral rotation in the opposite TMJ.

The TMJ does not behave like a rigid joint as those on articulators (mechanical devices used by dentists to simulate jaw movement and reference positions). Because soft tissues cover the two articulating bones and an intervening disk composed of soft tissue is present, some resilience is to be expected in the TMJs. In addition to resilience, normal, healthy TMJs have flexibility, allowing small posterolateral movements of the condyles. In healthy TMJs, the movements are restricted to slightly less than 1 mm laterally and a few tenths of a millimeter posteriorly.

When morphologic changes occur in the hard and soft tissues of a TMJ because of disease, the disk–condyle relationship is possibly altered in many ways, including distortion, perforation, or tearing of the disk, and remodeling of the soft tissue articular surface coverings or their bony support. Diseased TMJs have unusual disk–condyle relationships, different geometry, and altered jaw movements and reference positions. Textbooks on TMJ disorders and occlusion should be consulted for information concerning the evaluation of diseased joints.[12] The remainder of this description of the movement and position of the mandible is based on normal, healthy TMJs and may not apply to diseased joints.

Review of Normal Masticatory Muscle Function and Mandibular Movement

The masticatory muscles work together to allow controlled, subtle movements of the mandible. The relative amount of muscle activity depends on the interarch relationships of maxillary and mandibular teeth as well as the amount of resistance to movement.[13-16] Primary muscles involved in mandibular movements include the anterior temporalis, middle temporalis, posterior temporalis, superficial masseter, deep masseter, superior lateral pterygoid, inferior lateral pterygoid, medial pterygoid, and digastric muscles.[14,15,17] The suprahyoid, infrahyoid, mylohyoid, and geniohyoid muscles also are involved in mandibular movements but not usually included in routine clinical examinations.[15,18] The relative amount of muscle activity of the various muscles has been identified through the use of electromyographic technology, in which electrodes were placed in the evaluated muscles,[14,15,19] as well as on the skin immediately adjacent to the muscles of interest.[5,9,14,15,17,18-27] The strategic three-dimensional arrangement of the muscles and the corresponding force vectors allow for the complete range of finely controlled mandibular movements. Consult an appropriate human anatomy textbook to identify the location, size, shape, three-dimensional orientation, and bony insertion of the various muscles discussed in this section.

Simple jaw opening requires the activation of digastric and inferior lateral pterygoid muscles.[14,15,19] Fine control of opening is accomplished by simultaneous mild antagonistic activity of the medial pterygoid.[14,15] When resistance is applied to jaw opening, mild masseter activation allows further stabilization and fine control.[14,15]

Jaw closure requires activation of the masseter and medial pterygoid.[15] Once teeth come into contact, the temporalis (anterior, middle, and posterior) muscles activate as well.[14,15] Clenching involves maximum activation of the masseter and temporalis, moderate activation of the medial pterygoid and superior lateral pterygoid, and recruitment of the inferior lateral pterygoid, digastric, and mylohyoid muscles.[14,15,19] In general, the superficial masseter has slightly higher activity than the deep masseter during clenching.[17] Coactivation of cooperating and antagonistic muscles allows for controlled force to be applied to teeth.[14]

Protrusion requires maximum bilateral activation of the inferior lateral pterygoid, with moderate activation of the medial pterygoid, masseter, and digastric muscles. During protrusion minimal activation of the temporalis and superior lateral pterygoid occurs. The superior lateral pterygoid has muscle fibers that insert into the temporomandibular disc as well as the neck of the mandibular condyle (see Fig. 1-44).[19] It is important to note that minimal activation of the superior lateral pterygoid is necessary if the temporomandibular disc is to rotate to the top of the condylar head as the condyle translates down the articular eminence during mandibular protrusive or excursive movements.[14]

Incisal biting with posterior disclusion requires maximum bilateral activity of the superficial masseter to force the incisors toward each other, as well as maximum activity of the inferior lateral pterygoid to maintain the protruded position of the condylar head down the slope of the articular eminence.[14] Incisal biting also requires moderate activity of the anterior temporalis, medial pterygoid, anterior digastric, and superior lateral pterygoid.[14] Note that the shift in the level of activity of the superior lateral pterygoid from protrusion to incisal biting indicates a dual role in condylar positioning and temporomandibular disc positioning or stabilization. The middle and posterior temporalis regions have minimal activity during incisal biting.[15]

Retrusion of the mandible requires bilateral maximum activation of the posterior and middle temporalis as well as moderate activity of the anterior temporalis and anterior digastric.[14,15] The superior lateral pterygoid is maximally active when the mandible is retruded and the posterior teeth are clenched.[14] The masseter has minimal activity in retrusion.[14] The inferior lateral pterygoid and the medial pterygoid have minimal to no activity during retrusion.[14,15]

Movement of the mandible to the right requires moderate to maximal activity of the left inferior lateral pterygoid and medial pterygoid muscles as well as the right posterior temporalis, middle temporalis, and anterior digastric.[14-16] In addition to these, the right superior lateral pterygoid, right anterior temporalis, and left anterior digastric are minimally to moderately active.[14-16] Activation of the right superior lateral pterygoid provides resistance to right condyle distalization as well positional support of the right temporomandibular disc. The right superficial masseter, right inferior lateral pterygoid, right medial pterygoid, left superior lateral pterygoid, left anterior temporalis, left middle temporalis, left posterior temporalis, and left superficial masseter all have minimal activity.[14-16] Minimal activity of the left superior lateral pterygoid allows the disk to shift distally, as needed, to remain between the condylar head and the articular eminence while translation and rotation of the left condylar head occurs. Activation of the elevator muscles on the left side provides for the translating left condyle–disk complex to remain in contact with the articular eminence. Movement of the mandible to the left follows the same pattern of coordinated muscle activity except in reverse.

Wide opening requires bilateral moderate to maximal activity of the inferior lateral pterygoid and anterior digastric muscles.[14] In addition to these the medial pterygoid muscles are minimally to moderately active.[14] The temporalis, masseter, and superior lateral pterygoid muscles have minimal to no activity during wide opening.[14,15]

During mastication, the typical mandibular movement involves opening with corresponding bilateral anterior, inferior, and rotating condylar motion.[9,28] As closure begins, the entire mandible moves laterally.[9] As closure continues, the working side condyle shifts back to its terminal hinge position before the teeth occlude and remains nearly stationary.[9] As the closure continues, the working side condyle shifts medially while the nonworking side condyle shifts superiorly, distally, and laterally to its terminal hinge position.[9] The medial shift of the working side condyle may be caused by the influence of the superior lateral pterygoid muscle contraction. The opening and closing paths of the incisors vary from individual to individual and also depend on the consistency of the food being masticated.[9] The realistic normal lower limit for the incisal opening in patients between 10 and 70 years of age is 40 mm.[29]

To describe mandibular motion, its direction and length must be specified in three mutually perpendicular planes. By convention, these planes are sagittal, coronal (frontal), and transverse (horizontal) (see Fig. 1-44, *A*). The mid-sagittal plane is a vertical (longitudinal) plane that passes through the center of the head in an anteroposterior direction. A vertical plane off the center line, such as a section through the TMJ, is termed *parasagittal plane.* The coronal plane is a vertical plane perpendicular to the sagittal plane. The transverse plane is a horizontal plane that passes from anterior to posterior and is perpendicular to the sagittal and frontal planes. Mandibular motion is described in each of these planes.

Types of Motion

Centric relation (CR) is the position of the mandible when the condyles are positioned superiorly in the fossae in healthy TMJs. In this position, the condyles articulate with the thinnest avascular portion of the disks and are in an anterosuperior position against the shapes of the articular eminences. This position is independent of tooth contacts.

Rotation is a simple motion of an object around an axis (see Fig. 1-44, *C*). The mandible is capable of rotation about an axis through centers located in the condyles. The attachments of the disks to the poles of the condyles permit the condyles to rotate under the disks. Rotation with the condyles positioned in CR is termed *terminal hinge (TH) movement.* TH is used in dentistry as a reference movement for construction of restorations and dentures. Initial contact between teeth during a TH closure provides a reference point termed *centric*

occlusion (CO). Many patients have a small slide from CO to MI, referred to as *slide in centric,* which may have forward and lateral components, resulting in a slight superior mandibular movement. Maximum rotational opening in TH is limited to approximately 25 mm measured between the incisal edges of anterior teeth.

Translation is the bodily movement of an object from one place to another (see Fig. 1-44, *D*). The mandible is capable of translation by the anterior movement of the disk–condyle complex from the TH position forward and down the articular eminence and back. Simultaneous, direct anterior movement of both condyles, or mandibular forward thrusting, is termed *protrusion.* The pathway followed by anterior teeth during protrusion may not be smooth or straight because of contact between anterior teeth and sometimes posterior teeth. (See the superior border of Posselt's diagram in Fig. 1-45, *A*.) Protrusion is limited to approximately 10 mm by the ligamentous attachments of masticatory muscles and the TMJs.

Fig. 1-44, *E*, illustrates complex motion, which combines rotation and translation in a single movement. Most mandibular movement during speech, chewing, and swallowing consists of rotation and translation. The combination of rotation and translation allows the mandible to open 50 mm or more.

Fig. 1-44, *F*, illustrates the left lateral movement of the mandible. It is the result of forward translation of the right condyle and rotation of the left condyle. Right lateral movement of the mandible is the result of forward translation of the left condyle and rotation of the right condyle.

Capacity of Motion of the Mandible

In 1952, Posselt recorded mandibular motion and developed a diagram (termed *Posselt's diagram*) to illustrate it (see Fig. 1-45, *A*).[30] By necessity, the original recordings of mandibular movement were done outside of the mouth, which magnified the vertical dimension but not the horizontal dimension. Modern systems using digital computer techniques can record mandibular motion in actual time and dimensions and then compute and draw the motion as it occurred at any point in the mandible and teeth.[9] This makes it possible to accurately reconstruct mandibular motion simultaneously at several points. Three of these points are particularly significant clinically—incisor point, molar point, and condyle point (Fig. 1-46, *A*).[31] The incisor point is located on the midline of the mandible at the junction of the facial surface of mandibular central incisors and the incisal edge. The molar point is the tip of the mesiofacial cusp of the mandibular first molar on a specified side. The condyle point is the center of rotation of the mandibular condyle on the specified side.

Limits of Mandibular Motion: The Borders

In Fig. 1-45, *A*, the limits for movement of the incisor point are illustrated in the sagittal plane. The mandible is not drawn to scale with the drawing of the sagittal borders. Also, in this particular diagram, CO coincides with MI. (As mentioned earlier, in some patients, a small slide may occur from CO to MI.) The starting point for this diagram is CO, the first contact of teeth when the condyles are in CR. The posterior border of the diagram from CO to *a* in Fig. 1-45, *A*, is formed by the

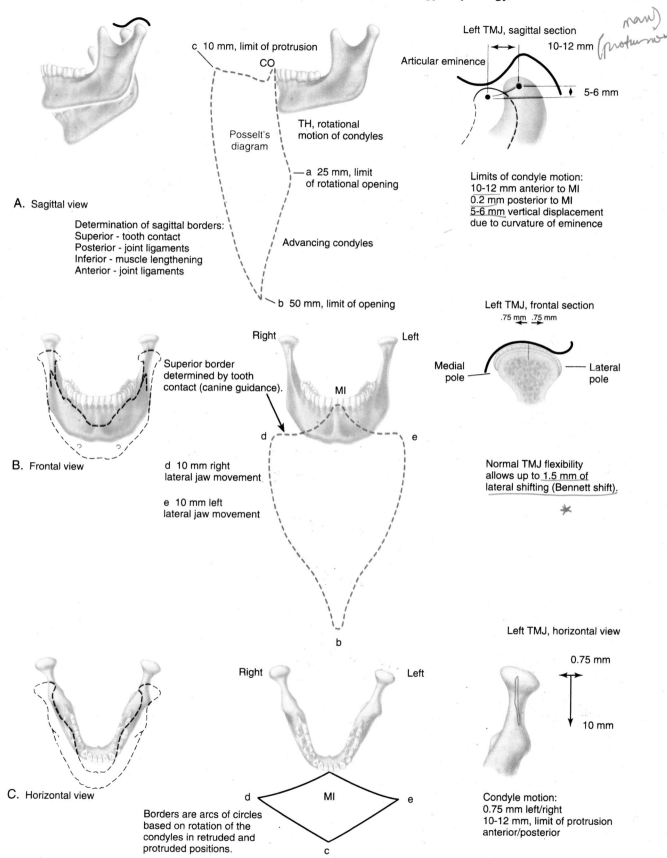

A. Sagittal view

c 10 mm, limit of protrusion

CO

Posselt's diagram

TH, rotational motion of condyles

a 25 mm, limit of rotational opening

Advancing condyles

b 50 mm, limit of opening

Determination of sagittal borders:
Superior - tooth contact
Posterior - joint ligaments
Inferior - muscle lengthening
Anterior - joint ligaments

Left TMJ, sagittal section   10-12 mm   (protrusion)

Articular eminence

5-6 mm

Limits of condyle motion:
10-12 mm anterior to MI
0.2 mm posterior to MI
5-6 mm vertical displacement
due to curvature of eminence

B. Frontal view

Right   Left

MI

Superior border determined by tooth contact (canine guidance).

d

e

d 10 mm right lateral jaw movement

e 10 mm left lateral jaw movement

b

Left TMJ, frontal section
.75 mm .75 mm

Medial pole

Lateral pole

Normal TMJ flexibility allows up to 1.5 mm of lateral shifting (Bennett shift).

C. Horizontal view

Right   Left

Borders are arcs of circles based on rotation of the condyles in retruded and protruded positions.

d   MI   e

c

Left TMJ, horizontal view

0.75 mm

10 mm

Condyle motion:
0.75 mm left/right
10-12 mm, limit of protrusion anterior/posterior

Fig. 1-45 Capacity of mandibular movement. (Mandible drawings are not to scale with border diagrams.)

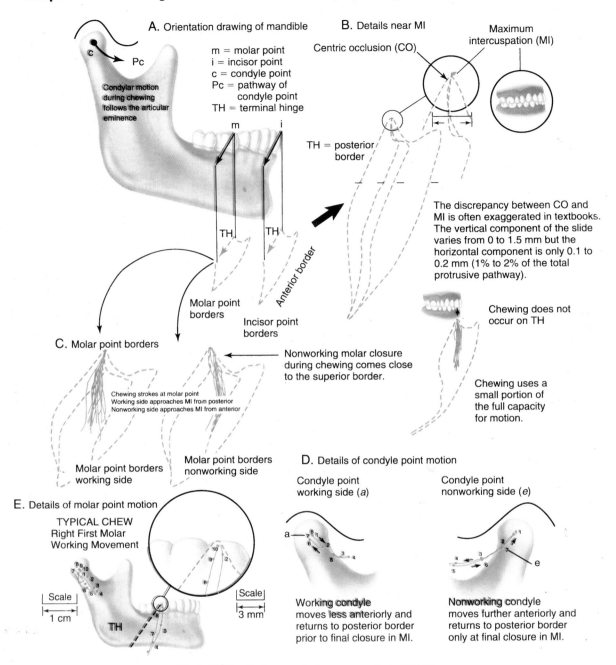

A. Orientation drawing of mandible

m = molar point
i = incisor point
c = condyle point
Pc = pathway of condyle point
TH = terminal hinge

Condylar motion during chewing follows the articular eminence

B. Details near MI

Centric occlusion (CO)

Maximum intercuspation (MI)

TH = posterior border

The discrepancy between CO and MI is often exaggerated in textbooks. The vertical component of the slide varies from 0 to 1.5 mm but the horizontal component is only 0.1 to 0.2 mm (1% to 2% of the total protrusive pathway).

Chewing does not occur on TH

Chewing uses a small portion of the full capacity for motion.

Molar point borders

Incisor point borders

Nonworking molar closure during chewing comes close to the superior border.

C. Molar point borders

Chewing strokes at molar point
Working side approaches MI from posterior
Nonworking side approaches MI from anterior

Molar point borders working side

Molar point borders nonworking side

D. Details of condyle point motion

Condyle point working side (*a*)

Condyle point nonworking side (*e*)

Working condyle moves less anteriorly and returns to posterior border prior to final closure in MI.

Nonworking condyle moves further anteriorly and returns to posterior border only at final closure in MI.

E. Details of molar point motion

TYPICAL CHEW
Right First Molar
Working Movement

Scale
1 cm

Scale
3 mm

Fig. 1-46 Mandibular capacity for movement: sagittal view.

rotation of the mandible around the condyle points. This border from CO to *a* is the TH movement. *Hinge axis* is the term used to describe an imaginary line connecting the centers of rotation in the condyles (condyle points) and is useful for reference to articulators. Hinge-axis closure is a reference movement used in prosthetic dentistry and is valid only when the TMJs are properly positioned in the fossae. The inferior limit to this hinge opening occurs at approximately 25 mm and is indicated by *a* in Fig. 1-45, *A*. The superior limit of the posterior border occurs at the first tooth contact and is identified by CO. In many healthy adults, a sliding tooth contact movement positions the mandible slightly anteriorly or slightly anterolaterally from CO into MI (see Fig. 1-46, *B*).

This anterior or anterolateral movement is termed *slide in centric.*

At point *a* in Fig. 1-45, *A*, further rotation of the condyles is impossible because of the stretch limits of the joint capsule, ligamentous attachments to the condyles, and the mandible-opening muscles. Further opening can be achieved only by translation of the condyles anteriorly, producing the line *a-b*. Maximum opening (point *b*) in adults is approximately 50 mm. These measures are important diagnostically. Mandibular opening limited to 25 mm suggests blockage of condylar translation, usually the result of a disc derangement. Limitation of opening in the 35 to 45 mm range suggests masticatory muscle hypertonicity. The line CO-*a-b* represents the maximum retruded opening path. This is the posterior border, or the posterior limit of mandibular opening. The line *b-c* represents the maximum protruded closure. This is achieved by a forward thrust of the mandible that keeps the condyles in their maximum anterior positions, while arching the mandible closed.

Retrusion, or posterior movement of the mandible, results in the irregular line *c*-CO. The irregularities of the superior border are caused by tooth contacts; the superior border is a tooth-determined border. Protrusion is a reference mandibular movement starting from CO and proceeding anteriorly to point *c*. Protrusive mandibular movements are used by dentists to evaluate occlusal relationships of teeth and restorations. The complete diagram, CO-*a-b-c*-CO, represents the maximum possible motion of the incisor point in all directions in the sagittal plane. The area of most interest to dentists is the superior border produced by tooth contact. (Mandibular movement in the sagittal plane is illustrated in more detail in Fig. 1-46.)

The motion of the condyle point during chewing is strikingly different from the motion of the incisor point. Motion of the condyle point is a curved line that follows the articular eminence. The maximum protrusion of the condyle point is 10 to 12 mm anteriorly when following the downward curve of the articular eminence. The condyle point does not drop away from the eminence during mandibular movements. Chewing movements in the sagittal plane are characterized by a nearly vertical up-and-down motion of the incisor point, whereas the condyle points move anteriorly and then return posteriorly over a curved surface (see Fig. 1-46, *B*).

In the frontal view shown in Fig. 1-45, *B*, the incisor point and chin are capable of moving about 10 mm to the left or right. This lateral movement—or excursion—is indicated by the lines MI-*d* to the right and MI-*e* to the left. Points *d* and *e* indicate the limit of the lateral motion of the incisor point. Lateral movement is often described with respect to only one side of the mandible for the purpose of defining the relative motion of mandibular teeth to maxillary teeth. In a left lateral movement, the left mandibular teeth move away from the midline, and the right mandibular teeth move toward the midline. → Laterotrusion

Mandibular pathways directed away from the midline are termed *working* (synonyms include *laterotrusion*, *functional*), and mandibular pathways directed toward the midline are termed *nonworking* (synonyms include *mediotrusion*, *nonfunctional*, and *balancing*). The terms *working* and *nonworking* are based on observations of chewing movements in which the mandible is seen to shift during closure toward the side of the mouth containing the food bolus. The working side is used to crush food, whereas the nonworking side is without a food bolus.

The left lateral mandibular motion indicated by the line MI-*e* (see Fig. 1-45, *B*) is the result of rotation of the left condyle (working side condyle) and translation of the right condyle (nonworking side condyle) to its anterior limit (see Fig. 1-44, *F*). The translation of the nonworking condyle in a right lateral motion of the mandible can be seen in the horizontal view in Figure 1-47, *A* and *B*. The line *e-b* in Figure 1-45, *B*, is completed by mandibular opening that is the result of rotation of both condyles and translation of the working condyle to its maximum anterior position. The line *b-d*-MI represents similar motions on the right side.

The vertical displacement in the incisor point line from MI to *e* or *d*, shown in Fig. 1-45, *B*, is the result of teeth, usually canines, gliding over each other. Vertical displacement of the mandible secondary to gliding contact of canine teeth is termed *canine guidance* and has significance for restorative procedures. The gliding tooth contact supplied by canine guidance provides some of the vertical separation of posterior teeth during lateral jaw movements and prevents potentially damaging collisions of their cusps secondary to the increased elevator muscle activity that occurs when posterior teeth come into contact. When the canine guidance is shallow, the occlusal surface of posterior teeth must be altered to prevent potentially damaging contacts in lateral movements. An articulator aids in the evaluation of the relationships of posterior teeth during fabrication of indirect posterior restorations.

Flexibility in the TMJs allows the condyles to move slightly to the working side during the closing stroke. This lateral shift of the condylar head, illustrated in the frontal view of a right TMJ in Fig. 1-45, *B*, is termed *Bennett shift* or *lateral shift* and varies from patient to patient (see Figs. 1-47, *B–D*). The magnitude of the shift in normal TMJs varies from 0 to 1.5 and normally has little effect on posterior teeth. Excessive lateral shift may be associated with morphologic changes of the TMJs. Excessive lateral condylar shifting coupled with shallow canine guidance poses a significant problem, however, for restorative procedures because the resulting lateral mandibular movements are flat; consequently, little separation of posterior teeth occurs, resulting in increased contact of posterior teeth.

In Fig. 1-45, *C*, the horizontal view illustrates the capability of the mandible to translate anteriorly. Extreme left lateral motion is indicated by MI-*e* produced by rotation of the left condyle (working condyle) and translation of the right condyle (non-working condyle) to its anterior limit. From point *e*, protrusion of the left condyle moves the incisor point to *c*, the maximum protruded position where both condyles have translated.

Sagittal View

In Fig. 1-46, the drawing of the mandible is used to orient the sagittal border diagrams. Projected below the mandible are diagrams of the incisor point (*i*) and molar point (*m*) borders (see Fig. 1-46, *A*). The molar point borders are similar to the incisor point diagram but are shorter in the vertical dimension because the molar point is closer to the TMJ. Closure of the jaw on the posterior border is termed *TH closure*. TH closure is a simple arc of a circle with a radius equal to the length from the incisor point to the center of the hinge axis (condyle point *c*). The area near MI is enlarged to illustrate the details of the TH closure (see Fig. 1-46, *B*). CO and MI are located close to each other. In the magnified view, teeth can be seen to guide the mandible from CO to MI. The gliding (sliding) contact typically is 1 to 2 mm long and can occur on any of the posterior teeth. The horizontal component of this slide is only a few tenths of a millimeter in healthy joints but may position the condyle(s) on the slope of the articular eminence, a position which requires protrusive muscle activity to maintain.[14,19]

The clinical significance of the shift between CO and MI has been a source of debate in dentistry, resulting in extensive literature on the topic.[32,33] Clinical ramifications may include

posterior teeth may contact the opposing tooth during mandibular movements. In Fig. 1-52, *D*, the opposing surfaces of molar teeth are divided into five areas:

1. *Inner incline of the nonsupporting (noncentric) cusp.* This area has the potential for undesirable contact in working side movements by contacting the outer aspect of the supporting (centric) cusp (area 5).
2. *Fossa or marginal ridge contact area.* This is the main holding contact (or centric stop) area for the opposing supporting cusp.
3. *Inner incline of the supporting (centric holding) cusp.* This area has the potential for undesirable contact during nonworking movements.
4. *Contact area of the supporting (centric holding) cusp.* This is the main cusp contact area.
5. *Outer aspect of the supporting (centric holding) cusp.* This area sometimes participates in working side movements by contacting the inner incline of the nonsupporting (noncentric) cusp (area 1).

Anterior Tooth Contacts

During anterior movement of the mandible (i.e., protrusion), the lower anterior teeth glide along the lingual surfaces of maxillary anterior teeth (see Figs. 1-52, *E* and *F*). The combination of the anterior guidance (slope and vertical overlap of anterior teeth) and the slope of the articular eminence (horizontal condylar guidance on the articulator) determines the amount of vertical separation of the posterior teeth as the mandible moves anteriorly. Some texts refer to this separation as *disocclusion* (or *disclusion*) of the posterior teeth. Multiple contacts between the opposing dental arches on anterior teeth are desirable in protrusion movements. With protrusion, multiple contacts serve to prevent excessive force on any individual pair of gliding teeth. Posterior tooth contact during protrusion is not desirable because it may overload the involved teeth secondary to the increased elevator muscle activity that occurs when posterior teeth come into contact. It has been shown that when anterior teeth are in contact and posterior teeth are discluded, elevator muscles are less active.[13-16,20,24,27,44]

Articulator-mounted casts can be used to assess the superior border near MI, which is the critical zone for tooth contact. This information is useful during the fabrication of indirect restorations because the position and height of the restored cusps can be evaluated and adjusted in the laboratory, which minimizes the chairside time and effort required to adjust the completed restorations.

Posterior Tooth Contacts

In idealized occlusal schemes designed for restorative dentistry, posterior teeth should contact only in MI such that the force which results from maximum activation of the elevator muscles is distributed evenly over multiple teeth.[13-16,20,24,25,27,44] Any movement of the mandible should result in the separation of posterior teeth by the combined effects of anterior guidance and the slope of the articular eminence (horizontal condylar guidance on the articulator). This separation of posterior teeth during protrusion or excursion results in a decrease in the level of activity and force being generated by the elevator muscles.[13,15,16,18,20,24,27,44]

Forceful contact of individual posterior tooth cusps during chewing and clenching may lead to muscle discomfort, damage to teeth and supporting structures, or both in some patients. In patients with shallow anterior guidance or open bite, restoration is more difficult without the introduction of undesirable tooth contacts. Articulator-mounted casts may be used to assess and solve restorative problems that are difficult to manage by direct intraoral techniques.

The side of the jaw where the bolus of food is placed is termed *the working side*. Working side also is used in reference to jaws or teeth when the patient is not chewing (e.g., in guided test movements directed laterally). The term also can identify a specific side of the mandible (i.e., the side toward which the mandible is moving). During chewing, the working side closures start from a lateral position and are directed medially to MI. Test movements are used by dentists to assess the occlusal contacts on the working side; for convenience, these movements are started in MI and are continued laterally. The working side test movement follows the same pathway as the working side chewing closure but occurs in the opposite direction. The preferred occlusal relationship for restorative purposes is one that limits the working side contact to canines only. This is directly related to the observation that compared with canine guidance alone, guidance from canines *and* posterior teeth will allow greater activation of the anterior temporalis muscle and longer activation of the masseter and temporalis muscles during excursive movements.[24,27,44]

Tooth contact posterior to the canine on the working side may occur naturally in worn dentitions. As canines are shortened by wear, separation of the posterior teeth diminishes. Lateral mandibular movements in worn dentitions successively bring into contact more posterior teeth as the heights of the canines decrease. Multiple tooth contacts during lateral jaw movements are termed *group function*. Right-sided group function is illustrated in Fig. 1-52, *E*, compared with left canine guidance contact in Fig. 1-52, *F*. Because the amount of torque and wear imposed on teeth increases closer to the muscle attachments on the mandible, molar contact in group function is undesirable. Group function occurs naturally in a worn dentition. Group function may be a therapeutic goal when the bony support of canines is compromised by periodontal disease or Class II occlusions in which canine guidance is impossible.

The nonworking side is opposite the working side and normally does not contain a food bolus during chewing. During chewing closures, mandibular teeth on the nonworking side close from an anteromedial position and approach MI by moving posterolaterally. Contact of the molar cusps on the nonworking side may overload these teeth, compromise the ipsilateral TMJ, or both because of a resultant increase in the activity of the masseter, anterior temporalis, and posterior temporalis muscles and the ipsilateral superior lateral pterygoid.[13-15,17] Each of these muscles counteracts the action of the nonworking side inferior lateral pterygoid, which is responsible (along with the contralateral posterior temporalis and digastric muscles) for effecting the down and forward translation of the nonworking side condyle. Additional activity of the ipsilateral superior lateral pterygoid muscle should not occur during condylar translation when the TMJ disk needs to rotate posteriorly toward the top of the condylar head to maintain its position between the condyle and the articular eminence. Even in light of this normal physiologic muscle response to nonworking side tooth contact, it has been observed that the presence of a nonworking side contact does not necessarily mean that it is an interference to mandibular function.[45] Great variation exists among patients in the level of masticatory system tolerance to nonworking side contacts. An understanding of the neuromuscular response to nonworking side posterior contacts leads to the conclusion that avoidance of these contacts is an important goal for restorative procedures on molars. Undesirable nonworking side contacts are illustrated in Fig. 1-52, *F*.

Neurologic Correlates and Control of Mastication

This summary of neurologic control is based on an excellent review by Lund.[46] The control of mastication depends on sensory feedback. Sensory feedback serves to control the coordination of the lips, tongue, and mandibular movement during manipulation of the food bolus through all stages of mastication and preparation for swallowing. Physiologists divide an individual chewing cycle into three components: *opening, fast-closing,* and *slow-closing.* The slow-closing segment of chewing is associated with the increased forces required for crushing food. The central nervous system receives several types of feedback from muscle spindles, periodontal receptors, and touch receptors in the skin and mucosa. This feedback controls the mandibular closing muscles during the slow-closing phase. Sensory feedback often results in inhibition of movement (e.g., because of pain). During mastication, some sensory feedback from teeth is excitatory, causing an increase in the closing force as the food bolus is crushed. An upper limit must, however, be present where inhibition occurs; this prevents the buildup of excessive forces on teeth during the occlusal stage.

A group of neurons in the brainstem produces bursts of discharges at regular intervals when excited by oral sensory stimuli. These bursts drive motor neurons to produce contractions of the masticatory muscles at regular intervals, resulting in rhythmic mandibular movement. The cluster of neurons in the brainstem that drives the rhythmic chewing is termed the *central pattern generator.* The chewing cycles illustrated in Figures 1-46, 1-47, and 1-48 are caused by central pattern generator rhythms. Oral sensory feedback can modify the basic central pattern generator pattern and is essential for the coordination of the lips, tongue, and mandible. Sensory input from the periodontal and mucosal receptors maintains the rhythmic chewing. During opening, the mandibular opening muscles are contracted, and the closing muscles are inhibited. During closing, the mandibular closing muscles are activated, but the opening muscles are not inhibited. Coactivation of the opening and closing muscles serves to protect the dentition from excessively forceful contact, makes the mandible more rigid, and probably serves to brace the condyles while the food is crushed.

References

1. Digka A, Lyroudia K, Jirasek T, et al: Visualisation of human dental pulp vasculature by immunohistochemical and immunofluorescent detection of CD34: A comparative study. *Aust Endod J* 32:101–106, 2006.
2. Garberoglio R, Brännström M: Scanning electron microscopic investigation of human dentinal tubules. *Arch Oral Biol* 21:355–362, 1976.
3. Scott JH, Symons NBB: *Introduction to dental anatomy,* ed 9, Philadelphia, 1982, Churchill Livingstone.
4. Craig RG, Powers JM: *Restorative dental materials,* ed 12, St Louis, 2006, Mosby.
5. Brännström M: *Dentin and pulp in restorative dentistry,* London, 1982, Wolfe Medical.
6. Michelich V, Pashley DH, Whitford GM: Dentin permeability: Comparison of function versus anatomic tubular radii. *J Dent Res* 57:1019–1024, 1978.
7. Sturdevant JR, Pashley DH: Regional dentin permeability of Class I and II cavity preparations (abstract no. 173). *J Dent Res* 68:203, 1989.
8. Mohl ND, Zarb GA, Carlsson GE, et al: The dentition. In Mohl ND, Zarb GA, Carlsson GE, et al, editors: *A textbook of occlusion,* Chicago, 1988, Quintessence.
9. Gibbs CH, Messerman T, Reswick JB, et al: Functional movements of the mandible. *J Prosthet Dent* 26(5):604–620, 1971.
10. Angle EH: Classification of malocclusion. *Dent Cosmos* 41:248–264, 350–357, 1899.
11. Kraus BS, Jorden E, Abrams L: *Dental anatomy and occlusion,* ed 1, Baltimore, 1969, Williams & Wilkins.
12. Dawson PE: *Functional occlusion: From TMJ to smile design,* St Louis, 2007, Mosby.
13. Belser UC, Hannam AG: The influence of altered working-side occlusal guidance on masticatory muscles and related jaw movement. *J Prosthet Dent* 53(3):406–413, 1985.
14. Gibbs CH, Mahan PE, Wilkinson TM, et al: EMG activity of the superior belly of the lateral pterygoid muscle in relation to other jaw muscles. *J Prosthet Dent* 51(5):691–702, 1984.
15. Vitti M, Basmajian JV: Integrated actions of masticatory muscles: Simultaneous EMG from eight intramuscular electrodes. *Anat Rec* 187:173–190, 1976.
16. Williamson EH, Lundquist DO: Anterior guidance: Its effect on electromyographic activity of the temporal and masseter muscles. *J Prosthet Dent* 49(6):816–823, 1983.
17. Santana U, Mora MJ: Electromyographic analysis of the masticatory muscles of patients after complete rehabilitation of occlusion with protection by non-working side contacts. *J Oral Rehabil* 22:57–66, 1995.
18. Valenzuela S, Baeza M, Miralles R, et al: Laterotrusive occlusal schemes and their effect on supra- and infrahyoid electromyographic activity. *Angle Orthod* 76(4):585–590, 2006.
19. Mahan PE, Wilkinson TM, Gibbs CH, et al: Superior and inferior bellies of the lateral pterygoid muscle and EMG activity at basic jaw positions. *J Prosthet Dent* 50(5):710–718, 1983.
20. Borromeo GL, Suvinen TI, Reade PC: A comparison of the effects of group function and canine guidance interocclusal device on masseter muscle electromyographic activity in normal subjects. *J Prosthet Dent* 74(2):174–180, 1995.
21. Graham GS, Rugh JD: Maxillary splint occlusal guidance patterns and electrographic activity of the jaw-closing muscles. *J Prosthet Dent* 59(1):73–77, 1988.
22. Hannam AG, De Cou RE, Scott JD, et al: The relationship between dental occlusion, muscle activity and associated jaw movement in man. *Arch Oral Biol* 22:25–32, 1977.
23. Leiva M, Miralles R, Palazzi C, et al: Effects of laterotrusive occlusal scheme and body position on bilateral sternocleidomastoid EMG activity. *J Craniomandibular Practice* 21(2):99–109, 2003.
24. Manns A, Chan C, Miralles R: Influence of group function and canine guidance on Electromyographic activity of elevator muscles. *J Prosthet Dent* 57(4):494–501, 1987.
25. Manns A, Miralles R, Valdivia J, et al: Influence of variation in anteroposterior occlusal contacts on electromyographic activity. *J Prosthet Dent* 61:617–623, 1989.
26. Rugh JD, Drago CJ: Vertical dimension: A study of clinical rest position and jaw muscle activity. *J Prosthet Dent* 45(6):670–675, 1981.
27. Shupe RJ, Mohamed SE, Christensen LV, et al: Effects of occlusal guidance on jaw muscle activity. *J Prosthet Dent* 51(6):811–818, 1984.
28. Huang BY, Whittle T, Peck CC, et al: Ipsilateral interferences and working-side condylar movements. *Arch Oral Biol* 51:206–214, 2006.
29. Solberg WK, Woo MW, Houston JB: Prevalence of mandibular dysfunction in young adults. *J Am Dent Assoc* 98:25–34, 1979.
30. Posselt U: Studies in the mobility of the mandible. *Acta Odont Scand* 10(Suppl 10), 1952.
31. Gibbs CH, Lundeen HC: Jaw movements and forces during chewing and swallowing and their clinical significance. In Lundeen HC, Gibbs CH, editors: *Advances in occlusion,* Bristol, 1982, John Wright PSG.
32. Celenza FV, Nasedkin JN: *Occlusion: The state of the art,* Chicago, 1978, Quintessence.

33. Keshvad A, Winstanley RB: An appraisal of the literature on centric relation. *J Oral Rehabil* 28:55–63, 2001.

34. Crawford SD: Condylar axis position, as determined by the occlusion and measured by the CPI instrument, and signs and symptoms of temporomandibular dysfunction. *Angle Orthod* 69(2):103–116, 1999.

35. Landi N, Manfredini D, Tognini F, et al: Quantification of the relative risk of multiple occlusal variables for muscle disorders of the stomatognathic system. *J Prosthet Dent* 92:190–195, 2004.

36. Pahkala R, Qvarnstrom M: Can temporomandibular dysfunction signs be predicted by early morphological or functional variables? *Eur J Orthod* 26(4):367–373, 2004.

37. Griffiths RH: Report of the president's conference on the examination, diagnosis, and management of temporomandibular disorders. *J Am Dent Assoc* 106:75–77, 1983.

38. Kim SK, Kim KN, Chang IT, et al: A study of the effects of chewing patterns on occlusal wear. *J Oral Rehabil* 28:1048–1055, 2001.

39. Mongelli de Fantini S, Batista de Paiva J, Neto JR, et al: Increase of condylar displacement between centric relation and maximal habitual intercuspation after occlusal splint therapy. *Braz Oral Res* 19(3):176–182, 2005.

40. Lundeen HC, Wirth CG: Condylar movement patterns engraved in plastic blocks. *J Prosthet Dent* 30:866–875, 1973.

41. Lundeen HC, Shryock EF, Gibbs CH: An evaluation of mandibular border movements: their character and significance. *J Prosthet Dent* 40:442–452, 1978.

42. Lundeen TF, Mendosa MA: Comparison of Bennett shift measured at the hinge axis and an arbitrary hinge axis position. *J Prosthet Dent* 51:407–410, 1984.

43. Lundeen TF, Mendosa MA: Comparison of two methods for measurement of immediate Bennett shift. *J Prosthet Dent* 51:243–245, 1984.

44. Akoren AC, Karaagaclioglu L: Comparison of the electromyographic activity of individuals with canine guidance and group function occlusion. *J Oral Rehabil* 22:73–77, 1995.

45. Tipton RT, Rinchuse DJ: The relationship between static occlusion and functional occlusion in a dental school population. *Angle Orthod* 61(1):57–66, 1990.

46. Lund JP: Mastication and its control by the brain stem. *Crit Rev Oral Biol Med* 2:33–64, 1991.

Chapter 2

Dental Caries: Etiol[...]
Clinical Characteris[...]
Assessment, and Ma[...]

André V. Ritter, R. Scott Eidson, Terrence E. Donovan

Handwritten margin note:
- No. & type of microbial flora
- Diet
- Oral hygiene
- Genetics
- Dental Anatomy
- Use of Flourides
- Use of chemo therapeutic agents
- salivary flow
- Buffering capacity
- Inherent resistance of tooth surface

This chapter presents basic definitions and information on dental caries, clinical characteristics of the caries lesion, caries risk assessment, and caries management, in the context of clinical operative dentistry.

What is Dental Caries?

Dental caries is a multifactorial, transmissible, infectious oral disease caused primarily by the complex interaction of cariogenic oral flora (biofilm) with fermentable dietary carbohydrates on the tooth surface over time. Traditionally, this tooth-biofilm-carbohydrate interaction has been illustrated by the classical Keyes-Jordan diagram (Fig. 2-1).[1] However, dental caries onset and activity are, in fact, much more complex than this three-way interaction, as not all persons with teeth, biofilm, and consuming carbohydrates will have caries over time. Several modifying risk and protective factors influence the dental caries process, as will be discussed later in this chapter.

At the tooth level, caries activity is characterized by localized demineralization and loss of tooth structure (Figs. 2-2 and 2-3). Cariogenic bacteria in the biofilm metabolize refined carbohydrates for energy and produce organic acid by-products. These organic acids, if present in the biofilm ecosystem for extended periods, can lower the pH in the biofilm to below a critical level (5.5 for enamel, 6.2 for dentin). The low pH drives calcium and phosphate from the tooth to the biofilm in an attempt to reach equilibrium, hence resulting in a net loss of minerals by the tooth, or *demineralization*. When the pH in the biofilm returns to neutral and the concentration of soluble calcium and phosphate is supersaturated relative to that in the tooth, mineral can then be added back to partially demineralized enamel, in a process called *remineralization*. At the tooth surface and sub-surface level, therefore, dental caries results from a dynamic process of attack (demineralization)

and restitution (remineralization) of the tooth matter. These events take place several times a day over the life of the tooth and are modulated by many factors, including number and type of microbial flora in the biofilm, diet, oral hygiene, genetics, dental anatomy, use of fluorides and other chemotherapeutic agents, salivary flow and buffering capacity; and inherent resistance of the tooth structure and composition that will differ from person to person, tooth to tooth, and site to site. The balance between demineralization and remineralization has been illustrated in terms of pathologic factors (i.e., those favoring demineralization) and protective factors (i.e., those favoring remineralization) (Fig. 2-4).[2] Individuals in whom the balance tilts predominantly toward protective factors (remineralization) are much less likely to develop dental caries than those in which the balance is tilted toward pathologic factors (demineralization). ***Understanding the balance between demineralization and remineralization is key to caries management.***

Repeated demineralization events may result from a predominantly pathologic environment causing the localized dissolution and destruction of the calcified dental tissues, evidenced as a caries lesion or a "cavity." Severe demineralization of enamel results in the formation of a cavitation in the enamel surface. Severe demineralization of dentin results in the exposure of the protein matrix, which is denatured initially by host matrix metalloproteinases (MMPs) and is subsequently degraded by MMPs and other bacterial proteases. Demineralization of the inorganic phase and denaturation and degradation of the organic phase result in dentin cavitation.[3]

It is essential to understand that caries lesions, or cavitations in teeth, are signs of an underlying condition, an imbalance between protective and pathologic factors favoring the latter. In clinical practice, it is very easy to lose sight of this fact and focus entirely on the restorative treatment of caries lesions, failing to treat the underlying cause of the disease

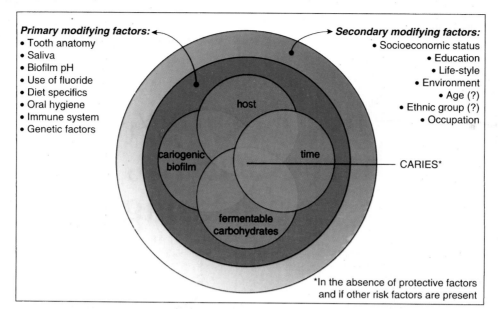

Fig. 2-1 Modified Keyes-Jordan diagram. As a simplified description, dental caries is a result of the interaction of cariogenic oral flora (biofilm) with fermentable dietary carbohydrates on the tooth surface (host) over time. However, dental caries onset and activity are, in fact, much more complex, as not all persons with teeth, biofilm, and who are consuming carbohydrates will have caries over time. Several modifying risk factors and protective factors influence the dental caries process. *(Modified from Keyes PH, Jordan HV: Factors influencing initiation, transmission and inhibition of dental caries. In Harris RJ, editor: Mechanisms of hard tissue destruction, New York, 1963, Academic Press.)*

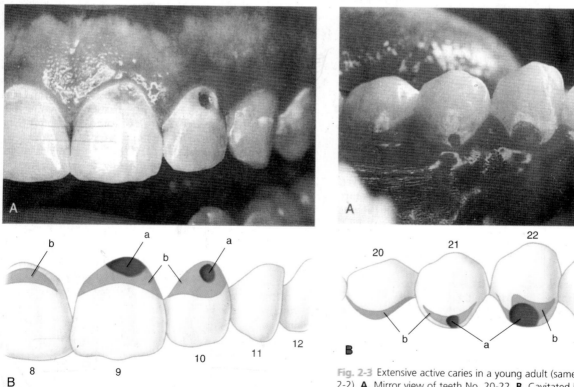

Fig. 2-2 A, Young adult with multiple active caries lesions involving teeth No. 8-10. **B,** Cavitated areas (*a*) are surrounded by areas of extensive demineralization that are chalky and opaque (*b*). Some areas of noncavitated caries have superficial stain.

Fig. 2-3 Extensive active caries in a young adult (same patient as in Fig. 2-2). **A,** Mirror view of teeth No. 20-22. **B,** Cavitated lesions (*a*) are surrounded by extensive areas of chalky, opaque demineralized areas (*b*). The presence of smooth-surface lesions such as these is associated with rampant caries. Occlusal and interproximal smooth-surface caries usually occur in advance of facial smooth-surface lesions. The presence of these types of lesions should alert the dentist to the possibility of extensive caries activity elsewhere in the mouth. The interproximal gingiva is swollen red and would bleed easily on probing. These gingival changes are the consequence of long-standing irritation from the plaque adherent to the teeth.

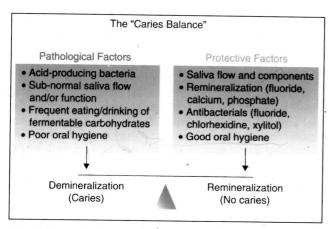

Fig. 2-4 The caries balance. The balance between demineralization and remineralization is illustrated in terms of pathologic factors (i.e., those favoring demineralization) and protective factors (i.e., those favoring remineralization). *(Modified from Featherstone JDB: Prevention and reversal of dental caries: Role of low level fluoride,* Community Dent Oral Epidemiol *27:31–40, 1999.)*

Table 2-1 Caries Management Based on the Medical Model

Primary Etiology	Cariogenic Biofilm (Infection)
Symptoms	Demineralization lesions in teeth
Treatment, symptomatic	Restoration of cavitated lesions
Treatment, therapeutic	Improvement of host resistance by (1) biofilm control, (2) elevating biofilm pH, and (3) enhancing remineralization
Post-treatment assessment, symptomatic	Examination of teeth for new lesions
Post-treatment assessment, therapeutic	Re-evaluation of etiologic conditions and primary and secondary risk factors; and continuous management based on findings

(Table 2-1). Although symptomatic treatment is important, failure to identify and treat the underlying causative factors allows the disease to continue. This chapter emphasizes the components of a caries management program that is based first on risk assessment and then on modifying the biofilm ecology to enhance protective factors and minimize pathologic factors.[4]

This chapter also presents information on clinical characteristics of caries lesion as they relate to clinical operative dentistry. Use of correct and consistent terms when referring to caries lesions is important. Box 2-1 summarizes the most common terms used in this textbook to define caries lesions based on their location, cavitation status, and activity status.

Ecologic Basis of Dental Caries: The Role of the Biofilm

Dental plaque is a term historically used to describe the soft, tenacious film accumulating on the surface of teeth.

Box 2.1 Caries Lesion Definitions

This box summarizes the most common terms used in this textbook to define caries lesions based on their location, cavitation status, and activity status.

- **Caries lesion**. Tooth demineralization as a result of the caries process. Other texts may use the term *carious lesion*. Laypeople may use the term *cavity*.
- **Smooth-surface caries**. A caries lesion on a smooth tooth surface.
- **Pit-and-fissure caries**. A caries lesion on a pit-and-fissure area.
- **Occlusal caries**. A caries lesion on an occlusal surface.
- **Proximal caries**. A caries lesion on a proximal surface.
- **Enamel caries**. A caries lesion in enamel, typically indicating that the lesion has not penetrated into dentin. (Note that many lesions detected clinically as enamel caries may very well have extended into dentin histologically.)
- **Dentin caries**. A caries lesion into dentin.
- **Coronal caries**. A caries lesion in any surface of the anatomic tooth crown.
- **Root caries**. A caries lesion in the root surface.
- **Primary caries**. A caries lesion not adjacent to an existing restoration or crown.
- **Secondary caries**. A caries lesion adjacent to an existing restoration, crown, or sealant. Other term used is *caries adjacent to restorations and sealants (CARS)*. Also referred to as *recurrent caries*, implying that a primary caries lesion was restored but that the lesion reoccurred.
- **Residual caries**. Refers to carious tissue that was not completely excavated prior to placing a restoration. Sometimes residual caries can be difficult to differentiate from secondary caries.
- **Cavitated caries lesion**. A caries lesion that results in the breaking of the integrity of the tooth, or a *cavitation*.
- **Non-cavitated caries lesion.** A caries lesion that has not been cavitated. In enamel caries, non-cavitated lesions are also referred to as "white spot" lesions.

  (Clinically, the distinction between a cavitated and a non-cavitated caries lesion is not as simple as it may seem. Although historically any roughness detectable with a sharp explorer has been considered a cavitated lesion, more recent caries detection guidelines establish that only lesions in which a blunt probe (e.g., WHO[World Health Organization]/CPI[Communty Periodonatal Index]/PSR[Periodontal Screening and Recording] probe) penetrates are to be considered cavitated. This distinction has important implications on lesion management.)
- **Active caries lesion.** A caries lesion that is considered to be biologically active, that is, lesion in which tooth demineralization is in frank activity at the time of examination.
- **Inactive caries lesion.** A caries lesion that is considered to be biologically inactive at the time of examination, that is, in which tooth demineralization caused by caries may have happened in the past but has stopped and is currently stalled. Also referred to as *arrested caries*, meaning that the caries process has been arrested but that the clinical signs of the lesion itself are still present.
- **Rampant caries.** Term used to describe the presence of extensive and multiple cavitated and active caries lesions in the same person. Typically used in association with "baby bottle caries," "radiation therapy caries," or "meth-mouth caries." These terms refer to the etiology of the condition.

Dental plaque has been more recently referred to as a *plaque biofilm*, or simply biofilm, which is a more complete and accurate description of its composition (bio) and structure (film).[5] Biofilm is composed mostly of bacteria, their by-products, extracellular matrix, and water (Figs. 2-5 to 2-9). Biofilm is not adherent food debris, as is widely and erroneously thought, nor does it result from the haphazard collection of opportunistic microorganisms. The accumulation of biofilm on teeth is a highly organized and ordered sequence of events. Many of the organisms found in the mouth are not found elsewhere in nature. Survival of microorganisms in the oral environment depends on their ability to adhere to a surface. Free-floating organisms are cleared rapidly from the mouth by salivary flow and frequent swallowing. Only a few specialized organisms, primarily streptococci, are able to adhere to oral surfaces such as the mucosa and tooth structure.

Significant differences exist in the biofilm communities found in various habitats (ecologic environments) within the oral cavity (Fig. 2-10). Teeth normally have a biofilm community dominated by *Streptococcus sanguis* and *S. mitis*. The population size of mutans streptococci (MS) on teeth varies. Normally, it is a small percentage of the total biofilm population, but it can be one-half the facultative streptococcal

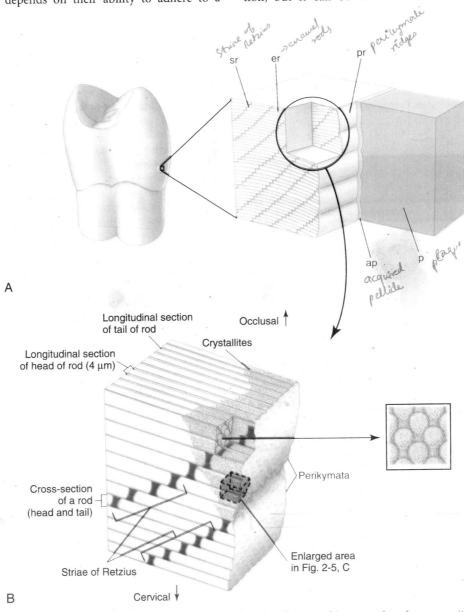

Fig. 2-5 **A,** Composite diagram illustrating the relationship of plaque biofilm (*p*) to the enamel in a smooth-surface noncavitated lesion. A relatively cell-free layer of precipitated salivary protein material, the acquired pellicle (*ap*), covers the perikymata ridges (*pr*). The plaque bacteria attach to the pellicle. Overlapping perikymata ridges can be seen on surface of enamel (see Fig. 2-6). Figs. 2-7 to 2-9 are photomicrographs of cross-sections of plaque biofilm. The enamel is composed of rod-like structures (*er*) that course from the inner dentinoenamel junction (DEJ) to the surface of the crown. Striae of Retzius (*sr*) can be seen in cross-sections of enamel. **B,** Higher power view of the cutout portion of enamel in *A*. Enamel rods interlock with each other in a head-to-tail orientation. The rod heads are visible on the surface as slight depressions on the perikymata ridges. The enamel rods comprise tightly packed crystallites. The orientation of the crystallites changes from being parallel to the rod in the head region to being perpendicular to the rod axis in the tail end. Striae of Retzius form a descending diagonal line, descending cervically.

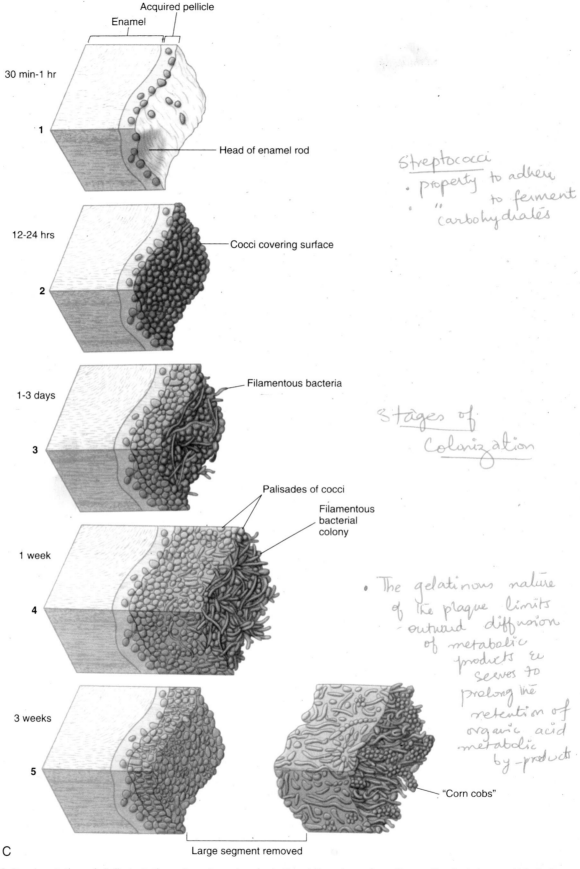

Enamel

Acquired pellicle

30 min–1 hr

1

Head of enamel rod

St. sanguis
St. mitis

Streptococci
• property to adhere
• " to ferment carbohydrates

12-24 hrs

2

Cocci covering surface

1-3 days

3

Filamentous bacteria

Stages of Colonization

Palisades of cocci

Filamentous bacterial colony

1 week

4

• The gelatinous nature of the plaque limits outward diffusion of metabolic products & serves to prolong the retention of organic acid metabolic by-products.

3 weeks

5

"Corn cobs"

C

Large segment removed

Fig. 2-5, cont'd **C,** Drawings 1 through 5 illustrate the various stages in colonization during plaque formation on the shaded enamel block shown in *B*. The accumulated mass of bacteria on the tooth surface may become so thick that it is visible to the unaided eye. Such plaques are gelatinous and tenaciously adherent; they readily take up disclosing dyes, aiding in their visualization for oral hygiene instruction. Thick plaque biofilms (*4* and *5*) are capable of great metabolic activity when sufficient nutrients are available. The gelatinous nature of the plaque limits outward diffusion of metabolic products and serves to prolong the retention of organic acid metabolic byproducts.

flora in other biofilms. Mature plaque biofilm communities have tremendous metabolic potential and are capable of rapid anaerobic metabolism of any available carbohydrates (Fig. 2-11).

Many distinct habitats may be identified on individual teeth, with each habitat containing a unique biofilm community (Table 2-2). Although the pits and fissures on the crown may harbor a relatively simple population of streptococci, the root surface in the gingival sulcus may harbor a complex community dominated by filamentous and spiral bacteria. Facial and lingual smooth surfaces and proximal surfaces also may harbor vastly different biofilm communities. The mesial surface of a molar may be carious and have a biofilm dominated by large populations of MS and lactobacilli, whereas

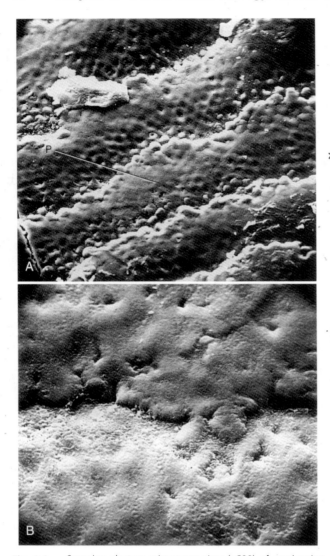

Fig. 2-6   Scanning electron microscope view (×600) of overlapping perikymata (P) in sound enamel from unerupted molar. **B,** Higher power view (×2300) of overlapped site rotated 180 degrees. Surface of non-cavitated enamel lesions has "punched-out" appearance. *(From Hoffman S: Histopathology of caries lesions. In Menaker L, editor: The biologic basis of dental caries, New York, 1980, Harper & Row.)*

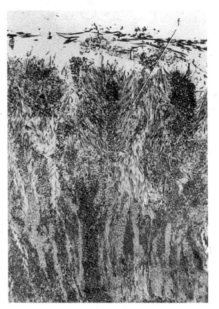

Fig. 2-8 Plaque biofilm formation at 1 week. Filamentous bacteria (*f*) appear to be invading cocci microcolonies. Plaque near gingival sulcus has fewer coccal forms and more filamentous bacteria (×860). *(From Listgarten MA, Mayo HE, Tremblay R: Development of dental plaque on epoxy resin crowns in man. A light and electron microscopic study, J Periodontol 46(1):10–26, 1975.)*

Fig. 2-7 Photomicrograph of one-day old plaque biofilm. This plaque biofilm consists primarily of columnar microcolonies of cocci (C) growing perpendicular to crown surface (S) (×1350). *(From Listgarten MA, Mayo HE, Tremblay R: Development of dental plaque on epoxy resin crowns in man. A light and electron microscopic study, J Periodontol 46(1):10–26, 1975.)*

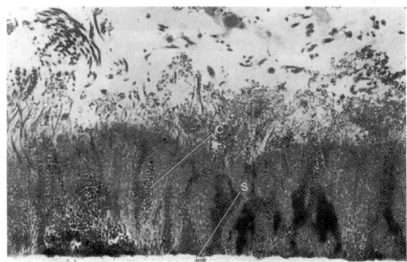

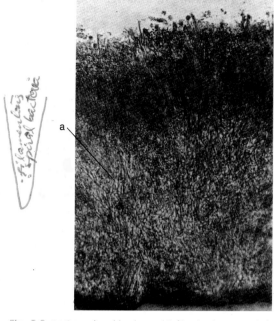

Fig. 2-9 At 3 weeks old, plaque biofilm is almost entirely composed of filamentous bacteria. Heavy plaque formers have spiral bacteria (a) associated with subgingival plaque (¥660). *(From Listgarten MA, Mayo HE, Tremblay R: Development of dental plaque on epoxy resin crowns in man. A light and electron microscopic study, J Periodontol 46(1):10–26, 1975.)*

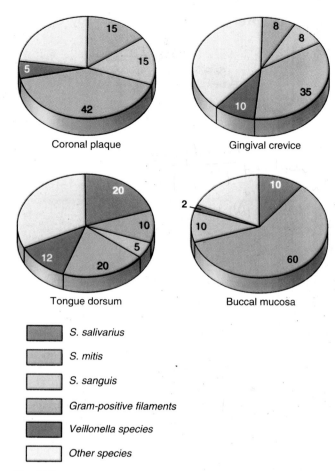

Coronal plaque

Gingival crevice

Tongue dorsum

Buccal mucosa

- *S. salivarius*
- *S. mitis*
- *S. sanguis*
- *Gram-positive filaments*
- *Veillonella species*
- *Other species*

Fig. 2-10 Approximate proportional distribution of predominant cultivable flora of four oral habitats. *(Redrawn from Morhart R, Fitzgerald R: Composition and ecology of the oral flora. In Menaker L, editor: The biologic basis of dental caries, New York, 1980, Harper & Row.)*

Table 2-2 Oral Habitats*

Habitat	Predominant Species	Environmental Conditions within Plaque
Mucosa	*S. mitis* ✓ *S. sanguis* ✓ *S. salivarius* ✓	Aerobic pH approximately 7 Oxidation-reduction potential positive
Tongue	*S. salivarius* *S. mutans* *S. sanguis*	Aerobic pH approximately 7 Oxidation-reduction potential positive
Teeth (non-carious)	*S. sanguis*	Aerobic pH 5.5 Oxidation-reduction negative
Gingival crevice	*Fusobacterium* ✓ *Spirochaeta* *Actinomyces* *Veillonella* ✓	Anaerobic pH variable Oxidation-reduction very negative
Enamel caries	*S. mutans*	Anaerobic pH <5.5 Oxidation-reduction negative
Dentin caries	*S. mutans* *Lactobacillus*	Anaerobic pH <5.5 Oxidation-reduction negative
Root caries	*Actinomyces* ✓	Anaerobic pH <5.5 Oxidation-reduction negative

*The micro-environmental conditions in the habitats associated with host health are generally aerobic, near neutrality in pH, and positive in oxidation-reduction potential. Significant micro-environmental changes are associated with caries and periodontal disease. The changes are the result of the plaque community metabolism.

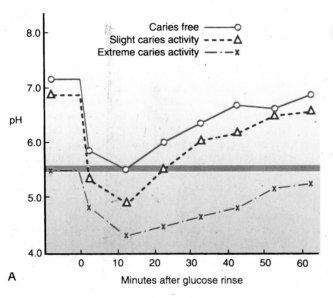

A

Effect of Frequency of Ingestion of
Sugary Foods on Caries Activity

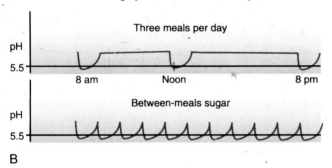

B

Changes in Mineral Content Over Time

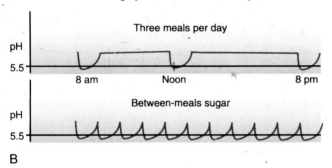

C

the distal surface may lack these organisms and be caries-free. Generalization about biofilm communities is difficult. Nevertheless, the general activity of biofilm growth and maturation is predictable and sufficiently well known to be of therapeutic importance in the prevention of caries.

Professional tooth cleaning is intended to control biofilm (plaque) and prevent disease. After professional removal of all organic material and bacteria from the tooth surface, a new coating of organic material begins to accumulate immediately. Within 2 hours, a cell-free, structureless organic film, the acquired enamel pellicle (AEP, see Figs. 2-5, *A* and *C*), can cover the previously denuded area completely. The pellicle is formed primarily from the selective precipitation of various components of saliva. The functions of the pellicle are believed to be as follows: (1) to protect the enamel, (2) to reduce friction between teeth, and (3) possibly to provide a matrix for remineralization.[6]

Tooth Habitats for Cariogenic Biofilm

The tooth surface is unique because it is not protected by the surface shedding mechanisms (continual replacement of epithelial cells) used throughout the remainder of the alimentary canal. The tooth surface is stable and covered with the pellicle of precipitated salivary glycoproteins, enzymes, and immunoglobulins. It is the ideal surface for the attachment of many oral streptococci. If left undisturbed, biofilm rapidly builds up to sufficient depth to produce an anaerobic environment adjacent to the tooth surface. Tooth habitats favorable for harboring pathogenic biofilm include (1) pits and fissures (Fig. 2-12); (2) the smooth enamel surfaces immediately gingival to the proximal contacts and in the gingival third of the facial and

Fig. 2-11 **A,** Mature plaque biofilm communities have tremendous metabolic potential and are capable of rapid anaerobic metabolism of any available carbohydrates. Classic studies by Stephan show this metabolic potential by severe pH drops at the plaque-enamel interface after glucose rinse. It is generally agreed that a pH of 5.5 is the threshold for enamel demineralization. Exposure to a glucose rinse for an extreme caries activity plaque results in a sustained period of demineralization (pH 5.5). Recording from a slight caries activity plaque shows a much shorter period of demineralization. **B,** The frequency of sucrose exposure for cariogenic plaque greatly influences the progress of tooth demineralization. The top line illustrates pH depression, patterned after Stephan's curves in *A.* Three meals per day results in three exposures of plaque acids, each lasting approximately 1 hour. The plaque pH depression is relatively independent of the quantity of sucrose ingested. Between-meal snacks or the use of sweetened breath mints results in many more acid attacks, as illustrated at the bottom. The effect of frequent ingestion of small quantities of sucrose results in a nearly continuous acid attack on the tooth surface. The clinical consequences of this behavior can be seen in Fig. 2-35. **C,** In active caries, a progressive loss of mineral content subjacent to the cariogenic plaque occurs. Inset illustrates that the loss is not a continuous process. Instead, alternating periods of mineral loss (demineralization) occur, with intervening periods of remineralization. The critical event for the tooth is cavitation of the surface, marked by the vertical dashed line. This event marks an acceleration in caries destruction of the tooth and irreversible loss of tooth structure. For these reasons, restorative intervention is required. *(A, adapted and redrawn from Stephan RM: Intra-oral hydrogen-ion concentration associated with dental caries activity, J Dent Res 23:257, 1944.)*

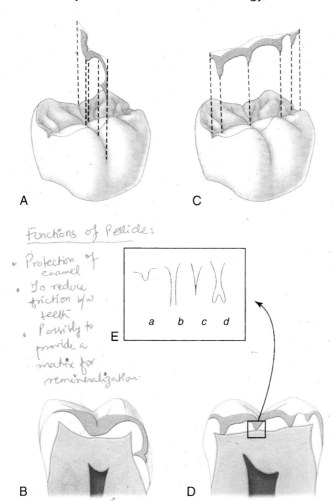

operulum

Functions of Pellicle:

• Protection of enamel
• To reduce friction b/w teeth
• Possibly to provide a matrix for remineralization

Fig. 2-12 Developmental pits, grooves, and fissures on the crowns of the teeth can have complex and varied anatomy. **A** and **B,** The facial developmental groove of the lower first molar often terminates in a pit. The depth of the groove and the pit varies. **C** and **D,** The central groove extends from the mesial pit to the distal pit. Sometimes grooves extend over the marginal ridges. **E,** The termination of pits and fissures may vary from a shallow groove (*a*) to complete penetration of the enamel (*b*). The end of the fissure may end blindly (*c*) or open into an irregular chamber (*d*).

lingual surfaces of the clinical crown (Fig. 2-13); (3) root surfaces, particularly near the cervical line; and (4) subgingival areas (Fig. 2-14). These sites correspond to the locations where caries lesions are most frequently found.

Pits and Fissures

Pits and fissures are particularly susceptible surfaces for caries initiation (see Fig. 2-12; Figs. 2-15 to 2-19; see also Fig. 2-12). The pits and fissures provide excellent mechanical shelter for organisms and harbor a community dominated by *S. sanguis* and other streptococci. The relative proportion of MS most probably determines the cariogenic potential of the pit-and-fissure community. The appearance of MS in pits and fissures is usually followed by caries 6 to 24 months later. In susceptible patients, sealing the pits and fissures just after tooth

eruption may be the most important event in their resistance to caries.

Smooth Enamel Surfaces

The proximal enamel surfaces immediately gingival to the contact area are the second most susceptible areas to caries (Figs. 2-20 and 2-21; see also Figs. 2-14 and 2-18). These areas are protected physically and are relatively free from the effects of mastication, tongue movement, and salivary flow. The types and numbers of organisms composing the proximal surface biofilm community vary. Important ecologic determinants for the biofilm community on the proximal surfaces are the topography of the tooth surface, the size and shape of the gingival papillae, and the oral hygiene of the patient. A rough surface (caused by caries, a poor-quality restoration, or a structural defect) restricts adequate biofilm removal. This situation favors the occurrence of caries or periodontal disease at the site.

What is FLUTING?

Root Surfaces

The proximal root surface, particularly near the cemento-enamel junction (CEJ), often is unaffected by the action of hygiene procedures such as flossing because it may have concave anatomic surface contours (fluting) and occasional roughness at the termination of the enamel. These conditions, when coupled with exposure to the oral environment (as a result of gingival recession), favor the formation of mature, cariogenic biofilm and proximal root-surface caries. Likewise, the facial or lingual root surfaces (particularly near the CEJ), when exposed to the oral environment (because of gingival recession), are often both neglected in hygiene procedures and usually not rubbed by the bolus of food. Consequently, these root surfaces also frequently harbor cariogenic biofilm. Root-surface caries is more common in older patients because of niche availability and other factors sometimes associated with senescence, such as decreased salivary flow and poor oral hygiene as a result of lowered digital dexterity and decreased motivation. Caries originating on the root is alarming because (1) it has a comparatively rapid progression, (2) it is often asymptomatic, (3) it is closer to the pulp, and (4) it is more difficult to restore.

↑ because dentin is attacked initially.

Oral Hygiene and Its Role in the Caries Process

Oral hygiene, accomplished primarily by proper tooth brushing and flossing, is another ecologic determinant of caries onset and activity. Careful mechanical cleaning of teeth disrupts the biofilm and leaves a clean enamel surface. The cleaning process does not destroy most of the oral bacteria but merely removes them from the surfaces of teeth. Large numbers of these bacteria subsequently are removed from the oral cavity during rinsing and swallowing after flossing and brushing, but sufficient numbers remain to recolonize teeth. Some fastidious organisms and obligate anaerobes may be killed by exposure to oxygen during tooth cleaning. No single species is likely to be entirely eliminated, however. Although all the species that compose mature biofilm continue to be present, most of these are unable to initiate colonization on the clean tooth surface.

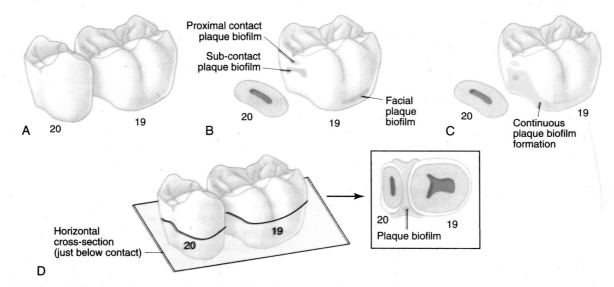

Fig. 2-13 Plaque biofilm formation on posterior teeth and associated caries lesions. **A,** Teeth No. 19 and No. 20 in contacting relationship. **B,** The crown of tooth No. 20 has been removed at the cervix. The proximal contact and subcontact plaque can be seen on the mesial surface of tooth No. 19. A facial plaque also is illustrated. **C,** During periods of unrestricted growth, the mesial and facial plaques become part of a continuous ring of plaque around teeth. **D,** A horizontal cross-section through teeth No. 19 and No. 20 with heavy plaque. Inset shows the interproximal space below the contact area filled with gelatinous plaque. This mass of interproximal plaque concentrates the effects of plaque metabolism on the adjacent tooth smooth surfaces. All interproximal surfaces are subject to plaque accumulation and acid demineralization. In patients exposed to fluoridated water, most interproximal lesions become arrested at a stage before cavitation.

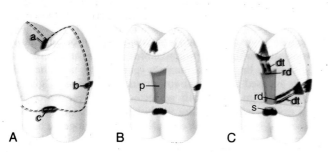

Fig. 2-14 A, Caries may originate at many distinct sites: pits and fissures (*a*), smooth surface of crown (*b*), and root surface (*c*). Proximal surface lesion of crown is not illustrated here because it is a special case of smooth-surface lesion. Histopathology and progress of facial (or lingual) and proximal lesions are identical. Dotted line indicates cut used to reveal cross-sections illustrated in *B* and *C*. **B,** In cross-section, the three types of lesions show different rates of progression and different morphology. Lesions illustrated here are intended to be representative of each type. No particular association between three lesions is implied. Pit-and-fissure lesions have small sites of origin visible on the occlusal surface but have a wide base. Overall shape of a pit-and-fissure lesion is an inverted "V." In contrast, a smooth-surface lesion is V-shaped with a wide area of origin and apex of the V directed toward pulp (*p*). Root caries begins directly on dentin. Root-surface lesions can progress rapidly because dentin is less resistant to caries attack. **C,** Advanced caries lesions produce considerable histologic change in enamel, dentin, and pulp. Bacterial invasion of lesion results in extensive demineralization and proteolysis of the dentin. Clinically, this necrotic dentin appears soft, wet, and mushy. Deeper pulpally, dentin is demineralized, but not invaded by bacteria, and is structurally intact. This tissue appears to be dry and leathery in texture. Two types of pulp–dentin response are illustrated. Under pit-and-fissure lesions and smooth-surface lesions, odontoblasts have died, leaving empty tubules called dead tracts (*dt*). New odontoblasts have been differentiated from pulp mesenchymal cells. These new odontoblasts have produced reparative dentin (*rd*), which seals off dead tracts. Another type of pulp-dentin reaction is sclerosis (*s*)—occlusion of the tubules by peritubular dentin. This is illustrated under root-caries lesion.

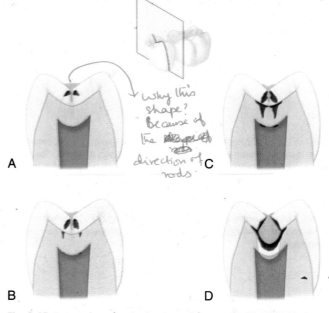

Fig. 2-15 Progression of caries in pits and fissures. **A,** The initial lesions develop on the lateral walls of the fissure. Demineralization follows the direction of the enamel rods, spreading laterally as it approaches the dentinoenamel junction (DEJ). **B,** Soon after the initial enamel lesion occurs, a reaction can be seen in the dentin and pulp. Forceful probing of the lesion at this stage can result in damage to the weakened porous enamel and accelerate the progression of the lesion. Clinical detection at this stage should be based on observation of discoloration and opacification of the enamel adjacent to the fissure. These changes can be observed by careful cleaning and drying of the fissure. **C,** Initial cavitation of the opposing walls of the fissure cannot be seen on the occlusal surface. Opacification can be seen that is similar to the previous stage. Remineralization of the enamel because of trace amounts of fluoride in the saliva may make progression of pit-and-fissure lesions more difficult to detect. **D,** Extensive cavitation of the dentin and undermining of the covering enamel darken the occlusal surface (see Fig. 2-16).

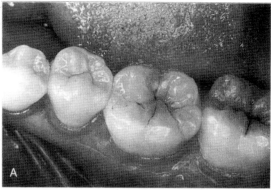

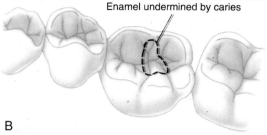

Fig. 2-16 **A,** Mandibular first molar has undermined discolored enamel owing to extensive pit-and-fissure caries. The lesion began as illustrated in Fig. 2-15 and has progressed to the stage illustrated in Fig. 2-15, *D.* **B,** Discolored enamel is outlined by broken line in the central fossa region.

Saliva: Nature's Anticaries Agent

Saliva is an extremely important substance for the proper digestion of foods, and it also plays a key role as a natural anticaries agent (Table 2-3). Many medications are capable of reducing salivary flow and increasing caries risk (Table 2-4). The importance of saliva in the maintenance of the oral health is illustrated dramatically by observing changes in oral health after therapeutic radiation to the head and neck. After radiation, salivary glands become fibrotic and produce little or no saliva, leaving the patient with an extremely dry mouth, a condition termed *xerostomia* (*xero*, dry; *stoma*, mouth). Such patients may experience near-total destruction of the teeth in just a few months after radiation treatment.[8,9] Salivary protective mechanisms that maintain the normal oral flora and tooth surface integrity include bacterial clearance, direct antibacterial activity, buffers, and remineralization.[10]

Bacterial Clearance

Secretions from various salivary glands pool in the mouth to form whole or mixed saliva. The amount of saliva secreted varies greatly over time. When secreted, saliva remains in the mouth for a short time before being swallowed. While in the mouth, saliva lubricates oral tissues and bathes teeth and the biofilm. The secretion rate of saliva may have a bearing on caries susceptibility and calculus formation. Adults produce 1-1.5 L of saliva a day, very little of which occurs during sleep. The flushing effect of this salivary flow is, by itself, adequate to remove virtually all microorganisms not adherent to an oral

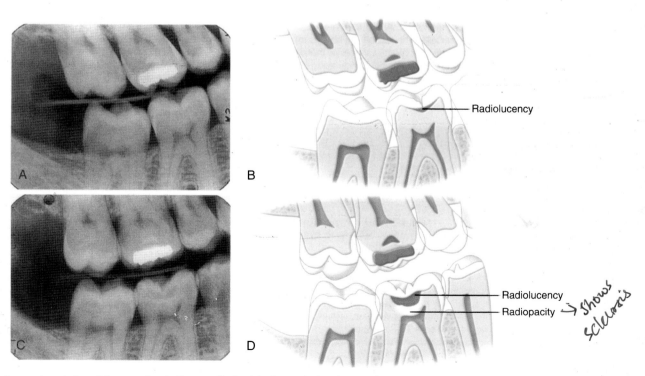

Fig. 2-17 Progression of pit-and-fissure caries. **A,** The mandibular right first molar (tooth No. 30) was sealed. Note radiolucent areas under the occlusal enamel in *A* and *B*. The sealant failed, and caries progressed slowly during the next 5 years; the only symptom was occasional biting-force pain. **C** and **D,** Note the extensive radiolucency under the enamel and an area of increased radiopacity below the lesion, suggesting sclerosis.

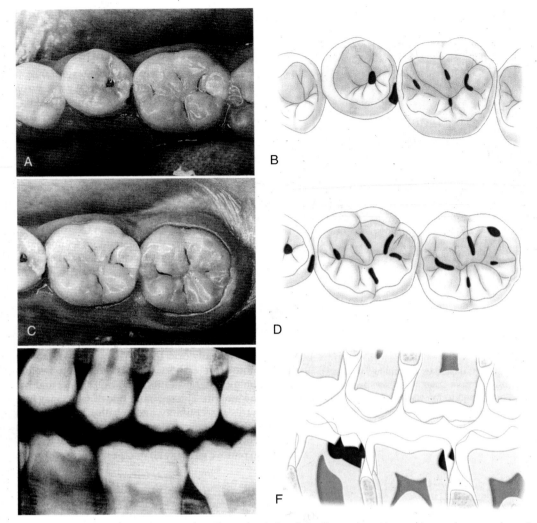

Fig. 2-18 A young patient with extensive caries. **A** and **B,** The occlusal pits of the first molar and second premolar are carious. An interproximal caries lesion is seen on the second premolar. The second premolar is rotated almost 90 degrees, bringing the lingual surface into contact with the mesial surface of the first molar. Normally, the lingual surfaces of mandibular teeth are rarely attacked by caries, but here, the tooth rotation makes the lingual surface a proximal contact and, consequently, produces an interproximal habitat, which increases the susceptibility of the surface to caries. **C** and **D,** The first and second molars have extensive caries in the pits and fissures. **E** and **F,** On the bitewing radiograph, not only can the extensive nature of the caries in the second premolar be seen but also seen is a lesion on the distal aspect of the first molar, which is not visible clinically. (Dark areas in *B, D,* and *F* indicate caries.)

Table 2-3 Elements of Saliva that Control Plaque Biofilm Communities

Names	Action	Effects on Plaque Biofilm Community
SALIVARY ENZYMES		
Amylase	Cleaves—1,4 glucoside bonds	Increases availability of oligosaccharides
Lactoperoxidase	Catalyzes hydrogen peroxide–mediated oxidation; adsorbs to hydroxyapatite in active form	Lethal to many organisms: suppresses plaque formation on tooth surfaces
Lysozyme	Lyses cells by degradation of cell walls, releasing peptidoglycans; binds to hydroxyapatite in active conformation	Lethal to many organisms; peptidoglycans activate complement; suppresses plaque formation on tooth surfaces
Lipases	Hydrolysis of triglycerides to free fatty acids and partial glycerides	Free fatty acids inhibit attachment and growth of some organisms
NON-ENZYME PROTEINS		
Lactoferrin	Ties up free iron	Inhibits growth of some iron-dependent microbes
Secretory immunoglobulin A(IgA) (smaller amounts of IgM, IgG)	Agglutination of bacteria inhibits bacterial enzymes	Reduces numbers in saliva by precipitation; slows bacterial growth
Glycoproteins (mucins)	Agglutination of bacteria	Reduces numbers in saliva by precipitation

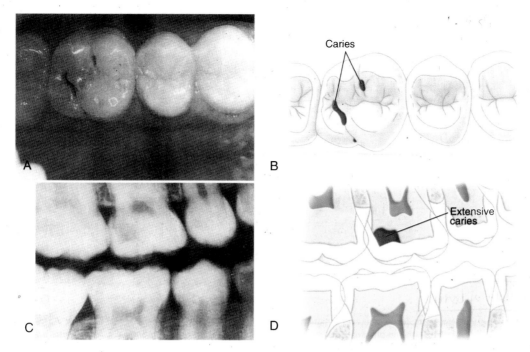

Fig. 2-19 Example of occlusal caries that is much more extensive than is apparent clinically. **A** and **B,** Clinical example. **C** and **D,** A bitewing radiograph further reveals an extensive area of demineralization undermining the distofacial cusp.

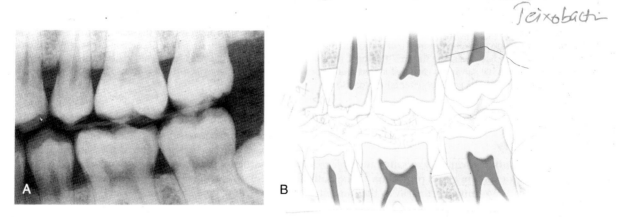

Fig. 2-20 Bitewing radiograph of normal teeth, free from caries. Note the uniform density of the enamel on the interproximal surfaces. A third molar is impacted on the distal aspect of the lower second molar. The interproximal bone levels are uniform and located slightly below the cementoenamel junctions, suggesting a healthy periodontium.

surface. The flushing is most effective during mastication or oral stimulation, both of which produce large volumes of saliva. Large volumes of saliva also can dilute and buffer biofilm acids.

Direct Antibacterial Activity

Salivary glands produce an impressive array of antimicrobial products (see Table 2-3). Lysozyme, lactoperoxidase, lactoferrin, and agglutinins possess antibacterial activity. These salivary proteins are not part of the immune system but are part of an overall protection scheme for mucous membranes that occurs in addition to immunologic control. These protective proteins are present continuously at relatively uniform levels,

have a broad spectrum of activity, and do not possess the "memory" of immunologic mechanisms. The normal resident oral flora apparently has developed resistance to most of these antibacterial mechanisms.

Although the antibacterial proteins in saliva play an important role in the protection of soft tissue in the oral cavity from infection by pathogens, they have little effect on caries because similar levels of antibacterial proteins can be found in caries-active and caries-free individuals.[11,12] It is suggested that caries susceptibility in healthy individuals is not related to saliva composition. Individuals with decreased salivary production (owing to illness, medication, or irradiation) may have significantly higher caries susceptibility (see Table 2-4).

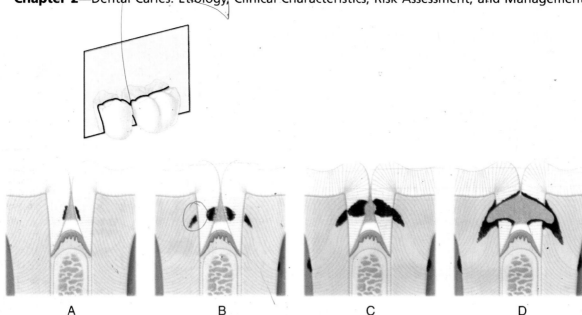

Fig. 2-21 Longitudinal sections (see inset for *A*) showing initiation and progression of caries on interproximal surfaces. **A,** Initial demineralization (indicated by the shading in the enamel) on the proximal surfaces is not detectable clinically or radiographically. All proximal surfaces are demineralized to some degree, but most are remineralized and become immune to further attack. The presence of small amounts of fluoride in the saliva virtually ensures that remineralization and immunity to further attack will occur. **B,** When proximal caries first becomes detectable radiographically, the enamel surface is likely still to be intact. An intact surface is essential for successful remineralization and arrest of the lesion. Demineralization of the dentin (indicated by the shading in the dentin) occurs before cavitation of the surface of the enamel. Treatment designed to promote remineralization can be effective up to this stage. **C,** Cavitation of the enamel surface is a critical event in the caries process in proximal surfaces. Cavitation is an irreversible process and requires restorative treatment and correction of the damaged tooth surface. Cavitation can be diagnosed only by clinical observation. The use of a sharp explorer to detect cavitation is problematic because excessive force in application of the explorer tip during inspection of the proximal surfaces can damage weakened enamel and accelerate the caries process by creating cavitation. Separation of the teeth can be used to provide more direct visual inspection of suspect surfaces. Fiberoptic illumination and dye absorption also are promising new evaluation procedures, but neither is specific for cavitation. **D,** Advanced cavitated lesions require prompt restorative intervention to prevent pulpal disease, limit tooth structure loss, and remove the nidus of infection of odontopathic organisms.

Buffer Capacity

The volume and buffering capacity of saliva available to tooth surfaces have major roles in caries protection.[13] The buffering capacity of saliva is determined primarily by the concentration of bicarbonate ion. Buffering capacity can be estimated by titration techniques and may be a useful method for assessment of saliva in caries-active patients. The benefit of the buffering is to reduce the potential for acid formation.

In addition to buffers, saliva contains molecules that contribute to increasing biofilm pH. These include urea and sialin, which is a tetrapeptide that contains lysine and arginine. Hydrolysis of either of these basic compounds results in production of ammonia, causing the pH to increase.

Because saliva is crucial in controlling the oral flora and the mineral content of teeth, salivary testing should be done on patients with high caries activity. A portion of the salivary sample also may be used for bacteriologic testing, as will be described later in this chapter.

Remineralization

Saliva and biofilm fluid are supersaturated with calcium and phosphate ions. Without a means to control precipitation of these ions, the teeth literally would become encrusted with mineral deposits. Saliva contains statherin, a proline-rich peptide that stabilizes calcium and phosphate ions and prevents excessive deposition of these ions on teeth.[14] This supersaturated state of the saliva provides a constant opportunity for remineralizing enamel and can help protect teeth in times of cariogenic challenges.

Diet and Caries

High-frequency exposure of fermentable carbohydrates such as sucrose may be the most important factor in producing cariogenic biofilm and, ultimately, caries lesions. Frequent ingestion of fermentable carbohydrates begins a series of changes in the local tooth environment that promotes the growth of highly acidogenic bacteria and eventually leads to caries. In contrast, when ingestion of fermentable carbohydrates is severely restricted or absent, biofilm growth typically does not lead to caries. Dietary sucrose plays a leading role in the development of pathogenic biofilms and may be the most important factor in disruption of the normal healthy ecology of dental biofilm communities. Because the eventual metabolic product of cariogenic diet is acid, and the acid leads to the development of caries, the exposure to acidity from other sources (e.g., dried fruits, fruit drinks, or other acidic foods and drinks) also may result in caries. The dietary emphasis must include all intakes that result in acidity, not just sucrose.

Table 2-4 Medications with Potential to Cause Hyposalivation or Dry Mouth (Xerostomia)

Action/Medication Group	Medicaments	Action/Medication Group	Medicaments
SYMPATHOMIMETIC		**ANTICHOLINERGIC, DEHYDRATION**	
Antidepressants	Ventafaxine Duloxetine Reboxetine Bupropion	Diuretics	Furosemide Bumetanide Torsemide Ethacrynic acid
ANTICHOLINERGIC		**SYMPATHOMIMETIC**	
Tricyclic antidepressants	Amitriptyline Clomiparamine Amoxapine Protripyline Doxepin Impramine Trimiparamine Nortriptyline Desiparamine	Antihypertensive agents	Metroprolol Monoxidine Rilmenidine
		Appetite suppressants	Fenfluoramine Sibutramine Phentermine
Muscarinic receptor antagonists	Oxybutynin	Decongestants	Pseudoephedrine
Alpha-receptor antagonists	Tamsulosin Terazosin	Bronchodilators	Tiotripium
		Skeletal muscle relaxants	Tizanidine
		Antimigraine agents	Rizatriptan
Antipsychotics	Promazine Triflupromazine Mesoridazine Thioridazine Clozapine Olanzapine	**SYNERGISTIC MECHANISM**	
		Opioids, hypnotics	Opium Cannabis Tramadol Diazepam
		UNKNOWN	
Antihistamines	Azaridine Brompheniramine Chlorpheniramine Cyproheptadine Dexchlopheniramine Hydroxyzine Phenindamine Cetirizine Loratidine	H2 antagonists, proton pump inhibitors	Cimetidine Ranitidine Famotidine Nizatidine Omeprazole
		Cytotoxic drugs	Fluorouracil
		Anti-HIV drugs, protease inhibitors	Didanosine

(Adapted from the Kois Center, Support Materials, Always Pages, http://koiscenter.com/store/supmatlist.aspx, accessed January 13, 2012.)

Clinical Characteristics of the Caries Lesion

The caries lesion is the product of disequilibrium between the demineralization and remineralization processes discussed previously. When the tooth surface becomes cavitated, a more retentive surface area becomes available to the biofilm community. The cavitation of the tooth surface produces a synergistic acceleration of the growth of the cariogenic biofilm community and the expansion of the demineralization with ensuing expanded cavitation. This situation results in a rapid and progressive destruction of the tooth structure. When enamel caries penetrates to the dentinoenamel junction (DEJ), rapid lateral expansion of the caries lesion occurs because dentin is much less resistant to acid demineralization. This sheltered, highly acidic, and anaerobic environment provides an ideal niche for cariogenic bacteria.

Clinical Sites for Caries Initiation

The characteristics of a caries lesion vary with the nature of the surface on which the lesion develops. There are three distinctly different clinical sites for caries initiation: (1) developmental pits and fissures of enamel, which are the most susceptible sites; (2) smooth enamel surfaces that shelter cariogenic biofilm; and (3) the root surface (see Fig. 2-14). Each of these areas has distinct surface topography and environmental conditions. Consequently, each area has a distinct biofilm population. The diagnosis, treatment, and prevention of these different lesion types should take into account the different etiologic factors operating at each site.

Pits and Fissures

Bacteria rapidly colonize the pits and fissures of newly erupted teeth. The type and nature of the organisms prevalent in the oral cavity determine the type of organisms colonizing pits and fissures and are instrumental in determining the outcome of the colonization. Large variations exist in the microflora found in pits and fissures, suggesting that each site can be considered a separate ecologic system. Numerous gram-positive cocci, especially *S. sanguis*, are found in the pits and fissures of newly erupted teeth, whereas large numbers of MS usually are found in carious pits and fissures.

The shape of the pits and fissures contributes to their high susceptibility to caries. The long, narrow fissure prevents adequate biofilm removal (see Fig. 2-12). Considerable morphologic variation exists in these structures. Some pits and fissures end blindly, others open near the dentin, and others penetrate entirely through the enamel.

Pit-and-fissure caries expands as it penetrates into the enamel. The entry site may appear much smaller than the actual lesion, making clinical diagnosis difficult. Caries lesions of pits and fissures develop from attack on their walls (see Fig. 2-15, A through C). Progression of the dissolution of the walls of a pit-and-fissure lesion is similar in principle to that of the smooth-surface lesion because a wide area of surface attack extends inward, paralleling the enamel rods. A lesion originating in a pit or fissure affects a greater area of the DEJ than does a comparable smooth-surface lesion. In cross-section, the gross appearance of a pit-and-fissure lesion is an inverted "V" with a narrow entrance and a progressively wider area of involvement closer to the DEJ (see Fig. 2-15, D).

Smooth Enamel Surfaces

The smooth enamel surfaces of teeth present a less favorable site for cariogenic biofilm attachment. Cariogenic biofilm usually develops only on the smooth surfaces that are near the gingiva or are under proximal contacts. The proximal surfaces are particularly susceptible to caries because of the extra shelter provided to resident cariogenic biofilm owing to the proximal contact area immediately occlusal to it (Fig. 2-22). Lesions starting on smooth enamel surfaces have a broad area of origin and a conical, or pointed, extension toward the DEJ. The path of ingress of the lesion is roughly parallel to the long axis of the enamel rods in the region. A cross-section of the enamel portion of a smooth-surface lesion shows a V-shape, with a wide area of origin and the apex of the V directed toward the DEJ. After caries penetrates the DEJ, softening of dentin spreads rapidly laterally and pulpally (see Fig. 2-21).

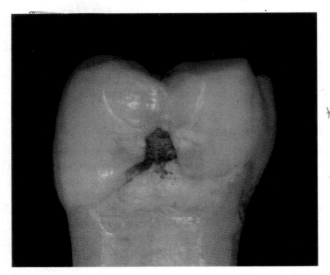

Fig. 2-22 Extracted tooth showing extensive caries lesion just gingival to the proximal contact area. (Note the slightly "flat" contact area adjacent to marginal ridge.)

Root Surfaces

*[handwritten: ⌐ * U-shaped in cross-section.]*

The root surface is rougher than enamel and readily allows cariogenic biofilm formation in the absence of good oral hygiene. The cementum covering the root surface is extremely thin and provides little resistance to caries attack. In addition, the critical pH for dentin is higher than for enamel, so demineralization is likely to start even before the pH reaches the critical level for enamel (pH = 5.5). Root caries lesions have less well-defined margins, tend to be U-shaped in cross-section, and progress more rapidly because of the lack of protection from an enamel covering. In recent years, the prevalence of root caries has increased significantly because of the increasing number of older persons who retain more teeth, experience gingival recession, and usually have cariogenic biofilm on the exposed root surfaces.[15-18]

Progression of Caries Lesions

The progression and morphology of the caries lesion vary, depending on the site of origin and the conditions in the mouth (see Figs. 2-14, 2-15, and 2-21). The time for progression from non-cavitated caries to clinical caries (*cavitation*) on smooth surfaces is estimated to be 18 months ± 6 months.[19] Peak rates for the incidence of new lesions occur 3 years after the eruption of the tooth. Occlusal pit-and-fissure lesions develop in less time than smooth-surface caries. Poor oral hygiene and frequent exposures to sucrose-containing or acidic food can produce noncavitated ("white spot") lesions (first clinical evidence of demineralization) in 3 weeks. Radiation-induced *xerostomia* (dry mouth) can lead to clinical caries development in 3 months from the onset of the radiation. Caries development in healthy individuals is usually slow compared with the rate possible in compromised persons.

Enamel Caries

An understanding of the enamel composition and histology is helpful to understand enamel caries histopathology (see Chapter 1 (Figs. 2-23 to 2-25). On clean, dry teeth, the earliest evidence of caries on the smooth enamel surface of a crown is a white spot (Fig. 2-26; see also Figs. 2-2 and 2-3). These lesions usually are observed on the facial and lingual surfaces of teeth. White spots are chalky white, opaque areas that are revealed only when the tooth surface is desiccated and are termed *noncavitated enamel caries lesions*. These areas of enamel lose their translucency because of the extensive subsurface porosity caused by demineralization. Care must be exercised in distinguishing white spots of noncavitated caries from developmental white spot hypocalcifications of enamel. Noncavitated (white spot) caries partially or totally disappears visually when the enamel is hydrated (wet), whereas hypocalcified enamel is affected less by drying and wetting (Table 2-5). Hypocalcified enamel does not represent a clinical problem except for its esthetically objectionable appearance. The surface texture of a non-cavitated lesion is unaltered and is undetectable by tactile examination with an explorer. A more advanced lesion develops a rough surface that is softer than the unaffected, normal enamel. Softened chalky enamel that can be chipped away with an explorer is a sign of active caries. Injudicious use of an explorer tip can cause actual cavitation

Table 2-5 Clinical Characteristics of Normal and Altered Enamel

	Hydrated	Desiccated	Surface Texture	Surface Hardness
Normal enamel	Translucent	Translucent	Smooth	Hard
Hypocalcified enamel	Opaque	Opaque	Smooth	Hard
Noncavitated caries	Translucent	Opaque	Smooth	Softened
Active caries	Opaque	Opaque	Cavitated	Very soft
Inactive caries	Opaque, dark	Opaque, dark	Roughened	Hard

Timings:
Smooth surface:
18 months ± 6 months
Pits & fissures:
6-24 months
Radiation-induced xerostomia:
3 months.

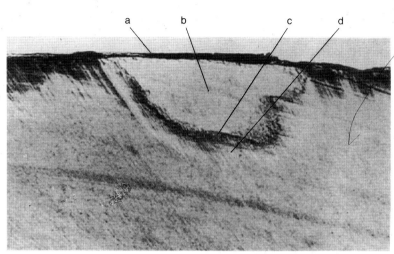

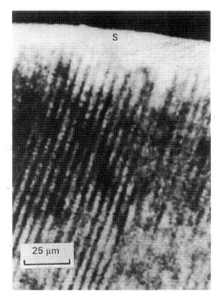

Fig. 2-23 Cross-section of small caries lesion in enamel examined in quinoline by transmitted light (×100). Surface (*a*) appears to be intact. Body of lesion (*b*) shows enhancement of striae of Retzius. Dark zone (*c*) surrounds body of lesion, whereas translucent zone (*d*) is evident over entire advancing front of lesion. *(From Silverstone LM et al, editors: Dental caries, London and Basingstoke, 1981, Macmillan, Ltd.)*

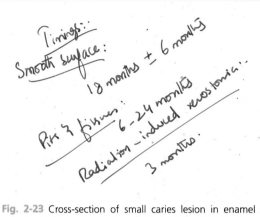

Fig. 2-24 Microradiograph (×150) of cross-section of small caries lesion in enamel. Well-mineralized surface (*s*) is evident. Alternating radiolucent and radiopaque lines indicate demineralization between enamel rods. *(From Silverstone LM et al, editors: Dental caries, London and Basingstoke, 1981, Macmillan, Ltd.)*

in a previously noncavitated area, requiring, in most cases, restorative intervention. Similar noncavitated lesions occur on the proximal smooth surfaces, but usually are undetectable by visual or judicious tactile (explorer) examination. Noncavitated enamel lesions sometimes can be seen on radiographs as a faint radiolucency that is limited to the superficial enamel. When a proximal lesion is clearly visible radiographically, the lesion may have advanced significantly, and histologic alteration of the underlying dentin probably already has occurred, whether the lesion is cavitated or not (Fig. 2-27).

It has been shown experimentally and clinically that noncavitated caries of enamel can remineralize.[20-21] Table 2-5 and Table 2-6 list the characteristics of enamel at various stages of demineralization. Noncavitated enamel lesions retain most of the original crystalline framework of the enamel rods, and the etched crystallites serve as nucleating agents for remineralization. Calcium and phosphate ions from saliva can penetrate the enamel surface and precipitate on the highly reactive crystalline surfaces in the enamel lesion. The supersaturation of saliva with calcium and phosphate ions serves as the driving force for the remineralization process. Artificial and natural caries lesions of human enamel have been shown to regress to earlier histologic stages after exposure to conditions that promote remineralization. The presence of trace amounts of fluoride ions during this remineralization process greatly enhances the precipitation of calcium and phosphate, resulting in the remineralized enamel becoming more

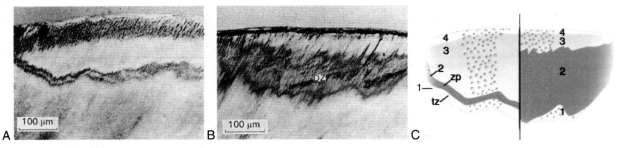

Fig. 2-25 A, Cross-section of small caries lesion in enamel examined in quinoline with polarized light (×100). Advancing front of lesion appears as a dark band below body of lesion. **B,** Same section after exposure to artificial calcifying solution examined in quinoline and polarized light. Dark zone (*DZ*) covers a much greater area after remineralization has occurred (×100). **C,** Schematic diagram of Figs. 2-25, *A* and *B*. Left side indicates small extent of zones 1 and 2 before remineralization. Small circles indicate relative sizes of pores in each zone. Right side indicates increase in zone 2, the dark zone, after remineralization. This micropore system must have been created where previously the pores were much larger. *(Redrawn from Silverstone LM et al, editors:* Dental caries, *London and Basingstoke, 1981, Macmillan, Ltd., C was redrawn)*

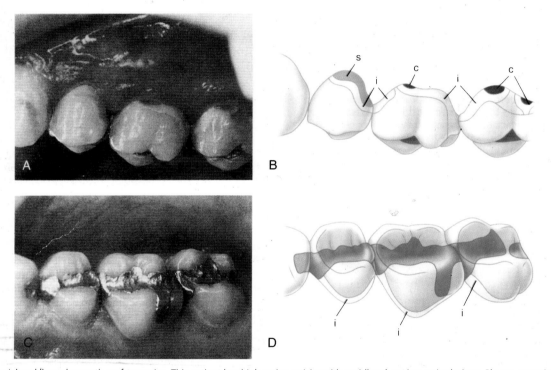

Fig. 2-26 Facial and lingual smooth-surface caries. This patient has high caries activity with rapidly advancing caries lesions. Plaque, containing mutans streptococci (MS), extends entirely around the cervical areas of the posterior teeth. Several levels of caries involvement can be seen, including cavitation (*c*); non-cavitated white spot lesions (*i*); and stained, roughened, partially remineralized non-cavitated lesions (*s*).

Table 2-6 Clinical Significance of Enamel Lesions

	Plaque Biofilm	Enamel Structure	Non-restorative, Therapeutic Treatment (e.g., remineralization, antimicrobial, pH control)	Restorative Treatment
Normal enamel	Normal	Normal	Not indicated	Not indicated
Hypocalcified enamel	Normal	Abnormal, but not weakened	Not indicated	Only for esthetics
Noncavitated caries	Cariogenic	Porous, weakened	Yes	Not indicated
Active caries	Cariogenic	Cavitated, very weak	Yes	Yes
Inactive caries	Normal	Remineralized, strong	Not indicated	Only for esthetics

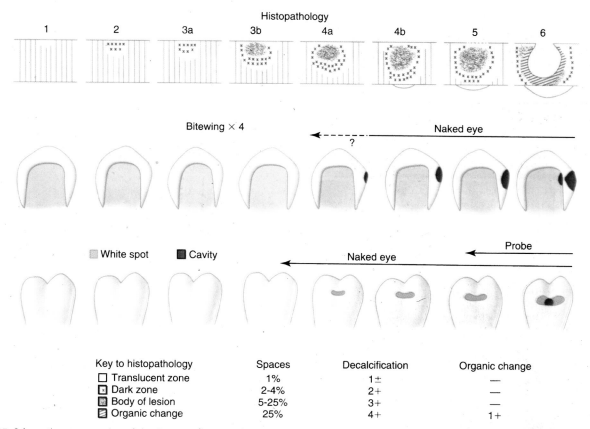

Key to histopathology	Spaces	Decalcification	Organic change
☐ Translucent zone	1%	1±	—
▨ Dark zone	2-4%	2+	—
▦ Body of lesion	5-25%	3+	—
▨ Organic change	25%	4+	1+

Fig. 2-27 Schematic representation of developmental stages of enamel caries lesion correlated with radiographic and clinical examination. Cavitation occurs late in development of the lesion and before cavitation remineralization is possible. *(Redrawn from Darling AI: The pathology and prevention of caries, Br Dent J 107:287–302, 1959.)*

Discoloration in arrested caries? → By trapped organic debris & metallic ions within the enamel

resistant to subsequent caries attack because of the incorporation of more acid-resistant fluorapatite (Fig. 2-28). Remineralized (arrested) lesions can be observed clinically as intact, but discolored, usually brown or black, spots (Fig. 2-29). The change in color is presumably caused by trapped organic debris and metallic ions within the enamel. These discolored, remineralized, arrested caries areas are intact and are more resistant to subsequent caries attack than the adjacent unaffected enamel. They should not be restored unless they are esthetically objectionable.

Cavitated enamel lesions can be initially detected as subtle breakdown of the enamel surface. These lesions are very sensitive to probing, and can be easily enlarged by using sharp explorers and excessive probing force. More advanced cavitated enamel lesions are more obviously detected as enamel breakdown. Although some cavitated enamel lesions can be arrested and may not progress to larger lesions, most cavitated caries lesions require restorative treatment.

Dentin Caries

An understanding of the dentin composition and histology is helpful to understand the histopathology of dentin caries (see Chapter 1 (Fig. 2-30). Progression of caries in dentin is different from progression in the overlying enamel because of the structural differences of dentin (Figs. 2-31 to 2-33; see also

Local mechanism of enamel adaptation to the cariogenic challenge

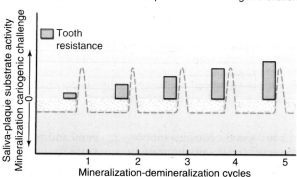

Fig. 2-28 Diagrammatic representation of enamel adaptation reaction. Enamel interacts with its fluid environment in periods of undersaturation and supersaturation, presented here as periodic cycles. Undersaturation periods dissolve most soluble mineral at the site of cariogenic attack, whereas periods of supersaturation deposit most insoluble minerals if their ionic components are present in immediate fluid environment. As a result, under favorable conditions of remineralization, each cycle could lead toward higher enamel resistance to a subsequent challenge. *(Redrawn from Koulourides T: In Menaker L, editor: The biologic basis of dental caries, New York, 1980, Harper & Row.)*

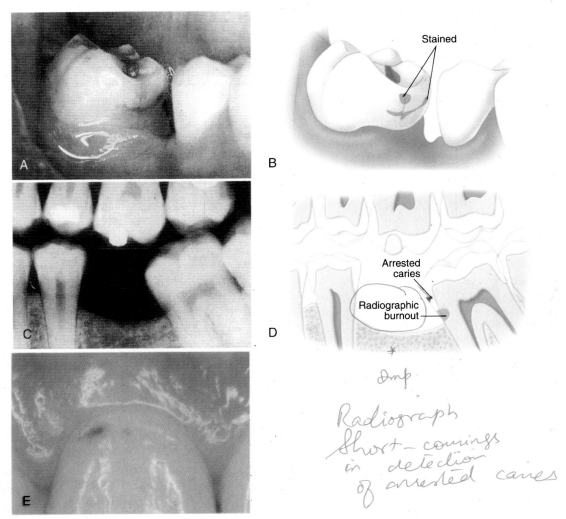

Fig. 2-29 A and **B,** Example of arrested caries on the mesial surface of a mandibular second molar. The area below the proximal contact (*A* and *B,* mirror view of tooth No. 18) is partly opaque and stained. Clinically the surface is hard and intact, yet the area is more radiolucent than the enamel above or below the stain. **C** and **D,** In a different clinical case, caries diagnosis based only on the radiograph would lead to a false-positive diagnosis (i.e., caries present when it is not). The radiolucency is caused by the broad area of subsurface demineralization that extends from the facial to the lingual line angles. The x-ray beam was directed parallel to the long axis of demineralization and consequently produced a sharply demarcated zone of radiolucency in the enamel. This example illustrates the shortcomings of radiographic diagnosis. Were there not visual access to the mesial surface of the second molar, it would be easy to diagnose active caries incorrectly and consequently restore the tooth. **E,** Cavitated inactive (arrested) enamel caries lesion on the cervical one third of a central incisor of a 27-year-old patient with low caries risk. This lesion, if not esthetically offensive, does not require a restoration and should be monitored.

Fig. 2-30). Dentin contains much less mineral and possesses microscopic tubules that provide a pathway for the ingress of bacteria and egress of minerals. The DEJ has the least resistance to caries attack and allows rapid lateral spreading when caries has penetrated the enamel (see Figs. 2-15 and 2-21). Because of these characteristics, dentinal caries is V-shaped in cross-section with a wide base at the DEJ and the apex directed pulpally. Caries advances more rapidly in dentin than in enamel because dentin provides much less resistance to acid attack owing to less mineralized content. Caries produces a variety of responses in dentin, including pain, sensitivity, demineralization, and remineralization.

Often, pain is not reported even when caries invades dentin except when deep lesions bring the bacterial infection close to the pulp. Episodes of short-duration pain may be felt occasionally during earlier stages of dentin caries. The pain is caused by stimulation of pulp tissue by the movement of fluid through the dentinal tubules that have been opened to the oral environment by cavitation. When bacterial invasion of the dentin is close to the pulp, toxins and possibly a few bacteria enter the pulp, resulting in inflammation of the pulpal tissues and, thus, pulpal pain.

The pulp–dentin complex reacts to caries attacks by attempting to initiate remineralization and blocking off the open tubules. These reactions result from odontoblastic activity and the physical process of demineralization and remineralization. Three levels of dentinal reaction to caries can be recognized: (1) reaction to a long-term, low-level acid demineralization associated with a slowly advancing lesion; (2) reaction to a moderate-intensity attack; and (3) reaction to severe, rapidly advancing caries characterized by very high acid levels. Dentin can react defensively (by repair) to low-intensity and

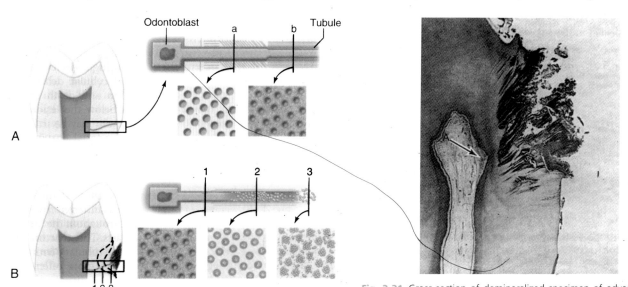

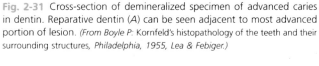

Fig. 2-30 Normal and carious dentin. **A,** Normal dentin has characteristic tubules that follow a wavy path from the external surface of dentin, below enamel or cementum, to the inner surface of dentin in the pulp tissue of the pulp chamber or pulp canal. Dentin is formed from the external surface and grows inward. As dentin grows, odontoblasts become increasingly compressed in the shrinking pulp chamber, and the number of associated tubules becomes more concentrated per unit area. The more recently formed dentin near the pulp (a) has large tubules with little or no peritubular dentin and calcified intertubular dentin filled with collagen fibers. Older dentin, closer to the external surface (b), is characterized by smaller, more widely separated tubules and a greater mineral content in intertubular dentin. The older dentin tubules are lined by a uniform layer of mineral termed *peritubular dentin*. These changes occur gradually from the inner surface to the external surface of the dentin. Horizontal lines indicate predentin; diagonal lines indicate increasing density of minerals; darker horizontal lines indicate densely mineralized dentin and increased thickness of peritubular dentin. The transition in mineral content is gradual, as indicated in Fig. 2-25. **B,** Carious dentin undergoes several changes. The most superficial infected zone of carious dentin (3) is characterized by bacteria filling the tubules and granular material in the intertubular space. The granular material contains very little mineral and lacks characteristic cross-banding of collagen. As bacteria invade dentinal tubules, if carbohydrates are available, they can produce enough lactic acid to remove peritubular dentin. This doubles or triples the outer diameter of the tubules in infected dentin zone. Pulpal to (below) the infected dentin is a zone where the dentin appears transparent in mounted whole specimens. This zone (2) is affected (not infected) carious dentin and is characterized by loss of mineral in the intertubular and peritubular dentin. Many crystals can be detected in the lumen of the tubules in this zone. The crystals in the tubule lumen render the refractive index of the lumen similar to that of the intertubular dentin, making the zone transparent. Normal dentin (1) is found pulpal to (below) transparent dentin.

Fig. 2-31 Cross-section of demineralized specimen of advanced caries in dentin. Reparative dentin (A) can be seen adjacent to most advanced portion of lesion. *(From Boyle P: Kornfeld's histopathology of the teeth and their surrounding structures, Philadelphia, 1955, Lea & Febiger.)*

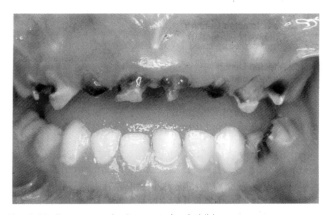

Fig. 2-32 Rampant caries in a preschool child. *(From Dean JA, Avery DR, McDonald RE: McDonald and Avery's dentistry for the child and adolescent, ed 9, St Louis, 2011, Mosby.)*

moderate-intensity caries attacks as long as the pulp remains vital and has an adequate blood circulation.

In slowly advancing caries, a vital pulp can repair demineralized dentin by remineralization of the intertubular dentin and by apposition of peritubular dentin. Early stages of caries or mild caries attacks produce long-term, low-level acid demineralization of dentin. Direct exposure of the pulp tissue to microorganisms is not a prerequisite for an inflammatory response. Toxins and other metabolic byproducts, especially hydrogen ion, can penetrate via the dentinal tubules to the pulp. Even when the lesion is limited to enamel, the pulp can be shown to respond with inflammatory cells.[22,23] Dentin responds to the stimulus of its first caries demineralization episode by deposition of crystalline material in the lumen of the tubules and the intertubular dentin of affected dentin in front of the advancing infected dentin portion of the lesion (see Fig. 2-30, *B*). Hypermineralized areas may be seen on radiographs as zones of increased radiopacity (often S-shaped following the course of the tubules) ahead of the advancing, infected portion of the lesion. This repair occurs only if the tooth pulp is vital.

Dentin that has more mineral content than normal dentin is termed *sclerotic dentin*. Sclerotic dentin formation occurs ahead of the demineralization front of a slowly advancing lesion and may be seen under an old restoration. Sclerotic dentin is usually shiny and darker in color but feels hard to the explorer tip. By contrast, normal, freshly cut dentin lacks

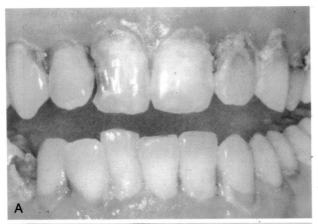

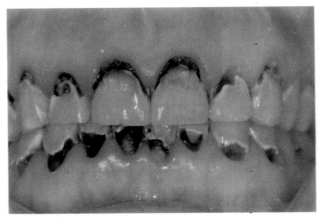

Fig. 2-37 Advance cavitated active caries lesions on a 35-year-old patient with high caries risk. (Courtesy of Dr. Ayesha Swarn, DDS, Operative Dentistry Graduate Program at UNC School of Dentistry.)

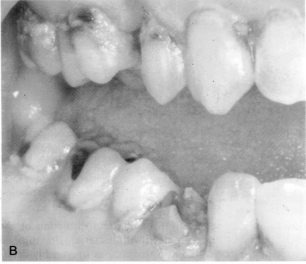

Fig. 2-36 Acute, rampant caries in both anterior (A) and posterior (B) teeth.

hydroxide liner can be used on the deepest portions of the excavation to enhance the formation of reparative dentin.

Advanced Caries Lesions

Increasing demineralization of the body of the enamel lesion results in the weakening and eventual collapse of the surface enamel. The resulting cavitation provides an even more protective and retentive habitat for the cariogenic biofilm, accelerating the progression of the lesion. The DEJ provides less resistance to the carious process than either enamel or dentin. The resultant lateral spread of the lesion at the DEJ produces the characteristic second cone of caries activity in dentin. Figures 2-30, 2-32, and 2-36 and Figure 2-37 illustrate advanced lesions with infected dentin.

Necrotic dentin is recognized clinically as a wet, mushy, easily removable mass. This material is structureless or granular in histologic appearance and contains masses of bacteria. Occasionally, remnants of dentinal tubules may be seen in histologic preparations. Removal of the necrotic material uncovers deeper infected dentin (turbid dentin), which appears dry and leathery. Leathery dentin is easily removed by hand instruments and flakes off in layers parallel to the

DEJ. Microscopic examination of this material reveals distorted dentinal tubules engorged with bacteria. Clefts coursing perpendicular to the tubules also are seen in leathery dentin. Apparently, these clefts represent the rest lines formed during the original deposition of dentin and are more susceptible to caries attack. Further excavation uncovers increasingly harder dentin. If the lesion is progressing slowly, a zone of hard, hypermineralized sclerotic dentin may be present, as a result of remineralization of what formerly was affected (or transparent) dentin (zone 2). When sclerotic dentin is encountered, it represents the ideal final excavation depth because it is a natural barrier that blocks the penetration of toxins and acids.

Removal of the bacterial infection is an essential part of all operative procedures. Because bacteria never penetrate as far as the advancing front of the lesion, it is not necessary to remove all of the dentin that has been affected by the caries process. In operative procedures, it is convenient to term dentin as either *infected*, which requires removal, or *affected*, which does not require removal. Affected dentin is softened, demineralized dentin that is not yet invaded by bacteria. Infected dentin is softened and contaminated with bacteria. It includes superficial, granular necrotic tissue and softened, dry, leathery dentin. The outer layer (infected dentin) can be selectively stained in vivo by caries detection solutions such as 1% acid red 52 (acid rhodamine B or food red 106) in propylene glycol.[35] This solution stains the irreversibly denatured collagen in the outer carious layer but not the reversibly denatured collagen in the inner carious layer.[36] Clinical use of this staining technique may provide a more conservative tooth preparation because the boundary between the two layers differentiated by this technique cannot easily be detected in a tactile manner.

Caries Risk Assessment and Management

In Chapter 3, the clinical examination process for diagnosis and detection of caries lesions is discussed in detail. Although it is very important to detect caries lesions, this is a tooth-centered process. It is critical to remember that clinicians treat the entire patient and not just individual teeth and caries lesions. As noted earlier in this chapter, dental caries is a multi-factorial medical disease process, and the caries lesions are the expression of that disease process involving the patient as a whole. Equally important in the management of caries as a disease entity is the ability to individualize caries diagnosis and treatment or interventions for each patient. To do this, the clinician must formulate a caries risk assessment profile that is based on the patient's risk factors and risk indicators currently present (A *risk factor* is defined as an environmental, behavioral, or biologic factor that directly increases the probability that a disease will occur and, the absence or removal of which reduces the possibility of disease)[37,38] Risk factors are part of the causal chain of the disease process, or they expose the host to the causal chain; but once the disease occurs, removal of a risk factor may not always result in the disease process being halted. Any definition of risk factor must clearly establish that the exposure has occurred before the outcome or before the conditions are established that make the outcome likely. This means that longitudinal studies are necessary to demonstrate risk factors. Terms such as *risk indicators* and *risk markers* are also used in the caries literature to refer to risk factors, putative risk factors, or something else entirely. For example, *risk indicators* can refer to existing signs of the disease process, or signs that the disease process has occurred, but are not part of the disease causal chain. For example, existing caries lesions would be risk indicators, as they indicate a risk status, but are not per se part of the causal chain. Multiple risk factors (and indicators) have been studied, reviewed, and validated in the assessment of risk for development of future caries disease, but caries risk assessment is not an exact science. Because caries is a complex multi-factorial disease, no single risk factor (or indicator, or marker) is highly predictive of future caries. However, caries risk assessment is necessary to inform what (if any) interventions are needed to lower the patient's caries risk and activity—which is the ultimate goal of caries management in a medical model.[39,40] A discussion of different risk factors will be included in this section of this chapter.

(Caries risk assessments are specific for adults and adolescents older than 6 years and children under 6 years of age). It is very important to spend the time with the patient to uncover all relevant risk factors and indicators currently present. Some risk factors and protective factors can be adjusted and modified by either the patient or the clinician, such as sucrose intake and fluoride exposure; other risk factors are not modifiable, such as xerostomia as the result of a needed medication. Understanding and controlling risk factors and protective factors can be very important in the prevention of new caries lesions and to slow down or arrest the progression of existing caries lesions.

No consensus exists on exactly how to define the risk categories for caries risk assessments. Terms used are "at risk," "low risk," "medium risk," "high risk," and so on. Assignment of these terms is typically based on the subjective judgment of the clinician with general rules applied, based on the clinician's previous clinical experiences and training. If a clinician finds no detectable or active caries lesions and minimum or no identifiable risk factors, that patient would be assigned a *low caries risk*. In this situation, in the current state of the patient's health, the protective factors for not developing

caries lesions outweigh the risk factors that could lead to new caries lesions. The strongest predictor for caries risk for patients in the *at risk* and *high risk* categories are the number of caries lesions being detected for the patient over the last 2 to 3 years along with past history of caries lesions in the patient's lifetime.[39]

Historically, dentistry has used a surgical model for the management of dental caries, which mainly contemplated the biomechanical excision of caries lesions and the restoration of the resultant *tooth preparation* to form and function with a restorative material. Management of caries disease by a surgical model consisted of waiting until cavitations were detected and treating the cavitations with restorations. Eventually, it became apparent that dealing only with the end result of the disease and not addressing its etiology for each individual patient was not successful in controlling the caries disease process. Since surgical management alone was not successful, a system has been developed using caries management strategies. This system looks at individualized caries risk assessments and uses this information to design treatment plans according to the risk assessment findings. These assessments look at each patient's unique set of pathologic factors and protective factors. Caries management by risk assessment represents a management philosophy that manages the caries disease process using a medical model. This process provides an individualized evaluation of a patient's pathologic factors and protective factors and assesses the patient's risk for developing future disease. The risk assessment is then used to develop an *individualized* evidence-based caries management plan that would involve all aspects of nonsurgical therapeutics and dental surgical interventions. Both risk assessment and patient-centered interventions are based on the concept of caries balance as discussed earlier in this chapter (see Fig. 2-1). The caries balance model is based on minimizing pathologic factors while maximizing protective factors to attain a balance that favors no disease occurring, or health. With the use of caries management by risk assessment for patient management, mounting evidence suggests that early damage to teeth may be reversed and that the incidences of disease manifestations can be significantly reduced or prevented. Caries management by risk assessment is evolving into the standard of care in caries management. In the United States, one of the most widely used systems is CAMBRA (caries management by risk assessment).[4,41]

· Risk Management
· Patient-centered interventions

Caries Risk Assessment

In Chapter 3, the examination process and formulation of the diagnosis, prognosis, and treatment planning related to caries management and operative dentistry interventions are reviewed. The caries risk assessment is an important part of this overall process of patient care. The clinician must gather all appropriate data from both the interview with the patient and the clinical examination for caries detection to formulate an individualized caries risk assessment. Part of the caries risk assessment identifies the causative factors, called *risk factors*, but does not predict the caries outcome. Risk factors can exist for a patient without the disease being expressed at the current point in time. The predictive model part of the risk assessment looks at the assessment of caries progression in the future. The term *risk factor* is associated with the variables studied that have value for prediction purposes, which means that the risk factor is present *before* the disease occurs. As discussed above, risk indicators are existing signs of the disease process. They are examples of what is happening with the patient's current state of oral health, not how disease occurred. They are clinical observations and detection modalities used to identify risk-level status. Examples include visible cavitations in pits and fissures or in proximal surfaces of teeth, brown spots, active white spots, or cavitated lesions on free smooth surfaces, as well as any restorations in the past 3 years. The ideal caries risk assessment model should be inexpensive and easy to use but at the same time have high degrees of accuracy in predictive value. It should be valuable in decision making for caries management in the use of nonsurgical therapeutics and surgical interventions that serve the patient in a cost-effective and health-promoting manner.

One of the roles of caries risk assessments in caries management is to assist in determining the current caries lesion activity. Caries lesions can be detected much before frank cavitation occurs. The diagnosis of caries lesions should include whether they are actively progressing. An inactive lesion may be visible clinically or radiographically. However, an inactive caries lesion does not progress over time. With a positive shift in protective factors, change in oral hygiene, reduction of negative risk factors, it is possible for caries lesions to change in density, size, hardness and show increased sheen compared with the previous matte surface texture. These inactive lesions may remineralize and not require operative intervention. Assessment by the clinician of all the risk factors and protective factors in the patient's current history can greatly aid in the decision regarding current activity. Looking at all the possible risk factors with a thorough risk assessment allows for a more predictive analysis of current and future disease activity and assists in deciding on nonsurgical or surgical interventions. Caries risk assessments help the clinician to identify the etiologic causes of the disease for a specific patient at a specific point in time. Risk assessments are important in determining the frequency of recare visits and the treatment protocols for follow-up visits. Restorative decisions in terms of material used and cavity preparation design are also influenced by the information gathered in the risk assessments. The data gathered establish an important baseline for use in future reassessments to help the clinician and the patient measure the effectiveness of the caries management treatment protocol used for the patient. The systematic use of risk assessment profiles is essential in uncovering risk factors that are present before expression of the disease. This information can be useful in the prevention of caries lesions in patients who have risk factors present but no disease expression and then experience a lifestyle change that adds additional risk factors. This new risk factor then becomes a tipping point for the caries balance equation toward disease expression. For instance, a patient who has the risk factor of frequent consumption of high-sugar soft drinks during the day suddenly is prescribed a xerostomia-inducing medication that increases his caries risk. The informed patient would have the option of making the decision to eliminate a modifiable risk factor (soft drinks) before expression of the disease and before the introduction of the xerostomia-producing medication to his risk assessment.

The incorporation of risk assessments in routine patient care and in each patient's caries management program is necessary because of the multi-factorial nature of caries. No one

factor can be used to predict the probability of a patient developing caries lesions. Looking at the whole patient in developing a preventive and restorative caries management plan is essential to successful outcomes. In addition, having recorded specific risk assessment profiles provides patients with an educational tool that empowers them to be an important part of managing their disease. Finally, risk assessments provide a means for both the clinician and the patient to monitor and measure the proposed caries management protocols over time and evaluate and adjust the protocols as needed. Risk assessments lead to better treatment outcomes for patients.

Knowing certain factors pertaining to the patient's history are key in establishing a caries risk assessment. Such factors that have been identified as contributing to caries risk include age, gender, fluoride exposure, home care, smoking habits, alcohol intake, medications, dietary habits, economic and educational status, and general health. Increased smoking, alcohol consumption, use of medications, and sucrose intake result in increased risks for caries development.[42] Children and older adults have increased risks. Decreased fluoride exposure, lower economic status, and lower educational attainment also increase risk. Poor general health also increases the risk. A strong body of evidence suggests that past caries experience is the best predictor of future caries activity.[43] Information that is important and obtained in the patient history interview would be biologic and environmental factors that include, but are not limited to, medical history including current and past diseases, current medications, and history of xerostomia from medications or conditions; dental history including past history of dental caries, dental phobias, and history of dental conditions; current home care practices and how well this is done; current diet and exposure to sucrose and other fermentable carbohydrates; and current exposure to topical fluoride products in toothpaste, mouth rinses, and fluoridated water supply. Some of these factors are explored in more detail in the following sections.

Figure 2-38, *A* and *B*, present two examples of Caries Risk Assessment forms that can be used as part of the initial caries diagnosis process, and Figure 2-38, *C*, is an example of a Caries Assessment form that can be used to facilitate communication of the findings with patients; this Caries Assessment form is a useful tool to measure changes and determine the effectiveness of caries management procedures. All of these forms can be incorporated into an electronic patient management system for increased efficiency.

Social, Economic, and Education Status

Social status and economic status are not directly involved in the disease process but are important because they affect the expression and management of the caries disease. The socioeconomic status and educational status of the patient have implications on the necessary compliance and behavioral changes that can decrease risk for caries in patients. These are predictive at the population level but are generally inaccurate at the individual level.

Dietary Analysis

Sugar intake in the form of fermentable carbohydrates and increased frequency of intake are conditions that increase risk for caries. The use of candies and lozenges frequently during

Caries Risk Assessment Form (Age >6)

Patient Name: Score:

Birth Date: Date:

Age: Initials:

		Low Risk (0)	Moderate Risk (1)	High Risk (10)	Patient Risk
Contributing Conditions					
I.	**Fluoride Exposure** (through drinking water, supplements, professional applications, toothpaste)	Yes	No		
II.	**Sugary Foods or Drinks** (including juice, carbonated or non-carbonated soft drinks, energy drinks, medicinal syrups)	Primarily at mealtimes		Frequent or prolonged between meal exposures/day	
III.	**Caries Experience of Mother, Caregiver** and/or other **Siblings** (for patients ages 6-14)	No carious lesions in last 24 months	Carious lesions in last 7-23 months	Carious lesions in last 6 months	
IV.	**Dental Home**: established patient of record, receiving regular dental care in a dental office	Yes	No		
General Health Conditions					
I.	**Special Health Care Needs***	No	Yes (over age 14)	Yes (ages 6-14)	
II.	**Chemo/Radiation Therapy**	No		Yes	
III.	**Eating Disorders**	No	Yes		
IV.	**Medications that Reduce Salivary Flow**	No	Yes		
V.	**Drug/Alcohol Abuse**	No	Yes		
Clinical Conditions					
I.	**Cavitated or Non-Cavitated** (incipient) **Carious Lesions or Restorations** (visually or radiographically evident)	No new carious lesions or restorations in last 36 months	1 or 2 new carious lesions or restorations in last 36 months	3 or more carious lesions or restorations in last 36 months	
II.	**Teeth Missing Due to Caries** in past 36 months	No		Yes	
III.	**Visible Plaque**	No	Yes		
IV.	**Unusual Tooth Morphology** that compromises oral hygiene	No	Yes		
V.	**Interproximal Restorations - 1 or more**	No	Yes		
VI.	**Exposed Root Surfaces** Present	No	Yes		
VII.	**Restorations with Overhangs** and/or **Open Margins**; **Open Contacts** with Food Impaction	No	Yes		
VIII.	**Dental/Orthodontic Appliances** (fixed or removable)	No	Yes		
IX.	**Severe Dry Mouth (Xerostomia)**	No		Yes	
				TOTAL:	

Patient Instructions:

*Patients with developmental, physical, medical or mental disabilities that prevent or limit performance of adequate oral health care by themselves or caregivers.

A

Fig. 2-38 **A,** Example of a Caries Risk Assessment form recommended by the American Dental Association.

Caries Risk Initial Assessment

Name_____

Date_____

Risk	Low Risk	At Risk	High Risk
Risk Rating Score	≤ 3	≥4 and ≤8	≥9

Patient Interview Assessment
Dental History   Risk Rating
1. Had non emergency dental care in last year   yes   no   -1
2. Brushes teeth at least twice daily   yes   no   -3
3. Uses fluoridated toothpaste or product daily   yes   no   -3
4. New caries lesions within the last 3 years   yes   no   8
5. Patient has teeth sensitive to hot, cold, sweets yes no   3
6. Patient avoids brushing any part of mouth   yes   no   3

Supplemental notes for dental history

Dietary Assessment
1. Water supply currently fluoridated   yes   no   -2
2. Frequent snacking with sugary foods,
   acidic foods, fermentable carb foods   yes   no   8
3. Sugary drinks including soft drinks,
   juice, sports drinks, medicinal syrups   yes   no   8
4. Tobacco use of any kind   yes   no   3
5. Excessive alcohol or recreational drug use   yes   no   8
6. Eating disorders   yes   no   5

Supplemental notes for dietary assessment

Xerostomia Assessment
1. Patient is aware of dry mouth or reduced saliva yes no   10
2. Medications taken that reduce salivary flow   yes no   8
3. Medical conditions affecting salivary flow/content yes no   8
4. Saliva flow or content visibly abnormal   yes no   10

Xerostomia Assessments with scores of 8-10 indicate baseline salivary testing is required

Patient Clinical Assessment
Clinical Oral Findings
1. Readily visible biofilm/plaque   yes   no   5
2. Visible cavitated lesions   yes   no   10
3. Interproximal enamel lesions or radiolucencies yes   no   10
4. Visible white spots   yes   no   5
5. Visible brown spots or non cavitated caries lesions yes no 3
6. Deep pits or grooves   yes   no   5
7. Radiographic cavitated lesions   yes   no   10
8. Restorations with overhangs
   and/or margin concerns or open contacts   yes   no   3
9. Prosthesis ortho, fixed, or removable   yes   no   3

Clinical Assessments with scores of 10 indicate that baseline bacterial testing is required

Risk Rating Total =

10. Clinician's impression of patient's risk   low   at risk   high

This is clinician's impression of patient's risk if different than would be indicated by risk factors marked. Describe in box below.

Patient Compliance Assessment
Patient's attitude and general assessment of patient's ability to comply for each of the following categories:

Oral hygiene compliance patient limitations   yes   no
Dietary recommendation patient limitations   yes   no
Therapeutic homecare products limitations   yes   no

Special needs health care (physical or mental compliance issues)   yes   no

This is clinician's assessment of any perceived limitations for the patient to comply with oral hygiene, dietary, or using home care products. Could be lifestyle, physical, or economic reasons. Describe in box below.

Patient Clinical In Office Tests Indicated From Risk Score

Cariscreen Meter   completed   at risk   low risk   reading _____
GC America Saliva Check   completed   at risk   low risk
GC America Strep Mutans   completed   at risk   low risk
GC America Plaque Indicator completed   at risk   low risk
UNC Biologic Testing Lab   completed   at risk   low risk

Notes from oral findings, patient's attitude, office tests, special circumstances that would influence caries risk or management

B

Fig. 2-38, cont'd B, Example of a Caries Risk Assessment form used by the University of North Carolina, Department of Operative Dentistry.

Caries Assessment Testing Results

Name_____

Date_____

_____.

Your Risk Scores: Risk predicts your likelihood of developing future disease. Green is low risk and means you are unlikely to develop a cavity whereas red means you are very likely to develop a cavity unless your risk factors are managed. We will use these results to work with you to develop an individualized plan to control your disease.

Existing Dental Conditions

Your dental condition score is based on current areas of decay, number of cavities in the last three years, exposed root surfaces, crowns and fillings that are defective. Your score will also be higher if you wear partial dentures or other appliances.

Saliva Assessment Testing

Saliva pH Testing

>6.8   6.0-6.6   <5.8

Saliva Flow and Buffering

Normal   Abnormal

Your saliva is the main protective factor in the caries risk disease state equation. Yellow and Red results can produce an increased incidence of cavities. If the pH of the saliva is low, it sets the stage for the bacteria to grow that cause cavities to form in your mouth. If the quantity of the saliva is below normal, the healing ability of the saliva to remineralize your teeth after acidic food and beverages is greatly reduced. This can, in most incidences, result in a dry mouth that is uncomfortable when eating and lead to an increase in cavities on the roots and other surfaces of your teeth. Any change in saliva content, amount, or pH can increase your risk for cavities to form even if you have not had cavities in the past. New medications and medical conditions can cause your saliva to change rapidly.

Plaque Assessment Testing

Plaque pH Testing

>6.8   6.0-6.6   <5.8

Biofilm Activity

<1500   1500-2000   >2000

Visible Plaque

Low   High

Plaque or biofilm is the mass of bacteria that is always changing and clings to the surfaces of your teeth. Plaque is one of the main risk factors that result in cavities. For plaque to produce the acid that dissolves your teeth and form cavities, it has to be in an acidic state, or in other words, have a low pH. The more acidic, the more damage that can result. The type of bacteria in the plaque also influences how easy it is for the damage to occur. The biofilm activity measures the amount of the "bad" bacteria present in the plaque. The higher the number, the more bacteria are present that cause the cavities to form. The amount of plaque on your teeth means more bacteria are present in your mouth. More bacteria produce higher amounts of acid to demineralize your teeth and cause them to decay.

Dietary Habits

Frequency of Snacking

< 1   2-3   >3

Frequency of sweetened beverages and sport drinks

< 1   2-3   >3

A key factor in how you control your disease and prevent cavities is how you eat and what beverages you consume. Snacking with sweet foods or high carbohydrate foods that can form sugars causes the plaque to become acidic. This results in more bacteria forming that produce even more acid. All of this acid dissolves your teeth and forms the cavities. Sweetened drinks or drinks high in acid content also produce low pH plaque and more bacteria. Soft drinks and sports drinks like Gatorade are very low in pH. The more you drink, the more acid the plaque and bacteria produce to cause the cavities in your teeth.

C

Fig. 2-38, cont'd **C,** Another caries Assessment form used by the University of North Carolina, Department of Operative Dentistry. This form is very useful for patient communication and compliance. (**A,** Copyright 2009, 2011 the American Dental Association.)

the day or night increases the risk. Acidic beverages, including sport drinks, fruit juices, and soft drinks, all contribute to increasing risk by providing energy to the acidogenic and aciduric bacteria and by influencing the pH of the biofilm to support cariogenic bacteria. Frequency of snacking and the frequency of consuming these foods and beverages all support an increase in biologic caries risk factors by modifying the biofilm to support a lower pH environment.

Salivary Analysis

Salivary flow rate, buffering capacity, and pH all can be measured by different tests and means. The predictive value for these tests for caries is not supported by the highest evidence in all circumstances. Patients with good saliva flow and adequate buffering can still have caries. In cases of dry mouth, or xerostomia, a salivary analysis is a predictive risk factor for root caries in older patients with recession and for increased caries in general in other populations. As discussed previously, saliva has numerous effects in protection against caries, including inhibition of bacteria, diluting and eliminating bacteria and their substrates, buffering bacterial acids, and offering a reparative environment with necessary calcium and phosphate minerals after bacteria-induced demineralization. Since all of these benefits are missing when patients have salivary hypofunction, patients with dry mouth are at higher risk for caries. These patients are more susceptible to dietary changes that are associated with lower pH foods and beverages or foods and beverages containing fermentable carbohydrates, since the protective factors of saliva are diminished in patients with xerostomia.

Dental Clinical Analysis (Dental Exam)

The dental examination determines risk indicators more than risk factors. This is also important as many of the indicators are directly related to the current caries activity. The indicators and current caries activity drive the decision making process for the type of intervention that the clinician would prescribe. Visible cavitated caries lesions, white spots on teeth, and brown spots on teeth are all indicators for caries risk. Visible plaque or biofilm can be considered a risk factor for caries development. Other examination findings that would influence increased risk for caries are exposed root surfaces, deep pits or grooves, fixed, removable prosthesis, or orthodontic appliances used, poor quality existing restorations with open contacts, open margins, or overhangs.

Bacterial Biofilm Analysis

Use of supplemental tests to analyze the bacterial component of the biofilm can help determine the patient's risk level. However, the evidence is weaker with some potential for bias by the examiners for these tests being predictive of future caries. For example, the presence of S. mutans or lactobacilli in saliva or plaque as a sole predictor for caries in primary teeth was shown to have low sensitivity but high specificity. Other means of bacterial testing still being evaluated is the measurement of adenosine triphosphate (ATP) activity of the biofilm bacteria as a surrogate measure of caries activity. Although these bacterial tests can be useful for communication with the patient and can provide insight into the type of

bacteria present and the type of biofilm environment present, predictive evidence for caries from these tests need to be further studied and improved.

Risk Considerations for Children Under 6 Years Old

In addition to all the above risk factors for adults and adolescents, age-specific risk factors and indicators that should be considered for children under 6 years old include presence of active caries in the primary caregiver in the past year; feeding on demand past 1 year of age; bedtime bottle or sippy cup with anything other than water; no supervised brushing; and severe enamel hypoplasia.

Caries risk assessment is only effective if used in conjunction with a corresponding caries management program. The caries prevention or management program should comprise a menu of prevention therapies and interventions that should be recommended on the basis of the level of caries risk (Table 2-7 and Box 2-2). However, as was discussed in the previous section, no caries risk assessment system is perfect. Therefore, in addition to the outcome of the caries risk assessment tool, the clinician needs to use the best clinical judgment, coupled with the best available research evidence, to design a preventive or therapeutic program that works for the patient. Needless to say, this is a dynamic process, so monitoring and periodic reassessment and re-evaluation of the disease activity and prevention or management program are critical.

Caries Management and Protocols or Strategies for Prevention

Management of dental caries and its consequences remains the predominant activity of dentists. Preventive and diagnostic services are, however, increasing.[44,45] Although these activities relate to a variety of dental problems, diagnosis and prevention of caries are major parts of these increases. In a modern practice model, the restoration of a caries lesion should no longer be considered a cure for dental caries. Rather, the practitioner must identify patients who have active caries lesions and patients at high risk for caries and institute appropriate preventive and treatment measures. This section presents some measures that can reduce the likelihood of a patient developing caries lesions. Depending on the risk status of the patient, the dentist must decide which of these to institute. In the future, dentistry will focus increasing effort on limiting the need for restorative treatment.

Preventive treatment methods are designed to limit tooth demineralization caused by cariogenic bacteria, preventing cavitated lesions. These methods include (1) limiting pathogen growth and altering metabolism, (2) increasing the resistance of the tooth surface to demineralization, and (3) increasing biofilm pH. A caries prevention and management program is a complex process involving multiple interrelated factors (Table 2-7; Tables 2-8, 2-9, 2-10 and 2-11; see also Table 2-7 and Box 2-2). The primary goals of a caries prevention program are to reduce the numbers of cariogenic bacteria and to create an environment conducive to remineralization. Prevention should start with a consideration of the overall resistance of the patient to infection by the cariogenic bacteria. Although the general health of the patient, fluoride exposure

1/1 %/5000 ppm NaF

Table 2-7 Suggested Risk-Based Interventions for Adults*

Caries Risk Category	Office-Based Interventions	Home-Based Interventions
HIGH	3-month recare examination and oral prophylaxis Fluoride varnish at each recare visit Individualized oral hygiene instructions and use of specialized cleaning aids (e.g., powered toothbrush, Waterpik) Dietary counseling Bitewing radiographs every 6–12 months[†]	Brush with prescription fluoride dentifrice, e.g. 1/1%/5000 ppm NaF Use sugar substitutes (e.g., xylitol, sorbitol) Apply calcium-phosphate compounds (e.g., MI Paste) Use antimicrobial agents (e.g., xylitol gum or lozenge, chlorhexidine rinse) If xerostomic, increase salivary function (e.g., xylitol gum, rinses, oral moisturizers)
MODERATE	4–6 month recare examination and oral prophylaxis Fluoride varnish at each recall Reinforce proper oral hygiene Dietary counseling	Brush with fluoride dentifrice (e.g., 1450 ppm fluoride) OTC fluoride rinse (e.g., 0.05% NaF)
LOW	9-12 month recare examination and oral prophylaxis Reinforce good oral hygiene	Brush with fluoride dentifrice

*These are general guidelines, and should be customized based on the specific patient's needs and on weight of individual risk factors uncovered with a caries risk assessment instrument.

[†]Data from U.S. Department of Health and Human Services, Public Health Service, Food and Drug Administration; and American Dental Association, Council on Dental Benefit Programs, Council on Scientific Affairs. The selection of patients for dental radiographic examinations. Rev. ed. 2004. Available at: "www.ada.org/prof/resources/topics/radiography.asp". Accessed January 20, 2012.

NaF, sodium fluoride; *OTC*, over the counter; *ppm*, parts per million.

(Modified from Shugars DA, Bader JD: MetLife Quality Resource Guide: Risk-based management of dental caries in adults, *MetLife Quality Resource Guide*, ed 3, Metropolitan Life Insurance, Co., Bridgewater NJ; 2009-2012, p. 6)

Box 2.2 Sample Preventive Protocol for a High-Risk Patient with Cavitated Caries Lesions

1. A comprehensive oral and radiographic evaluation is conducted charting caries lesions, periodontal pocket probing, existing restorations, and oral cancer exam; the medical and dental histories are reviewed. In this hypothetical patient, multiple caries lesions, poor oral hygiene, and generalized marginal gingivitis are noted.

2. A caries risk assessment is completed with emphasis on discovering the risk factors that are contributing to the causative aspect of the caries problem and discovering the risk factors for the patient that are predictors of future caries risk. A discussion of these risk factors with the patient is essential for understanding of the caries disease process and the patient's role and the provider's role in controlling the disease.

3. Diagnosis and treatment planning procedures are completed and discussed with the patient.

4. Nonoperative and operative treatments will be completed in three phases: (i) A control phase, (ii) a definitive treatment phase, (iii) a maintenance re-assessment phase.

5. CONTROL PHASE (2–4 weeks):

   a. Oral hygiene procedures are explained and reviewed at each patient visit. The frequency of the visits in this initial phase is determined by severity of the disease. This could be weekly or more frequent, depending on the provider's evaluation. When attempting behavior modification, repetition is essential. Review of patient's current home care techniques and frequency of home care are reviewed along with lifestyle issues that might impede compliance. Use of a powered toothbrush and an oral irrigator for possibly improving patient compliance and technique are discussed. Evaluation of the patient's motivation along with the person's mental and physical capacity to comply with recommendations for home care must be noted and considered by the provider.

   Specific recommendations are listed for the patient to use at home, and the patient agrees that this is practical for his or her life situation.

   b. Prescription fluoride toothpaste is prescribed (5000 parts per million [ppm]) and the patient is instructed to brush with it three times per day and to use according to given instructions (do not rinse after use, only expectorate excess). Any products used for home care should be carefully reviewed for the pH of the product. Products with pH lower than 6.0 should be carefully considered whether their use would contribute to the pH shift of the biofilm to pathologic for caries lesion formation.

   c. A diet analysis is completed, analyzed, and reviewed with the patient. Cariogenic foods and beverages are identified and alternatives suggested. Also, acidic foods and beverages that are contributing to the pH shift to a lower oral pH environment are identified and discussed. Options for foods that have impact to raise the oral pH are suggested, such as foods rich in arginine. Again the patient's motivation and abilities to fit the necessary diet modifications into his or her lifestyle must be evaluated and discussed.

   d. A microbiologic survey is completed, using either the adenosine triphosphate (ATP) chairside device or formal saliva samples to identify specific mutans streptococci (MS) and lactobacilli counts. This will serve as baseline data to determine the effectiveness of the prevention protocol for both the provider and the patient and can serve as a motivation for the patient.

   e. A saliva analysis is conducted to determine stimulated flow rate, salivary pH and buffering capacity, and viscosity. Treatment protocols for xerostomia are recommended for patients with an analysis that indicates deficiencies in the above

Continued

Box 2.2 Sample Preventive Protocol for a High-Risk Patient with Cavitated Caries Lesions, cont'd

areas. Patients with low salivary pH would need to use baking soda rinses during the day and use xylitol gum or other recommended products to raise pH levels, increase flow, and increase buffering capacity.

f. Caries control (described elsewhere in this chapter) is completed. This involves partial caries removal and sealing of all cavitated caries lesions, usually during one appointment and sealing the cavities with glass ionomer. This is critical to prevent re-inoculation of the oral cavity with MS from the caries lesions.

g. The patient is instructed to rinse twice a day with either a chlorhexidine (CHX) mouth rinse preferably without alcohol or sodium hypochlorite mouth rinse. If CHX is used, an SLS free prescription toothpaste should be used. The goal is to substantially reduce the numbers of MS in saliva.

h. A prophylaxis is performed and 5% sodium fluoride (NaF) varnish is applied to all teeth.

i. The microbiologic testing is repeated 2 to 4 weeks after initiation of treatment. If the numbers of circulating MS are significantly reduced, the patient will then receive definitive restorative treatment. If the numbers are not reduced, use of the therapeutic mouth rinses is continued until the counts are lowered. Diet analysis is followed up and reviewed again. Successes in diet modifications are positively reinforced. Shortcomings in diet modifications are discussed and options explored with the patient to rectify diet issues, where needed. Home care regimens are reviewed again with patients and refined. It is important to listen to the patient and work to incorporate diet and home care into the patient's lifestyle and abilities to mentally and physically comply with the recommendations.

6. DEFINITIVE TREATMENT PHASE:

a. The glass ionomer provisional restorations are replaced (usually by quadrants) with definitive restorations.

b. Oral hygiene procedures are reinforced at each visit. Flossing and brushing three times per day with prescription toothpaste is recommended.

c. The patient is instructed to chew xylitol chewing gum with at least one gram of xylitol per piece three to six times per day, preferably after meals and snacks.

d. The patient is instructed to apply casein phosphopeptide–amorphous calcium phosphates (CPP-ACP) to teeth after brushing and flossing prior to retiring to bed.

e. If reduced salivary flow rates are considered to be a major etiologic factor, the patient should be instructed to chew sugar-free mints several times a day or use other recommended products for xerostomia treatment. Prescribing pilocarpine or other salivary stimulant should be considered.

f. When all definitive restorations are completed, the patient then enters the maintenance reassessment phase.

7. MAINTENANCE REASSESSMENT PHASE:

a. The patient should be recalled every 3 months. Oral hygiene and home care procedures are reviewed and evaluated. Recommendations for improvement and modifications to home care are evaluated and discussed.

b. Prophylaxis followed by fluoride varnish application is accomplished.

c. Caries risk assessment is completed again; changes are noted in risk factors that have been controlled and those risk factors still listed as causative and predictive factors.

d. Diet analysis and recommendations from previous visits are reviewed and evaluated.

e. Patient continues use of prescription 5000 ppm toothpaste, CPP-ACP paste, and xylitol chewing gum. Any other recommendations to changes or additions to the product protocols are reviewed, discussed, and implemented.

f. Every 6 months, salivary and microbiologic evaluations are repeated.

g. Bitewing radiographs are taken on an annual basis or more frequently if new lesions continue to be detected.

h. It is critical for the patient to understand that caries is a disease that is only controlled and not "cured." The protocol that is determined to be currently successful may have to be periodically reviewed, updated, and changed. More importantly, the patient will be much like a patient with diabetes, requiring lifetime medication and therapy, diet control, and lifestyle management for disease stability, and will need to be dedicated to a lifetime of careful management of caries risk factors to keep the disease controlled.

Table 2-8 Health History Factors Associated with Increased Caries Risk

History Factor	Risk-Increasing Observations
Age	Childhood, adolescence, senescence
Fluoride exposure	No fluoride in public water supply No fluoride toothpaste
Smoking	Risk increases with amount smoked
Alcohol	Risk increases with amount consumed
General health	Chronic illness and debilitation decreases ability to give self-care
Medication	Medications that reduce salivary flow

history, and function of the immune system and salivary glands have a significant impact on the patient's caries risk, the patient may have little control over these factors. The patient usually is capable of controlling other factors such as diet, oral hygiene, use of antimicrobial agents, and dental care (which may include use of sealants and restorations). This section presents a variety of factors that may have an impact on the prevention of caries.

General Health

The patient's general health has a significant impact on overall caries risk. Declining health signals the need for increased preventive measures, including more frequent recalls. Every patient has an effective surveillance and destruction system for

secondary caries can be difficult around old restorations. Discoloration of the enamel adjacent to a restoration suggests secondary caries. This condition appears as a localized opalescent area next to the restoration margins. (*Exception*: A bluish color of facial or lingual enamel that directly overlies an old, otherwise acceptable, amalgam restoration does not indicate replacement unless for improvement of esthetics. Such a discoloration may be caused by the amalgam itself.) Because metallic restorations are radiopaque, the radiolucency of secondary caries may be masked. The placement of restorations is preventive only in the sense of removing large numbers of cariogenic organisms and some of the sites in which they may be protected. The placement of a restoration into a cavitated carious tooth does not cure the carious process.

Although diagnostic and preventive measures have been improved and are more widely used, the repair of destruction caused by the carious process still is necessary for many patients. The treatment regimen is dictated by the patient's caries status. If the patient is at high risk for caries development, treatment should consist of restorative procedures and many of the preventive measures described previously. The damage done by caries can be repaired, and the patient's risk status for further caries attacks can be reduced. Sometimes, patients present with acute caries lesions in numerous teeth. Because these teeth may be in jeopardy and because of the large numbers and sites of cariogenic bacteria, restorative treatment for caries control may be indicated, as described later in this section. This procedure rapidly gets rid of the caries lesions, providing better assessment of the pulpal responses of some teeth and greater success of the preventive measures instituted. Later, teeth can be restored with placement of more definitive restorations.

Once caries has produced cavitation of the tooth surface, preventive measures usually are inadequate to prevent further progression of the lesion because it is impossible to adequately remove cariogenic biofilm from a cavitated caries lesion. Excision of the lesion (tooth preparation) and proper tooth restoration is the most effective method to control the progression of active, cavitated lesions.

Caries-Control Restorations

The term *caries control* refers to an operative procedure in which multiple teeth with acute threatening caries are treated quickly by (1) removing the infected tooth structure, (2) medicating the pulp, if necessary, and (3) restoring the defect(s) with a temporary material. With this technique, most of the infecting organisms and their protecting sites are removed, limiting further acute spread of caries throughout the mouth. The caries-control procedure must be accompanied by other preventive measures (Table 2-14). Teeth rapidly treated by caries-control procedures subsequently are treated by using routine restorative techniques, if appropriate pulpal responses are obtained. Also, the intent of caries-control procedures is immediate, corrective intervention in advanced caries lesions to prevent and assess pulpal disease and avoid possible sequelae such as toothache, root canal therapy, or more complex ultimate restorations.

OBJECTIVES AND INDICATIONS

Active, rapidly progressing caries requires urgent clinical treatment when dentin softening has progressed at least half the

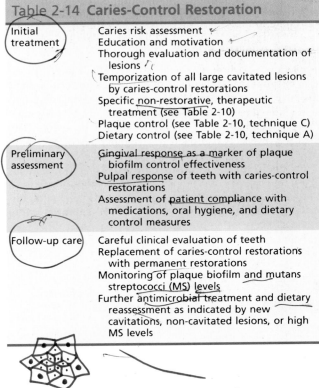

Table 2-14 Caries-Control Restoration

Initial treatment	Caries risk assessment Education and motivation Thorough evaluation and documentation of lesions Temporization of all large cavitated lesions by caries-control restorations Specific non-restorative, therapeutic treatment (see Table 2-10) Plaque control (see Table 2-10, technique C) Dietary control (see Table 2-10, technique A)
Preliminary assessment	Gingival response as a marker of plaque biofilm control effectiveness Pulpal response of teeth with caries-control restorations Assessment of patient compliance with medications, oral hygiene, and dietary control measures
Follow-up care	Careful clinical evaluation of teeth Replacement of caries-control restorations with permanent restorations Monitoring of plaque biofilm and mutans streptococci (MS) levels Further antimicrobial treatment and dietary reassessment as indicated by new cavitations, non-cavitated lesions, or high MS levels

distance from the DEJ to the pulp. Acute caries may progress rapidly without operative intervention. Conventional restorative treatment techniques may not address acute problems with sufficient rapidity to prevent pulpal infection or death of the pulp.

The treatment objective for caries control is to remove the infected tooth matter from all of the advanced caries lesions, place appropriate pulpal medication (if needed), and restore the tooth in the most expedient manner. Provisional restorative materials (intermediate restorative material, a strong glass-ionomer material such as Fuji IX, or amalgam) are usually the treatment materials of choice. Caries control is an intermediate step in restorative treatment and has several other indications. Teeth with questionable pulpal prognosis should be treated with a caries-control approach. In this way, the progression of demineralization of the dentin is stopped, and the response of the pulp can be determined before making a commitment to a permanent restoration. Another clinical situation in which caries control is a useful approach is during an operative procedure when a tooth is unexpectedly found to have extensive caries. Caries-control technique provides the busy practitioner the flexibility to respond rapidly to stop the carious process in that tooth without causing major changes in the daily schedule. The caries-control procedure allows quick removal of the caries, placement of a temporary restoration, and the rescheduling of the patient for a more time-consuming, permanent restoration. Before placement of a permanent restoration, a caries-control procedure also provides a suitable delay that gives the pulp some time to recover, allowing a better assessment of the pulpal status. A caries-control procedure is indicated when (1) the caries is extensive enough that adverse pulpal sequelae are likely to occur soon, (2) the goal of treatment is to remove the nidus of caries infection in the patient's mouth, or (3) a tooth has extensive carious involvement that cannot or should not be permanently restored because of inadequate time or questionable pulpal prognosis.

CARIES-CONTROL TECHNIQUE

The following description involves only a single tooth, for the sake of simplicity. Caries control of multiple teeth in a single sitting is a practical clinical procedure and is simply an extension of the procedure for a single tooth. Figure 2-44 is a schematic representation of the caries-control procedure, and Figure 2-45, *A*, is a preoperative radiograph of the tooth described in the following sections.

Anesthesia for the affected area is usually indicated, unless a test preparation for pulpal vitality is to be performed. Because pulpal necrosis may occur when oral fluids contaminate exposure sites during excavation of advanced caries lesions, the operating site must be isolated. The rubber dam provides an excellent means of isolation and protection of the

excavation site from contamination by oral fluids during the operative procedure and should be used routinely in most caries-control procedures.

The primary objective of the caries-control tooth procedure is to provide adequate visual and mechanical access to

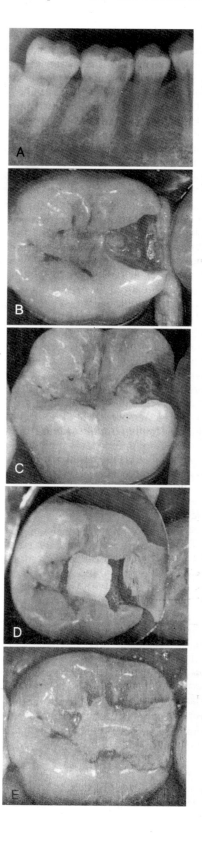

Fig. 2-44 Schematic representation of caries-control procedure. **A** and **B,** Faciolingual (*A*) and mesiodistal (*B*) cross-sections of mandibular first molar show extensive preoperative occlusal and proximal caries lesions. **C,** Tooth after excavation of extensive caries. Note remaining unsupported enamel. **D,** Temporary amalgam restoration inserted after appropriate liner or base.

Fig. 2-45 **A,** Preoperative clinical radiograph illustrating extensive caries lesion in the proximal and occlusal regions of the mandibular right first molar. Initial caries excavation of tooth. **B,** Remaining caries requires further excavation. Also, note the wedge in place, protecting rubber dam and soft tissue; it has been lightly shaved by a bur. **C,** Remaining unsupported enamel under mesiolingual cusp. **D,** Tooth ready for placement of temporary restoration. Carious involvement required further extension than that seen in *B* and *C*. Liner or base material has been applied to deepest excavated areas, and matrix, appropriately wedged, has been placed. **E,** Temporary restoration completed for caries-control procedure. Caries has been eliminated, the pulp adequately protected, and interarch and intra-arch positions of tooth maintained by caries-control procedure.

Labels in Fig. 2-44:
- Enamel
- Extensive carious lesion
- Dentin
- Pulp
- Excavated area
- Temporary restoration
- Base/liner

facilitate the removal of infected dentin. The initial opening of the tooth is made with the largest carbide bur that can be used. A high-speed handpiece with an air-water spray is the most practical instrument for this procedure (see Fig. 2-45, *B* and *C*). Retaining unsupported enamel is permissible in caries-control procedures because this tooth structure, although undermined, assists in the retention of the restorative material. Removal of unsupported enamel occurs when the final restoration is placed at a later date. Retaining sound portions of old restorative material also may enhance the temporary restoration and reduce the risk of pulpal exposure. Care must be exercised, however, when deciding not to remove all old restorative material because it may mask residual infected dentin.

When access has been gained, the identification and removal of caries depends primarily on the dentist's interpretation of tactile stimuli. Color differences cannot be used as a reliable index for complete caries removal, although caries-indicating solutions may provide color guides. In rapidly advancing lesions, softened dentin shows little or no color change, whereas more slowly advancing lesions have more discoloration. Dentin that appears leathery, peels off in small flakes, or can be judiciously penetrated by a sharp explorer should be removed.

Because fine tactile discrimination is required for complete removal of caries, the use of a high-speed handpiece at full speed is contraindicated for the removal of deep caries. Effective caries removal can be accomplished with (1) hand instrumentation using spoon excavators, (2) a slow-speed handpiece with a large round bur, or (3) a high-speed handpiece using a round bur operated just above stall-out speed (low speed). The use of spoon excavators may result in larger amounts of softened dentin being peeled off than intended and may result in inadvertent pulp exposure. Hand excavation requires great skill and sharp instruments. Rotary instruments provide good control and require less skill. The high-speed handpiece, when running just above stalling speed, provides good control. A simple technique is to run the handpiece slowly enough that the bur stalls shortly after contacting dentin. Repeated applications of the bur remove dentin in small increments and allow the operator to monitor carefully changes in hardness and color. After removal of softened dentin, it is helpful to evaluate the excavated area carefully with a sharp explorer to determine if the remaining dentin is hard and sound. Extreme care must be used with the explorer to prevent penetration into the pulp. Penetration of the explorer into the pulp may cause pulpal infection, increasing the possibility of pulpal death.

Usually, all softened, infected dentin is removed during caries-control procedures. In asymptomatic teeth that have deep lesions (in which complete excavation of softened dentin is anticipated to produce pulpal exposure), softened, affected dentin nearest the pulp may be left. The deliberate retention of softened dentin near the tooth pulp and medication of the remaining dentin is termed *indirect pulp capping* and will be discussed in the next section. The goals of the caries-control and indirect pulp capping procedures are to prevent pulp exposure and aid pulpal recovery by medication.

If the pulp is penetrated by an instrument during the operative procedure, a decision must be made whether to proceed with root canal therapy or do a direct pulp capping. Direct pulp capping is a technique for treating a pulp exposure with a material that seals over the exposure site and promotes reparative dentin formation. If the exposure site is the consequence of infected dentin extending into the pulp, termed *carious pulpal exposure*, infection of the pulp already has occurred, and removal of the tooth pulp is indicated. If, however, the pulp exposure occurs in an area of normal dentin (usually as a result of operator error or misjudgment), termed *mechanical pulpal exposure*, and bacterial contamination from salivary exposure does not occur, the potential success of the direct pulp capping procedure is enhanced. With either type of exposure, a more favorable prognosis for the pulp after direct pulp capping may be expected if any of the following findings are present:

1. The tooth has been asymptomatic (no spontaneous pain, normal response to thermal testing, and vital) before the operative procedure.
2. The exposure is small (<0.5mm in diameter).
3. The hemorrhage from the exposure site is easily controlled.
4. The exposure occurred in a clean, uncontaminated field (such as that provided by rubber dam isolation).
5. The exposure was relatively atraumatic, and little desiccation of the tooth occurred, with no evidence of aspiration of blood into dentin (dentin blushing).

A deep caries excavation close to the pulp, which may result in either an undetected pulpal exposure or a visible pulpal exposure, should be covered with a calcium hydroxide liner that can stimulate formation of dentin bridges (reparative dentin) over the exposure.[99] If used, the calcium hydroxide liner should always be covered with a glass ionomer or resin-modified glass ionomer liner before the tooth is restored. Deep excavations not encroaching on the pulp should be covered with a glass-ionomer material and then restored with either a definitive or a temporary restorative material. Alternatively, a reinforced glass ionomer material (such as Fuji IX) can be used for caries-control restorations, which eliminates the need for liners or bases in cases where no pulp exposure has occurred. The selection of a caries-control restorative material depends on the amount of missing tooth structure and the expected length of service anticipated for this temporary restoration. Amalgam, Fuji IX, and intermediate restorative material are the most frequently used materials for caries-control procedures.

If a long interval is anticipated between the caries-control procedure and the permanent restoration, amalgam ensures better maintenance of tooth position and proper contour. If significant portions of the proximal or occlusal surfaces are missing, an amalgam temporary restoration maintains the adjacent and occlusal tooth contact better than other weaker restorative materials. The extent of the access preparation and tooth structure loss indicates the need for a matrix application before placement of the restorative material (see Fig. 2-45, *D*). Matrix choice and application are described in subsequent chapters. Condensation and carving should be accomplished in the conventional manner. Precise anatomic form is unnecessary for temporary restorations. Proper proximal contacts and contours should be established, however, to maintain satisfactory dimension of the embrasures to foster interdental papilla health (see Fig. 2-45, *E*). Teeth lacking interproximal contacts may drift, making subsequent restoration more difficult. Also, a condensation technique that exerts less pressure (i.e., using a spherical amalgam) reduces the chance of pulpal perforation.

Different opinions exist concerning various aspects of the caries-control technique. Some practitioners advocate removal of all caries in all teeth initially, regardless of the size of the lesion. This approach is undoubtedly the most effective for controlling the infection from dental caries. This approach has disadvantages, however, because it necessitates the excavation of all lesions, which is very laborious. Limiting caries-control procedures to pulp-threatening advanced caries lesions is advocated in this text as a more practical procedure. Caries-control restorations can be replaced after the remaining small- to moderate-sized lesions are completely restored. The interval between the caries-control restoration and its replacement with a permanent restoration provides time to complete the following: assessment of the pulpal response to excavation and medication, treatment of the cariogenic infection with prescribed anti-caries measures, assessment of the patient's ability to perform oral hygiene procedures, assessment of the patient's compliance with dietary changes, and assessment of caries activity elsewhere in the mouth. The outcome of these factors may have an important bearing on the choice of materials and techniques for the final restoration of teeth. Regardless of the caries-control concept endorsed, advanced caries lesions should be treated without delay to minimize the potential for adverse pulpal reaction and to provide time for assessment of the pulpal response to therapy.

Some controversy exists concerning the medication material to place over deeply excavated areas. Although most practitioners recognize the potential for stimulating reparative dentin formation with the use of calcium hydroxide materials, this is not universally accepted. More importantly, no consensus exists with regard to the mechanism of action of calcium hydroxide liners. One group of practitioners supports the concept that a calcium hydroxide liner must be in direct contact with pulpal tissue to cause reparative dentin formation. These practitioners believe that the use of calcium hydroxide liners in any situation other than a direct pulpal exposure would not stimulate reparative dentin formation. Other practitioners believe, however, that the calcium hydroxide material is soluble and is transmitted by the fluid in the dentinal tubules to the pulp and, consequently, causes reparative dentin formation.

Finally, minor controversy, or at least confusion, exists about the terminology related to this procedure. Although this section has termed the procedure *caries-control restorative treatment*, other terms such as *interim restoration*, *treatment restoration*, or *temporary restoration* may be used. All of these descriptions have validity when applied to the technique of removing acute caries without delay and temporarily restoring the involved tooth or teeth.

Partial Caries Excavation and Indirect Pulp Capping

Teeth that have large caries lesions but no overt pulpal or periapical pathology should be managed conservatively. It is generally not advisable to initiate definitive root canal therapy for asymptomatic teeth with a healthy pulp and healthy periapical area. Growing clinical and scientific evidence indicates that large carious lesions with healthy pulpal and periapical tissues should be managed via *partial caries excavation* and *indirect pulp capping*. Aggressive complete caries removal that invades the pulp space and forces a decision of definitive root canal treatment or extraction in the context of caries control is to be avoided. Partial caries excavation followed by indirect pulp capping via placement of a sedative restoration has significant benefits. For the individual patient, it might allow retention of the tooth through the control phase without root canal therapy—thereby avoiding the time, expense, and necessary deferral of treatment for other teeth (including those with a better prognosis)—and it also avoids the problem of performing endodontic therapy on a tooth that might be recommended for extraction in the definitive phase of treatment. The complexity and cost of treatment increase several-fold once the pulp is exposed. For many patients, this can mean a death sentence for the tooth. From a public health perspective, teeth should not be extracted merely for financial reasons but should be maintained to provide some level of esthetics, function, and preservation of oral health, especially in patients with limited financial resources.

One of the major motivations in performing partial caries excavation and indirect pulp capping is to ensure that large caries lesions are treated as a priority, thus reducing the overall bacterial load and arresting or stopping lesion progression, which, in effect, is caries control as described in the preceding section. The philosophy behind this approach is that when the tooth is vital and no signs or symptoms of irreversible pulpitis are present, it is better to simply seal partially demineralized dentin from the oral environment and arrest the decay process than to engage in more complex and expensive procedures. When successful, the benefits in reduced cost and postoperative pain are obvious. Ample literature exists to support this approach as being more successful than the removal of all caries even if it means pulp exposure.[28-34,100-123]

It is appropriate to use partial caries excavation and indirect pulp capping in the context of caries control on any tooth with a large caries lesion (or multiple teeth with moderately large lesions) that is deemed restorable and for which the pulpal and periapical areas are deemed healthy (no irreversible pulpitis or pulpal necrosis). Teeth that are restorable only with full-coverage restoration generally are not appropriate for this approach because of the difficulty of evaluating the tooth for possible failures such as continuing caries activity under the full-coverage restoration. Another concern is the cost of rectifying failures.

The following four steps summarize the partial caries excavation clinical protocol:

1. Preliminary assessment of pulpal and periapical health and restorability of teeth being considered for partial caries excavation and indirect pulp capping should be done. *(At the subsequent restorative steps, pulpal diagnosis and restorability may be reassessed.)* Partial caries excavation and indirect pulp capping are used only for teeth determined to be vital and to have a healthy periapical area. At worst, these teeth would have symptoms consistent with reversible pulpitis. If the tooth is found to be nonvital, if symptoms are consistent with irreversible pulpitis, or if apical periodontitis of endodontic origin is present, partial caries excavation and indirect pulp capping are contraindicated.

2. The restorability of the tooth is assessed at the beginning of the restorative appointment. Restorability must be definitively confirmed after completion of all peripheral caries removal (i.e., a caries-free DEJ should be established around the entire periphery of the cavity preparation). Partial caries excavation and indirect pulp capping are used only for teeth that are restorable with a direct restoration (glass ionomer, resin-modified glass ionomer, composite, amalgam, foundation) and teeth that have a fair to good restorative prognosis. A treatment plan should be made for the extraction of teeth that are found to be nonrestorable.

3. Caries is completely excavated peripherally to a sound, caries-free DEJ. Axially and pulpally, caries will be excavated to within approximately 1 mm of the pulp. The goal is to stop removing caries when the first of either of these two situations occurs: (1) All caries has been removed; or (2) all caries has been removed from all the walls except the axial or pulpal walls, where demineralized dentin still remains and approximately 1 mm of dentin thickness remains. If all caries has been removed (option 1), a definitive direct restoration may be placed, if recommended. If all caries has not been removed (option 2), a glass ionomer (e.g., Fuji IX) sedative restoration is placed. The sedative restoration is left in place for approximately 12 weeks.

   a. Use of calcium hydroxide or other liner or base material after caries excavation and before use of the sedative restoration is not required, but it is permitted.

   b. Use of a definitive restoration when all caries has not been removed (option 2) can be considered as well. The rationale behind this approach is that subsequent appointments, which require patient compliance, would not be necessarily required, and therefore, the tooth is more properly restored should the patient not follow up with subsequent appointments. Additionally, the placement of a definitive restoration at the time of the partial caries excavation may eliminate the need for a subsequent intervention in the tooth.

4. The treated tooth is re-evaluated approximately 12 weeks after the restorative appointment. Teeth that are vital and asymptomatic at this visit are restored with a direct restoration (either amalgam or composite). *The glass ionomer caries control restoration is **not** removed to facilitate the removal of caries left at the first appointment.* Rather, it is cut back pulpally and axially to serve as a base, and a definitive direct restoration (e.g., amalgam, composite resin) is placed. Strong evidence indicates that re-entering an asymptomatic, vital tooth significantly increases the likelihood of pulp exposure without increasing favorable outcomes.[26,27,29,31,34,122] Re-evaluation of the remaining tooth structure prior to placement of a definitive direct restoration may sometimes result in a decision to place a full-coverage restoration. If that is the case, the glass ionomer may be removed, at the discretion of the operator, to facilitate the removal of any residual partially demineralized dentin and a foundation for a crown is placed. If pulp exposure occurs, the tooth should be treated endodontically. At the follow-up appointment, teeth that still have symptoms consistent with a reversible pulpitis or are found to be necrotic are recommended for endodontic therapy or extraction. The dentist does have flexibility to extend the observation period and schedule one additional re-evaluation, but this is discouraged unless it is strongly believed that the status of the pulp will change dramatically.

The pulpal diagnoses outlined as part of the partial caries excavation and indirect pulp capping protocol rely on signs and symptoms of pulp pathology determined by using the best diagnostic tools available. However, actual pulpal status is difficult to determine clinically—bacteria and toxins progressing ahead of caries can cause areas of undetectable pulp necrosis or irreversible pulpitis.[99] This protocol calls for the use of glass ionomer (e.g., Fuji IX) as the indirect pulp capping or sedative restoration material because evidence indicates that it provides a good seal, which is critical to arresting the decay. Use of a material other than glass ionomer for the sedative restoration is permitted at the discretion of the dentist.

Root Caries Management

It is clear that the "baby boom" generation of North America is aging. In the year 1900, 3% of the U.S. population was over 60 years of age, whereas in the year 2000, 13% of the population was over 60 years old.[124] In the year 2030, it is estimated that at least 20% of the population will be 60 years or older. Root caries is a pervasive problem in a high percentage of older patients.[125,126] Many of these patients have had extensive restorative dentistry done in their lifetimes. Approximately 38% of patients between the ages of 55 and 64 years have root caries, and 47% of those between 65 and 74 years have experienced root caries.[127] The incidence of root caries in old-older adults (over 75 years) is even higher.[128]

One of the primary etiologic factors for these patients is their use of prescription drugs for a wide variety of systemic medical problems. It has been estimated that 63% of the 200 most commonly prescribed medications have dry mouth as an adverse effect. It is the subsequent reduction in salivary flow rates and concomitant diminished buffering capacity resulting from use of these medications that is primarily responsible for the increase in root caries in older patients.

The critical pH of dentin (pH at which dentin begins to demineralize) is between 6.2 and 6.7, whereas that of enamel is about 5.5.[129] As a result, root dentin will demineralize in very weak acids, and root caries progresses at about twice the rate of coronal caries. Thus, it is critical that all older patients receive thorough clinical and radiographic examinations on a regular basis.

As described previously in this chapter, a caries risk assessment should be carried out for all older patients. Risk factors for root caries include the following:

1. Gingival recession
2. Poor oral hygiene
3. Cariogenic diet
4. Presence of multiple restorations or multiple missing teeth
5. Existing caries

6. Xerogenic medications
7. Compromised salivary flow rates

Once it has been determined that a patient is at high risk for root caries, an aggressive preventive protocol as described previously should be considered. This protocol is based upon four primary strategies for the prevention of root caries. The *first* strategy is to try to improve salivary flow rates and increase the buffering capacity. The *second* strategy is to try to reduce the numbers of cariogenic bacteria (*S. mutans*) in the oral cavity. The *third* strategy is to reduce the quantity and numbers of exposures of ingested refined carbohydrates, and the *fourth* is to attempt to remineralize noncavitated lesions and prevent new lesions from developing. In addition to following the aforementioned protocol, two additional considerations are important:

1. *Recommend the use of powered toothbrushes.* It is critical that patients susceptible to root caries practice meticulous oral hygiene. However, many of these patients have physical and visual deficiencies, and this makes it difficult for them to adequately cleanse the mouth. For these patients, a powered toothbrush may be advantageous. If the patient can use a water irrigation device (Waterpik, Water Pik Inc., Fort Collins, CO), daily use of the device will be beneficial. Although it will not remove plaque, studies have shown that daily use will change the composition of the plaque in a beneficial way.

2. *Restore all root caries lesions with a fluoride-releasing material.* All Fuji IX restorations should be removed, and all active caries removed. Resin-modified glass ionomer materials are preferred for definitive restorations primarily because they bond effectively to both enamel and dentin and they act as reservoirs for fluoride which can be re-released into the oral cavity.[130,131] They are effective as anti-caries materials *only* if patients reload the material a minimum of three times a day by brushing with fluoride-containing toothpaste or by using other fluoride-containing products. Educating patients of the necessity for three exposures to fluoride per day and for reloading the fluoride-releasing materials can assist in motivating them to improved levels of compliance.

In summary, many older patients are experiencing an epidemic of root caries, primarily as a result of the xerogenic effects of medications prescribed for systemic illnesses. Many root caries lesions occur in locations that make them difficult, if not impossible, to restore. The dental profession has a strong track record of prevention, and it is clear that with root caries, prevention is much better than restoration.

Summary

Much of the remainder of this textbook presents information on when and how to restore tooth defects. Many tooth defects are the result of caries activity. As stated previously, the restoration of a caries lesion does not cure the carious process. Only implementation of appropriate caries-preventive measures reduces the probability that caries lesions will recur. Tooth restorations are preventive in the sense that they remove numerous cariogenic organisms in the affected site and

eliminate a protected habitat for other cariogenic bacteria; however, they primarily repair the tooth damage caused by caries and have only a limited impact on the patient's overall caries risk.

In managing caries, the objective is to focus on the diagnosis (identifying individuals at high risk for caries via caries risk assessment protocols), preventive or therapeutic measures, and treatment modalities. Caries management efforts must be directed not at the tooth level (traditional or surgical treatment) but at the total-patient level (medical model of treatment). Restorative treatment does not cure the caries process. Instead, identifying and eliminating the causative factors for caries must be the primary focus, in addition to the restorative repair of damage caused by caries.

References

1. Keyes PH: Research in dental caries. *J Am Dent Assoc* 76(6):1357–1373, 1968.
2. Featherstone JD: The caries balance: The basis for caries management by risk assessment. *Oral Health Prev Dent* 2(Suppl 1):259–264, 2004.
3. Chaussain-Miller C, Fioretti F, Goldberg M, et al: The role of matrix metalloproteinases (MMPs) in human caries. *J Dent Res* 85(1):22–32, 2006.
4. Young DA, Kutsch VK, Whitehouse J: A clinician's guide to CAMBRA: A simple approach. *Compend Contin Educ Dent* 30(2):92–94, 96, 98, passim, 2009.
5. Marsh PD: Dental plaque as a biofilm and a microbial community— implications for health and disease. *BMC Oral Health* 6(Suppl 1):S14, 2006.
6. Hannig C, Hannig M: The oral cavity—a key system to understand substratum-dependent bioadhesion on solid surfaces in man. *Clin Oral Invest* 13(2):123–139, 2009.
7. Juhl M: Three-dimensional replicas of pit and fissure morphology in human teeth. *Scand J Dent Res* 91(2):90–95, 1983.
8. Brown LR: Effects of selected caries preventive regimes on microbial changes following radiation-induced xerostomia in cancer patients. *Microbiol Abstr Spec Suppl* 1:275, 1976.
9. Dreizen SBL: Xerostomia and dental caries. *Microbiol Abstr Spec Suppl* 1263, 1976.
10. Mandel ID: Salivary factors in caries prediction, *Sp. Suppl. Microbiology Abstracts.* In Bibby BG, Shern RJ, editors: *Proceedings "Methods of Caries Prediction",* ed 4, Arlington, Va, 1978, Information Retrieval, Inc, pp 147–162.
11. Arnold RR, Russell, JE, Devine SM, et al: Antimicrobial activity of the secretory innate defense factors lactoferrin, lactoperoxidase, and lysozyme. In Guggenheim B, editor: *Cariology today,* Basel, 1984, Karger, pp. 75–88.
12. Mandel I, Ellison SA: Naturally occurring defense mechanism in saliva. In Tanzer JM, editor: *Animal models in cariology (supplement to Microbiology Abstracts),* Washington, DC, 1981, Information Retrieval.
13. van Houte J: Microbiological predictors of caries risk. *Adv Dent Res* 7(2):87–96, 1993.
14. Hay DI: Specific functional salivary proteins. In Guggenheim B, editor: *Cariology today,* Basel, 1984, Karger.
15. Ritter AV, Shugars DA, Bader JD: Root caries risk indicators: A systematic review of risk models. *Community Dent Oral Epidemiol* 38(5):383–397, 2010.
16. Du M, Jiang H, Tai B, et al: Root caries patterns and risk factors of middle-aged and elderly people in China. *Community Dent Oral Epidemiol* 37(3):260–266, 2009.
17. Saunders RH, Jr, Meyerowitz C: Dental caries in older adults. *Dent Clin North Am* 49(2):293–308, 2005.
18. Berry TG, Summitt JB, Swift EJ, Jr: Root caries. *Oper Dent* 29(6):601–607, 2004.
19. Parfitt GJ: The speed of development of the carious cavity. *Br Dent J* 100:204–207, 1956.
20. Backer DO: Posteruptive changes in dental enamel. *J Dent Res* 45:503, 1966.
21. Silverstone LM: In vitro studies with special reference to the enamel surface and the enamel-resin interface. In Silverstone LM, Dogon IC, editors: *Proceedings of an international symposium on the acid etch tecnique,* St Paul, MN, 1975, North Central.
22. Baum LJ: Dentinal pulp conditions in relation to caries lesions. *Int Dent J* 20:309–337, 1970.

23. Brannstrom M, Lind PO: Pulpal response to early dental caries. *J Dent Res* 44(5):1045–1050, 1965.
24. Pashley DH: Clinical correlations of dentin structure and function. *J Prosthet Dent* 66(6):777–781, 1991.
25. Ogawa K, Yamashita Y, Ichijo T, et al: The ultrastructure and hardness of the transparent layer of human carious dentin. *J Dent Res* 62(1):7–10, 1983.
26. Hayashi M, Fujitani M, Yamaki C, et al: Ways of enhancing pulp preservation by stepwise excavation—a systematic review. *J Dent* 39(2):95–107, 2011.
27. Bjorndal L, Reit C, Bruun G, et al: Treatment of deep caries lesions in adults: Randomized clinical trials comparing stepwise vs. direct complete excavation, and direct pulp capping vs. partial pulpotomy. *Eur J Oral Sci* 118(3):290–297, 2010.
28. Ricketts DN, Pitts NB: Novel operative treatment options. *Monogr Oral Sci* 21:174–187, 2009.
29. Hilton TJ: Keys to clinical success with pulp capping: a review of the literature. *Oper Dent* 34(5):615–625, 2009.
30. Thompson V, Craig RG, Curro FA, et al: Treatment of deep carious lesions by complete excavation or partial removal: A critical review. *J Am Dent Assoc* 139(6):705–712, 2008.
31. Bjorndal L: Indirect pulp therapy and stepwise excavation. *J Endod* 34(7 Suppl):S29–S33, 2008.
32. Oen KT, Thompson VP, Vena D, et al: Attitudes and expectations of treating deep caries: A PEARL Network survey. *Gen Dent* 55(3):197–203, 2007.
33. Miyashita H, Worthington HV, Qualtrough A, et al: Pulp management for caries in adults: Maintaining pulp vitality. *Cochrane Database Syst Rev* (2):CD004484, 2007.
34. Maltz M, Oliveira EF, Fontanella V, et al: Deep caries lesions after incomplete dentine caries removal: 40-month follow-up study. *Caries Res* 41(6):493–496, 2007.
35. Fusayama T: Two layers of carious dentin: Diagnosis and treatment. *Oper Dent* 4(2):63–70, 1979.
36. Kuboki Y, Liu CF, Fusayama T: Mechanism of differential staining in carious dentin. *J Dent Res* 62(6):713–714, v, 1983.
37. Beck JD, Kohout F, Hunt RJ: Identification of high caries risk adults: Attitudes, social factors and diseases. *Int Dent J* 38(4):231–238, 1988.
38. Beck JD: Risk revisited. *Community Dent Oral Epidemiol* 26(4):220–225, 1998.
39. Fontana M, Zero DT: Assessing patients' caries risk. *J Am Dent Assoc* 137(9):1231–1239, 2006.
40. Steinberg S: Understanding and managing dental caries: A medical approach. *Alpha Omegan* 10(3):127–134, 2007.
41. Steinberg S: Adding caries diagnosis to caries risk assessment: The next step in caries management by risk assessment (CAMBRA). *Compend Contin Educ Dent* 30(8):522, 24–26, 28 passim, 2009.
42. Domejean-Orliaguet S, Gansky SA, Featherstone JD: Caries risk assessment in an educational environment. *J Dent Educ* 70(12):1346–1354, 2006.
43. Hausen H: Caries prediction—state of the art. *Community Dent Oral Epidemiol* 25(1):87–96, 1997.
44. Riley JL, 3rd, Gordan VV, Rindal DB, et al: General practitioners' use of caries-preventive agents in adult patients versus pediatric patients: Findings from the dental practice-based research network. *J Am Dent Assoc* 141(6):679–687, 2010.
45. Riley JL, 3rd, Gordan VV, Rindal DB, et al: Preferences for caries prevention agents in adult patients: Findings from the dental practice-based research network. *Community Dent Oral Epidemiol* 38(4):360–370, 2010.
46. Kidd EA: The use of diet analysis and advice in the management of dental caries in adult patients. *Oper Dent* 20(3):86–93, 1995.
47. Löe H: Human research model for the production and prevention of gingivitis. *J Dent Res* 50:256, 1971.
48. Krase B: *Caries risk*, Chicago, 1985, Quintessence.
49. Klock B, Krasse B: Effect of caries-preventive measures in children with high numbers of S. mutans and lactobacilli. *Scand J Dent Res* 86(4):221–230, 1978.
50. Gorur A, Lyle DM, Schaudinn C, et al: Biofilm removal with a dental water jet. *Compend Contin Educ Dent* 30(Spec No 1):1–6, 2009.
51. Brown LJ, Lazar V: The economic state of dentistry. Demand-side trends. *J Am Dent Assoc* 129(12):1685–1691, 1998.
52. HHS US Department of Health & Human Services: New Assessments & Actions on Fluoride: Accessed 06/07/2011: http://www.hhs.gov/news/press/2011pres/01/20110107a.html.
53. American Dental Association Sc: *Key dental facts*, Chicago, 2004, American Dental Association.
54. Populations receiving optimally fluoridated public drinking water—United States, 1992-2006. *MMWR Morb Mortal Wkly Rep* 57(27):737–741, 2008.
55. Svanberg M, Westergren G: Effect of SnF2, administered as mouthrinses or topically applied, on *Streptococcus mutans*, *Streptococcus sanguis* and lactobacilli in dental plaque and saliva. *Scand J Dent Res* 91(2):123–129, 1983.
56. Beltran-Aguilar ED, Goldstein JW, Lockwood SA: Fluoride varnishes. A review of their clinical use, cariostatic mechanism, efficacy and safety. *J Am Dent Assoc* 131(5):589–596, 2000.
57. Centers for Disease Control and Prevention: Recommendations for using fluoride to prevent and control dental caries in the United States. *MMWR Morb Mortal Wkly Rep* 50(RR-14) 1:30, 2001.
58. Newbrun E: Topical fluorides in caries prevention and management: A North American perspective. *J Dent Educ* 65(10):1078–1083, 2001.
59. Weintraub JA: Fluoride varnish for caries prevention: Comparisons with other preventive agents and recommendations for a community-based protocol. *Spec Care Dentist* 23(5):180–186, 2003.
60. Borutta A, Kunzel W, Rubsam F: The caries-protective efficacy of 2 fluoride varnishes in a 2-year controlled clinical trial [translation]. *Dtsch Zahn Mund Kieferheilkd Zentralbl* 79(7):543–549, 1991.
61. Borutta A, Reuscher G, Hufnagl S, et al: Caries prevention with fluoride varnishes among preschool children [translation]. *Gesundheitswesen* 68(11):731–734, 2006.
62. Castellano JB, Donly KJ: Potential remineralization of demineralized enamel after application of fluoride varnish. *Am J Dent* 17(6):462–464, 2004.
63. Haugejorden O, Nord A: Caries incidence after topical application of varnishes containing different concentrations of sodium fluoride: 3-year results. *Scand J Dent Res* 99(4):295–300, 1991.
64. Seppa L: Effects of a sodium fluoride solution and a varnish with different fluoride concentrations on enamel remineralization in vitro. *Scand J Dent Res* 96(4):304–309, 1988.
65. Hutter JW, Chan JT, Featherstone JD, et al: Professionally applied topical fluoride. Executive summary of evidence-based clinical recommendations. *J Am Dent Assoc* 137(8):1151–1159, 2006.
66. Alaluusua S, Kleemola-Kujala E, Gronroos L, et al: Salivary caries-related tests as predictors of future caries increment in teenagers. A three-year longitudinal study. *Oral Microbiol Immunol* 5(2):77–81, 1990.
67. Professionally applied topical fluoride: Evidence-based clinical recommendations. *J Am Dent Assoc* 137(8):1151–1159, 2006.
68. Lehner T, Challacombe SJ, Caldwell J: An immunological investigation into the prevention of caries in deciduous teeth of rhesus monkeys. *Arch Oral Biol* 20(5-6):305–310, 1975.
69. Taubman MA, Smith DJ: Effects of local immunization with glucosyltransferase fractions from *Streptococcus mutans* on dental caries in rats and hamsters. *J Immunol* 118(2):710–720, 1977.
70. Sreebny LM, Schwartz SS: A reference guide to drugs and dry mouth—2nd edition.. *Gerodontology* 14(1):33–47, 1997.
71. Swarn K, Ritter AV, Donovan T, et al: Caries risk evaluation: Correlation between chair-side, laboratory and clinical tests. *J Dent Res*, 89(Special Issue B, USB of abstracts #4272), 2010.
72. Barkvoll P, Rolla G, Svendsen K: Interaction between chlorhexidine digluconate and sodium lauryl sulfate in vivo. *J Clin Periodontol* 16(9):593–595, 1989.
73. Emilson CG: Potential efficacy of chlorhexidine against mutans streptococci and human dental caries. *J Dent Res* 73(3):682–691, 1994.
74. Slot DE, Vaandrager NC, Van Loveren C, et al: The effect of chlorhexidine varnish on root caries: A systematic review. *Caries Res* 45(2):162–173, 2011.
75. Ashley P: Effectiveness of chlorhexidine varnish for preventing caries uncertain. *Evid Based Dent* 11(4):108, 2010.
76. Santos A: Evidence-based control of plaque and gingivitis. *J Clin Periodontol* 30(Suppl 5):13–16, 2003.
77. Sharma NC, Charles CH, Qaqish JG, et al: Comparative effectiveness of an essential oil mouthrinse and dental floss in controlling interproximal gingivitis and plaque. *Am J Dent* 15(6):351–355, 2002.
78. Tanzer JM: Xylitol chewing gum and dental caries. *Int Dent J* 45(1 Suppl 1):65–76, 1995.
79. Trahan L: Xylitol: A review of its action on mutans streptococci and dental plaque–its clinical significance. *Int Dent J* 45(1 Suppl 1):77–92, 1995.
80. Edgar WM: Saliva and dental health. Clinical implications of saliva: Report of a consensus meeting. *Br Dent J* 169(3–4):96–98, 1990.
81. Hayes C: The effect of non-cariogenic sweeteners on the prevention of dental caries: A review of the evidence. *J Dent Educ* 65(10):1106–1109, 2001.
82. Deshpande A, Jadad AR: The impact of polyol-containing chewing gums on dental caries: A systematic review of original randomized controlled trials and observational studies. *J Am Dent Assoc* 139(12):1602–1614, 2008.

83. Tung MS, Eichmiller FC: Amorphous calcium phosphates for tooth mineralization. *Compend Contin Educ Dent* 25(9 Suppl 1):9–13, 2004.

84. Chow LC, Takagi S, Vogel GL: Amorphous calcium phosphate: The contention of bone. *J Dent Res* 77(1):6; author reply 7, 1998.

85. Cai F, Shen P, Morgan MV, et al: Remineralization of enamel subsurface lesions in situ by sugar-free lozenges containing casein phosphopeptide-amorphous calcium phosphate. *Aust Dent J* 48(4):240–243, 2003.

86. Morgan MV, Adams GG, Bailey DL, et al: The anticariogenic effect of sugar-free gum containing CPP-ACP nanocomplexes on approximal caries determined using digital bitewing radiography. *Caries Res* 42(3):171–184, 2008.

87. Reynolds EC: Remineralization of enamel subsurface lesions by casein phosphopeptide-stabilized calcium phosphate solutions. *J Dent Res* 76(9):1587–1595, 1997.

88. Reynolds EC, Cai F, Shen P, et al: Retention in plaque and remineralization of enamel lesions by various forms of calcium in a mouthrinse or sugar-free chewing gum. *J Dent Res* 82(3):206–211, 2003.

89. Yengopal V, Mickenautsch S: Caries preventive effect of casein phosphopeptide-amorphous calcium phosphate (CPP-ACP): A meta-analysis. *Acta Odontol Scand* 67(6):1–12, 2009.

90. Llena C, Forner L, Baca P: Anticariogenicity of casein phosphopeptide-amorphous calcium phosphate: A review of the literature. *J Contemp Dent Pract* 10(3):1–9, 2009.

91. Simonsen RJ: Cost effectiveness of pit and fissure sealant at 10 years. *Quintessence Int* 20(2):75–82, 1989.

92. Tinanoff N, Douglass JM: Clinical decision making for caries management in children. *Pediatr Dent* 24(5):386–392, 2002.

93. Ahovuo-Saloranta A, Hiiri A, Nordblad A, et al: Pit and fissure sealants for preventing dental decay in the permanent teeth of children and adolescents. *Cochrane Database Syst Rev* (3):CD001830, 2004.

94. Beauchamp J, Caufield PW, Crall JJ, et al: Evidence-based clinical recommendations for the use of pit-and-fissure sealants: A report of the American Dental Association Council on Scientific Affairs. *J Am Dent Assoc* 139(3):257–268, 2008.

95. Bader JD, Shugars DA, Bonito AJ: Systematic reviews of selected dental caries diagnostic and management methods. *J Dent Educ* 65(10):960–968, 2001.

96. Simonsen RJ: Pit and fissure sealant: Review of the literature. *Pediatr Dent* 24(5):393–414, 2002.

97. Paris S, Meyer-Lueckel H: Masking of labial enamel white spot lesions by resin infiltration—a clinical report. *Quintessence Int* 40(9):713–718, 2009.

98. Paris S, Meyer-Lueckel H: Inhibition of caries progression by resin infiltration in situ. *Caries Res* 44(1):47–54, 2010.

99. Swift EJ: Treatment options for the exposed vital pulp. *Pract Periodontics Aesthet Dent* 11:735–739, 1999.

100. Banerjee A, Watson TF, Kidd EA: Dentine caries: Take it or leave it? *Dent Update* 27(6):272–276, 2000.

101. Bjorndal L: Buonocore Memorial Lecture. Dentin caries: Progression and clinical management. *Oper Dent* 27(3):211–217, 2002.

102. Bjorndal L: Indirect pulp therapy and stepwise excavation. *Pediatr Dent* 30(3):225–229, 2008.

103. Bjorndal L, Kidd EA: The treatment of deep dentine caries lesions. *Dent Update* 32(7):402–404, 407–410, 413, 2005

104. Bjorndal L, Larsen T: Changes in the cultivable flora in deep carious lesions following a stepwise excavation procedure. *Caries Res* 34(6):502–508, 2000.

105. Bjorndal L, Larsen T, Thylstrup A: A clinical and microbiological study of deep carious lesions during stepwise excavation using long treatment intervals. *Caries Res* 31(6):411–417, 1997.

106. Bjorndal L, Thylstrup A: A practice-based study on stepwise excavation of deep carious lesions in permanent teeth: A 1-year follow-up study. *Community Dent Oral Epidemiol* 26(2):122–128, 1998.

107. Foley J, Evans D, Blackwell A: Partial caries removal and cariostatic materials in carious primary molar teeth: A randomised controlled clinical trial. *Br Dent J* 197(11):697–701; discussion 689, 2004.

108. Innes NP, Evans DJ, Stirrups DR: The Hall Technique; a randomized controlled clinical trial of a novel method of managing carious primary molars in general dental practice: Acceptability of the technique and outcomes at 23 months. *BMC Oral Health* 7:18, 2007.

109 Kidd EA: How "clean" must a cavity be before restoration? *Caries Res* 38(3):305–313, 2004.

110. Kidd EA, Fejerskov O: What constitutes dental caries? Histopathology of carious enamel and dentin related to the action of cariogenic biofilms. *J Dent Res* 83(Spec No C):C35–C38, 2004.

111. Leksell E, Ridell K, Cvek M, Mejare I: Pulp exposure after stepwise versus direct complete excavation of deep carious lesions in young posterior permanent teeth. *Endod Dent Traumatol* 12(4):192–196, 1996.

112. Maltz M, de Oliveira EF, Fontanella V, et al: A clinical, microbiologic, and radiographic study of deep caries lesions after incomplete caries removal. *Quintessence Int* 33(2):151–159, 2002.

113. Mertz-Fairhurst EJ, Adair SM, Sams DR, et al: Cariostatic and ultraconservative sealed restorations: Nine-year results among children and adults. *ASDC J Dent Child* 62(2):97–107, 1995.

114. Mertz-Fairhurst EJ, Curtis JW, Jr, Ergle JW, et al: Ultraconservative and cariostatic sealed restorations: Results at year 10. *J Am Dent Assoc* 129(1):55–66, 1998.

115. Mertz-Fairhurst EJ, Schuster GS, Fairhurst CW: Arresting caries by sealants: Results of a clinical study. *J Am Dent Assoc* 112(2):194–197, 1986.

116. Mertz-Fairhurst EJ, Schuster GS, Williams JE, et al: Clinical progress of sealed and unsealed caries. Part II: Standardized radiographs and clinical observations. *J Prosthet Dent* 42(6):633–637, 1979.

117. Mertz-Fairhurst EJ, Schuster GS, Williams JE, et al: Clinical progress of sealed and unsealed caries. Part I: Depth changes and bacterial counts. *J Prosthet Dent* 42(5):521–526, 1979.

118. Mjor IA: Pulp-dentin biology in restorative dentistry. Part 7: The exposed pulp. *Quintessence Int* 33(2):113–135, 2002.

119. Pinheiro SL, Simionato MR, Imparato JC, et al: Antibacterial activity of glass-ionomer cement containing antibiotics on caries lesion microorganisms. *Am J Dent* 18(4):261–266, 2005.

120. Ricketts D: Management of the deep carious lesion and the vital pulp dentine complex. *Br Dent J* 191(11):606–610, 2001.

121. Ricketts DN, Kidd EA, Innes N, et al: Complete or ultraconservative removal of decayed tissue in unfilled teeth. *Cochrane Database Syst Rev* 3:CD003808, 2006.

122. Uribe S: Partial caries removal in symptomless teeth reduces the risk of pulp exposure. *Evid Based Dent* 7(4):94, 2006.

123. van Amerongen WE: Dental caries under glass ionomer restorations. *J Public Health Dent* 56(3 Spec No):150–154; discussion 161–163, 1996.

124. Shay K: The evolving impact of aging America on dental practice. *J Contemp Dent Pract* 5(4):101–110, 2004.

125. Leake JL: Clinical decision-making for caries management in root surfaces. *J Dent Educ* 65(10):1147–1153, 2001.

126. Thomson WM: Dental caries experience in older people over time: What can the large cohort studies tell us? *Br Dent J* 196(2):89–92; discussion 87, 2004.

127. Winston AE, Bhaskar SN: Caries prevention in the 21st century. *J Am Dent Assoc* 129(11):1579–1587, 1998.

128. Berkey DB, Berg RG, Ettinger RL, et al: The old-old dental patient: The challenge of clinical decision-making. *J Am Dent Assoc* 127(3):321–332, 1996.

129. Surmont PA, Martens LC: Root surface caries: An update. *Clin Prev Dent* 11(3):14–20, 1989.

130. Burgess JO, Gallo JR: Treating root-surface caries. *Dent Clin North Am* 46(2):385–404, vii–viii, 2002.

131. Haveman CW, Redding SW: Dental management and treatment of xerostomic patients. *Tex Dent J* 115(6):43–56, 1998.

Chapter 3

Patient Assessment, Examination and Diagnosis, and Treatment Planning

R. Scott Eidson, Daniel A. Shugars

Primum non nocere

This chapter provides an overview of the process through which a clinician completes patient assessment, clinical examination, diagnosis, and treatment plan for operative dentistry procedures. The chapter assumes that the reader has a background in oral medicine and an understanding of how to perform complete extraoral hard and soft tissue examinations along with intraoral cancer screening, as well as an understanding of the etiology, characteristics, risk assessment, and nonoperative management of dental caries as presented in Chapter 2. It is not in the scope of this chapter to incorporate the details of other aspects of a complete dental examination, including periodontal examination, occlusal examination, and esthetic evaluation.

Any discussion of diagnosis and treatment must begin with an appreciation of the role of the dentist in helping patients maintain their oral health. This role is summarized by the Latin phrase "primum non nocere," which means "do no harm." This phrase represents a fundamental principle of the healing arts over many centuries.

The implication of this concept for operative dentistry is that before we recommend treatment, we must be reasonably confident that the patient will be better off as a result of our intervention. However, how can we be reasonably confident when we realize that few, if any, of the tests we perform or the assessments of risk that we make are completely accurate? To make matters even more challenging, none of the treatments we provide is without adverse outcomes and none will likely last for the life of the patient. The answer is that we must acknowledge that the information or evidence we have is not perfect and that we must be clear about the possible consequences of our decisions. If we are as informed and clear about the options and their consequences, then we reduce the chances of doing any harm.

The success of operative treatment depends heavily on an appropriate plan of care, which, in turn, is based on a comprehensive analysis of the patient's reasons for seeking care and on a systematic assesssment of the patient's current conditions and risk for future problems. This information is then combined with the best available evidence on the approaches to managing the patient's needs so that an appropriate plan of care can be offered to the patient.

The collection of this information and the determinations based on these findings should be comprehensive and occur in a stepwise manner. Simply put, skipping steps can lead to overlooking potentially important parts of the patient's individual needs. These steps include reasons for seeking care, medical and dental histories, clinical examination for the detection of abnormalities, establishing diagnoses, assessing risk, and determining prognosis. All of these steps must occur before a sound and appropriate plan of care can be recommended.

Growing attention to using only the most effective and appropriate treatment has spawned interest in numerous activities. Research that provides information on treatments that work best in certain situations is expanding the knowledge base of dentistry and has led to an interest in translating the results of that research into practice activities and enhanced care for patients. This movement has been termed *evidence-based dentistry* and is defined as the "conscientious, explicit, and judicious use of current best evidence in making decisions about the care of individual patients."[1] Systematic reviews emerging from the focus on evidence-based dentistry will provide practitioners with a distillation of the available knowledge about various conditions and treatments. Currently, the American Dental Association (ADA) has developed a Web site (http://ebd.ada.org/) that can be used by dental professionals for evidence-based dentistry decision making. This Web site helps clinicians identify systematic reviews, describes the preferred method for assembling the best available scientific evidence, and provides an appraisal of the evidence through critical summaries. As evidence-based dentistry continues to expand, professional associations will become more active in the development of guidelines to assist dentists and their patients in making informed and appropriate decisions.

Patient Assessment

General Considerations

Clinical examination is the "hands-on" process of observing the patient's oral structures and detecting signs and symptoms of abnormal conditions or disease. This information is used to formulate diagnoses, which are a determination or judgment of health versus disease and variations from normal. During the clinical examination, the dentist must be keenly sensitive to subtle signs, symptoms, and variations from normal to detect pathologic conditions and etiologic factors. Meticulous attention to detail generates a base of information for assessing the patient's general physical health and diagnosing specific dental problems.

Chief Concern

Before initiating any treatment, the patient's chief concerns, or the problems that initiated the patient's visit, should be obtained. Concerns are recorded essentially verbatim in the dental record. The patient should be encouraged to discuss all aspects of the current problems, including onset, duration, symptoms, and related factors. This information is vital to establishing the need for specific diagnostic tests, determining the cause, selecting appropriate treatment options for the concerns, and building a sound relationship with the patient.

Medical History

The patient or legal guardian completes a standard, comprehensive medical history form. This form is an integral part of the pre-examination patient interview, which helps identify conditions that could alter, complicate, or contraindicate proposed dental procedures. The practitioner should identify (1) communicable diseases that require special precautions, procedures, or referral; (2) allergies or medications, which can contraindicate the use of certain drugs; (3) systemic diseases, cardiac abnormalities, or joint replacements, which require prophylactic antibiotic coverage or other treatment modifications; and (4) physiologic changes associated with aging, which may alter clinical presentation and influence treatment. The practitioner also might identify a need for medical consultation or referral before initiating dental care. All of this information is carefully detailed in the patient's permanent record and is used, as needed, to shape subsequent treatment.

Dental History

The dental history is a review of previous dental experiences and current dental problems. Review of the dental history often reveals information about past dental problems, previous dental treatment, and the patient's responses to treatments. Frequency of dental care and perceptions of previous care may be indications of the patient's future behavior. If a patient has difficulty tolerating certain types of procedures or has encountered problems with previous dental care, an alteration of the treatment or environment might help avoid future complications. Also, this discussion might lead to identification of other problems such as areas of food impaction, inability to floss, areas of pain, and broken restorations or tooth structure. It is crucial to understand past experiences to

provide optimal care in the future. Finally, the date and type of available radiographs should be recorded to ascertain the need for additional radiographs and to minimize the patient's exposure to unnecessary ionizing radiation.

Magnifaction in Operative Dentistry

Clinical dentistry often requires the viewing and evaluation of small details in teeth, intraoral and perioral tissues, restorations, and study casts. Unaided vision is often inadequate to view details needed to make treatment decisions. Magnification aids such as loupes provide a larger image size for improved visual acuity, while allowing proper upright posture to be maintained with less eye fatigue.

When choosing loupes, several parameters should be considered.[2,3,4] Magnification (power) describes the increase in image size. Most dentists use magnifications of 2× to 4×. The lower power systems of 2× to 2.5× allow multiple quadrants to be viewed, whereas the higher power systems of 3× to 4× enable viewing of several teeth or a single tooth. In general, higher magnification systems are heavier, have a narrower field of view, are more expensive, and require more light than lower power systems. The use of small, lightweight LED (light-emitting diode) headlamps attached to the eyeglass frame or attached to a headband offer the considerable visual advantage of added illumination when used with loupes.

Working distance (focal length) is the distance from the eye to the object when the object is in focus. This parameter should be considered carefully before selecting loupes because the desired working distance depends on the dentist's height, arm length, and seating preferences. Dentists of average height typically choose a working distance of 13 to 14 inches (33–35 cm), whereas tall dentists and those who prefer to work farther away from the patient use working distances of 14 to 16 inches (35–40 cm).

Depth of focus, or the difference between the far and near focus limits of the working distance, depends on the magnification. Typically, the lower the magnification, the greater is the depth of focus.

Many choices of magnification loupes are currently available for dentistry. The simplest magnifiers are the diopter single-lens loupes, which are single-piece plastic pairs of lenses that clip onto eyeglass frames. These loupes are inexpensive and lightweight and can provide magnification of up to 2.5×. However, images can be distorted, and working lengths can be less than ideal. The more commonly used dental loupe is the binocular loupe with lenses mounted on an eyeglass frame. Binocular loupes typically have Galilean and prismatic optics that provide 2× to 3.5× magnification or even 4× and greater magnification. Prescription lenses can be fitted in the eyeglass frames for all loupe types. Most models also have side shields or a wraparound design for universal precautions and ease of infection control. Two mounting systems are currently available for binocular loupes: (1) flip-up and (2) fixed or through-the-lens.

Previously limited primarily to endodontic practices, dental microscopes now are being used in some restorative dentistry practices. Compared with high-powered loupes, dental microscopes allow the clinician to view intraoral structures at a higher level of magnification while maintaining a broader field of view. Because very small areas can be seen, microscopes are used in detail-oriented procedures such as the

probabilities that a given condition is sound or at risk for further breakdown. At least 11 distinct conditions might be encountered when amalgam restorations are evaluated: (1) amalgam "blues," (2) proximal overhangs, (3) marginal ditching, (4) voids, (5) fracture lines, (6) lines indicating the interface between abutted restorations, (7) improper anatomic contours, (8) marginal ridge incompatibility, (9) improper proximal contacts, (10) improper occlusal contacts, and (11) recurrent caries lesions.

Discolored areas or "amalgam blues" are often seen through the enamel in teeth that have amalgam restorations. This bluish hue results either from the leaching of amalgam corrosion products into the dentinal tubules or from the color of underlying amalgam seen through translucent enamel. The latter occurs when the enamel has little or no dentin support, such as in undermined cusps, marginal ridges, and regions adjacent to proximal margins. When other aspects of the restoration are sound, amalgam blues do not indicate caries, do not warrant classifying the restoration as defective, and require no further treatment. Replacement of the restoration may be considered, however, for elective improvement of esthetics or for areas under heavy functional stress that may require a cusp capping restoration to prevent possible tooth fracture.

Proximal overhangs are diagnosed visually, tactilely, and radiographically (Fig. 3-6). The amalgam–tooth junction is evaluated by moving the explorer back and forth across it. If the explorer stops at the junction and then moves outwardly onto the amalgam, an overhang is present. Overhangs also can be confirmed by the catching or tearing of dental floss. Such an overhang can provide an obstacle to good oral hygiene and result in inflammation of adjacent soft tissue. If it causes problems, an overhang should be corrected, and this often indicates the need for restoration replacement.

Marginal gap or ditching is the deterioration of the amalgam–tooth interface as a result of wear, fracture, or improper tooth preparation (Fig. 3-7, A). It can be diagnosed visually or by the explorer dropping into an opening as it crosses the margin. Shallow ditching less than 0.5 mm deep usually is not a reason for restoration replacement because such a restoration usually looks worse than it really is.[21] The eventual self-sealing property of amalgam allows the restoration to continue serving adequately if it can be satisfactorily cleaned and maintained. If the ditch is too deep to be cleaned or jeopardizes the integrity of the remaining restoration or tooth structure, the restoration should be replaced.[12] In addition, secondary caries is frequently found around marginal gaps near the gingival wall and warrants replacement.[22]

Voids that are usually localized and are caused by poor condensation of the amalgam can also occur at the margins of amalgam restorations. If the void is at least 0.3 mm deep and is located in the gingival third of the tooth crown, the restoration is judged as defective and should be repaired or replaced. Accessible small voids in other marginal areas where the enamel is thicker may be corrected by recontouring or repairing with a small restoration.

A careful clinical examination detects any fracture line across the occlusal portion of an amalgam restoration. A line that occurs in the isthmus region generally indicates fractured amalgam, and the defective restoration that must be replaced (Fig. 3-8, A). Care must be taken to correctly evaluate any such line, however, especially if it is in the mid-occlusal area because this may be an interface line, a manifestation of two abutted restorations accomplished at separate appointments (see Fig. 3-8, B). If other aspects of the abutted restorations are satisfactory, replacement is unnecessary.

Amalgam restorations should duplicate the normal anatomic contours of teeth. Restorations that impinge on soft tissue, have inadequate embrasure form or proximal contact, or prevent the use of dental floss should be classified as defective, indicating recontouring or replacement (see Fig. 3-7, B).

The marginal ridge portion of the amalgam restoration should be compatible with the adjacent marginal ridge. Both ridges should be at approximately the same level and display correct occlusal embrasure form for passage of food to the facial and lingual surfaces and for proper proximal contact area. If the marginal ridges are incompatible and are associated with poor tissue health, food impaction, or the inability of the patient to floss, the restoration is defective and should be recontoured or replaced.

The proximal contact area of an amalgam restoration should touch the adjacent tooth (a "closed" contact) at the proper contact level and with correct embrasure form and possess the proper size. If the proximal contact of any restoration is suspected to be inadequate, it should be evaluated with dental floss or visually by trial angulations of a mouth mirror (held lingually when viewing from the facial aspect) to reflect light and see if a space at the contact ("open" contact) is present. For this viewing, the contact must be free of saliva. If the contact is open and is associated with poor interproximal tissue health, food impaction, or both, the restoration should be classified as defective and should be replaced or repaired. An open contact typically is annoying to the patients, so correcting the problem usually is an appreciated service.

Recurrent caries at the marginal area of the restoration is detected visually, tactilely, or radiographically and is an indication for repair or replacement (see Figs. 3-5, D, and 3-7, C). The same criteria for initial proximal and occlusal caries lesions apply for the diagnosis of and intervention for recurrent caries lesions around restorations.

Improper occlusal contacts on an amalgam restoration may cause deleterious occlusal loading, undesirable tooth movement, or both. Premature occlusal contacts can be seen as a "shiny" spot on the surface of the restoration or detected by occlusal marking paper. Such a condition warrants correction or replacement.

Clinical Examination of Indirect Restorations

Indirect restorations should be evaluated clinically in the same manner as amalgam restorations. If any aspect of the restoration is not satisfactory or is causing harm to tissue, it should

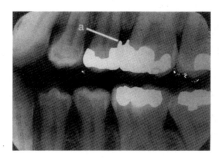

Fig. 3-6 Proximal overhang (a) can be diagnosed radiographically.

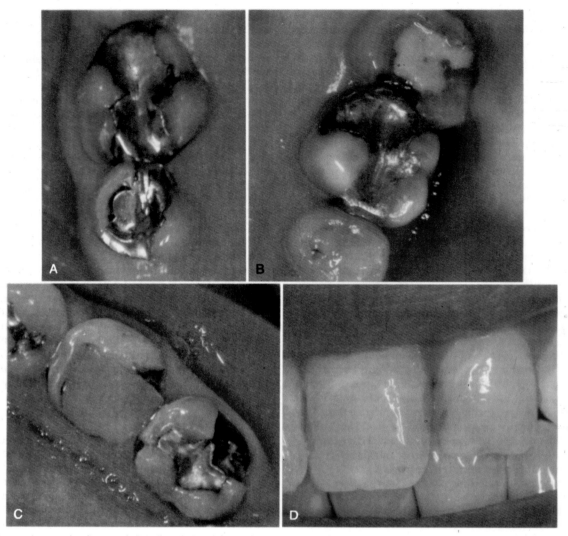

Fig. 3-7 Restorations can be diagnosed clinically as being defective by observing the following. **A,** Significant marginal ditching. **B,** Improper contour. **C,** Recurrent caries. **D,** Esthetically unappealing dark staining (*d*).

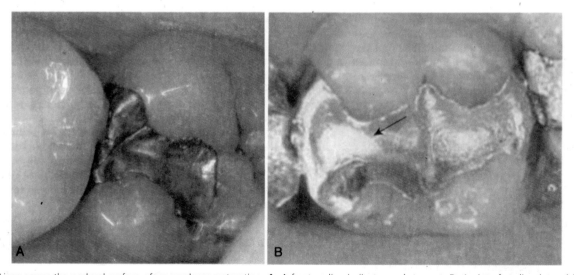

Fig. 3-8 Lines across the occlusal surface of an amalgam restoration. **A,** A fracture line indicates replacement. **B,** An interface line (arrow) indicates two restorations placed at separate appointments, which, by itself, is insufficient indication for replacement.

be classified as defective and considered for recontouring, repair, or replacement.

Clinical Examination of Composite and Other Tooth-Colored Restorations

Tooth-colored restorations should be evaluated clinically in the same manner as amalgam and cast-metal restorations. In the presence of an improper contour or proximal contact, an overhanging margin, recurrent caries, or other condition that impairs cleaning or harms the soft tissue, the restoration is considered defective. Corrective procedures include recontouring, polishing, repairing, or replacing.

One of the main concerns with anterior teeth is esthetics. If a tooth-colored restoration has dark marginal staining or is discolored to the extent that it is esthetically unappealing and the patient is unhappy with the appearance, the restoration should be judged defective (see Fig. 3-7, *D*). Marginal staining that is judged noncarious may be corrected by a small repair restoration along the margin. Occasionally, the staining is superficial and can be removed by resurfacing.

Clinical Examination of Dental Implants and Implant-Supported Restorations

Existing dental implants and implant restorations should be examined and evaluated on the basis of the same parameters for fit and seal as in the case of natural teeth. However, evaluation differences exist between implant restorations and restored natural teeth. Implant restorations in the molar area are generally one implant to replace a tooth with two or three large natural roots. This results in a large crown on a small root and may create issues for the restoration to re-establish a form with acceptable proximal contours. Often, pre-treatment vertical loss of bone support prior to implant placement makes it difficult to establish proper contours and vertical space and can create difficulties in managing the ratios for the vertical height of the crown to the length of the implant. When this happens, it can result in the same problems of long-term stability that poor crown–root ratios in natural teeth present. Therefore, it is important to evaluate implant restortions not only for fit and seal but also for contours that allow food to pack or plaque to easily build up in inaccessible areas. All of this increases risk for problems with the implant, the implant restoration, and with adjacent teeth.

Peri-implantitis is a concern that can affect implant survival along with survival of the implant restoration. Peri-implantitis is a multifactorial problem, and when this occurs, successful treatment can result in a guarded prognosis for the survival of the dental implant. Occlusion for implant restorations must be managed very carefully because dental implants lack the cushioning effect of natural teeth with periodontal ligaments. Restorations must be examined for careful placement of contacts in a single central area and to limit any deflective loading contacts or occlusal interferences.

Clinical Examination for Additional Defects

A thorough clinical examination occasionally discloses localized intact, hard white areas on the facial (Fig. 3-9) or lingual surfaces or on the cusp tips of teeth. Generally, these are hypocalcified areas of enamel resulting from childhood fever,

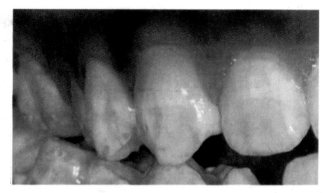

Fig. 3-9 Non-hereditary hypocalcified areas on facial surfaces. These areas may result from numerous factors but do not warrant restorative intervention unless they are esthetically offensive or cavitation is present.

trauma, or fluorosis that occurred during the developmental stages of tooth formation. Another cause of hypocalcification is arrested and remineralized incipient caries, which leaves an opaque, discolored, and hard surface. When smooth and cleanable, such areas do not warrant restorative intervention unless they are esthetically offensive to the patient. These areas remain visible whether the tooth is wet or dry. The smooth-surface incipient caries lesion also is opaque white when dried. Care must be exercised in distinguishing early enamel lesion from non-hereditary developmental enamel hypocalcification.

Chemical erosion is the loss of surface tooth structure by chemical action in the continued presence of demineralizing agents with low pH (Fig. 3-10). The resulting defective surface is usually smooth. Although these agents are predominant causative factors, it is thought that toothbrushing may be a contributing factor. It is necessary to document the severity of the erosion and the areas of teeth that are affected by the erosion. The areas of teeth affected can be important in helping the clinician determine the possible source of the chemical actions contributing to the erosive process. If the defect is only on the lingual of upper teeth, the diagnosis would be different from finding erosion on the occlusal surfaces of lower molars. Exogenous acidic agents such as lemon juice (through sucking on lemons) may cause crescent-shaped or dished defects (rounded as opposed to angular) on the surfaces of exposed teeth (see Fig. 3-10, *A*), whereas endogenous acidic agents such as gastric fluids cause generalized erosion on the lingual, incisal, and occlusal surfaces (see Fig. 3-10, *B*). The latter defective surfaces are associated with the binge–purge syndrome in bulimia, or with gastroesophageal reflux disease (GERD). Many patients with GERD are often not aware of their gastric symptoms or do not associate them with the problems with their teeth. Consultation with a physician to obtain a proper diagnosis of GERD can assist in the diagnosis and management of erosion. The flow and buffering capacity of saliva are factors in chemical erosion when other factors are present. Other sources of erosion can be use of sports drinks, herbal teas, and vomiting associated with chemotherapy, and, in the case of alcoholism, the presence of stomach contents in the mouth during periods of excessive alcohol consumption. It is necessary to document the erosion process as it occurs over a progressive period. It is possible to use accurate study models and photography to document

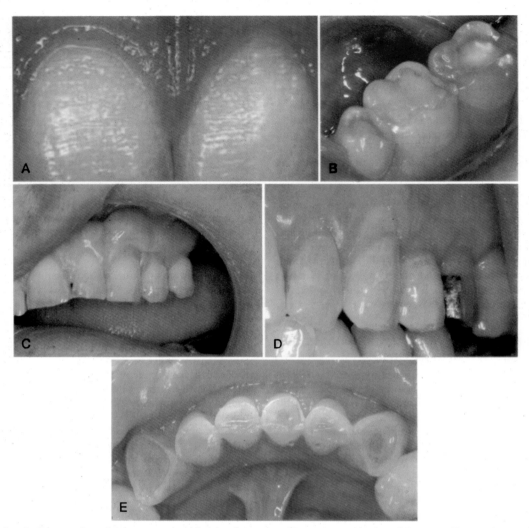

Fig. 3-10 Erosion. **A,** Crescent-shaped defects on enamel facial surfaces caused by exogenous demineralizing agent (from sucking on lemons several years previous to the time of the photograph). **B,** Generalized erosion caused by endogenous fluids. **C,** Idiopathic erosion lesion at the dentinoenamel junction is hypothesized to be associated with abnormal occlusal force. **D,** Wedge-shaped lesions caused by abrasion from toothbrush. **E,** Generalized attrition caused by excessive functional or parafunctional mandibular movements.

increasing erosion. Risk assessments for erosion would be included in the assessment of the patient, as indicated.

In contrast to chemical erosion, abfraction lesions are cervical, wedge-shaped defects (angular as opposed to rounded) similar to the defects customarily associated with toothbrush abrasion (discussed next) but in which one of the possible causative factors is heavy force in eccentric occlusion, resulting in flexure of the tooth and frequently associated with a wear facet (see Fig. 3-10, *C*). It is hypothesized further that the flexural force produces tension stress in the affected wedge-shaped region on the tooth side away from the tooth-bending direction, resulting in loss of the surface tooth structure by microfractures, which is termed *abfracture*.[23] Proponents of this hypothesis add that the microfractures can foster loss of tooth structure from toothbrush abrasion and from acids in the diet, plaque, or both. The resulting defect has smooth surfaces.

Abrasion is abnormal tooth surface loss resulting from direct frictional forces between teeth and external objects or from frictional forces between contacting teeth in the presence of an abrasive medium. Such wear is caused by improper brushing techniques or habits such as holding a pipe stem between teeth, tobacco chewing, and chewing on hard objects such as pens or pencils. Toothbrush abrasion is the most common example and is usually seen as a sharp wedge-shaped notch in the gingival portion of the facial aspects of teeth (see Fig. 3-10, *D*). The surface of the defect is smooth. The presence of such defects does not automatically warrant intervention. It is important to determine and eliminate the cause.

Attrition is mechanical wear of the incisal or occlusal tooth structure as a result of functional or parafunctional movements of the mandible. Although a certain degree of attrition is expected with age, it is important to note abnormally advanced attrition (see Fig. 3-10, *E*). If significant abnormal attrition is present, the patient's functional movements should be evaluated, and inquiry needs to be made about any habits creating this problem, such as tooth grinding, or *bruxism*, usually resulting from stress, airway issues, or sleep apnea. In some older patients, the enamel of the cusp tips (or incisal edges) is worn off, resulting in cupped-out areas because the exposed, softer dentin wears faster than the surrounding enamel. Sometimes, these areas are an annoyance because of food retention or the presence of peripheral, ragged, sharp enamel edges. Slowing such wear by appropriate restorative treatment is indicated. The sharp edges can result in tongue or cheek biting; rounding these edges does not completely resolve the problem but does improve comfort.

Complete cusp fracture is a common occurrence in posterior teeth. In general, the most frequently fractured cusps are the nonholding cusps. Specifically, the most frequently fractured teeth are mandibular molars and second premolars, with the lingual cusps fracturing more often than the facial cusps. Maxillary premolars also frequently fractured, but in contrast to mandibular teeth, the facial cusps fracture more often than the lingual cusps. The mesiofacial and distolingual cusps are the most commonly fractured cusps in maxillary molars.

A study of fracture severity found that 95% of the fractures exposed dentin, 25% were below the CEJ, and 3% resulted in pulp exposure. The consequences of posterior tooth fracture were found to vary, with maxillary premolar and mandibular molar fractures being generally more severe. Most fractures were treated with direct or indirect restorations or recontouring and polishing; 3% were extracted, and 4% received endodontic treatment.[24] Risk factors for nontraumatic fracture of posterior teeth were found to be the presence of a fracture line in enamel and an increase in the proportion of the volume of the natural tooth crown occupied by a restoration.[25,26]

Fracture or "craze lines" in a tooth are often visible, especially with advancing age, and should be considered potential cleavage planes for possible future fractures. Appropriate dye materials or transillumination aid in detecting fracture lines. Any tooth that has an extensive restoration and weakened cusps should be identified as being susceptible to future fracture (Fig. 3-11) and should be considered for a cusp-protecting restoration. Deep developmental fissures across marginal or cusp ridges are cleavage planes, especially in a tooth weakened by caries or previous restoration. The dental examination also may reveal dental anomalies that include variations in size, shape, structure, or number of teeth—such as dens in dente, macrodontia, microdontia, gemination, concrescence, dilaceration, amelogenesis imperfecta, and dentinogenesis imperfecta. An in-depth discussion of these anomalies is beyond the scope of this text. The reader should consult an oral pathology textbook for additional information.

Radiographic Examination of Teeth and Restorations

Radiographs are an indispensable part of the contemporary dentist's diagnostic armamentarium. The use of diagnostic ionizing radiation is, however, not without risks. Cumulative exposure to ionizing radiation potentially can result in adverse effects. The diagnostic yield or potential benefit that could be gained from a radiograph must be weighed against the financial costs and the potential adverse effects of exposure to radiation. Several technologies, particularly digital radiography, are now available and are designed to enhance diagnostic yield and reduce radiation exposure.

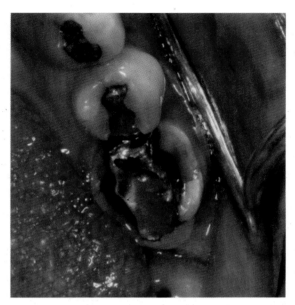

Fig. 3-11 Extensively restored teeth with weakened and fractured cusps. Note the distal developmental fissure in the second molar, which further predisposes the distal cusps to fracture.

The American Dental Association (ADA), in collaboration with the FDA, developed guidelines for the prescription of dental radiographic examinations to serve as an adjunct to the dentist's professional judgment with regard to the best use of diagnostic imaging. Radiographs help the dental practitioner evaluate and definitively diagnose many oral diseases and conditions. However, the dentist must weigh the benefits of taking dental radiographs against the risk of exposing a patient to radiographs, the effects of which accumulate from multiple sources over time. The dentist, being aware of the patient's health history and vulnerability to oral disease, is in the best position to make this judgment. For this reason, the guidelines are intended to serve as a resource for the practitioner and are not intended to be standards of care nor requirements or regulations. The ADA/FDA guidelines help direct the type and frequency of radiographs needed according to patient condition and risk factors (Table 3-1).[27]

Generally, patients at higher risk for caries or periodontal disease should receive more frequent and more extensive radiographic surveys. A systematic review of methods of diagnosing dental caries lesions found that although radiographs were useful in detecting lesions, they do have limitations.[28] For the examination of occlusal surfaces, radiographs had moderate sensitivity and good specificity for diagnosing dentinal lesions; however, for enamel lesions, the sensitivity was poor, and the specificity was reduced. Studies of the radiographic examination of proximal surfaces found that there was moderate sensitivity and good specificity for the detection of cavitated lesions and low to moderate sensitivity and moderate to high specificity for enamel or dentinal lesions. Before rendering a diagnosis and deciding on treatment, information obtained from radiographs should be confirmed or augmented with other examination findings. In addition, the consequences of false positives, which may prompt unneeded treatment, and false negatives, which may leave disease undetected, as well as an understanding of the typically slow

Table 3-1 Guidelines for Prescribing Dental Radiographs

The recommendations in this chart are subject to clinical judgment and may not apply to every patient. They are to be used by dentists only after reviewing the patient's health history and completing a clinical examination. Because every precaution should be taken to minimize radiation exposure, protective thyroid collars and aprons should be used, whenever possible. This practice is strongly recommended for children, women of childbearing age, and pregnant women.

Type of Encounter	Patient Age and Dental Developmental Stage				
	Child with Primary Dentition (Prior to Eruption of First Permanent Tooth)	Child with Transitional Dentition (After Eruption of First Permanent Tooth)	Adolescent with Permanent Dentition (Prior to Eruption of Third Molars)	Adult, Dentate or Partially Edentulous	Adult, Edentulous
New patient* being evaluated for dental diseases and dental development	Individualized radiographic exam consisting of selected periapical/occlusal views and/or posterior bitewings if proximal surfaces cannot be visualized or probed. Patients without evidence of disease and with open proximal contacts may not require a radiographic exam at this time.	Individualized radiographic exam consisting of posterior bitewings with panoramic exam or posterior bitewings and selected periapical images.	Individualized radiographic exam consisting of posterior bitewings with panoramic exam or posterior bitewings and selected periapical images. A full mouth intraoral radiographic exam is preferred when the patient has clinical evidence of generalized dental disease or a history of extensive dental treatment.		Individualized radiographic exam, based on clinical signs and symptoms.
Recall patient* with clinical caries or at increased risk for caries**	Posterior bitewing exam at 6–12 month intervals if proximal surfaces cannot be examined visually or with a probe.	Posterior bitewing exam at 6–12 month intervals if proximal surfaces cannot be examined		Posterior bitewing exam at 6–18 month intervals	Not applicable
Recall patient* with no clinical caries and not at increased risk for caries**	Posterior bitewing exam at 12–24 month intervals if proximal surfaces cannot be examined visually or with a probe	Posterior bitewing exam at 18-36 month intervals		Posterior bitewing exam at 24–36 month intervals	Not applicable
Recall patient* with periodontal disease	Clinical judgment as to the need for and type of radiographic images for the evaluation of periodontal disease. Imaging may consist of, but is not limited to, selected bitewing and/or periapical images of areas where periodontal disease (other than nonspecific gingivitis) can be identified clinically.				Not applicable
Patient for monitoring of growth and development	Clinical judgment as to need for and type of radiographic images for evaluation and/or monitoring of dento-facial growth and development		Clinical judgment as to need for and type of radiographic images for evaluation and/or monitoring of dento-facial growth and development. Panoramic or periapical exam to assess developing third molars	Usually not indicated	

Patient with other circumstances including, but not limited to, proposed or existing implants, pathology, restorative/endodontic needs, treated periodontal disease and caries remineralization	Clinical judgment as to need for and type of radiographic images for evaluation and/or monitoring in these circumstances.

(From American Dental Association, US Food and Drug Administration. The Selection of Patients for Dental Radiograph Examinations. Available on www.ada.org. Document created November 2004.)

*Clinical situations for which radiographs may be indicated include but are not limited to:

A. Positive Historical Findings
1. Previous periodontal or endodontic treatment
2. History of pain or trauma
3. Familial history of dental anomalies
4. Postoperative evaluation of healing
5. Remineralization monitoring
6. Presence of implants or evaluation for implant placement

B. Positive Clinical Signs/Symptoms
1. Clinical evidence of periodontal disease
2. Large or deep restorations
3. Deep carious lesions
4. Malposed or clinically impacted teeth
5. Swelling
6. Evidence of dental/facial trauma
7. Mobility of teeth
8. Sinus tract ("fistula")
9. Clinically suspected sinus pathology
10. Growth abnormalities
11. Oral involvement in known or suspected systemic disease
12. Positive neurologic findings in the head and neck
13. Evidence of foreign objects
14. Pain and/or dysfunction of the temporomandibular joint
15. Facial asymmetry
16. Abutment teeth for fixed or removable partial prosthesis
17. Unexplained bleeding
18. Unexplained sensitivity of teeth
19. Unusual eruption, spacing, or migration of teeth
20. Unusual tooth morphology, calcification, or color
21. Unexplained absence of teeth
22. Clinical erosion

**Factors increasing risk for caries may include but are not limited to:
1. High level of caries experience or demineralization
2. History of recurrent caries
3. High titers of cariogenic bacteria
4. Existing restoration(s) of poor quality
5. Poor oral hygiene
6. Inadequate fluoride exposure
7. Prolonged nursing (bottle or breast)
8. Frequent high sucrose content in diet
9. Poor family dental health
10. Developmental or acquired enamel defects
11. Developmental or acquired disability
12. Xerostomia
13. Genetic abnormality of teeth
14. Many multi-surface restorations
15. Chemotherapy/radiation therapy
16. Eating disorders
17. Drug/alcohol abuse
18. Irregular dental care

progressing nature of caries lesions should factor into the diagnosis and management strategy.

For diagnosis of proximal surface caries, restoration overhangs, or poorly contoured restorations, posterior bitewing and anterior periapical radiographs are most helpful. When interpreting the radiographic presentation of proximal tooth surfaces, it is necessary to know the normal anatomic picture presented in a radiograph before any abnormalities can be diagnosed. In a radiograph, a proximal caries lesion usually appears as a dark area or a radiolucency in the enamel at or apical to the contact (see Fig. 3-5, A). This radiolucency is typically triangular and has its apex toward the dentinoenamel junction (DEJ).

Moderate-to-deep occlusal caries lesions may be seen as a radiolucency extending into dentin (see Fig. 3-5, C). Because the specificity of radiographs for detecting dentinal lesions on occlusal surfaces is relatively good at 80% (very few false positives), when a radiolucency is apparent beneath the occlusal enamel surface emanating from the DEJ a diagnosis of caries is appropriate. However, because the sensitivity of radiographs for dentinal lesions on the occlusal surface is rather low (50%), the absence of a radiolucency does not mean that a lesion is not present. In these situations, the clinician should rely more on the results of the visual–tactile examination and the findings of any adjunctive tests (discussed later).

Some defective aspects of restorations, including improper contour, overhangs (see Fig. 3-6), and recurrent caries lesions gingival to restorations (see Fig. 3-5, D), may also be identified radiographically. Pulpal abnormalities such as pulp stones and internal resorption may be identified in anterior periapical radiographs. The height and integrity of the marginal periodontium may be evaluated from bitewing radiographs. Periapical radiographs are helpful in diagnosing changes in the periapical periodontium such as periapical abscesses, dental granulomas, or cysts. Impacted third molars, supernumerary teeth, and other congenital or acquired abnormalities also may be discovered on periapical radiographic examination. The sensitivity and specificity of dental radiographs vary, however, according to the diagnostic task (e.g., surface of the tooth being examined, proximal versus occlusal, and depth, enamel vs. dentin).

Dental radiographs should always be interpreted cautiously. One limitation imposed when interpreting a dental radiograph is that the image is a two-dimensional representation of a three-dimensional mass. In addition, the interpretation of dental radiographs can produce a certain number of false-positive and false-negative diagnoses. Misdiagnosis can occur when cervical burnout (the radiographic picture of the normal structure and contour of the cervical third of the crown) mimics a caries lesion. A Class V lesion or a radiolucent tooth-colored restoration may be radiographically superimposed on the proximal area, mimicking a proximal caries lesion. Finally, although a caries lesion may be more extensive clinically than it appears radiographically, it is estimated that over half of the teeth with what appear to be radiographic proximal caries lesions in the outer half of dentin are likely to be non-cavitated and treatable with remineralization measures.[29] Although radiographs are an excellent diagnostic tool, they do have certain limitations. To guard against these limitations, clinical and radiographic findings should be correlated continually and the implications of their limitations should be understood when formulating a diagnosis and deciding on treatment.

Adjunctive Aids for Examining Teeth and Restorations

Study casts are helpful in evaluating a patient's clinical status in many situations. Study casts can be useful, as they provide an understanding of occlusal relationships, help in developing the treatment plan, and serve as a tool for educating the patient. Accurately mounted study casts provide an opportunity for a thorough evaluation of the tooth interdigitation, the functional occlusion, and any occlusal abnormalities that may need treatment. Study casts allow further evaluation of the plane of occlusion; tilted, rotated, or extruded teeth; crossbites; plunger cusps; wear facets and defective restorations; coronal contours; proximal contacts; and embrasure spaces between teeth. Combined with clinical and radiographic findings, study casts allow the practitioner to develop a treatment plan without the patient present, thus saving valuable chair time. When a proposed treatment plan is discussed with the patient, study casts can be a valuable educational medium in helping the patient understand and visualize existing conditions and the need for the proposed treatment.

Radiographs aid in determining the relationship between the margins of existing or proposed restorations and bone. A biologic width of at least 2 mm is required for the junctional epithelium and the connective tissue attachments located between the base of the sulcus and the alveolar bone crest (Fig. 3-12, A). In addition to this physiologic dimension, the restoration margin should be placed occlusally as far away as possible from the base of the sulcus to foster gingival health. Encroachment on this biologic width may cause an inflammatory response in gingival tissue, causing redness, swelling, and bleeding on probing or flossing in the area of the violation of biologic width. It is possible that breakdown and apical migration of the attachment apparatus can also occur. The attachment breakdown and apical migration are in response to the inflammatory process caused by bacterial plaque that accumulates at the inaccessible restoration margins. The final position of a proposed gingival margin, which is dictated by the existing restoration, caries, or retention features, must be estimated to determine if crown-lengthening procedures are indicated before restoration (see Fig. 3-12, B). Another possible correction for biologic width violations is to orthodontically extrude the tooth to make room for the distance between the restoration margin and bone. Surgical crown lengthening procedures involve the surgical removal of the gingiva, bone, or both to create a longer clinical crown and provide more tooth structure for placing the restoration margin and for increasing retention form. Because of the obvious importance of the periodontium, operative procedures must be performed continually with respect, understanding, and concern for the periodontium.

Examination of Occulusion

Several reasons exist for completing a thorough occlusal examination, such as developing an analysis and understanding of the patient's occlusion before initiating restorative care. First, the clinician can establish the patient's presenting condition before any alterations are attempted. This documentation includes the identification of signs of occlusal trauma such as enamel cracks or tooth mobility and notation of occlusal abnormalities that contribute to pathologic conditions such

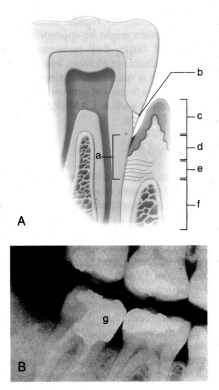

Fig. 3-12 **A,** Biologic width (*a*) is the physiologic dimension needed for the junctional epithelium (*d*) and the connective tissue attachment (*e*), which is measured from the base of the sulcus (*c*) to the level of the bone crest (*f*). The margin of the restoration (*b*) must not violate this dimension. **B,** Tooth with an existing restoration (*g*) that encroaches on the biologic width requires crown-lengthening procedures before placement of a new restoration.

as bone loss. Second, the potential effect of the proposed restorative treatment on the occlusion can be assessed. The potential of the proposed restoration to provide a beneficial and harmonious occlusion must be determined. Third, the effect of the current occlusal scheme on the proposed restorative treatment can be identified, and the existing occlusion can be altered, if needed, before placement of restorations.

The static and dynamic occlusion must be examined carefully (see Chapter 1). Not all occlusal variances from normal require treatment, mostly because the patient's ability to adapt to the abnormalities without pathologic symptoms. However, the clinician must be able to identify deviations from normal and be prepared to treat, refer, or make allowances for these problems in any planned therapy. A description of the patient's static anatomic occlusion in maximum intercuspation, including the relationship between molars and canines (Angle's Classes I, II, or III), and the amount of vertical overlap (overbite) and horizontal overlap (overjet) of anterior teeth should be recorded. The presence of missing teeth and the relationship of the maxillary and mandibular midlines should be determined. The appropriateness of the occlusal plane and the positions of malposed teeth should be identified. Supererupted teeth, spacing, fractured teeth, and marginal ridge discrepancies should be noted. The dynamic functional occlusion in all movements of the mandible (right, left, forward, and all excursions in between) should be evaluated. This evaluation also includes assessing the relationship of teeth in

centric relation, which is the orthopedic position of the joint where the condyle head is in its most anterior and superior position against the articular eminence within the glenoid fossa. Functional movements of the mandible are evaluated to determine if canine guidance or group function exists. The presence and amount of anterior guidance is evaluated to note the degree of potential posterior disclusion. Nonworking-side contacts are recorded so that any planned restorative care for the involved teeth would not perpetuate these contacts. Any mobility of teeth or fremitus during function is identified and classified as primary or secondary occlusal traumatism. Movement of the mandible from maximum intercuspation to maximum opening is observed; any clicking or popping of the joint during such movement could be a nonsymptomatic variation from normal or be an indication of a possible pathologic condition. A load test for the joint and palpatation of the joint would be completed to further test for joint tenderness to determine joint pathology that is symptomatic.

Teeth are examined for abnormal wear patterns that are excessive and not age appropriate. If signs of abnormal or premature wear are present, the patient is queried as to the presence of any contributing habits such as nocturnal bruxism or parafunctional habits. The examination also should disclose possible unfavorable occlusal relationships such as a plunger cusp, which is a pointed cusp "plunging" deep into the occlusal plane of the opposing arch. A plunger cusp might contact the lower of two adjacent marginal ridges of different levels, contacting directly between two adjacent marginal ridges in maximum intercuspation, or positioned in a deep fossa. These may result in food impaction and tooth or restoration fracture.

The results of the occlusal analysis should be included in the dental record and considered in the restorative treatment plan. Acceptable aspects of the occlusion must be preserved and not altered during treatment. When possible, improvement of the occlusal relationship is desirable; abnormalities must not be perpetuated in the restorative treatment.

Examination for Esthetic Considerations

Examination of esthetic considerations can be described as the evaluation of tooth color, tooth display, and ideal tooth position in relation to the face. An important part of the evaluation is a discussion of what would be realistic esthetic expectations when discussing treatment options with the patient. Esthetic predisposing conditions for a patient are defined as the clinical conditions presented by the patient that might adversely affect the clinician's ability to meet the patient's esthetic expectations and vision. Attaining the desired esthetic outcomes may be complicated by maximum tooth display and excessive or uneven tissue display. Risk can be lowered primarily by establishing ideal intrafacial tooth position and secondarily, by establishing intra-arch tooth position. Tooth color evaluation becomes a factor as teeth are more visible when smiling or at the resting position of lips. Darker colored teeth, teeth with enamel intrinsic staining, and conditions such as tetracycline staining all increase the risk for not satisfying the esthetic expectations of patients with tooth color concerns. Gingival symmetry also becomes very important in maximum display situations, and lack of symmetry increases the risk of not meeting the patient's esthetic expectations. Presence of multiple risk factors would require more aggressive treatment options to meet the patient's overall esthetic expectations. These treatment options may not be appropriate if they satisfy a patient's esthetic expectations but negatively affect the long-term health of teeth. In many of these situations, conservative direct or indirect enamel-supported restorations are more appropriate for long-term risk management than are more aggressive preparations that remove more tooth structure.

Risk Profiles

After the examination and data collection are completed, the next step is to assess the risk or likelihood of future problems, given the patient's current behaviors, clinical conditions, and so on. In relation to operative dentistry, risk assessments are made for caries and structural problems of teeth such as fractures and erosion. However, in addition to caries risk assessments, risk assessment profiles should be established in other areas of patient care, such as tooth structural concerns, periodontal disease, functional occlusal and temporomandibular joint (TMJ) issues, and for the "risk" involved in satisfying the patient's esthetic expectations. Taken together, these assessments provide a risk profile that helps guide the preventive and operative recommendations that are made to the patient with the goal of mitigating as many risk factors as possible.

The CAMBRA guidelines were developed over several years as an evidence-based approach to preventing, reversing, and, when necessary, repairing early damage to teeth caused by caries. Refer to Chapter 2 for more information on how CAMBRA is used to determine caries risk and how this determination helps the clinician in the decision-making process for surgical or nonsurgical therapeutic interventions.

Risk assessments help organize the data on multiple causative factors. Few diseases or dental conditions are caused by a single factor. Rather, most diseases and dental conditions have been shown to be associated with numerous behavioral or sociodemographic, physical or environmental, microbiologic, or host factors. In addition, every patient has a different set of risk factors. This presents a challenge to determining the likelihood that a disease or condition would occur in the future or that some form of dental treatment or therapeutics would decrease the chances of disease occurrence. Many risk assessments use terms such as *low risk*, *medium risk*, and *high risk* to associate a level of risk to a category. This is sometimes expressed by using colors: red for high risk, yellow for medium risk, and green for low risk. This helps simplify the concept for the patient, as this is easily understood while discussing assessments and their implications for treatment recommendations. All treatment for patients should be designed to lower their risks for problems in each of these areas. The clinician must understand the concepts of risk management thoroughly. Dental treatment in any one of the above areas may improve risk status in that area but at a cost of increased risk in another area. For example, preparation of teeth for full-coverage crowns might reduce occlusal or esthetic risk but at a cost of increasing risk for future caries or tooth fracture.

Risk assessments are highly useful in managing patients who are candidates for operative dentistry. Patients who possess risk factors and risk indicators should be considered to be at risk for dental caries.[6,30] The assessments are used to guide treatment. A patient at high risk for dental caries should receive aggressive intervention to remove or alter as many risk factors as possible. Alternatively, regular monitoring and reassessment of the condition might be appropriate for a patient at low risk for dental caries. Risk assessment is a relatively young science in the dental profession, but as more research is completed, evidence is quickly validating this approach to patient care. Approaches to patient care using risk assessments and disease management such as CAMBRA are becoming the recognized standard of care.

Prognosis

Prognosis is the term used to describe the prediction of the probable course and outcome of a disease or condition as well as the outcome expected from an intervention, be it preventive or operative. Prognosis can also be used to estimate the likelihood of recovery from a disease or condition. In operative dentistry, prognosis can be used to describe the likelihood of success of a particular treatment procedure in terms of time of service, functional value to the patient, comfort for the patient, and esthetic value for the patient. A prognosis can be described as *excellent*, *good*, *fair*, *poor*, or even *hopeless*. Prognosis for a disease or condition is largely dependent on the risk factors and disease indicators that are present in the patient. However, other factors such as the skill of the dentist and the current status of the disease before beginning treatment also have an effect on the prognosis. For example, a patient with severe caries may be willing to eliminate all of the modifiable risk factors, but if the disease is too advanced, the long-term prognosis for the affected teeth may still be poor. Therefore, it is important for the clinician to take in account the entire risk profile of the patient in all areas of the person's medical and dental health when trying to establish a prognosis. It is also important to consider the skill level of the treating dentist and the current state of the disease or conditions before evaluating possible treatment options. Once the dentist and the patient have a good understanding of the patient's risk profile and the present disease state and conditions, they can work as a team to decide the best treatment options and alternatives to fit the patient's needs.

Treatment Planning
General Considerations

A treatment plan is a carefully sequenced series of services designed to eliminate or control etiologic factors, repair existing damage, and create a functional, maintainable environment. An appropriate treatment plan depends on thorough evaluation of the patient, the expertise of the dentist, and a prediction of the patient's response to treatment. An accurate prognosis for each tooth and for the patient's overall oral health is central to a successful treatment plan.

The development of a dental treatment plan for a patient often consists of four steps: (1) examination, problem identification, and risk assessment; (2) decision to recommend intervention; (3) identification of treatment alternatives; and (4) selection of treatment with the patient's involvement. Step one, examination, diagnosis, and risk assessment, which was discussed in detail in the first part of this chapter, results in the listing of the patient's dental problems. For step two, the decision to intervene surgically or non-surgically depends on the determination that a tooth is diseased, a restoration is defective, or the tooth or restoration is at some increased risk of further deterioration if the intervention does not occur. If any of these conditions exists, intervention is recommended to the patient. Step three, identification of treatment alternatives, involves establishing a list of one or more reasonable interventions from the set of possible alternatives. Treatment alternatives for a specific condition may include, for example, periodic re-evaluation to monitor the condition, chemotherapeutics (e.g., applications of fluoride to promote remineralization or antimicrobials to reduce bacteria), recontouring defective restorations or irregular tooth surfaces, repair of an existing restoration, and restoration. This list of reasonable treatment alternatives is based on current evidence of the effectiveness of treatments, the prevailing standards of care, and clinical and nonclinical patient factors. Step four, selection of the treatment, is conducted in consultation with the patient. The patient is advised of the reasonable treatment alternatives and their related risks and benefits. After the patient is fully informed, the dentist and patient can select a course of action that is most appropriate.

Treatment plans are influenced by many factors, including patient preferences, motivation, systemic health, emotional status, and financial resources. The treatment plan is influenced by the dentist's knowledge, experience, and training; laboratory support; dentist–patient compatibility; availability of specialists; and the patient's functional, esthetic, and technical demands. Finally, a treatment plan is not a static list of services. Rather, it is often a multi-phase and dynamic series of activities. The success of the treatment plan is determined by its ability to meet the patient's initial and long-term needs. A treatment plan should allow for re-evaluation and be adaptable to meet the changing needs, preferences, and health conditions of the patient.

Treatment Plan Sequencing

Proper sequencing is a crucial component of a successful treatment plan. Certain treatments must follow others in a logical order, whereas other treatments can or must occur concurrently and require coordination. Complex treatment plans often are sequenced in phases, including an urgent phase, a control phase, a re-evaluation phase, a definitive phase, and a recare or re-assessment phase.[31] For most patients, the first three phases are accomplished as a single phase. Generally, the principle of "greatest need" guides the order in which treatment is sequenced. This principle suggests that what the patient needs most is performed first—with pain, bleeding, and swelling at one end of the continuum to elective esthetic procedures on the other.

Urgent Phase

The urgent phase of care begins with a thorough review of the patient's medical condition and history. A patient presenting with swelling, pain, bleeding, or infection should have these problems managed as soon as possible, before initiation of subsequent phases.

Control Phase

Most patients will not need a formal control phase. A control phase is appropriate when the patient presents with multiple pressing problems and extensive active disease or when the prognosis is unclear. The goals of this phase are to remove etiologic factors and stabilize the patient's dental health. These goals are accomplished by (1) eliminating active disease such as caries and inflammation, (2) removing conditions preventing maintenance, (3) eliminating potential causes of disease, and (4) beginning preventive activities. Examples of control phase treatment include extractions; endodontics; periodontal debridement and scaling; occlusal adjustment; caries removal; replacement or repair of defective restorations such as those with gingival overhangs; and use of caries control measures, as discussed in Chapter 2.

As part of the control phase, the dentist should develop a plan for the management and prevention of dental caries. After the patient's caries status and caries risk have been determined, chemical, surgical, behavioral, mechanical, and dietary techniques can be used to improve host resistance and alter the oral flora.[30,32] Chapter 2 presents a detailed discussion of caries diagnosis, prevention, treatment, and control.

Re-evaluation Phase

This phase allows time between the control and definitive phases for resolution of inflammation and healing. Home care habits are reinforced, motivation for further treatment is assessed, and initial treatment and pulpal responses are re-evaluated before definitive care is begun.

Definitive Phase

After the dentist reassesses initial treatment and determines the need for further care, the patient enters the corrective or definitive phase of treatment. This phase may include endodontic, periodontal, orthodontic, and surgical procedures before fixed or removable prosthodontic treatment. This phase is discussed in detail in the section on interdisciplinary considerations in operative treatment planning.

Recare and Re-assessment Phase

The re-assessment phase includes regular re-evaluation examinations that (1) may reveal the need for adjustments to prevent future breakdown and (2) provide an opportunity to reinforce home care. The frequency of re-evaluation examinations during the maintenance phase depends, in large part, on the patient's risk for dental disease. A patient who has stable periodontal health, has a recent history of no caries lesions, and is at low risk, may have longer intervals (e.g., 9–12 months) between recall visits. In contrast, patients at high risk for dental caries or periodontal problems should be examined much more frequently (e.g., 3–4 months).

Interdisciplinary Considerations in Operative Treatment Planning

When an operative procedure is performed during the control or definitive phases, general guidelines help determine when the operative treatment should occur relative to other forms of care. Following is a discussion on sequencing operative care with endodontic, periodontal, orthodontic, surgical, and prosthodontic treatments.

Endodontics

All teeth to be restored with large restorations should have a pulpal or periapical evaluation. If indicated, teeth should have endodontic treatment before restoration is completed. Also, a tooth previously endodontically treated that shows no evidence of healing or has an inadequate filling or a filling exposed to oral fluids should be evaluated for re-treatment before restorative therapy is initiated.[33]

Periodontics

Generally, periodontal treatment should precede operative care, especially when improved oral hygiene, initial scaling, and root planing procedures can create a more desirable environment for performing operative treatment. A tooth with a questionable periodontal prognosis should not receive an extensive restoration until periodontal treatment provides a more favorable prognosis. If a tooth has a good periodontal prognosis, however, operative treatment can occur before or after periodontal therapy, as long as the operative treatment is not compromised by the existing tissue condition. Treatment of deep carious lesions often requires caries control, foundations, or temporization or root canal therapy or both before periodontal therapy. The correction of gross restorative defects in restoration contours (e.g., open contacts, gingival overhangs, and poor embrasure form) is considered a part of initial periodontal therapy, and such corrections enhance a favorable tissue response. If periodontal surgical procedures are required, permanent restorations such as inlays or onlays, crowns, and prostheses should be delayed until the surgical phase is completed. Teeth planned for cast restorations can, however, be prepared and temporized before periodontal surgery. This approach permits confirmation of the restoration prognosis before surgery and allows improved access for the surgical procedure.

Patients with gingivitis and early periodontitis generally respond favorably to improved oral hygiene and scaling or root planing procedures. Patients with more advanced periodontitis might require surgical pocket elimination or reduction procedures or various regenerative procedures. If indicated, an increase in the zones of attached gingiva and the elimination of abnormal frenal tension should be achieved by corrective periodontal surgical procedures around teeth receiving restorations with subgingival margins. In addition, any teeth requiring restorations that may encroach on the biologic width of the periodontium should have appropriate crown-lengthening surgical procedures performed before the final restoration is placed. Usually, a minimum of 6 weeks is required after the surgery before final restorative procedures are undertaken.

Orthodontics

Orthodontic therapy may include extrusion or realignment of teeth to provide favorable interdental spacing, stress distribution, function, and esthetics. All teeth should be caries-free before orthodontic banding. Treatment of caries may include the placement of amalgam and composite restorations. Few indications exist for cast restorations before orthodontic treatment is completed. In addition, patients undergoing orthodontic treatment should receive more intense caries prevention measures.

Oral Surgery

In most instances, impacted, unerupted, and hopelessly involved teeth should be removed before operative treatment. This recommendation especially applies when second molars that are to be restored might be damaged or dislodged during the removal of third molars. In addition, soft-tissue lesions, complicating exostoses, and improperly contoured ridge areas should be eliminated or corrected before final restorative care.

Occlusion

The occlusion should be evaluated, and several essential keys for acceptable functional occlusion should be present in the patient. Functional movements of the mandible and occlusion of teeth are necessary for chewing food and even talking. First, all movements and terminal closure of the mandible must be compatible for harmonious temporomandibular joint (TMJ) function. The envelope of function must create efficient use of opening and closing muscle movements. The envelope of function must not cause a premature loading of teeth which could result in excess tooth wear, mobility, or temporomandibular disorders. Maximum intercuspation should be as close as possible to providing equal bilateral simultaneous contacts of teeth on closure of the mandible. If these conditions are achieved, and the patient history and examination does not reveal any other significant risk factors or symptoms, the patient would be diagnosed as having acceptable functional occlusion at the current point in time.

Fixed, Removable, and Implant Prosthodontics

Preferably, operative direct restorations should be completed before placing indirect restorations. Occasionally, a large amalgam or composite restoration is placed as a foundation to provide improved retention for a full crown. For use as a foundation, retention features must be placed well inside the restoration so that the material remains after tooth preparation for a crown. In removable prosthodontics, tooth preparations and restorations should allow for the design of the removable partial denture. This includes allowance for rests, guide planes, and clasps. The design of the operative restoration and the selection of appropriate restorative materials must be compatible with the design of the contemplated removable prosthesis. In cases where dental implants have been or will be placed, operative dentistry restorations should be planned and executed to allow for all the necessary parameters for successful implant restorations, including adequate space mesiodistally and vertically. Also, implant restorations may sometimes have unusual proximal contours, and adjacent amalgam or composite restorations should be designed to create the best proximal contact relationships possible.

Decision Making for Caries Management and Operative Treatment

As discussed in Chapter 2, dental caries is a multifactorial, transmissible, infectious oral disease caused primarily by the complex interaction of cariogenic oral flora (biofilm) with fermentable dietary carbohydrates on the tooth surface over time. *Caries lesions are the result of the caries disease process, not the cause.*

As described earlier in this chapter, the *first* step in managing dental caries is a thorough examination of teeth. This is accomplished by using all available diagnostic information to identify the location, size, depth, and activity of a caries lesion. The *second* step is to inventory existing risk factors or indicators using a systematic process as described in Chapter 2. The *third* step is the development of a preventive management treatment plan designed to reduce the patient's risk for future caries. The *fourth* step is to decide how best to manage the lesions that were detected. In making these decisions, the dentist should be mindful of the fact that except in cases of relatively large caries lesions, *the accuracy of the methods used to detect lesions (visual inspection, radiographs, caries detection devices, etc.) are all prone to inaccuracies* (Box 3-1). These inaccuracies result in false-positive and false-negative findings. This situation raises the question, "What are the implications of these inaccuracies for clinical decision making?" False-positives findings may result in the surgical treatment of a sound tooth, and false-negative findings will result in a diseased surface receiving remineralization treatment instead of operative treatment. The former situation is irreversible and should be avoided, whenever possible. In the latter situation, false negatives will be receiving remineralization therapy and regular monitoring so that they can be treated operatively at a later time, if needed. This approach is even sounder, considering that caries lesions generally do not progress rapidly.[34] Thus, the clinician should strive to reduce the number of false positives by making sure that strong diagnostic evidence supports the presence of cavitation or dentin penetration before recommending irreversible operative treatment.

As a general rule, remineralization therapies, as well as sealants in the case of pits and fissures, are the preferred methods of managing coronal lesions that are neither cavitated nor penetrated into the dentin. Remineralization is also recommended for root surface lesions, in which neither a break in the surface contour of the exposed root nor softening of the root surface occurs. However, it is very important to note that *remineralization requires a high level of patient compliance with the therapeutic regimen and frequent recall visits to assess the success of the treatment.* If lesion progression is detected at recall, then operative intervention is warranted.

However, there are exceptions to the general rule of managing noncavitated enamel lesions with remineralization. Because remineralization requires a shift in the delicate balance of the oral biofilm, it depends heavily on changes in patient behavior (improved home care, diet, etc.) and the timely application of antimicrobial agents, fluoride, and other remineralizing agents. Thus, when it is clear that the patient is unwilling or unable to follow the prescribed remineralization regimen of home care and professional care, it is often appropriate to treat these lesions with operative restorations.

If confirmed cavitation of the enamel or demineralization penetrating into the dentin on coronal surfaces is present or a break exists in the contour of exposed root and softening of the surface, then operative treatment is usually recommended. One exception to this general guideline is the lesion that is deemed arrested.

A paramount principle in dentistry, as was discussed earlier in this chapter, is to *do no harm.* Clinicians must have a sound knowledge of the current evidence on the risks and benefits of their treatment recommendations. In the context of planning dental treatment, the clinician should recommend invasive operative treatment only when the benefits outweigh the risks of adverse outcomes. As noted earlier, restorations which require permanent removal of tooth structure usually do not last forever. Studies have shown that the average lifespan of a restoration ranges from 5 to more than 15 years.[35] When a restoration is replaced, additional tooth structure usually is removed, regardless of how carefully the operator removes the existing restoration. This situation results in what has been termed *the cycle of re-restoration*, which leads to larger and more invasive restorations over the course of a patient's life.[36]

Esthetic Treatment

Interest in improved esthetics is growing among many segments of the population. As a result, a range of treatments has

---

Box 3-1 Assessing the Accuracy of a Diagnostic Test for Caries

Contingency Table for Diagnostic Test Evaluation

Histologic Gold Standard
Caries
No caries

Diagnostic Test
Caries
  True positive (TP)
  False positive (FP)
No caries
  False negative (FN)
  True negative (TN)

Desirable and Undesirable Outcomes Resulting from Diagnostic Tests with Low Sensitivity or Specificity

Example 1
Diagnosing 100 teeth (90 healthy and 10 carious) with a diagnostic test having a high sensitivity (0.80) and low specificity (0.50) would result in the following:
Desirable outcomes:
  Correctly detect 8 of 10 carious teeth (TP)
  Correctly diagnose 45 of 90 healthy teeth (TN)
Undesirable outcomes:
  Fail to detect 2 of 10 carious teeth (FN)
  Fail to diagnose 45 healthy teeth as carious (FP)

Example 2
Diagnosing 100 teeth (90 healthy and 10 carious) with a diagnostic test having low sensitivity (0.50) and high specificity (0.80) would result in the following:
Desirable outcomes:
  Correctly detect 5 of 10 carious teeth (TP)
  Correctly diagnose 72 of 90 healthy teeth (TN)
Undesirable outcomes:
  Fail to detect 5 of 10 carious teeth (FN)
  Fail to diagnose 18 healthy teeth as carious (FP)

been developed to manage a wide array of esthetic concerns. Chapter 12 describes these conservative esthetic treatments, which include esthetic recontouring of anterior teeth, vital bleaching, and microabrasion. These conservative approaches have well-documented outcomes. In addition to these conservative techniques, advances in direct composite restorations have permitted the closure of diastemas, recontouring of teeth, and other tooth additions by means other than extensive full-coverage restorations.

Treatment of Abrasion, Erosion, Abfraction, and Attrition

Abraded or eroded areas should be considered for restoration only if one or more of the following is true: (1) the area is affected by caries, (2) the defect is sufficiently deep to compromise the structural integrity of the tooth, (3) intolerable sensitivity exists and is unresponsive to conservative desensitizing measures, (4) the defect contributes to a periodontal problem, (5) the area is to be involved in the design of a removable partial denture, (6) the depth of the defect is judged to be close to the pulp, (7) the defect is actively progressing, or (8) the patient desires esthetic improvements. Areas of significant attrition that are worn into dentin and are sensitive or annoying should be considered for restoration. Before indirect restorations are used, however, a complete occlusal analysis and an in-depth interview with the patient regarding the etiology should be conducted to reduce contributing factors. Also, occlusal guard therapy should be considered.

Treatment of Root-Surface Caries

Root caries is common in older adults and in patients following periodontal treatments. Increases in the number of older patients in the patient population and tooth retention have contributed to this growing problem. Areas with root-surface caries usually should be restored when clinical or radiographic evidence of cavitation exists. Care must be exercised, however, to distinguish the active root-surface caries lesion from the root-surface lesion that once was active but has become inactive or arrested. The latter lesion shows sclerotic dentin that has darkened from extrinsic staining, is firm to the touch of an explorer, may be rough but is cleanable, and is seen in patients whose oral hygiene or diet has improved. Generally, these lesions should not be restored except when the patient wants restoration, probably for esthetic reasons. If it is determined that the lesion needs restoration, it can be restored with tooth-colored materials or amalgam. Adhesive materials have enhanced the restorative treatment of root-surface caries.

Prevention is preferred over restoration. It is recommended that appropriate preventive steps such as improvements in diet and oral hygiene and fluoride treatment with or without cementoplasty, be taken in hopes of avoiding carious breakdown and the need for restoration.[37]

Treatment of Root-Surface Sensitivity

It is not unusual for patients to complain of root-surface sensitivity, which is an annoying sharp pain usually associated with gingival recession and exposed root surfaces. The most widely accepted explanation of this phenomenon is *hydrodynamic theory*, which postulates that the pain results from indirect innervation caused by dentinal fluid movement in the tubules that stimulates the mechanoreceptors near the predentinal areas (see Chapter 1). Some causes of such fluid shifts are temperature change, air drying, and osmotic pressure. Any treatment that can reduce these fluid shifts by partially or totally occluding the tubules may help reduce the sensitivity.

Dentinal hypersensitivity is a particular problem for some patients that occurs immediately after periodontal surgery that results in the clinical exposure of root surfaces. Numerous forms of treatment have been used to provide relief, such as fluoride varnishes, oxalate solutions, resin-based adhesives, sealants, and desensitizing toothpastes that contain potassium nitrate. Although all of these methods have met with varying degrees of success, resin materials provide the best rate of success. When these conservative methods fail to provide relief, restorative treatment is indicated.

Repairing and Resurfacing Existing Restorations

Often amalgam, composite, or indirect restorations can be repaired or recontoured as opposed to complete removal and replacement. Growing evidence suggests that the removal and replacement result in the cycle of re-restoration, which leads to increasingly larger tooth preparations and the resultant trauma to the tooth and supporting structures.[36] In addition, resurfacing or repair of composites and repair of cast restorations have been shown to be effective.[28,38] Also, amalgam restorations with localized defects can be repaired with amalgam or with sealant resins.[22,38] If a restoration has an isolated defect, which, when explored operatively, can be confirmed, and if all carious tooth structure has been removed, it is acceptable and often preferable to repair or recontour. Reshaping of overcontoured restorations is an acceptable form of treatment.

Replacement of Existing Restorations

Generally, a restoration should not be replaced unless (1) it has significant marginal discrepancies, (2) the tooth is at risk for caries or fracture, or (3) the restoration is an etiologic factor to adjacent teeth or tissue.[39] In many instances, recontouring or resurfacing the existing restoration can delay replacement.

Indications for replacing restorations include the following: (1) marginal void, especially in the gingival one third, that cannot be repaired; (2) poor proximal contour or a gingival overhang that contributes to periodontal breakdown; (3) a marginal ridge discrepancy that contributes to food impaction; (4) over-contouring of a facial or lingual surface resulting in plaque gingival to the height of contour and resultant inflammation of gingiva overprotected from the cleansing action of food bolus or toothbrush; (5) poor proximal contact that is either open, resulting in interproximal food impaction and inflammation of impacted gingival papilla, or improper in location or size; (6) recurrent caries that cannot be treated adequately by a repair restoration; and (7) ditching deeper than 0.5 mm of the occlusal amalgam margin that is deemed carious or caries-prone. By itself, the presence of shallow ditching around an amalgam restoration is not an indication for replacement.

Indications for replacing tooth-colored restorations include (1) improper contours that cannot be repaired, (2) large voids, (3) deep marginal staining, (4) recurrent caries, and

(5) unacceptable esthetics. Restorations that have only light marginal staining and are deemed noncarious can be corrected by a shallow, narrow, marginal repair restoration.

Indication for Amalgam Restorations

Although its indications for use have decreased, dental amalgam still is recognized as a successful restorative material. The use of amalgam in dentistry has been the source of controversy. Although the use of amalgam is considered safe, as amalgam is removed from teeth, adverse environmental effects caused by mercury and amalgam waste do occur. Online Chapter 18 presents a more complete discussion of the issue, and Chapters 13 through 16 present the current indications for amalgam restorations.

Indications for Direct Composite and Other Tooth-Colored Restorations

Direct composite restorations are indicated for the treatment of many lesions in anterior and posterior teeth. Detailed indications for composite and other tooth-colored restorations are presented in Chapters 8 through 12.

Indications for Indirect Tooth-Colored Restorations

Partial-coverage indirect tooth-colored restorations may be indicated for Classes I and II restorations because of esthetics, strength, and other bonding benefits. Because of the potential of bonded restorations to strengthen remaining tooth structure, indirect tooth-colored restorations also may be selected for the conservative restoration of weakened posterior teeth in esthetically critical areas. Indirect tooth-colored restorations are covered in detail in Chapter 11.

Indications for Indirect Cast-Metal Restorations

Although indications for intracoronal cast restorations are few, a gold onlay that caps all of the cusps and includes some of the axial tooth line angles (see Chapter 17) is an excellent restoration. Cast metal restorations may be the treatment of choice for patients undergoing occlusal rehabilitation. Also, teeth with deep subgingival margins are appropriately treated with cast metal restorations because compared with direct restorations, they provide a better opportunity for control of proximal contours and for restoration of the difficult subgingival margin.

Treatment Considerations for Older Patients

In the past, older adults constituted a relatively minor proportion of the population. Older individuals used dental services infrequently because most were edentulous, had limited financial resources, and delayed unmet dental needs until they became symptomatic. Today, individuals 65 years and older represent a rapidly growing segment of the population. Older individuals today are better educated consumers, have greater financial resources, are more prevention minded, and have retained more teeth compared with their predecessors.[27] Older individuals are living with increasingly more complex medical, mental, emotional, and social conditions that affect their ability to care for their dentition and periodontium. These conditions must be considered when planning dental treatments for them. A comprehensive review of geriatric dentistry is beyond the scope of this chapter; rather, issues that are important for treatment planning for older patients are highlighted here.

Clear and effective communication is crucial. Because many older adults have hearing loss, the dentist must speak more distinctly and at a higher volume. Patients with memory loss appreciate written summaries and instructions that assist them in remembering details of the visit and planned treatment when they leave the dental office. The use of large simple fonts in written communications is particularly helpful to patients with diminished visual acuity.

An accurate medical history, risk assessment, and integration of dental and medical care are particularly important considerations for older patients. Many chronic diseases of the cardiovascular, respiratory, endocrine, renal, gastrointestinal, musculoskeletal, immune, and neurologic systems are associated with aging, influence dental disease, and complicate dental treatment decision making. Cardiovascular disease, Alzheimer's disease, depression, osteoarthritis, rheumatoid arthritis, osteoporosis, cancer, and diabetes are a few of the diseases that commonly affect older adults, and their medical management increases in complexity with advancing years. It is estimated that older individuals living in community settings take an average of four medications each day; six of the top 10 drugs prescribed in 2001 were used to treat age-related chronic conditions.[40] Many of these medications have adverse drug reactions, drug interactions, and oral adverse effects that include dry mouth (xerostomia), increased bleeding of tissues, lichenoid reactions, tissue overgrowth, and hypersensitivity reactions. The dentist must be aware of the impact these medications may have on dental treatment planning and management. Consultation with the patient's physician is highly recommended to fully understand these medical, mental, and emotional conditions and their potential impact on dental treatment. The dentist should recognize the use of xerostomic medications and discuss with the physician the potential substitution of medications with fewer xerostomic effects.

Oral changes associated with undernourishment, immunosuppression, dehydration, smoking, alcohol use, disease, medications, and dental problems lead to a depressed sense of taste and smell in older patients.[41] Perceptions of salty and bitter tastes and olfactory function decline with age, whereas perceptions of sweet and sour tastes do not. As a result, food can become tasteless and unappetizing, and more sugars, fats, and salts are added in an attempt to increase flavor. Undernourished individuals are encouraged to consume calorie-rich, complete-nutrition beverages, which also are rich in sugars. Smoking reduces the taste of foods by causing physical coating of the tongue and regression of the taste buds on the tongue and olfactory receptors in the roof of the nasal cavity over time. Inadequate fluid intake can lead to chronic dehydration and altered taste perception. These practices increase the risk of dental disease in this population. Dietary assessment and counseling are crucial in older patients to identify inadequate diets and suggest modifications that enhance taste and smell while lowering the risks of dental disease. Herb seasonings can enhance the flavor of foods in lieu of sugar and salt. Salivary stimulants, citric-flavored candies containing xylitol or other sugar replacements, tongue brushing or scraping, and smoking cessation are some additional measures that can promote taste and olfactory perception in older adults.

Dental and periodontal diseases can progress more rapidly in older adults.[42] Dental caries, particularly root caries, is the most significant reason for tooth loss in older adults. Ineffective plaque removal, xerostomia, soft sugar-rich diets, fixed and removable prostheses, abrasions at the CEJ, gingival recession, and bone loss from periodontal disease make root surfaces more prone to caries compared with other surfaces. Root-surface restorations are challenging to perform successfully and are at risk of recurrent decay in the future. Careful selection of restoration design, materials, and finishing can maximize the longevity and cleanability of restorations. Also, many dental practitioners prefer to intervene more aggressively with dental treatment rather than take a "watchful waiting" approach. As more teeth are being retained and have large restorations at risk of fracture or recurrent decay, attention must be placed on developing cost-effective and innovative means of restoring teeth, particularly for older individuals on a limited budget.

Prevention of dental disease increases in importance but becomes more challenging in older adults. Physical limitations such as arthritis, Parkinson's disease, vision impairment, and other chronic illnesses reduce the patients' ability to clean their teeth and periodontal tissues effectively. Powered rotation–oscillation toothbrushes and manual toothbrushes with larger handles for easier gripping are recommended to patients with decreased manual dexterity. Consistent use of fluoride-containing dentifrices and other remineralization products, antimicrobial mouth rinses, oral pH management, flossing, oral irrigation, and chewing of xylitol gum can reduce the risk of developing dental caries and periodontal infection.[41] Written reminders can serve as a key aid for older patients who forget to brush their teeth because of memory loss associated with Alzheimer's disease. Because many older individuals may have never been taught to clean their teeth effectively, the dentist must instruct them in proper oral hygiene procedures to be performed after each meal.

Financial and social barriers also prevent older individuals from seeking oral health care. Although as a group, older adults enjoy greater financial resources, many are on restricted budgets and are faced with tough decisions regarding the spending of limited resources. Transportation is another issue for older patients who no longer drive.

A unique aspect of aging is an increasing reliance on caregivers to assist with activities of daily living. As a result, the dentist must work with caregivers who provide dental care for patients in the home, assisted living facility, nursing home, and hospital settings. The dental professional may need to spend more time educating and training the caregiver, rather than the patient, in the importance of oral hygiene and effective plaque removal techniques.

Treatment Plan Approval

As mentioned earlier, informed consent has become an integral part of contemporary dental practice.[43] One aspect of informed consent is to provide patients with the necessary information about the alternative therapies available to manage their oral conditions. For nearly all conditions, usually more than one treatment alternative is available. These alternatives, with their advantages and disadvantages, should be presented to the patient. In addition, the patient should be informed of the risks associated with each alternative therapy. Often, a reasonable alternative is *not* to intervene but, instead, to monitor the condition or, in the case of caries lesions, attempt remineralization. Finally, the cost of treatment alternatives should be discussed with the patient. Treatment can proceed when the dentist is sure that the patient has a full and complete understanding of the alternative treatments, their associated risks and benefits, and the results of possible non-treatment.[44,45]

Summary

Proper diagnosis and treatment planning play a crucial role in the quality of dental care. Each patient must be evaluated individually in a thorough and systematic fashion. After the patient's condition is understood and recorded, a treatment plan can be developed and rendered. A successful treatment plan carefully integrates and sequences all necessary procedures indicated for the patient. Few absolutes exist in treatment planning; the available information must be considered carefully and incorporated into a plan that fits the needs of the individual. Patients should have an active role in the process; they should be informed of the findings, advised of the risks and benefits of the proposed treatment, and given the opportunity to decide the course of treatment. Examination, diagnosis, and treatment planning can be challenging but are rewarding for both the patient and the dentist if done thoroughly and properly with the patient's best interests in mind.

References

1. Sackett DL, Rosenberg WM, Gray JA, et al: Evidence-based medicine: What it is and what it isn't. *Br Med J* 312:71–72, 1996.
2. Christensen GJ: Magnification in dentistry: Useful tool or another gimmick? *J Am Dent Assoc* 134:1647–1650, 2003.
3. Fitch DR, Boyd WJ, McCoy RB, et al: Amalgam repair of cast gold crown margins: A microleakage assessment. *Gen Dent* 30:328–333, 1982.
4. Simons D, Brailsford SR, Kidd EA, et al: The effect of medicated chewing gums and oral health in frail elderly people: A one-year clinical trial. *J Am Geriatr Soc* 50:1348–1353, 2002.
5. Kidd EAM, Ricketts DN, Pitts NB: Occlusal caries diagnosis: A changing challenge for clinicians and epidemiologists. *J Dent* 21:323–331, 1993.
6. Lussi A: Validity of diagnostic and treatment decisions of fissure caries. *Caries Res* 25:296–303, 1991.
7. Penning C, van Amerongen JP, Seef RE, et al: Validity of probing for fissure caries diagnosis. *Caries Res* 26:445–449, 1992.
8. Pretty I, Maupome G: A closer look at diagnosis in clinical dental practice: Part 1. Reliablity, validity, specificity, and sensitivity of diagnostic procedures. *J Can Dent Assoc* 70:251–255, 2004.
9. Ekstrand K Qvist V, Thylstrup A: Light microscope study of the effect of probing occlusal surfaces. *Caries Res* 21:368–374, 1987.
10. Yassin OM: In vitro studies of the effect of a dental explorer on the formation of an artificial carious lesion. *J Dent Child* 62:111–117, 1995.
11. Ashley PF, Blinkhorn AS, Davies RM: Occlusal caries diagnosis: An in vitro histological validation of the Electronic Caries Monitor (ECM) and other methods. *J Dent* 26:83–88, 1998.
12. Kidd EA, Joyston-Bechal S, Beighton D: Diagnosis of secondary caries: A laboratory study. *Br Dent J* 176:135–139, 1994.

13. Bader JD, Shugars DA: Systematic review of selected dental caries diagnostic and management methods. *J Dent Educ* 65:960–968, 2001.
14. Hintze H, Wenzel A, Danielsen B, et al: Reliability of visual examination, fiber-optic transillumination, and bite-wing radiography, and reproducibility of direct visual examination following tooth separation for the identification of cavitated carious lesions in contacting approximal surfaces. *Caries Res* 32:204–209, 1998.
15. Forgie A: Magnification: What is available, and will it aid your clinical practice? *Dent Update* 28:125–130, 2001.
16. Katz RV: The clinical identification of root caries. *Gerodontology* 5:21–24, 1986.
17. Newwitter DS, Katz RV, Clive JM: Detection of root caries: Sensitivity and specificity of a modified explorer. *Gerodontics* 1:65–67, 1985.
18. Newbrun E: Problems in caries diagnosis. *Int Dent J* 43:133–142, 1993.
19. Ferreira-Zandona AG, Analoui M, Beiswanger BB, et al: An in vitro comparison between laser fluorescence and visual examination for detection of demineralization in occlusal pits and fissures. *Caries Res* 32:210–218, 1998.
20. Bader J, Shugars D: Systematic review of the performance of the DIAGNOdent device for caries detection. *J Am Dent Assoc* 135:1413–1426, 2004.
21. Kidd EAM, Joyston-Bechal S, Beighton D: Marginal ditching and staining as a predictor of secondary caries around amalgam restorations: A clinical and microbiological study. *J Dent Res* 74:1206–1211, 1995.
22. Mjor IA: Frequency of secondary caries at various anatomical locations. *Oper Dent* 10:88–92, 1985.
23. Grippo JO: Abfractions: A new classification of hard tissue lesions of teeth. *J Esthet Dent* 3:14–19, 1991.
24. Bader JD, Shugars DA, Sturdevant JR: Consequences of posterior cusp fracture. *Gen Dent* 52:128–131, 2004.
25. Bader JD, Shugars DA, Martin JA: Risk indicators for posterior tooth fracture. *J Am Dent Assoc* 135:883–892, 2004.
26. Fasbinder DJ: Treatment planner's toolkit. *Gen Dent* 47:35–39, 1999.
27. American Dental Association Council: *Access, Prevention and Interprofessional Relations: Providing dental care in long-term dental care facilities: A resource manual*, Chicago, 1997, American Dental Association.
28. Matteson SR, Joseph LP, Bottomley W, et al: The report of the panel to develop radiographic selection criteria for dental patients. *Gen Dent* 39:264–270, 1991.
29. Dove SB: Radiographic diagnosis of caries. *J Dent Educ* 65:985–990, 2001.
30. Axelsson P: *Diagnosis and risk prediction of dental caries*, Chicago, 2000, Quintessence Publishing.
31. Sturdevant JR, Bader JD, Shugars DA, et al: A simple method to estimate restoration volume as a possible predictor for tooth fracture. *J Prosthet Dent* 90:162–167, 2003.
32. American Dental Association Council: Access, Prevention and Interprofessional Relations: Caries diagnosis and risk assessment: A review of preventive strategies and management. *J Am Dent Assoc* 126(Special Suppl), 1995.
33. Madison M, Wilcox LR: An evaluation of coronal microleakage in endodontically-treated teeth: Part III. In vivo study. *J Endod* 14:455–458, 1998.
34. Hamilton JC, Dennison JB, Stoffers KW, et al: Early treatment of incipient carious lesions: a two-year clinical evaluation. *J Am Dent Assoc* 133:1643–1651, 2002.
35. Downer MC, Azli NA, Bedi R, et al: How long do routine dental restorations last? A systematic review. *Br Dent J* 187:432–439, 1999.
36. Brantley CF, Bader JD, Shugars DA, et al: Does the cycle of rerestoration lead to larger restorations? *J Am Dent Assoc* 126:1407–1413, 1995.
37. Strassler HE, Syme SE, Serio F, et al: Enhanced visualization during dental practice using magnification systems. *Compend Cont Educ Dent* 19:595–612, 1998.
38. Mertz-Fairhurst EJ, Call-Smith KM, Shuster GS, et al: Clinical performance of sealed composite restorations placed over caries compared with sealed and unsealed amalgam restorations. *J Am Dent Assoc* 115:689–694, 1987.
39. Anusavice K: Criteria for placement and replacement of dental restorations: An international consensus report. *Int Dent J* 38:193–194, 1988.
40. DeBiase CB, Austin SL: Oral health and older adults. *J Dent Hyg* 77:125–145, 2003.
41. Winkler S, Garg AK, Mekayarajjananonth T, et al: Depressed taste and smell in geriatric patients. *J Am Dent Assoc* 130:1759–1765, 1999.
42. Ettinger RL: The unique oral health needs of an aging population. *Dent Clin North Am* 41:633–649, 1997.
43. Sfikas PM: Informed consent and the law. *J Am Dent Assoc* 129:1471–1473, 1998.
44. Christensen GJ: Educating patients: A new necessity. *J Am Dent Assoc* 124:86–87, 1993.
45. Christensen GJ: Educating patients about dental procedures. *J Am Dent Assoc* 126:371–372, 1995.

Fundamental Concepts of Enamel and Dentin Adhesion

Jorge Perdigão, Edward J. Swift, Jr., Ricardo Walter

Basic Concepts of Adhesion

The American Society for Testing and Materials (specification D 907) defines adhesion as "the state in which two surfaces are held together by interfacial forces which may consist of valence forces or interlocking forces or both."[1] The word adhesion comes from the Latin *adhaerere* ("to stick to"). An adhesive is a material, frequently a viscous fluid, that joins two substrates together by solidifying and transferring a load from one surface to the other. Adhesion or adhesive strength is the measure of the load-bearing capacity of an adhesive joint.[2] Four different mechanisms of adhesion have been described, as follows:[3]

1. *Mechanical adhesion*—interlocking of the adhesive with irregularities in the surface of the substrate, or adherend
2. *Adsorption adhesion*—chemical bonding between the adhesive and the adherend; the forces involved may be primary (ionic and covalent) or secondary (hydrogen bonds, dipole interaction, or van der Waals) valence forces
3. *Diffusion adhesion*—interlocking between mobile molecules, such as the adhesion of two polymers through diffusion of polymer chain ends across an interface
4. *Electrostatic adhesion*—an electrical double layer at the interface of a metal with a polymer that is part of the total bonding mechanism

In dentistry, bonding of resin-based materials to tooth structure is a result of four possible mechanisms, as follows:[4]

1. *Mechanical*—penetration of resin and formation of resin tags within the tooth surface
2. *Adsorption*—chemical bonding to the inorganic component (hydroxyapatite) or organic components (mainly type I collagen) of tooth structure
3. *Diffusion*—precipitation of substances on the tooth surfaces to which resin monomers can bond mechanically or chemically
4. A *combination* of the previous three mechanisms

For good adhesion, close contact must exist between the adhesive and the substrate (enamel or dentin). The surface tension of the adhesive must be lower than the surface energy of the substrate. Failures of adhesive joints occur in three locations, which are generally combined when an actual failure occurs: (1) cohesive failure in the substrate; (2) cohesive failure within the adhesive; and (3) adhesive failure, or failure at the interface of substrate and adhesive.

A major problem in bonding resins to tooth structure is that all methacrylate-based dental resins shrink during free-radical addition polymerization.[5] Dental adhesives must provide a strong initial bond to resist the stresses of resin shrinkage.

Trends in Restorative Dentistry

The introduction of enamel bonding, the increasing demand for restorative and nonrestorative esthetic treatments, and the ubiquity of fluoride have combined to transform the practice of operative dentistry.[6,7] The classic concepts of tooth preparation were advocated in the early 1900s;[8] but these have changed drastically. This transformation in philosophy has resulted in a more conservative approach to tooth preparation, with regard to not only the basic concepts of retention form but also the resistance form of the remaining tooth structure. Bonding techniques allow more conservative tooth preparations, less reliance on macromechanical retention, and less removal of unsupported enamel.

The availability of new scientific information on the etiology, diagnosis, and treatment of carious lesions and the introduction of reliable adhesive restorative materials have substantially reduced the need for extensive tooth preparations. With improvements in materials, indications for resin-based

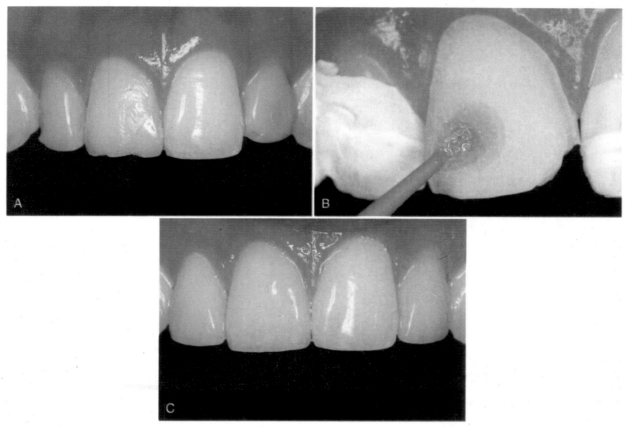

Fig. 4-1 **A,** Pre-operative view of anterior teeth in a 24-year-old patient with defective composite restorations. The treatment plan included bonded porcelain veneers on teeth #7, #8, and #10 to match the natural aspect of tooth #9. **B,** Porcelain veneers were bonded with a two-step etch-and-rinse adhesive and a light-activated resin cement. **C,** Final aspect 1 week after the bonding procedure.

materials have progressively shifted from the anterior segment only to posterior teeth as well. Adhesive restorative techniques currently are used to accomplish the following:

1. Restore Class I, II, III, IV, V, and VI carious or traumatic defects
2. Change the shape and the color of anterior teeth (e.g., with full or partial resin veneers)
3. Improve retention for porcelain-fused-to-metal (ceramometal) or metallic crowns
4. Bond all-ceramic restorations (Fig. 4-1)
5. Seal pits and fissures
6. Bond orthodontic brackets
7. Bond periodontal splints and conservative tooth-replacement prostheses
8. Repair existing restorations (composite, amalgam, ceramic, or ceramometal)
9. Provide foundations for crowns
10. Desensitize exposed root surfaces
11. Seal beneath or bond amalgam restorations to tooth structure
12. Impregnate dentin that has been exposed to the oral fluids, making it less susceptible to caries
13. Bond fractured fragments of anterior teeth (Fig. 4-2)
14. Bond prefabricated fiber or metal posts and cast posts
15. Reinforce fragile endodontically treated roots internally
16. Seal root canals during endodontic therapy
17. Seal apical restorations placed during endodontic surgery

Enamel Adhesion

Inspired by the industrial use of 85% phosphoric acid to facilitate adhesion of paints and resins to metallic surfaces, Buonocore envisioned the use of acids to etch enamel for sealing pits and fissures.[6] Since Buonocore's introduction of the acid-etch technique, many dental researchers have attempted to achieve methods for reliable and durable adhesion between resins and tooth structure.

Acid-etching transforms the smooth enamel into an irregular surface (Fig. 4-3) and increases its surface free energy. When a fluid resin-based material is applied to the irregular etched surface, the resin penetrates into the surface, aided by capillary action. Monomers in the material polymerize, and the material becomes interlocked with the enamel surface (Fig. 4-4).[9,10] The formation of resin microtags within the enamel surface is the fundamental mechanism of resin-enamel adhesion.[10-12] Figure 4-5 shows a replica of an etched enamel surface visualized through the extensions of resin that penetrated the irregular enamel surface. The acid-etch technique has revolutionized the practice of restorative dentistry.

Enamel etching results in three different micromorphologic patterns.[13,14] The type I pattern involves the dissolution of

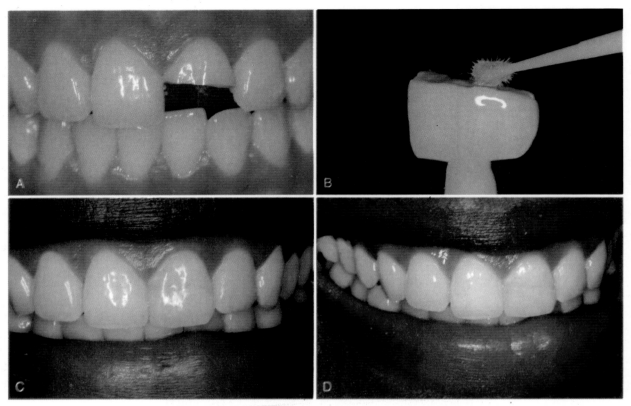

Fig. 4-2 **A,** Intraoral frontal view of a 20-year-old female presenting with complicated crown fracture on tooth #9 after endodontic treatment. The fracture extends subgingivally on the mesial aspect of the lingual surface. **B,** A total-etch, two-step, ethanol-based adhesive applied to the crown fragment and tooth. **C,** Extraoral view 6 months after rebonding. **D,** Extraoral view 3 years after rebonding. *(From Macedo GV, Ritter AV: Essentials of rebonding tooth fragments for the best functional and esthetic outcomes, Pediatr Dent 31(2):110–116, 2009.)*

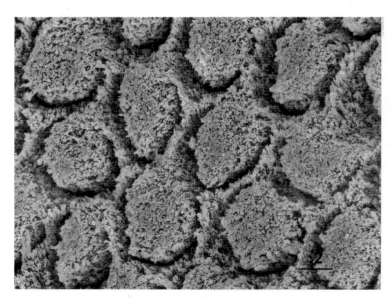

Fig. 4-3 Scanning electron micrograph (SEM) of enamel etched with 35% phosphoric acid for 15 seconds.

prism cores without dissolution of prism peripheries (Fig. 4-6, *A*). The type II etching pattern is the opposite of type I: the peripheral enamel is dissolved, but the cores are left intact (see Fig. 4-3). Type III etching is less distinct than the other two patterns. It includes areas that resemble the other patterns and

areas whose topography is not related to enamel prism morphology (see Fig. 4-6, *B*).

Beginning with Buonocore's use of 85% phosphoric acid, various concentrations of phosphoric acid have been used to etch enamel. Most current phosphoric acid gels have

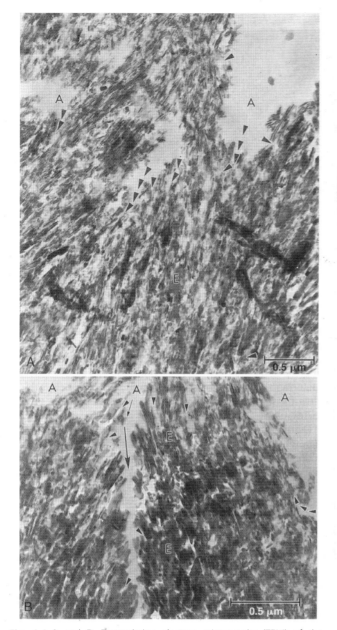

Fig. 4-4 **A** and **B,** Transmission electron micrographs (TEM) of the enamel-adhesive interface after application of Adper Single Bond (3M ESPE) as per manufacturer's instructions. Acid-etching with 35% phosphoric acid opened spaces between enamel prisms (*arrows*), allowing the permeation of resin monomers between the crystallites (*arrowheads*). *A*, adhesive; *E*, enamel.

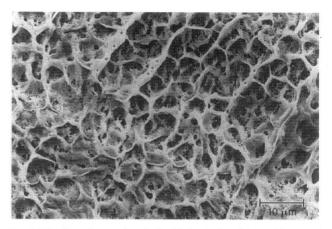

Fig. 4-5 Replica of enamel etched with 35% phosphoric acid. Enamel was dissolved completely in 6N hydrochloric acid for 24 hours. The resin extensions correspond to the interprismatic spaces (*asterisks*).

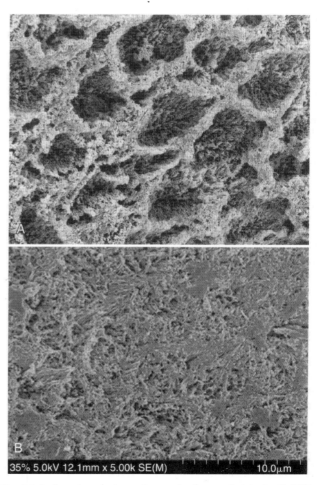

Fig. 4-6 **A,** Scanning electron micrograph of enamel etched with 35% phosphoric acid for 15 seconds, denoting a type I etching pattern. **B,** Scanning electron micrograph of enamel etched with 35% phosphoric acid for 15 seconds, denoting a type III etching pattern.

concentrations of 30% to 40%, with 37% being the most common, although some studies using lower concentrations have reported similar adhesion values.[15-17]

An etching time of 60 seconds originally was recommended for permanent enamel using 30% to 40% phosphoric acid. Although one study concluded that shorter etch times resulted in lower bond strengths, other studies using scanning electron microscopy (SEM) showed that a 15-second etch resulted in a similar surface roughness as that provided by a 60-second etch.[11,18-20] Other in vitro studies have shown similar bond

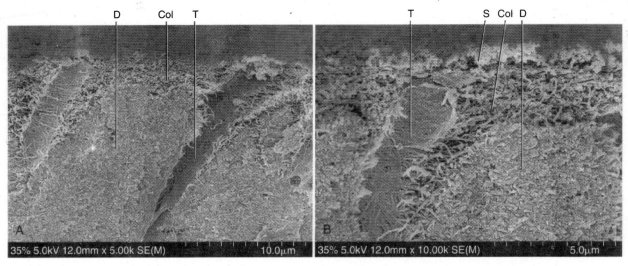

Fig. 4-7 A, Dentin etched with 35% phosphoric acid. **B,** Higher magnification view of etched dentin. *Col,* collagen exposed by the acid; *D,* normal dentin; *T,* dentinal tubule; *S,* residual silica particles used as acid gel thickener.

strengths and leakage for etching times of 15 and 60 seconds.[21-25]

As measured in the laboratory, shear bond strengths of composite to phosphoric acid-etched enamel usually exceed 20 megapascals (MPa) and can range up to over 50 MPa, depending on the test method used.[26-29] Such bond strengths provide adequate retention for a broad variety of procedures and prevent leakage around enamel margins of restorations.[24]

Dentin Adhesion

The classic concepts of operative dentistry were challenged in the 1980s and 1990s by the introduction of new adhesive techniques, first for enamel and then for dentin. Nevertheless, adhesion to dentin remains difficult. Adhesive materials can interact with dentin in different ways—mechanically, chemically, or both.[7,9,30-33] The importance of micromechanical bonding, similar to what occurs in enamel bonding, has become accepted.[30,34,35] Dentin adhesion relies primarily on the penetration of adhesive monomers into the network of collagen fibers left exposed by acid etching (Fig. 4-7).[35,36] However, for adhesive materials that do not require etching, such as glass ionomer cements and some phosphate-based self-etch adhesives, chemical bonding between polycarboxylic or phosphate monomers and hydroxyapatite has been shown to be an important part of the bonding mechanism.[32,37,38] Contemporary strategies for bonding to dentin are summarized in Table 4-1.

Challenges in Dentin Bonding
Substrate

Bonding to enamel is a relatively simple process, without major technical requirements or difficulties. Bonding to dentin presents a much greater challenge. Several factors account for this difference between enamel and dentin bonding. Enamel is a highly mineralized tissue composed of more than 90% (by volume) hydroxyapatite, whereas dentin contains a substantial proportion of water and organic material, primarily type I collagen (Fig. 4-8). Dentin also contains a dense network of tubules that connect the pulp with the

dentinoenamel junction (DEJ) (Fig. 4-9). A cuff of hypermineralized dentin called *peritubular dentin* lines the tubules. The less mineralized intertubular dentin contains collagen fibrils with the characteristic collagen banding (Fig. 4-10). Intertubular dentin is penetrated by submicron channels, which allow the passage of tubular liquid and fibers between neighboring tubules, forming intertubular anastomoses.

Dentin is an intrinsically hydrated tissue, penetrated by a maze of fluid-filled tubules. Movement of fluid from the pulp to the DEJ is a result of a slight but constant pulpal pressure.[39] Pulpal pressure has a magnitude of 25-30 mm Hg or 34 to 40 cm H_2O.[40,41]

Dentinal tubules enclose cellular extensions from the odontoblasts and are in direct communication with the pulp (Fig. 4-11). Inside the tubule lumen, other fibrous organic structures such as the lamina limitans are present, which substantially decreases the functional radius of the tubule. The relative area occupied by dentin tubules decreases with increasing distance from the pulp. The number of tubules decreases from about 45,000/mm^2 close to the pulp to about 20,000/mm^2 near the DEJ.[42] The tubules occupy an area of only 1% of the total surface near the DEJ, whereas they occupy 22% of the surface close to the pulp.[43] The average tubule diameter ranges from 0.63 μm at the periphery to 2.37 μm near the pulp.[44]

Adhesion can be affected by the remaining dentin thickness after tooth preparation. Bond strengths are generally less in deep dentin than in superficial dentin.[45-47] Nevertheless, some dentin adhesives, including one-step self-etch adhesives, do not seem to be affected by dentin depth.[48]

Whenever tooth structure is prepared with a bur or other instrument, residual organic and inorganic components form a "smear layer" of debris on the surface.[49,50] The smear layer fills the orifices of dentin tubules, forming "smear plugs" (Fig. 4-12), and decreases dentin permeability by nearly 90%.[51] The composition of the smear layer is basically hydroxyapatite and altered denatured collagen. This altered collagen can acquire a gelatinized consistency because of the friction and heat created by the preparation procedure.[52] Submicron porosity of the smear layer still allows for diffusion of dentinal fluid.[53] Removal of the smear layer and smear plugs with acidic

Table 4-1 Current Strategies for Adhesion of Resins to Dentin

	Etchant (E)	Primer (P)	Bonding Agent (B)
Three-step etch-and-rinse* E + P + B	Removes the smear layer Exposes intertubular and peritubular collagen Opens the tubules in a funnel configuration Decreases surface free energy	Includes bifunctional molecules (simultaneously hydrophilic and hydrophobic) Envelops the external surface of collagen fibrils Re-establishes surface free energy to levels compatible with a more hydrophobic restorative material	Includes monomers that are mostly hydrophobic, such as Bis-GMA; however, can contain a small percentage of hydrophilic monomers, such as HEMA Co-polymerizes with the primer molecules Penetrates and polymerizes into the interfibrillar spaces to serve as a structural backbone to the hybrid layer
Two-step etch-and-rinse E + [PB]	Removes the smear layer Exposes intertubular and peritubular collagen Opens tubules in a funnel configuration Decreases surface free energy	Penetrates into the dentin tubules to form resin tags The first coat applied on etched dentin works as a primer—it increases the surface free energy of dentin The second coat (and third, fourth, and so on) acts as the bonding agent used in three-step systems—it fills the spaces between the dense network of collagen fibers	
Two-step self-etch [EP] + B	Enamel etch is typically shallow The self-etching primer (SEP) does not remove the smear layer, but fixes it and exposes about 0.5–1 μm of intertubular collagen because of its acidity (pH = 1.2–2.0) The smear plug is impregnated with acidic monomers, but it is not removed; some SEP monomers bond chemically to dentin When it impregnates the smear plug, the SEP prepares the pathway for the penetration of the subsequently placed fluid resin into the microchannels that permeate the smear plug	Uses the same type of bonding agent included in the three-step, etch-and-rinse systems The resin tags form on resin penetration into the microchannels of the primer-impregnated smear plug	
One-step self-etch [EPB]	Etches enamel, but etch pattern is typically shallow Incorporates the smear layer into interface Being an aqueous solution of a phosphonated monomer, it demineralizes and penetrates dentin simultaneously, leaving a precipitate on the hybrid layer Forms a thin layer of adhesive, leading to low bond strengths; a multi-coat approach is recommended; an extra layer of a hydrophobic bonding resin improves bond strengths and clinical performance Incompatible with self-cure composite resins unless coated with an hydrophobic bonding resin		

*Although the meaning of the two terms is the same, the term "etch-and-rinse" is preferred over "total-etch."

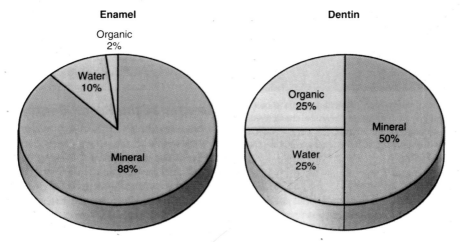

Fig. 4-8 Composition of enamel and dentin by volume percent.

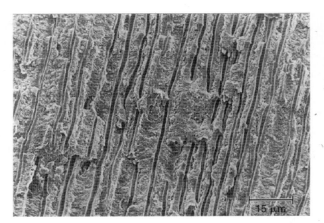

Fig. 4-9 Scanning electron micrograph of dentin that was fractured longitudinally to show dentinal tubules.

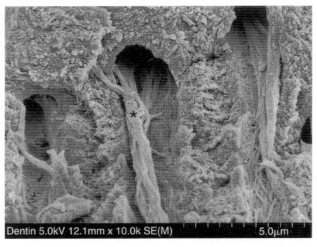

Fig. 4-11 Scanning electron micrograph of deep dentin displaying an odontoblastic process in a dentinal tubule (*asterisk*).

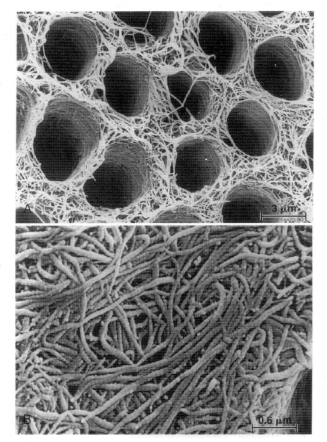

Fig. 4-10 **A,** Scanning electron micrograph of etched dentin showing exposed collagen fibers. **B,** Higher magnification shows the characteristic collagen banding in intertubular collagen. Superficial collagen was dissolved by collagenase to remove the most superficial collagen fibers that were damaged by tooth preparation.

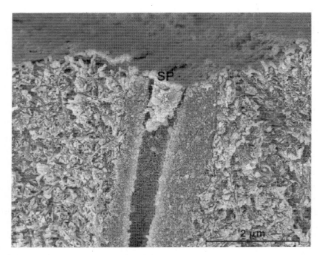

Fig. 4-12 Scanning electron micrograph of a smear plug blocking the entrance of a dentinal tubule. *SP,* smear plug.

pulpal pressure and fluid flow in the tubules, factors such as the radius and length of the tubules, the viscosity of dentin fluid, the pressure gradient, the molecular size of the substances dissolved in the tubular fluid, and the rate of removal of substances by the blood vessels in the pulp affect permeability. All of these variables make dentin a dynamic substrate and consequently a difficult substrate for bonding.[43,55]

Stresses at the Resin–Dentin Interface

Composites shrink as they polymerize, creating considerable stresses within the composite mass, depending on the configuration of the preparation.[56-59] When the composite is bonded to one surface only (e.g., for a direct facial veneer), stresses within the composite are relieved by flow from the unbonded surface. Stress relief within a three-dimensional bonded restoration is limited, however, by its configuration factor (C-factor).[60] In an occlusal preparation, composite is bonded to five tooth surfaces—mesial, distal, buccal, lingual, and pulpal. The occlusal surface of the composite is the only "free" or unrestrained surface. In such a situation, the ratio

solutions results in an increase of the fluid flow onto the exposed dentin surface. This fluid can interfere with adhesion because hydrophobic resins do not adhere to hydrophilic substrates, even if resin tags are formed in the dentin tubules.[49,54]

Several additional factors affect dentin permeability. Besides the use of vasoconstrictors in local anesthetics, which decrease between the number of bonded surfaces and the number of unbonded surfaces is 5 : 1, giving the restoration a configuration factor = 5. Stress relief is limited because flow can occur only from the single free surface.[60,61]

Unrelieved stresses in the composite contribute to internal bond disruption and marginal gaps around restorations that increase microleakage and potential postoperative sensitivity.[62] The C-factor might be partially responsible for the decrease in bond strengths observed when deep dentin is bonded as part of a three-dimensional preparation.[63]

It has been reported that immediate bond strengths of approximately 17 MPa are necessary to resist the contraction stresses that develop in the composite during polymerization, to prevent marginal debonding.[58,64] Water absorption by the resin might compensate for the effect of the polymerization shrinkage, as the resin might expand and seal off marginal gaps, but this occurs only over a relatively long time.[65] Water absorption is directly proportional to the resin content.[66]

Enamel bond strengths usually are sufficient to prevent the formation of marginal gaps by polymerization contraction stresses. These stresses might, however, be powerful enough to cause enamel defects at the margins.[67] Extension of the enamel cavosurface bevel helps improve the enamel peripheral seal.[56,68]

Each time a restoration is exposed to wide temperature variations in the oral environment (e.g., drinking coffee and eating ice cream), the restoration undergoes volumetric changes of different magnitude compared with those of the tooth structure. This occurs because the linear coefficient of thermal expansion of the composite is about four times greater than that of the tooth structure. Microleakage around dentin margins is potentiated by this discrepancy in linear coefficient of thermal expansion between the restoration and the substrate.[69]

Loading and unloading of restored teeth can result in transitional or permanent interfacial gaps.[70] Additionally, the tooth substrate itself might be weakened by cyclic loading.[71] A study found that 71% of Class V composite restorations in third molars with antagonists have significantly more leakage than restorations placed in teeth without opposing contact.[72] Another study found that cyclic loading and preparation configuration significantly reduced the bond strengths of self-etch and etch-and-rinse adhesives.[73,74]

Development
Beginning

During the 1950s, it was reported that a resin containing glycerophosphoric acid dimethacrylate (GPDM) could bond to a hydrochloric acid–etched dentin surface.[75] (*Note:* A complete listing of the chemical names mentioned in this chapter is provided in Table 4-2.) The bond strengths of this primitive adhesion technique were severely reduced by immersion in water. A few years before that report, another researcher had used the same monomer chemically activated with sulfinic acid, and that combination would later be known commercially as Sevriton Cavity Seal (Amalgamated Dental Company, London, England).[76,77]

First Generation

The development of the surface-active co-monomer NPG-GMA was the basis for Cervident (S.S. White Burs, Inc.,

Table 4-2 Abbreviations Commonly Used in Dentin/Enamel Adhesion Literature and in This Chapter

Abbreviation	Chemical Name
Bis-GMA	Bisphenol-glycidyl methacrylate
EDTA	Ethylenediamine tetra-acetic acid
GPDM	Glycerophosphoric acid dimethacrylate
HEMA	2-Hydroxyethyl methacrylate
10-MDP	10-Methacryloyloxy decyl dihydrogen phosphate
4-META	4-Methacryloxyethyl trimellitate anhydride
MMEP	Mono (2-methacryloxy) ethyl phthalate
NPG-GMA	N-phenylglycine glycidyl methacrylate
PENTA	Dipentaerythritol penta-acrylate monophosphate
Phenyl-P	2-(Methacryloxy) ethyl phenyl hydrogen phosphate

Lakewood, NJ), which is considered the first-generation dentin bonding system.[31,78] Theoretically, this comonomer could chelate with calcium on the tooth surface to generate water-resistant chemical bonds of resin to dentinal calcium.[79,80] The in vitro dentin bond strengths of this material were, however, in the range of only 2 to 3 MPa.[81] Likewise, the in vivo results were discouraging; Cervident had poor clinical results when used to restore non-carious cervical lesions without mechanical retention.[82]

Second Generation

In 1978, the Clearfil Bond System F[c] was introduced in Japan (Kuraray Co., Ltd., Osaka, Japan). Generally recognized as the first product of the second-generation of dentin adhesives, it was a phosphate-ester material (phenyl-P and hydroxyethyl methacrylate [HEMA] in ethanol). Its mechanism of action was based on the polar interaction between negatively charged phosphate groups in the resin and positively charged calcium ions in the smear layer.[81] The smear layer was the weakest link in the system because of its relatively loose attachment to the dentin surface. Examination of both sides of failed bonds revealed the presence of smear layer debris.[83]

Several other phosphate-ester dentin bonding systems were introduced in the early 1980s, including Scotchbond (3M EPSE Dental Products, St. Paul, MN), Bondlite (Kerr Corporation, Orange, CA), and Prisma·Universal Bond (DENTSPLY Caulk, Milford, DE). These second-generation dentin bonding systems typically had in vitro bond strengths of only 1 to 5 MPa, which was considerably below the 10 MPa value estimated as the threshold value for acceptable in vivo retention.[9,52] In addition to the problems caused by the loosely attached smear layer, these resins were relatively devoid of hydrophilic groups and had large contact angles on intrinsically moist surfaces.[84] They did not wet dentin well, did not penetrate the entire depth of the smear layer, and, therefore, could not reach the superficial dentin to establish ionic bonding or resin extensions into the dentinal tubules.[52]

Whatever bonding did occur was due to interaction with calcium ions in the smear layer.[85]

The in vitro performance of second-generation adhesives after 6 months was unacceptable.[86] The bonding material tended to peel from the dentin surface after water storage, indicating that the interface between dentin and some types of chlorophosphate ester–based materials was unstable.[86,87] The in vivo performance of these materials was found to be clinically unacceptable 2 years after placement in cervical tooth preparations without additional retention, such as beveling and acid-etching.[88,89]

Third Generation

The concept of phosphoric acid-etching of dentin before application of a phosphate ester-type bonding agent was introduced by Fusayama et al in 1979.[90] Because of the hydrophobic nature of the bonding resin, however, acid-etching did not produce a significant improvement in dentin bond strengths, despite the flow of the resin into the open dentinal tubules.[54,91] Pulpal inflammatory responses were thought to be triggered by the application of acid on dentin surfaces, providing another reason to avoid etching.[92,93] Nevertheless, continuing the etched dentin philosophy, Kuraray introduced Clearfil New Bond in 1984. This phosphate-based material contained HEMA and a 10-carbon molecule known as *10-MDP*, which includes long hydrophobic and short hydrophilic components.[79]

Most other third-generation materials were designed not to remove the entire smear layer but, rather, to modify it and allow penetration of acidic monomers, such as phenyl-P or PENTA. Despite promising laboratory results, some of the bonding mechanisms never resulted in satisfactory clinical results.[89,94]

Treatment of the smear layer with acidic primers was proposed using an aqueous solution of 2.5% maleic acid, 55% HEMA, and a trace of methacrylic acid (Scotchbond 2, 3M ESPE Dental Products).[79] Scotchbond 2 was the first dentin bonding system to receive "provisional" and "full acceptance" from the American Dental Association (ADA).[95] With this type of smear layer treatment, manufacturers effectively combined the dentin etching philosophy advocated in Japan with the more cautious approach advocated in Europe and the United States. The result was preservation of a modified smear layer with slight demineralization of the underlying intertubular dentin surface. Clinical results were mixed, with some reports of good performance and some reports of poor performance.[88,89]

The removal of the smear layer using chelating agents such as EDTA was recommended in the original Gluma system (Bayer Dental, Leverkusen, Germany) before the application of a primer solution of 5% glutaraldehyde and 35% HEMA in water. The effectiveness of this system might have been impaired, however, by the manufacturer's questionable recommendation of placing the composite over uncured unfilled resin.[89]

Current Options for Resin–Dentin Bonding
Three-Step Etch-and-Rinse Adhesives

Although the smear layer acts as a "diffusion barrier" that reduces the permeability of dentin, it also can be considered an obstacle that must be removed to permit resin bonding to the underlying dentin substrate.[51] Based on that consideration, a fourth generation of dentin adhesives was introduced for use on acid-etched dentin.[96] Removal of the smear layer via acid-etching led to significant improvements in the in vitro bond strengths of resins to dentin.[97-100] Because the clinical technique involves simultaneous application of an acid to enamel and dentin, this method was originally known as the "total-etch" technique. Now more commonly called *etch-and-rinse technique*, it was the most popular strategy for dentin bonding during the 1990s and remains somewhat popular today (Fig. 4-13).

Application of acid to dentin results in partial or total removal of the smear layer and demineralization of the underlying dentin.[90] Acids demineralize intertubular and peritubular dentin, open the dentin tubules, and expose a dense filigree of collagen fibers (see Fig. 4-7), increasing the microporosity of the intertubular dentin (Fig. 4-14).[35,101] Dentin is demineralized by up to approximately 7.5 μm, depending on the type of acid, application time, and concentration.[35,101]

Despite the obvious penetration of early adhesives into the dentinal tubules, etching did not result in a significant improvement in bond strengths, possibly as a result of the hydrophobic nature of the phosphonated resin.[91] On the basis of concerns about the potential for inflammatory pulpal responses, acids were believed to be contraindicated for direct application on dentin, and the total-etch technique was not readily accepted in Europe or the United States. Adhesive systems based on the total-etch philosophy have proved successful, however, in vitro and in vivo.[89,102-104] Laboratory shear bond strengths usually vary from 17 to 30 MPa, which are similar to the values typically obtained on enamel.

Adhesive systems such as All-Bond 2 and All-Bond 3 (Bisco, Inc., Schaumburg, IL), OptiBond FL (Kerr Corporation), and Scotchbond Multi-Purpose (3M ESPE) are described by some authors as fourth-generation adhesives. However, because they include three essential components that are applied sequentially, they are more accurately described as three-step etch-and-rinse systems. The three essential components are (1) a phosphoric acid–etching gel that is rinsed off; (2) a primer containing reactive hydrophilic monomers in ethanol, acetone, or water; and (3) an unfilled or filled resin bonding agent. Some authors refer to this third step as *adhesive*. It contains hydrophobic monomers such as Bis-GMA, frequently combined with hydrophilic molecules such as HEMA.

The acid-etching step not only alters the mineral content of the dentin substrate but also changes its surface free energy.[33,96] The latter is an undesirable effect because for good interfacial contact, any adhesive must have a low surface tension, and the substrate must have a high surface free energy.[34,52,87] Substrates are characterized as having low or high surface energy. Among dental materials, hydroxyapatite and glass ionomer cement filler particles are high-energy substrates, whereas collagen and composite have low-energy surfaces.[2] Consequently, dentin consists of two distinct substrates, one of high surface energy (hydroxyapatite) and one of low surface energy (collagen). After etching, the dense web of exposed collagen is a low surface energy substrate.[86] A correlation exists between the ability of an adhesive to spread on the dentin surface and the concentration of calcium on that same surface.[105] The primer in a three-step system is designed to increase the critical surface tension of dentin, and a direct correlation between

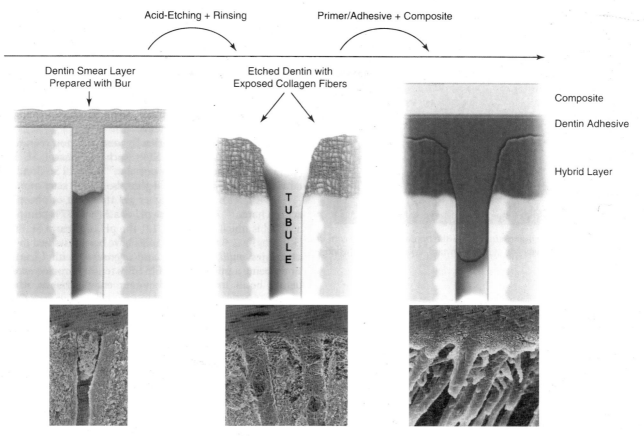

Acid-Etching + Rinsing   Primer/Adhesive + Composite

Dentin Smear Layer
Prepared with Bur

Etched Dentin with
Exposed Collagen Fibers

Composite

Dentin Adhesive

Hybrid Layer

TUBULE

Fig. 4-13 Bonding of resin to dentin using an etch-and-rinse technique.

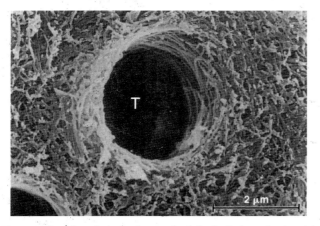

Fig. 4-14 Scanning electron micrograph of dentin that was kept moist after rinsing off the etchant. The abundant intertubular porosity serves as a pathway for the penetration of the dentin adhesive. *T*, dentinal tubule.

surface energy of dentin and shear bond strengths has been shown.[46]

When primer and bonding resin are applied to etched dentin, they penetrate the intertubular dentin, forming a resin–dentin interdiffusion zone, or hybrid layer. They also penetrate and polymerize in the open dentinal tubules, forming resin tags. For most etch-and-rinse adhesives, the ultramorphologic characterization of the transition between

the hybrid layer and the unaffected dentin suggests that an abrupt shift from hybrid tissue to mineralized tissue occurs, without any empty space or pathway that could result in leakage (Figs. 4-15 and 4-16). The demarcation line seems to consist of hydroxyapatite crystals embedded in the resin from the hybrid layer (see Fig. 4-16, *B*). For self-etch systems, the transition is more gradual, with a superficial zone of resin-impregnated smear residues and a deeper zone, close to the unaffected dentin, rich in hydroxyapatite crystals (Fig. 4-17).

Two-Step Etch-and-Rinse Adhesives

In vitro dentin bond strengths have improved so much that they approach the level of enamel bonding.[27] Therefore, much of the research and development (R&D) has focused on the simplification of the bonding procedure. A number of dental materials manufacturers are marketing a simplified, two-step etch-and-rinse adhesive system. Some authors refer to these as fifth-generation adhesives, and they are sometimes called "one-bottle" systems because they combine the primer and bonding agent into a single solution. A separate etching step still is required.

Numerous simplified bonding systems are available, including One-Step Plus (Bisco, Inc.), Prime & Bond NT (DENTSPLY Caulk), Adper Single Bond Plus (3M ESPE), OptiBond SOLO Plus (Kerr Corporation), PQ1 (Ultradent Products, South Jordan, UT), ExciTE (Ivoclar Vivadent, Schaan, Liechtenstein), Bond-1 (Pentron Clinical Technologies,

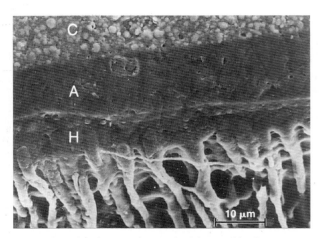

Fig. 4-15 Scanning electron micrograph of the transition between composite resin (*C*)–adhesive (*A*), adhesive–hybrid layer (*H*), and hybrid layer–dentin.

Wallingford, CT), One Coat Bond (Coltène/Whaledent Inc., Mahwah, NJ), and XP Bond (DENTSPLY Caulk).

Two-Step Self-Etch Systems

An alternative bonding strategy is the self-etch approach (Figs. 4-17 and 4-18). Some self-etch systems are most accurately described as nonrinsing conditioners or self-priming etchants. Examples include NRC Non-Rinse Conditioner (DENTSPLY DeTrey, Konstanz, Germany) and Tyrian SPE (Bisco, Inc.). NRC and Tyrian SPE required the subsequent application of a separate adhesive, the same used with the etch-and-rinse technique (Prime & Bond NT [DENTSPLY Caulk] with NRC, and One-Step Plus [Bisco, Inc.] with Tyrian SPE). Nonrinsing conditioners did not etch enamel to the same depth as phosphoric acid, and did not provide higher bond strengths or better clinical performance than phosphoric acid etchants.[106,107]

Another type of acidic conditioner was introduced in Japan—the self-etching primers (SEPs)—and has proved to be more successful. These acidic primers include a phosphonated resin molecule that performs two functions simultaneously—etching and priming of dentin and enamel. In contrast to conventional etchants, SEPs are not rinsed off. The bonding mechanism of SEPs is based on the simultaneous etching and priming of enamel and dentin, forming a continuum in the substrate and incorporating smear plugs into the resin tags (Fig. 4-19).[108,109] In addition to simplifying the bonding technique, the elimination of rinsing and drying steps reduces the possibility of over-wetting or over-drying, either of which can affect adhesion adversely.[98,99] Also, water is always a component of SEPs because it is needed for the acidic monomers to ionize and trigger demineralization of hard dental tissues; this makes SEPs less susceptible to variations in the degree of substrate moisture but more susceptible to chemical instability due to hydrolytic degradation.[110-112]

One disadvantage of SEPs that are currently available is that they do not etch enamel as well as phosphoric acid, particularly if the enamel has not been instrumented. The seal of enamel margins in vivo might be compromised.[113,114] When enamel bonds are stressed in the laboratory by thermal cycling, SEPs are more likely than etch-and-rinse systems to undergo deterioration.[115] This decrease in bond strengths with thermal fatigue might be a sign that a potential exists for enamel microleakage when SEPs are employed to bond to enamel. In a 10-year recall of an older generation SEP, 39 of 44 restorations had marginal discoloration.[116] The enamel bond strengths of some newer SEPs approach the enamel bond strengths of phosphoric acid–based adhesives, however, suggesting that SEPs are gradually being developed to replace etch-and-rinse adhesive systems.

Because they are user-friendly and do not require the etching and rinsing step, SEPs such as Clearfil SE Bond (Kuraray) have become very popular.[117] Clearfil SE Bond contains an aqueous mixture of a phosphoric acid ester monomer (10-MDP), with a much higher pH than that of phosphoric acid etchants.[118] Although the pH of a 34% to 37% phosphoric acid gel is much lower than 1.0, the pH of Clearfil SE Primer (Kuraray) is 1.9 to 2.0.[101,106] SEPs have been classified in three categories: *mild*, *moderate*, and *aggressive*, with Clearfil SE Bond being a mild SEP.[106] Mild SEPs tend to provide excellent dentin bond strengths and poorer enamel bonds, whereas more aggressive self-etch systems provide the reverse. Clearfil SE Bond resulted in 98% retention rate in Class V composite restorations at 8 years with or without separate enamel etching of the margins, which did improve marginal adaptation.[119] In posterior restorations, Clearfil SE Bond resulted in 100% retention rate at 2 years with a tendency for deterioration of the composite margins compared with the etch-and-rinse control Single Bond.[102] The clinical success of Clearfil SE Bond might be a result of its chemical composition, specifically the monomer 10-MDP. This monomer bonds chemically to hydroxyapatite by forming stable calcium-phosphate salts without causing strong decalcification. The chemical bonding formed by 10-MDP is more stable in water than that of other monomers used in the composition of self-etch adhesives, such as 4-META and phenyl-P.[120]

SEPs are less technique sensitive than are etch-and-rinse adhesives. Additionally, SEPs are less likely to result in a discrepancy between the depth of demineralization and the depth of resin infiltration because SEPs demineralize and infiltrate dentin simultaneously.[118] SEPs do not remove the smear layer from dentin completely (see Figs. 4-17 and 4-18), which is the main reason that they might result in less postoperative sensitivity compared with etch-and-rinse adhesives.[55,121]

Despite the prevailing opinion that SEPs cause less postoperative sensitivity compared with etch-and-rinse systems, the few clinical studies comparing these in posterior restorations have reported mixed results.[55,121] Nevertheless, recent clinical studies have shown no relationship between the type of adhesive and the occurrence of postoperative sensitivity.[123-129] One clinical study found no differences in postoperative sensitivity from 2 weeks to 6 months between an etch-and-rinse adhesive (Prime & Bond NT) and an SEP (Clearfil SE Bond) used in Class I and Class II composite restorations. These results suggest that the restorative technique is more important than the material itself.

One-Step Self-Etch Adhesives

Continuing the trend toward simplification, no-rinse, self-etching materials that incorporate the fundamental steps of etching, priming, and bonding into one solution have become increasingly popular. In contrast to conventional adhesive

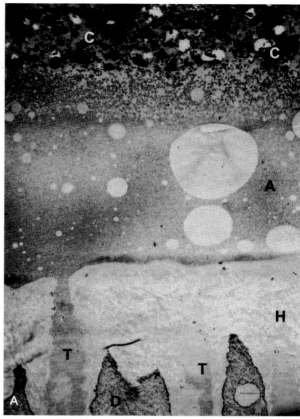

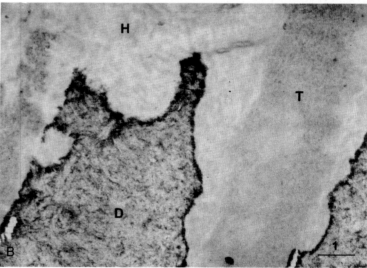

Fig. 4-16 Transmission electron micrograph of a resin–dentin interface formed by the etch-and-rinse adhesive Adper Single Bond Plus (3M ESPE). This specimen was not decalcified or stained; the unaltered dentin appears darker, and the hybrid layer appears lighter. **A,** General view showing the composite (*C*), the adhesive (*A*), the hybrid layer (*H*), a filled resin tag (*T*), and the unaffected dentin (*D*). **B,** Higher magnification of the transition between the hybrid layer and unaffected dentin. Note the filler in the resin tag as small dark dots (nanofiller).

systems that contain an intermediate light-cured, low-viscosity bonding resin to join the composite restorative material to the primed dentin–enamel substrate, these one-step self-etch or "all-in-one" adhesives contain uncured ionic monomers that contact the composite restorative material directly.[128,129] Their acidic unreacted monomers are responsible, in part, for the incompatibility between these all-in-one adhesives and self-cured composites (discussed later).[129] Additionally, one-step adhesives tend to behave as semi-permeable membranes, resulting in a hydrolytic degradation of the resin–dentin interface.[110] Because these adhesives must be acidic enough to be

able to demineralize enamel and penetrate dentin smear layers, the hydrophilicity of their resin monomers, usually organophosphates and carboxylates, also is high. Some of these resin monomers are too hydrophilic, which makes them liable to water degradation.[111,130]

Many one-step self-etch adhesives with etching, priming, and bonding functions delivered in a single solution are now available, including AdheSE One F (Ivoclar Vivadent), Adper Easy Bond (3M ESPE), All-Bond SE (Bisco Inc.), Bond Force (Tokuyama Dental, Tokyo, Japan), Clearfil S³ Bond (Kuraray), iBOND Self-Etch (Heraeus Kulzer, South Bend, IN),

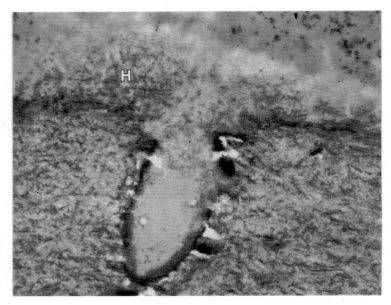

Fig. 4-17 Transmission electron micrograph of a resin–dentin interface formed with the two-step, self-etch adhesive Clearfil SE Bond (Kuraray). Residual hydroxyapatite crystals and residual components of the smear layer are embedded in the resin within the hybrid layer (*H*).

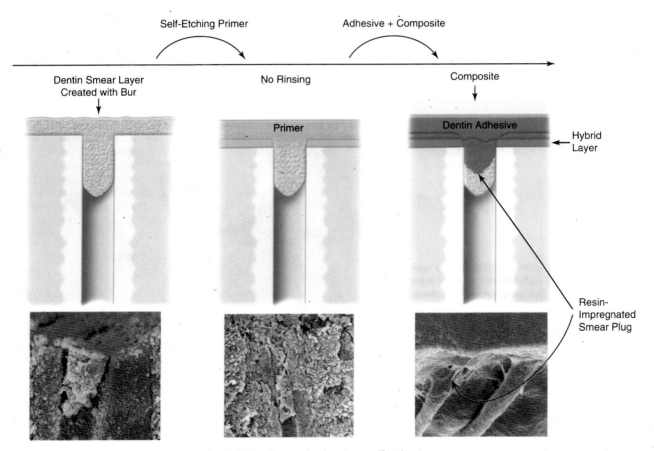

Fig. 4-18 Bonding to dentin using a self-etch primer.

OptiBond All-in-One (Kerr Corporation), and Xeno V+ (DENTSPLY DeTrey). As with the SEP systems, the pH of an all-in-one, self-etching adhesive affects its clinical properties. Also, application of multiple coats, such as four consecutive coats for Xeno III (DENTSPLY DeTrey) or five consecutive coats for iBond (Heraeus Kulzer), significantly increases

dentin bond strengths and decreases leakage, suggesting that some of the "all-in-one" adhesives might not coat the dentin surface uniformly.[131]

A clinical study of Adper Prompt L-Pop (3M EPSE) reported a 35% failure rate at 1 year in Class V restorations, although the material used in this study was an earlier version.[132] A

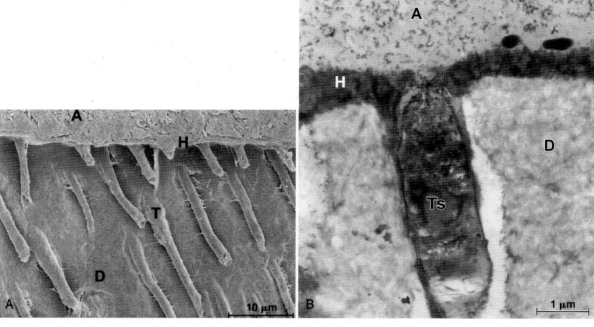

Fig. 4-19 **A,** Scanning electron micrograph of a resin–dentin interface formed with Clearfil SE Bond (Kuraray) on chemical dissolution of the superficial dentin. **B,** Transmission electron micrograph of a resin–dentin interface formed with Clearfil SE Bond on EDTA decalcification and staining with uranyl acetate and lead citrate. *A,* adhesive; *D,* residual dentin (appears gray in *B* because it was decalcified with EDTA); *H,* hybrid layer (appears dark in *B* because of decalcification followed by staining); *T,* resin tag; *Ts,* resin tag that incorporates the smear plug.

modified version of this material, Adper Prompt, had significantly worse marginal adaptation than Scotchbond Multi-Purpose in noncarious cervical lesions at 2 years.[133] Similar findings were reported for Adper Prompt L-Pop in another Class V clinical study. Although Adper Prompt L-Pop resulted in similar retention rates as Adper Single Bond at 3 years, the self-etch adhesive resulted in significantly higher incidence of marginal discoloration.[134]

For iBond, marginal discoloration and marginal adaptation were much less than ideal at 3 years.[135] Another clinical trial in noncarious Class V lesions compared different generations of dentin adhesives—three-step etch-and-rinse, two-step etch-and-rinse, two-step self-etch, and one-step (or all-in-one) self-etch.[136] Out of four different adhesives from the same manufacturer, only the three-step etch-and-rinse adhesive resulted in retention rate greater than 90% at 18 months necessary to fulfill the ADA requirement for full acceptance.[96] In a clinical study with posterior composite restorations, iBond resulted in a significant decrease in the quality of color match, marginal staining, and marginal adaptation at 2 years.[137]

The in vitro and clinical behavior of all-in-one (one-step) self-etch adhesives improves when the clinician adds an extra coat of a hydrophobic bonding layer.[138-140] In a recent clinical study in Class V lesions, the one-step self-etch adhesive Clearfil S3 Bond resulted in 77.3% retention rate at 18 months.[139] For the group to which an extra layer of a thick bonding resin was added (Scotchbond Multi-Purpose Adhesive), the retention rate increased to 93.4% at 18 months. In the same study, iBond, also a one-step self-etch adhesive, resulted in a 60% retention rate at 18 months. However, the retention increased to 83% when a coat of the same hydrophobic resin was applied

over the cured iBond, transforming it in a two-step system. This behavior of one-bottle self-etch adhesives may be related to their behavior as semi-permeable membranes in vitro and in vivo.[110,141] Simplified self-etch adhesives do not provide a hermetic seal for vital deep dentin as demonstrated by transudation of dentinal fluid across the polymerized adhesives to form fluid droplets on the surface of the adhesive.[111]

Moist versus Dry Dentin Surfaces with Etch-and-Rinse Adhesives

Because vital dentin is inherently wet, complete drying of dentin is difficult to achieve clinically.[99,142] Water has been considered an obstacle for attaining an effective adhesion of resins to dentin, so research has shifted toward the development of dentin adhesives that are compatible with humid environments. Many adhesives combine hydrophilic and hydrophobic monomers in the same bottle, dissolved in an organic solvent such as ethanol or acetone. The "moist bonding" technique used with etch-and-rinse adhesives prevents the spatial alterations (i.e., collagen collapse) that occur on drying demineralized dentin (Fig. 4-20; compare with Fig. 4-14).[99] Such alterations might prevent the monomers from penetrating the labyrinth of nanochannels formed by dissolution of hydroxyapatite crystals between collagen fibers.[143,144]

The use of etch-and-rinse adhesive systems on moist dentin is made possible by incorporation of the organic solvents acetone or ethanol in the primers or adhesives. Because the solvent can displace water from the dentin surface and the moist collagen network, it promotes the infiltration of resin monomers throughout the nanospaces of the dense collagen web. The moist bonding technique has been shown repeatedly to enhance bond strengths of etch-and-rinse adhesives because water preserves the porosity of collagen network available for monomer interdiffusion.[99,142,145] If the dentin surface is dried with air, the collagen undergoes immediate collapse and prevents resin monomers from penetrating (Fig. 4-21).[146,147]

Pooled moisture should not remain on the tooth because excess water can dilute the primer and render it less effective.[148,149] A glistening hydrated surface is preferred (Fig. 4-22).[150] Many clinicians still dry the tooth preparation, however, after rinsing off the etching gel to check for the classic etched enamel appearance. Because it is very difficult to dry enamel without simultaneously drying dentin, the dentin collagen collapses easily on air drying, resulting in the closing of the micropores in the exposed intertubular collagen.[36,149] For acetone-based, water-free bonding systems, the etched dentin surface must be re-wetted before applying the adhesive. Re-wetting the dried etched dentin with aqueous re-wetting agents has been shown to restore bond strength values and to raise the collapsed collagen network to a level similar to that in a "moist bonding" technique.[36,147,151] Some authors have suggested that the inclusion of water in the composition of some adhesives may result in re-wetting the collagen fibers in areas that are not left fully moist, opening the interfibrillar spaces to the infiltration of the priming resin.[149,152]

When etched dentin is dried using an air syringe, bond strengths decrease substantially, especially for acetone-based and (to a lesser extent) ethanol-based dentin adhesive systems.[98,147,149] When water is removed, the elastic characteristics of collagen may be lost. While in a wet state, wide gaps separate the collagen molecules from each other.[153] In a dry state, the molecules are arranged more compactly. This is because extrafibrillar spaces in hydrated type I collagen are filled with water, whereas dried collagen has fewer

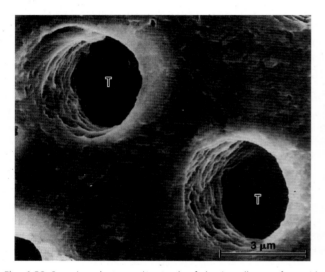

Fig. 4-20 Scanning electron micrograph of dentin collagen after acid etching with 35% phosphoric acid. Dentin was air-dried. The intertubular porosity disappeared as a consequence of the collapse of the collagen secondary to the evaporation of water that served as a backbone to keep collagen fibers raised.

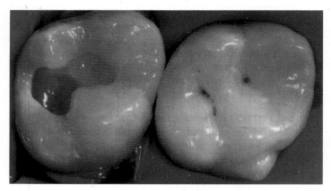

Fig. 4-22 Clinical aspect of moist dentin—a glistening appearance without accumulation of water. *(From Rubinstein S, Nidetz A: The art and science of the direct posterior restoration: Recreating form, color, and translucency, Alpha Omegan 100(1):30–35, 2007.)*

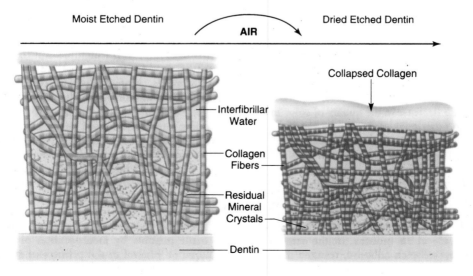

Fig. 4-21 Collapse of etched dentin by air-drying.

extrafibrillar spaces (see Fig. 4-1) open for the penetration of the monomers included in the adhesive systems.[154] During air drying, water that occupies the interfibrillar spaces previously filled with hydroxyapatite crystals is lost by evaporation, resulting in a decrease of the volume of the collagen network to about one third of its original volume.[146] Under the scanning electron microscope, the adhesive does not seem to penetrate etched intertubular dentin that has been dried.[147] Under the transmission electron microscope (TEM), collagen fibers coalesce into a structure without individualized interfibrillar spaces.[147] When air-dried demineralized dentin is re-wetted with water, the collagen matrix may re-expand and recover its primary dimensions to the levels of the original hydrated state.[144,146,155] This spatial re-expansion is a result of the spaces between fibers being refilled with water, but also re-expansion occurs because type I collagen itself is capable of undergoing expansion on rehydration.[156] The stiffness of decalcified dentin increases when the tissue is dehydrated chemically in water-miscible solvents or physically in air.[144] The increase in stiffness is reversed when specimens are rehydrated in water. Re-wetting dentin after air drying to check for the enamel frosty aspect is an acceptable clinical procedure.[36,157]

Recently, some in vitro research has evaluated the possibility of replacing water with ethanol in the etched dentin collagen network, a technique known as "ethanol wet-bonding."[158,159] When acid-etched dentin is saturated with 100% ethanol instead of water, the bond strengths of both hydrophilic and hydrophobic resins increase significantly.[158,159] Although ethanol wet-bonding appears promising, it involves an extra step of replacing rinsing water with 100% ethanol, and no clinical studies are available. Additionally, the time needed to replace water with ethanol in the dentin collagen network would make the technique difficult to implement in a clinical setting.

Clinically, it is difficult to assess or to standardize the amount of moisture that should be left on the dentin surface before the application of the etch-and-rinse adhesive system. Ideally, water should form a uniform layer without pooling (over-wet) and without dry areas (over-dried). Unless it is done very carefully, air drying with an air-water syringe after rinsing off the etching gel is not recommended because it cannot produce a uniform layer of water on the surface and can cause over-drying of the collagen-rich surface. Laboratory studies have shown that re-wetting over-dried dentin using aqueous solutions of HEMA can increase the wettability of etched dentin and return bond strengths to normal levels, especially when used with adhesives without HEMA in their composition.[147,160-162] A study showed that the excess water after rinsing the etching gel can be removed with a damp cotton pellet, high-volume suction, disposable brush, or laboratory tissue paper without adversely affecting bond strengths.[163,164]

Role of Water in Self-Etch Adhesives

Water plays different roles in the bonding mechanisms of self-etch adhesives and etch-and-rinse adhesives. Unlike etch-and-rinse adhesives, self-etch systems do not include separate acid-etching and rinsing steps. The functions of etching and priming are simultaneously performed by the acidic monomers. Water (10–30 weight percent [wt/%]) is added to the hydrophilic formulations to ionize the acidic methacrylate monomers (usually phosphate or carboxylic) and to solubilize calcium and phosphate ions that form from the interaction of the monomers with dentin and enamel.[165,166] When self-etching primers are formulated, a compromise must be made to provide sufficient water for adequate ionization of the acidic monomers without lowering the monomer concentration to levels that would jeopardize the bonding efficacy. Increasing the water concentration from 0 to 60 volume percent (vol%) resulted in improved acidic monomer ionization and increased depth of dentin demineralization created by the acidic monomers.[166] However, increasing the water concentration dilutes the concentration of the acidic monomer, thereby lowering the bonding efficacy of the respective adhesive system.

The mechanical properties of one-step self-etch adhesives might be significantly compromised in the presence of water, which is less likely to occur with two-step self-etch adhesives.[167] One-step self-etch adhesives have higher water absorption or solubility than two-step self-etch adhesives.[168]

Role of Proteins in Dentin Bonding

The partial removal of phospho-proteins from root lesions may enhance the remineralization potential of those lesions.[169] This observation is important because acid-etching demineralizes dentin and may leave a layer of exposed collagen at the bottom of the hybrid layer.[170,171] It has been reported that when demineralized dentin is restored with an adhesive system, the demineralized layer might undergo remineralization within 4 months.[172]

Some evidence suggests that phosphoric acid causes denaturation of collagen fibers in dentin.[52] Although evidence suggests that longer etching times might denature the collagen fiber, the normal 15-second etch does not change the spatial configuration of the collagen molecule. Etching for 15 seconds does not compromise the bonding substrate.[173]

Matrix metalloproteinases (MMPs) are zinc- and calcium-dependent endopeptidases capable of degrading all extracellular matrix components.[174-176] In 1999, one study suggested that the direct inhibition of the MMP activity by chlorhexidine might explain the beneficial effects of chlorhexidine in the treatment of periodontitis.[177] Chlorhexidine was first used in dentin bonding as a dentin disinfectant prior to the application of the dentin adhesive. SEM revealed that chlorhexidine debris remained on the dentin surface and within the tubules of etched dentin after rinsing, but chlorhexidine had no significant effect on the dentin shear bond strengths.[178]

More recently, research has shifted toward the preservation of the hybrid layer through the inhibition of specific dentin proteases capable of degrading collagen, using chlorhexidine as a protease inhibitor.[179] Collagen fibrils that are not encapsulated by resin might be vulnerable to degradation by endogenous MMPs after acid-etching.[174] Collagenolytic and gelatinolytic activities found in partially demineralized dentin imply the existence of MMP in human dentin.[178] Dentin contains gelatinases (MMP-2 and MMP-9), collagenase (MMP-8), and enamelysin MMP-20.[174-176] These enzymes are trapped within the mineralized dentin matrix during odontogenesis.[174,176]

Dentin collagenolytic and gelatinolytic activities can be overcome by protease inhibitors, indicating that MMP inhibition might preserve the integrity of the hybrid layer and reduce the rate of resin–dentin bond degradation within the first few months after restoration.[179,180] When chlorhexidine is used, the integrity of the hybrid layer and the magnitude of bond strengths are preserved in aged resin–dentin interfaces.[181,182] When phosphoric acid is applied without the subsequent application of chlorhexidine, it does not inhibit the collagenolytic activity of mineralized dentin. In contrast, the use of chlorhexidine after acid-etching—even in very low concentrations—strongly inhibits that activity.

However, the role of MMPs in dentin bonding is not completely clear for several reasons: (1) The immunoreactivity of MMP-2 is localized preferably in predentin and around the DEJ in teeth from subjects age 12 to 30 years; (2) MMP-2 and MMP-9 are both gelatinases and are unable to degrade the collagen fibrils directly, so the initial degradation step has to be performed by another mechanism; (3) MMPs do not inhibit the degradation of bonded interfaces created by self-etch adhesives; (4) preservation of the hybrid layer can occur even in the absence of MMP inhibitors.[183-185]

Microleakage and Nanoleakage

"Microleakage" is defined as the passage of bacteria and their toxins between restoration margins and tooth preparation walls. Clinically, microleakage becomes important when one considers that pulpal irritation is more likely caused by bacteria than by chemical toxicity of restorative materials.[186-188] An adhesive restoration might not bond sufficiently to etched dentin to prevent gap formation at margins.[189] The smear layer itself can serve as a pathway for leakage through the nanochannels within its core.[190]

Several studies have shown that the pulpal response to restorative materials is related to the degree of marginal leakage.[191-194] Bacteria are able to survive and proliferate within the fluid-filled marginal gaps under composite restorations. If the restoration is hermetically sealed, bacteria cannot survive.[186,193]

In some cases, pulpal inflammation may occur in the absence of bacteria. Some bacterial byproducts such as endotoxins, material from cell walls, and some elements derived from bacterial lipopolysaccharides can cause damage to the pulpal tissue. This damage is initiated when leukocytes migrate into the pulp, sometimes 72 hours after the pulp has been challenged.[191,195-198]

It is debatable whether the absence of marginal openings would result in a perfect seal between the resin and dentin.[199] Bonding the resin to a preparation with cavosurface margins in enamel is still the best way to prevent microleakage.[150]

The occurrence of gaps at the resin–dentin interface may not cause immediate debonding of the restoration. Despite having shown excellent marginal seal in vitro, OptiBond (Kerr Corporation) does not completely seal the interface in vivo.[62] Other reports showed excellent clinical retention of OptiBond and OptiBond FL in Class V lesions at 12 and 13 years, respectively.[62,103,104] If a dentin adhesive system does not adhere intimately to the dentin substrate, an interfacial gap eventually develops, and bacteria are able to penetrate through this gap.[200] Despite the probability of an incomplete dentin margin seal, Class V clinical studies using etch-and-rinse dentin adhesive systems reported no findings of pulpal inflammation or necrosis.[45,89] A plausible explanation for this apparent paradox is that a gap forms between the hybrid layer and the

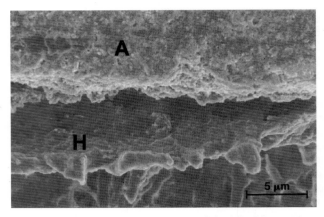

Fig. 4-23 Interfacial gap showing the top of the hybrid layer with tag filling the tubular space. **A,** adhesive; **H,** hybrid layer.

adhesive resin, leaving the tubules still plugged with resin tags (Fig. 4-23).[62]

In vitro microleakage studies generally involve Class V restorations. Specimens are usually thermocycled and sometimes mechanically loaded to simulate oral conditions.[201] It has been estimated that 10,000 thermal cycles correspond approximately to 1 year of thermal fatigue in vivo.[202] Hot water may accelerate hydrolysis of nonprotected collagen fibers and remove poorly polymerized monomers.[203,204] To quantify microleakage, specimens are immersed in a disclosing solution such as silver nitrate, basic fuchsin, or methylene blue. The dye penetrates the resin–dentin interface wherever gaps occurred. After the sectioning of teeth, the depth of dye penetration is usually measured and averaged for the sample size. The relationship between the laboratory testing and the oral cavity environment is, however, ambiguous at best. Silver nitrate penetration may be a particularly demanding test of marginal seal because silver ions are smaller than the bacteria that usually live in the oral cavity.[205] Some authors have speculated that in vivo leakage is less than the corresponding dye penetration in vitro.

Bond strengths decrease with time, and the resin–dentin interface undergoes ultrastructural changes that jeopardize adhesion.[203,206,207] When all margins of the restoration are in enamel, the quality and integrity of the bonds remain unchanged with time, at least in vitro.[208] Degradation of the bonds might result from hydrolysis, which occurs either in the adhesive resin or in the collagen fibers that are not fully enveloped by the adhesive in the hybrid layer, especially when margins are in dentin.[203,206,208] A nearly 50% reduction in bond strengths of the 24-hour control has been reported at 1 year with a one-step self-etching adhesive.[206] The water absorption (and resulting degradation) of two-step etch-and-rinse adhesives is more pronounced than that of three-step etch-and-rinse adhesives.[209]

The term "nanoleakage" has been used to describe small porosities in the hybrid layer or at the transition between the hybrid layer and the mineralized dentin that allow the penetration of minuscule particles of a silver nitrate dye.[210] When ammoniacal silver nitrate is used, silver deposits penetrate the hybrid layer formed by either etch-and-rinse or self-etch adhesive materials.[211] Penetration of ammoniacal silver nitrate results in two distinct patterns of nanoleakage: (1) a spotted

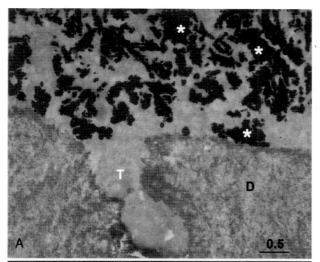

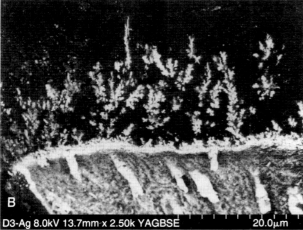

Fig. 4-24 Nanoleakage under the electron microscope. **A,** Spotted pattern in the hybrid layer formed by a one-step self-etch adhesive under the transmission electron microscope (TEM). **B,** Reticular pattern and "water trees" in the adhesive layer formed by a one-step self-etch adhesive under the scanning electron microscope (SEM) in backscattered mode.

pattern in the hybrid layer of self-etch adhesives, which might be caused by incomplete resin infiltration (Fig. 4-24, *A*), and (2) a reticular pattern that occurs in the adhesive layer, most likely caused by areas where water was not totally removed from the bonding area (see Fig. 4-24, *B*).[212]

The term "water trees" is associated with porosities in the polymerized adhesive layer.[212] Water trees might be one of the factors responsible for degradation of the bonding interface with time.[212] Silver uptake in hybrid layers formed by one-step self-etch adhesives is associated with areas of increased permeability within the polymerized resin from which water was incompletely removed. The residual water prevents complete polymerization.[212]

Biocompatibility

Besides demineralizing the dentin surface, phosphoric acid removes the smear layer and opens the orifices of the tubules (see Fig. 4-13).[35,213] Despite past apprehension about potential acid penetration into the dentin tubules and pulp

space, the interaction of etchants with dentin is limited to the superficial 1 to 7 μm.[35,101] It is unlikely that the acid is directly responsible for any injury to the pulp.[214,215] Acid penetration occurs primarily along the tubules, with penetration of intertubular dentin occurring at a lower rate.[215,216] The effects of etchants on dentin are limited by the buffering effect of hydroxyapatite and other dentin components, including collagen, which may act as a barrier that reduces the rate of demineralization.[217,218] Marshall et al elucidated the importance of pH with regard to the effects of acids on dentin surfaces.[215] Etching rates increase dramatically with lower pH. Small differences in pH between acidic gels of similar phosphoric acid concentration may be responsible for distinct depths of dentin demineralization. Manufacturers add thickeners to facilitate handling and other modifiers (e.g., buffers, surfactants, and colorants) to their etching gels, and these may contribute to that phenomenon.

Several early studies suggested that acidic components included in restorative materials such as silicate cements would trigger adverse pulp reactions.[92,219] For several decades, the development of adhesive systems was limited by the belief that acids applied to dentin during restorative procedures caused pulpal inflammation. The use of bases and liners was considered essential to protect the pulp from the toxicity of restorative materials. This concept has, however, changed over the years.[185,186,220,221]

Dentin adhesive systems are well tolerated by the pulp–dentin complex in the absence of bacterial infection.[221] To prevent bacterial infection, restorations must be hermetically sealed. The pulp response to dentin adhesives, when teeth are restored in an ideal clinical environment, has been studied using histologic assessment of animal pulps or in human premolars extracted for orthodontic reasons and in third molars extracted for surgical reasons.[188,220-227] Some clinical studies also have reported normal pulp responses after the application of adhesive on the dentin–pulp complex when the pulp is macroscopically exposed, although one report involved only one tooth.[106,228] Another study showed that the newest dentin adhesive systems are not harmful when applied to exposed pulps.[229] Several reports have shown, however, that etching the pulp and applying a dentin adhesive directly on the exposed pulp tissue results in severe inflammation and eventual formation of pulpal abscesses.[230-233] The solution for this disparity would be long-term follow-up of patients in whom the pulp was treated with acid and adhesive. Ethical concerns do not allow the routine use of pulpal etching in patients. It is known, however, that the thicker the remaining dentin left between the pulpal aspect of the preparation and the pulp, the better the prognosis for that specific pulp.[231] The concept of pulp capping remains a controversial topic.

Adverse pulpal reactions after a restorative procedure are not caused by the material used in that procedure but by bacteria remaining in, or penetrating, the preparation. In some cases, adverse reactions are caused by a combination of factors, as follows:

1. Bacterial invasion of the pulp, either from the tooth preparation or from an existing carious lesion
2. Bacterial penetration into the pulp caused by a faulty restoration
3. Pressure gradient caused by excessive desiccation or by excessive pressure during cementation[234,235]

4. Traumatic injuries
5. Iatrogenic tooth preparation—excessive pressure, heat, or friction[234]
6. Stress derived from polymerization contraction of composites and adhesives

With regard to the biocompatibility issue, tooth preparations with enamel peripheries are important. When all margins are in enamel, polymerization shrinkage stresses at the interface are counteracted by strong enamel adhesion. Marginal gaps are less likely to form, and the restoration is sealed against bacteria.

Relevance of In Vitro Studies

The laboratory parameter most often measured in dentin adhesion is shear bond strength. Flat dentin surfaces are prepared in extracted human or bovine teeth, the adhesive system is applied, and a composite is bonded to the adhesive using a matrix of some type. A shear force is applied at the resin–dentin interface, most often using a knife-edge rod. After testing, the specimens usually are evaluated to determine the nature of the fractures—adhesive, cohesive, or mixed.

The frequency of cohesive failures in the dentinal substrate increases with increasing bond strengths.[236] However, some misinterpretation of cohesive failures in dentin may occur.[237] A mean bond strength of 9.2 MPa has been reported to result in 82% of cohesive failures in dentin, whereas the intrinsic strength of dentin has been reported to be as high as 104 MPa.[238,239] Cohesive failures of dentin obtained during bond strength testing may result from anomalous stress distribution.[240]

A major disadvantage of shear bond strength testing is that it does not consider the three-dimensional geometry of tooth preparations and consequent variations in polymerization shrinkage vectors.[241,242] Additionally, it may not be a true representation of a shear force. In vitro shear bond strength studies are imprecise methods to evaluate the efficacy of dentin adhesive systems.[243,244]

Although these studies are only rough categorizing tools for evaluating the relative efficacy of bonding materials, they are excellent tools for screening new materials and for comparing the same parameter among different adhesive systems.[245] The results of in vitro bond strength tests have been validated with clinical results because improvements seen in the laboratory environment from the earlier generations to contemporary adhesive systems have been confirmed in clinical trials.[89] The combination of bond strength data with ultramorphologic analysis of adhesive interfaces supplies much useful information concerning the interaction of dentin bonding systems with dental substrates.[169]

A systematic analysis of the correlation between in vitro marginal adaptation and the outcome of clinical trials of Class V restorations revealed that the correlation is weak and only present for studies that used the same composite for the in vitro and in vivo evaluation.[246] Another systematic review found a correlation between bond strength data and clinical retention rates of Class V restorations, specifically when the bond strength specimens were aged prior to testing.[245] The clinical parameter in Class V restorations that is more directly related to bond strength data is marginal adaptation.[247]

One of the major concerns with laboratory bond strength testing is the wide range of results obtained for the same material in different testing sites. It is not an uncommon occurrence for the same dentin adhesive system to have average shear bond strengths of 20 MPa in one laboratory and bond strengths less than 10 MPa in another.[51,77] Also, some perplexity exists that no correlation can be established between bond strength and degree of resin penetration into the hybrid layer.[248,249] To illustrate this discrepancy, some reports have suggested that dentin adhesives do not penetrate the whole depth of the demineralized dentin layer but still result in bond strengths greater than 20 MPa.[250,251] In such cases, there would be good retention, despite a deficient seal over time, which could be a triggering factor for nanoleakage phenomena.[170] Intuitively, one would expect an inverse relationship between bond strength and microleakage, but that relationship has not been confirmed.[252]

Clinical studies with dentin adhesive systems are expensive for manufacturers and take at least 18 months to 3 years. Cost is a major concern, in part because of the constant developments in the area of adhesion, making new materials quickly obsolete. No financial incentive exists for the manufacturer to invest in a clinical study of a material that may not be on the market by the time the study is concluded. Consequently, in vitro studies are still used predominantly by manufacturers to anticipate the clinical behavior of their materials.

Several factors contribute to the questionable use of in vitro tests to predict clinical behavior. Among others, variables including age and storage conditions of the teeth used, dentin depth, degree of sclerosis, tooth surface to be bonded, dentin roughness, and type of test used frequently are not controllable.[4,5,237,253] According to some authors, one of the major drawbacks of laboratory bond strength testing is the usual lack of simulated pulpal pressure to replicate the pulpal pressure that occurs in vivo. Other authors have reported, however, that the pulpal pressure does not interfere significantly with bond strength results.[254]

A newer bond strength testing methodology has become popular in recent years.[255] This method, the microtensile test, allows for the assessment of bond strengths using bonded surfaces with a cross-sectional area in the range of 1 to 1.5 mm² or even less (Fig. 4-25). Microtensile testing has several advantages over conventional shear and tensile bond strength methods for the following reasons:

1. It permits the use of only one tooth to fabricate several bonded dentin–resin rods.
2. It allows for testing substrates of clinical significance, such as carious dentin, cervical sclerotic dentin, and enamel.[256]
3. It results in fewer defects occurring in the small-area specimens, as reflected in higher bond strengths.[257]

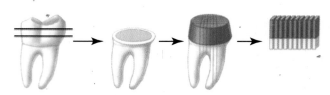

Fig. 4-25 Preparation of specimens for microtensile bond strength testing.

4. It allows for the testing of regional differences in bond strengths within the same tooth.[258]

Clinical Factors in Dentin Adhesion

Several clinical factors may influence the success of an adhesive restoration. The mineral content of dentin increases in different situations, including aged dentin; dentin beneath a carious lesion; and dentin exposed to the oral cavity in noncarious cervical lesions, in which the tubules become obliterated with tricalcium phosphate crystals.[255,259,260] The dentin that undergoes these compositional changes is called sclerotic dentin and is much more resistant to acid-etching than "normal" dentin.[97,261] Consequently, the penetration of a dentin adhesive is limited.[238,261,262] Irrespective of the use of an etch-and-rinse or a self-etch technique, bonding to sclerotic dentin in noncarious cervical lesions has resulted in low bond strengths.[260,263] Additionally, the clinical effectiveness of dentin adhesives is less in sclerotic cervical lesions than in normal dentin.[264,265] Nevertheless, some specific dentin adhesives may perform better in sclerotic dentin than in normal dentin.[266]

Some evidence suggests that masticatory forces not only might cause noncarious cervical lesions but also might contribute to the failure of Class V restorations.[263,267,268] Bruxism or any other eccentric movement may generate lateral forces that cause concentration of stresses around the cervical area of the teeth. Although this stress may be of very low magnitude, the fatigue caused by cyclic stresses may cause failure of bonds between resin and dentin.

The solvent used in the adhesive monomer solution has been shown to influence the clinical behavior of dentin adhesives. An acetone-based adhesive resulted in lower retention rate than an ethanol-based adhesive in a recent clinical study, which illustrates the technique sensitivity associated with acetone-based adhesives.[269]

The type of composite used might play an important role in clinical longevity of Class V restorations. Composites shrink as they polymerize, but the amount of shrinkage depends on the inorganic load of each specific composite. Microfilled composites have a low elastic (or Young's) modulus, which means that they are better able to relieve stresses caused by polymerization or by tooth flexure.[270,271] Materials that have a higher Young's modulus do not relieve stresses by flow; they are unable to compensate for the stresses accumulated during polymerization. These stresses subsequently might be transferred to the adhesive interface and cause debonding. As adhesives have improved, however, restorative material stiffness might be less important. A 2-year clinical study of a three-step, etch-and-rinse adhesive showed no difference in retention rates of Class V composite restorations based on stiffness of the restorative material.[272] Another clinical study reported that composite stiffness did not affect the clinical longevity of cervical composite restorations.[273]

Nevertheless, polymerization shrinkage stresses of composite remain a concern, and stress relief in a restoration is important. Polymerization is initiated on the surface of the restoration, close to the light source, eliminating this surface as a potential stress relief pathway.[274] Several methods have been advocated to improve the flow capacity of composites used in Class II tooth preparations. One of those methods is the use of a flowable composite between the composite and the tooth wall. Conceptually, this flowable low-modulus composite would serve as a shock absorber and simultaneously protect the interface against fatigue stresses.[241,275] Low-viscosity resins might decrease microleakage when used as part of dentin adhesive systems, but this has never been confirmed clinically.[276] The use of flowable composites as an intermediate layer in noncarious cervical lesions or as the gingival increment of Class II preparations, however, has not been proved effective clinically.[276-280]

Incompatibility Issues with Self-Cure and Dual-Cure Composites

Chemically activated and dual-activated composites still have significant use in restorative dentistry, especially in areas of preparations with limited access to light. Examples include crown foundations; bonded posts; and ceramic and composite inlays, onlays, and crowns.

Several studies have reported incompatibility between specific light-cured adhesives and chemically activated composite resins.[281-283] In one study, Prime & Bond NT (DENTSPLY Caulk), which contains PENTA, a monomer with an acidic phosphate group, did not bond to a self-cured composite unless the adhesive was mixed with a sulfinic acid activator.[283] In another study, the mean bond strength of adhesives decreased by 45% to 91% when self-cured composite was used instead of light-cured composite.[283] The most drastic reduction was associated with Prime & Bond NT. The inhibition of polymerization of the self-cured composites by adhesives with specific compositions seems to be related directly to the pH of the adhesive.[282] One-Step, which caused the least reduction in bond strengths between self-cured and light-cured composite, was the adhesive with the highest pH. Prime & Bond NT had the lowest (more acidic) pH.

Similarly, an adverse chemical interaction occurred between catalytic components of chemically cured composite and acidic one-step self-etch adhesives.[129,284] In contrast, despite the acidity of their primers, some two-step self-etch adhesives might be compatible with self-cure and dual-cure composites, owing to the presence of a thick resin layer that is less permeable and more hydrophobic than the layer formed with all-in-one systems.[129,284]

Expanded Clincal Indications for Dentin Adhesives
Desensitization

Dentin hypersensitivity is a common clinical condition that is difficult to treat because the treatment outcome is not consistently successful. Most authorities agree that the hydrodynamic theory best explains dentin hypersensitivity.[261] The equivalency of various hydrodynamic stimuli has been evaluated from measurements of the fluid movement induced in vitro and relating this to the hydraulic conductance of the same dentin specimen.[285]

Patients may complain of discomfort when teeth are subjected to temperature changes, osmotic gradients such as those caused by sweet or salty foods, or even tactile stimuli. Dentin hypersensitivity is a common problem and relatively high prevalence rates have been reported around the world. The cervical area of teeth is the most common site of hypersensitivity. Cervical hypersensitivity may be caused not only by chemical erosion but also by mechanical abrasion or even occlusal stresses.[286,287]

Theories about the transmission of pain stimuli in dentin sensitivity suggest that pain is amplified when the dentinal tubules are open to the oral cavity.[288,289] Dentin hypersensitivity can be a major problem for periodontal patients, who frequently have gingival recession and exposed root surfaces. The relationship between dentin hypersensitivity and the patency of dentin tubules in vivo has been established, and occlusion of the tubules seems to decrease that sensitivity.[290] It also has been suggested that the incorrect manipulation of some adhesive materials such as materials containing acetone might trigger postoperative sensitivity.[148,149] Clinicians have used many materials and techniques to treat dentin hypersensitivity, including specific dentifrices, carbon dioxide (CO_2) laser irradiation, dentin adhesives, antibacterial agents, aldehydes, resin suspensions, fluoride rinses, fluoride varnishes, calcium phosphate, potassium nitrate, and oxalates, among others.[281,291-299] More recently, dentin-desensitizing solutions also have been used under amalgam restorations and crowns to prevent postoperative sensitivity.[300] The use of a dentin desensitizer before cementing full-coverage crowns is supported by studies that showed dentin-desensitizing solutions do not interfere with crown retention, regardless of the type of luting cement used.[301,302]

The use of dentin adhesives to treat hypersensitive root surfaces has gained popularity.[303,304] Reductions in sensitivity can result from formation of resin tags and a hybrid layer when a dentin adhesive is used.[305] The precipitation of proteins from the dentinal fluid in the tubules also may account for the efficacy of desensitizing solutions.[306] Other factors may be involved, however, in the action of dentin desensitizing solutions.[307] The primers of the multi-bottle adhesive system All-Bond 2 have a desensitizing effect, even without consistent resin tag formation.[308] In a clinical study using the primer of the original GLUMA adhesive system (an aqueous solution of 5% glutaraldehyde and 35% HEMA, currently marketed as GLUMA Desensitizer [Heraeus Kulzer]), the desensitizing solution was applied to crown preparations.[309] The authors concluded that GLUMA primer reduced dentin sensitivity through a protein denaturation process with concomitant changes in dentin permeability. Glutaraldehyde has long been used as a fixative that cross-links proteins.[310] This theory has been supported by studies using confocal microscopy, which found the formation of transversal septa occluding the dentinal tubules after application of GLUMA Desensitizer.[311] Another study evaluated dentin permeability in dogs up to 3 months. At the end of this period, GLUMA Desensitizer had the lowest permeability value, providing a longer lasting tubule-occluding effect.[312] Another study used human molar dentin slices to compare in vitro the efficacy of five resin-based desensitizing agents, including GLUMA Desensitizer, and reported that all of the desensitizing agents greatly decreased dentin permeability.[313]

The same glutaraldehyde-based desensitizing agent has been suggested as a re-wetting agent on etched dentin to help prevent postoperative sensitivity under posterior composite restorations.[161] In spite of the favorable in vitro bond strengths, a clinical trial found that the operative technique might be more relevant to prevent postoperative sensitivity than the use of the glutaraldehyde-based desensitizer.[161,314,315]

Indirect Adhesive Restorations

Some current dentin adhesive systems are considered to be universal adhesives because they bond to various substrates besides dentin.[7,97,316-318] Developments in adhesion technology have led to new indications for bonding to tooth structure, such as indirect ceramic and resin-based restorations (crowns, inlays, onlays, and veneers). The use of a universal adhesive system in conjunction with a resin cement provides durable bonding of indirect restorations to tooth structure.[319]

Ceramic restorations (with the exception of alumina-core porcelains, such as In-Ceram High Strength Ceramic [Vita Zahnfabrik/Vident, Bäd Säckingen, Germany] and zirconia-core porcelain such as Lava [3M ESPE]) must be etched internally with 6% to 10% hydrofluoric acid for 1 to 2 minutes to create retentive microporosities (Fig. 4-26) analogous to those created in enamel by phosphoric acid etching. Hydrofluoric acid must be rinsed off thoroughly with running water. Some clinicians use sandblasting with aluminum oxide particles in the internal surface of the restoration. Mean bond strengths decrease, however, when hydrofluoric acid etching is not used.[320] After rinsing off the hydrofluoric acid and drying with an air syringe, a silane coupling agent is applied on the etched porcelain surface and air dried. The silane acts as a primer because it modifies the surface characteristics of etched

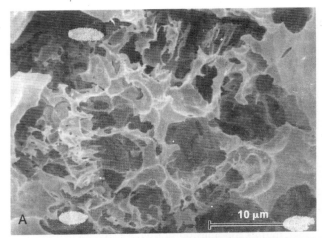

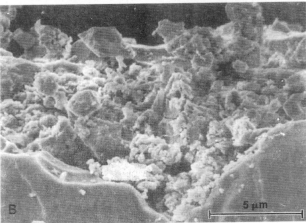

Fig. 4-26 Scanning electron micrograph of Vita (Vita/Vident) dental ceramic etched with 9.6% hydrofluoric acid for 2 minutes. **A,** Top view. **B,** Lateral view.

porcelain. Because etched porcelain is an inorganic substrate, silane makes this surface more receptive to organic materials, the adhesive system, and composite resin cement. Silane coupling agents were introduced in 1952 to bond organic with inorganic substances.[321] In 1962, this technology was transferred to dentistry to couple inorganic filler particles with Bis-GMA resin to form a composite.[322] The use of silanes might increase the bond between composite and porcelain in the range of 25%.[323-325]

The discovery of a transformation toughening phenomenon in zirconia (ZrO_2) has led to a new class of strong, tough, dense, relatively flaw-tolerant ceramics.[326-328] The high strength of zirconia-based ceramics is derived from a stress-induced transformation from the metastable tetragonal form to the stable monoclinic form ($t{\rightarrow}m$).[327,328] This $t{\rightarrow}m$ phase transformation can occur in the vicinity of a propagating crack, causing an increase in volume, thereby closing the crack tip and preventing further crack propagation.[326-328] Etching with hydrofluoric acid does not create retentive microporosities in alumina- and zirconia-core porcelain. However, sandblasting with simultaneous "silicatization" of zirconia improves bond strengths.[329] The use of primers containing a phosphonic acid monomer, a phosphate ester monomer, or a carboxylate monomer improves resin bonding to zirconia ceramic.[330,331]

Many resin cements are dual-cured, that is, they polymerize both chemically and by light activation. Some materials marketed as "dual-cure" do not polymerize efficiently in the absence of a curing light, however.[332-334] More recently, self-adhesive cements, a new category of resins, have become very popular to cement alumina- and zirconia-based ceramic restorations. Self-adhesive cements are dual-cured phosphate monomer-based resin cements (e.g., RelyX Unicem, 3M ESPE) that do not require any pretreatment of the tooth substrate. The acidic phosphate groups react with the filler and, simultaneously, etch enamel or dentin in the same manner as do self-etch adhesives. A chemical interaction between RelyX Unicem and hydroxyapatite has been reported.[335] The pH of some self-adhesive cements increases from 1 to 5 or 6 during their acid-base setting reaction.[336] The setting pH profiles of self-adhesive resin cements depend on the brand and mode of cure. In spite of their dual-curing ability, the physical properties improve significantly when light-activated.[335,337]

Summary

Reliable bonding of resins to enamel and dentin has revolutionized the practice of operative dentistry. Improvements in dentin bonding materials and techniques are likely to continue. Even as the materials themselves become better and easier to use, however, proper attention to technique and a good understanding of the bonding process remain essential for clinical success.

References

1. Packham DE: Adhesion. In Packham DE, editor: *Handbook of adhesion*, Essex, UK, 1992, Longman Scientific & Technical, pp 18–20.
2. Akinmade AO, Nicholson JW: Glass-ionomer cements as adhesives: Part I. Fundamental aspects and their clinical relevance. *J Mater Sci Mater Med* 4:95–101, 1993.
3. Allen KW: Theories of adhesion. In Packham DE, editor: *Handbook of adhesion*, Essex, UK, 1992, Longman Scientific & Technical, pp 473–475.
4. Söderholm K-JM: Correlation of in vivo and in vitro performance of adhesive restorative materials: A report of the ASC MD156 Task Group on test methods for the adhesion of restorative materials. *Dent Mater* 7:74–83, 1991.
5. Rueggeberg FA: Substrate for adhesion testing to tooth structure: Review of the literature. *Dent Mater* 7:2–10, 1991.
6. Buonocore MG: A simple method of increasing the adhesion of acrylic filling materials to enamel surfaces. *J Dent Res* 34:849–853, 1955.
7. Van Meerbeek B, Perdigao J, Lambrechts P, et al: The clinical performance of dentin adhesives. *J Dent* 26:1–20, 1998.
8. Black GV: *A work on operative dentistry in two volumes*, ed 3, Chicago, 1917, Medico-Dental Publishing Company.
9. Asmussen E, Munksgaard EC: Bonding of restorative materials to dentine: Status of dentine adhesives and impact on cavity design and filling techniques. *Int Dent J* 38:97–104, 1988.
10. Buonocore MG, Matsui A, Gwinnett AJ, et al: Penetration of resin into enamel surfaces with reference to bonding. *Arch Oral Biol* 13:61–70, 1968.
11. Barkmeier WW, Shaffer SE, Gwinnett AJ, et al: Effects of 15 vs 60 second enamel acid conditioning on adhesion and morphology. *Oper Dent* 11:111–116, 1986.
12. Gwinnett AJ, Matsui A: A study of enamel adhesives: The physical relationship between enamel and adhesive. *Arch Oral Biol* 12:1615–1620, 1967.
13. Gwinnett AJ: Histologic changes in human enamel following treatment with acidic adhesive conditioning agents. *Arch Oral Biol* 16:731–738, 1971.
14. Silverstone LM, Saxton CA, Dogon IL, et al: Variation in the pattern of acid etching of human dental enamel examined by scanning electron microscopy. *Caries Res* 9:373–387, 1975.
15. Gottlieb EW, Retief DH, Jamison HC: An optimal concentration of phosphoric acid as an etching agent: Part I. tensile bond strength studies. *J Prosthet Dent* 48:48–51, 1982.
16. Gwinnett AJ, Kanca J: Micromorphology of the bonded dentin interface and its relationship to bond strength. *Am J Dent* 5:73–77, 1992.
17. Soetopo, Beech DR, Hardwick JL: Mechanism of adhesion of polymers to acid-etched enamel: effect of acid concentration and washing on bond strength. *J Oral Rehabil* 5:69–80, 1978.
18. Mardaga WJ, Shannon IL: Decreasing the depth of etch for direct bonding in orthodontics. *J Clin Orthodont* 16:130–132, 1982.
19. Barkmeier WW, Gwinnett AJ, Shaffer SE, et al: Effects of enamel etching on bond strength and morphology. *J Clin Orthodont* 19:36–38, 1985.
20. Nordenvall K-J, Brännström M, Malmgren O: Etching of deciduous teeth and young and old permanent teeth: a comparison between 15 and 60 seconds of etching. *Am J Orthodont* 78:99–108, 1980.
21. Bastos PAM, Retief DH, Bradley EL, et al: Effect of etch duration on the shear bond strength of a microfill composite resin to enamel. *Am J Dent* 1:151–157, 1988.
22. Crim GA, Shay JS: Effect of etchant time on microleakage. *J Dent Child* 54:339–340, 1987.
23. Gilpatrick RO, Ross JA, Simonsen RJ: Resin-to-enamel bond strengths with various etching times. *Quintessence Int* 22:47–49, 1991.
24. Shaffer SE, Barkmeier WW, Kelsey WP, 3rd: Effects of reduced acid conditioning time on enamel microleakage. *Gen Dent* 35:278–280, 1987.
25. Barkmeier WW, Erickson RL, Kimmes NS, et al: Effect of enamel etching time on roughness and bond strength. *Oper Dent* 34:217–222, 2009.
26. De Munck J, Van Meerbeek B, Satoshi I, et al: Microtensile bond strengths of one- and two-step self-etch adhesives to bur-cut enamel and dentin. *Am J Dent* 16:414–420, 2003.
27. Swift EJ, Perdigao J, Heymann HO, et al: Enamel bond strengths of "one-bottle" adhesives. *Pediatr Dent* 20:259–262, 1998.
28. Senawongse P, Sattabanasuk V, Shimada Y, et al: Bond strengths of current adhesive systems on intact and ground enamel. *J Esthet Restor Dent* 16:107–115, 2004.
29. Barkmeier WW, Erickson RL, Latta MA, et al: Fatigue limits of enamel bonds with moist and dry techniques. *Dent Mater* 25:1527–1531, 2009.
30. Asmussen E, Hansen EK, Peutzfeldt A: Influence of the solubility parameter of intermediary resin on the effectiveness of the Gluma bonding system. *J Dent Res* 70:1290–1293, 1991.
31. Bowen RL: Adhesive bonding of various materials to hard tooth tissues: II. Bonding to dentin promoted by a surface-active comonomer. *J Dent Res* 44:895–902, 1965.
32. Nakabayashi N, Kojima N, Masuhara E, et al: The promotion of adhesion by the infiltration of monomers into tooth substrates. *J Biomed Mater Res* 16:265–273, 1982.
33. Yoshida Y, Van Meerbeek B, Nakayama Y, et al: Evidence of chemical bonding at biomaterial-hard tissue interfaces. *J Dent Res* 79:709–714, 2000.

34. Erickson RL: Surface interactions of dentin adhesive materials, *Oper Dent* 5(Suppl):81–94, 1992.

35. Van Meerbeek B, Ionkoshi S, Braem M, et al: Morphological aspects of the resin-dentin interdiffusion zone with different dentin adhesive systems. *J Dent Res* 71:1530–1540, 1992.

36. Tay FR, Gwinnett AJ, Wei SH, et al: Ultrastructure of the resin-dentin interface following reversible and irreversible rewetting. *Am J Dent* 10:77–82, 1997.

37. Lin A, McIntyre NS, Davidson RD: Studies on the adhesion of glass-ionomer cements to dentin. *J Dent Res* 71:1836–1841, 1992.

38. Tay FR, Smales RJ, Ngo H, et al: Effect of different conditioning protocols on adhesion of a GIC to dentin. *J Adhes Dent* 3:153–167, 2001.

39. Brännström M, Lindén LA, Johnson G, et al: Movement of dentinal and pulpal fluid caused by clinical procedures. *J Dent Res* 47:679–682, 1968.

40. Terkla LG, Brown AC, Hainisch AP, et al: Testing sealing properties of restorative materials against moist dentin. *J Dent Res* 66:1758–1764, 1987.

41. Van Hassel HJ: Physiology of the human dental pulp. *Oral Surg Oral Med Oral Pathol* 32:126–134, 1971.

42. Garberoglio R, Brännström M: Scanning electron microscopic investigation of human dentinal tubules. *Arch Oral Biol* 21:355–362, 1976.

43. Pashley DH: Dentin: A dynamic substrate—a review. *Scanning Microsc* 3:161–176, 1989.

44. Marchetti C, Piacentini C, Menghini P: Morphometric computerized analysis on the dentinal tubules and the collagen fibers in the dentine of human permanent teeth. *Bull Group Int Rech Sci Stomatol Odontol* 35:125–129, 1992.

45. Suzuki T, Finger WJ: Dentin adhesives: Site of dentin vs. bonding of composite resins. *Dent Mater* 4:379–383, 1988.

46. Rosales-Leal JI, Osorio R, Holgado-Terriza JA, et al: Dentin wetting by four adhesive systems. *Dent Mater* 17:526–532, 2001.

47. Sattabanasuk V, Shimada Y, Tagami J: The bond of resin to different dentin surface characteristics. *Oper Dent* 29:333–341, 2004.

48. Adebayo OA, Burrow MF, Tyas MJ: Bonding of one-step and two-step self-etching primer adhesives to dentin with different tubule orientations. *Acta Odontol Scand* 66:159–168, 2008.

49. Bowen RL, Eick JD, Henderson DA, et al: Smear layer: Removal and bonding considerations. *Oper Dent* 3(Suppl):30–34, 1984.

50. Ishioka S, Caputo AA: Interaction between the dentinal smear layer and composite bond strengths. *J Prosthet Dent* 61:180–185, 1989.

51. Pashley DH, Livingston MJ, Greenhill JD, et al: Regional resistances to fluid flow in a human dentine in vitro. *Arch Oral Biol* 23:807–810, 1978.

52. Eick JD, Cobb CM, Chappell RP, et al: The dentinal surface: its influence on dentinal adhesion: Part I. *Quintessence Int* 22:967–977, 1991.

53. Pashley DH: The effects of acid etching on the pulpodentin complex. *Oper Dent* 17:229–242, 1992.

54. Torney D: The retentive ability of acid-etched dentin. *J Prosthet Dent* 39:169–172, 1978.

55. Opdam NJ, Feilzer AJ, Roeters JJ, et al: Class I occlusal composite resin restorations: in vivo post-operative sensitivity, wall adaptation, and microleakage. *Am J Dent* 11:229–234, 1998.

56. Bowen RL, Nemoto K, Rapson JE: Adhesive bonding of various materials to hard tooth tissue: forces developing in composite materials during hardening. *J Am Dent Assoc* 106:475–477, 1983.

57. Davidson CL, Feilzer AJ: Polymerization shrinkage and polymerization shrinkage stress in polymer-based restoratives. *J Dent* 25:435–440, 1997.

58. Davidson CL, de Gee AJ, Feilzer A: The competition between the composite-dentin bond strength and the polymerization contraction stress. *J Dent Res* 63:1396–1399, 1984.

59. Hegdahl T, Gjerdet NR: Contraction stresses of composite filling materials. *Acta Odontol Scand* 35:191–195, 1977.

60. Feilzer A, De Gee AJ, Davidson CL: Setting stress in composite resin in relation to configuration of the restoration. *J Dent Res* 66:1636–1639, 1987.

61. Davidson CL, de Gee AJ: Relaxation of polymerization contraction stresses by flow in dental composites. *J Dent Res* 63:146–148, 1984.

62. Perdigão J, Lambrechts P, Van Meerbeek B, et al: The interaction of adhesive systems with dentin. *Am J Dent* 9:167–173, 1996.

63. Yoshikawa T, Sano H, Burrow MF, et al: Effects of dentin depth and cavity configuration on bond strength. *J Dent Res* 78:898–905, 1999.

64. Munksgaard EC, Irie M, Asmussen E: Dentin-polymer bond promoted by Gluma and various resins. *J Dent Res* 64:1409–1411, 1985.

65. Hansen EK, Asmussen E: Comparative study of dentin adhesives. *Scand J Dent Res* 93:280–287, 1985.

66. Oysaed H, Ruyter IE: Water sorption and filler characteristics of composites for use in posterior teeth. *J Dent Res* 65:1315–1318, 1986.

67. Kanca J, Suh BI: Pulse activation: Reducing resin-based composite contraction stresses at the enamel cavosurface margins. *Am J Dent* 12:107–112, 1999.

68. Hansen EK: Effect of Scotchbond dependent on cavity cleaning, cavity diameter and cavosurface angle. *Scand J Dent Res* 92:141–147, 1984.

69. Asmussen E: Clinical relevance of physical, chemical, and bonding properties of composite resins. *Oper Dent* 10:61–73, 1985.

70. Jørgensen KD, Matono R, Shimokobe H: Deformation of cavities and resin fillings in loaded teeth. *Scand J Dent Res* 84:46–50, 1976.

71. Tonami K, Takahashi H: Effects of aging on tensile fatigue strength of bovine dentin. *Dent Mater J* 16:156–169, 1997.

72. Qvist V: The effect of mastication on marginal adaptation of composite restorations in vivo. *J Dent Res* 62:904–906, 1983.

73. Nikaido T, Kunzelmann KH, Chen H, et al: Evaluation of thermal cycling and mechanical loading on bond strength of a self-etching primer system to dentin. *Dent Mater* 18:269–275, 2002.

74. Toledano M, Osorio R, Albaladejo A, et al: Effect of cyclic loading on the microtensile bond strengths of total-etch and self-etch adhesives. *Oper Dent* 31:25–32, 2006.

75. Brudevold F, Buonocore M, Wileman W: A report on a resin composition capable of bonding to human dentin surfaces. *J Dent Res* 35:846–851, 1956.

76. McLean JW: Bonding to enamel and dentin [letter]. *Quintessence Int* 26:334, 1995.

77. McLean JW, Kramer IRH: A clinical and pathological evaluation of a sulphinic acid activated resin for use in restorative dentistry. *Br Dent J* 93:255, 1952.

78. Barkmeier WW, Cooley RL: Laboratory evaluation of adhesive systems, *Oper Dent* 5(Suppl):50–61, 1992.

79. Albers HF: Dentin-resin bonding. *ADEPT Report* 1:33–42, 1990.

80. Alexieva C: Character of the hard tooth tissue-polymer bond: II. Study of the interaction of human tooth enamel and dentin with N-phenylglycine-glycidyl methacrylate adduct. *J Dent Res* 58:1884–1886, 1979.

81. Retief DH, Denys FR: Adhesion to enamel and dentin. *Am J Dent* 2:133–144, 1989.

82. Jendresen MD: Clinical performance of a new composite resin for Class V erosion (abstract 1057). *J Dent Res* 57:339, 1978.

83. Eick JD: Smear layer—materials surface. *Proc Finn Dent Soc* 88:225–242, 1992.

84. Baier RE: Principles of adhesion. *Oper Dent* 5(Suppl):1–9, 1992.

85. Causton BE: Improved bonding of composite restorative to dentine: A study in vitro of the use of a commercial halogenated phosphate ester. *Br Dent J* 156:93–95, 1984.

86. Huang GT, Söderholm K-JM: In vitro investigation of shear bond strength of a phosphate based dentinal bonding agent. *Scand J Dent Res* 97:84–92, 1989.

87. Eliades GC: Dentine bonding systems. In Vanherle G, et al, editors: *State of the art on direct posterior filling materials and dentine bonding*, Leuven, 1993, Van der Poorten, pp 49–74.

88. Tyas MJ, Burns GA, Byrne PF, et al: Clinical evaluation of Scotchbond: Three-year results. *Aust Dent J* 34:277–279, 1989.

89. Van Meerbeek B, Peumans M, Verschueren M, et al: Clinical status of ten adhesive systems. *J Dent Res* 73:1690–1702, 1994.

90. Fusayama T, Nakamura M, Kurosaki N, et al: Non-pressure adhesion of a new adhesive restorative resin. *J Dent Res* 58:1364–1370, 1979.

91. van Dijken JWV, Horstedt P: In vivo adaptation of restorative materials to dentin. *J Prosthet Dent* 56:677–681, 1986.

92. Retief DH, Austin JC, Fatti LP, et al: Pulpal response to phosphoric acid. *J Oral Pathol* 3:114–122, 1974.

93. Stanley HR, Going RE, Chauncey HH: Human pulp response to acid pretreatment of dentin and to composite restoration. *J Am Dent Assoc* 91:817–825, 1975.

94. Perdigão J, Swift EJ: Adhesion of a total-etch phosphate ester bonding agent. *Am J Dent* 7:149–152, 1994.

95. American Dental Association Council on Scientific Affairs: *Revised American Dental Association acceptance program guidelines: Dentin and enamel adhesives*, Chicago, 2001, American Dental Association, pp 1–9.

96. Eliades G: Clinical relevance of the formulation and testing of dentine bonding systems. *J Dent* 22:73–81, 1994.

97. Barkmeier WW, Suh B, Cooley RL, et al: Shear bond strength to dentin and Ni-Cr-Be alloy with the All-Bond universal adhesive system. *J Esthet Dent* 3:148–153, 1991.

98. Kanca J: Effect of resin primer solvents and surface wetness on resin composite bond strength to dentin. *Am J Dent* 5:213–221, 1992.

99. Kanca J: Resin bonding to wet substrate: I. Bonding to dentin. *Quintessence Int* 23:39–41, 1992.

100. Swift EJ, Triolo PT: Bond strengths of Scotchbond Multi-Purpose to moist dentin and enamel. *Am J Dent* 5:318–320, 1992.

101. Perdigão J, Lambrechts P, Van Meerbeek B, et al: Morphological field emission SEM study of the effect of six phosphoric acid etching agents on human dentin. *Dent Mater* 12:262–271, 1996.

102. Ermis RB, Kam O, Celik EU, et al: Clinical evaluation of a two-step etch & rinse and a two-step self-etch adhesive system in Class II restorations: Two-year results. *Oper Dent* 34:656–663, 2009.

103. Wilder AD, Swift EJ, Jr, Heymann HO, et al: A 12-year clinical evaluation of a three-step dentin adhesive in noncarious cervical lesions. *J Am Dent Assoc* 140:526–535, 2009.

104. Peumans M, De Munck J, Van Landuyt KL, et al: A 13-year clinical evaluation of two three-step etch-and-rinse adhesives in non-carious Class-V lesions. *Clin Oral Invest* Oct 8 2010 (e-pub ahead of print).

105. Panighi M, G'Sell C: Influence of calcium concentration on the dentin wettability by an adhesive. *J Biomed Mater Res* 26:1081–1089, 1992.

106. Pashley DH, Tay FR: Aggressiveness of contemporary self-etching adhesives: Part II: etching effects on unground enamel. *Dent Mater* 17:430–444, 2001.

107. Rosa BT, Perdigão J: Bond strengths of nonrinsing adhesives. *Quintessence Int* 31:353–358, 2000.

108. Perdigão J, Lopes L, Lambrechts P, et al: Effects of a self-etching primer on enamel shear bond strengths and SEM morphology. *Am J Dent* 10:141–146, 1997.

109. Watanabe I, Nakabayashi N, Pashley DH: Bonding to ground dentin by a Phenyl-P self-etching primer. *J Dent Res* 73:1212–1220, 1994.

110. Tay FR, Pashley DH, Suh B, et al: Single-step adhesives are permeable membranes. *J Dent* 30:371–382, 2002.

111. Tay FR, Pashley DH: Have dentin adhesives become too hydrophilic? *J Can Dent Assoc* 69:726–731, 2003.

112. Fukuoka A, Koshiro K, Inoue S, et al: Hydrolytic stability of one-step self-etching adhesives bonded to dentin. *J Adhes Dent* 13:243–248, 2011.

113. Ferrari M, Mannocci F, Vichi A, et al: Effect of two etching times on the sealing ability of Clearfil Liner Bond 2 in Class V restorations. *Am J Dent* 10:66–70, 1997.

114. Opdam NJ, Roeters FJ, Feilzer AJ, et al: Marginal integrity and postoperative sensitivity in Class 2 resin composite restorations in vivo. *J Dent* 26:555–562, 1998.

115. Miyazaki M, Sato M, Onose H: Durability of enamel bond strength of simplified bonding systems. *Oper Dent* 25:75–80, 2000.

116. Akimoto N, Takamizu M, Momoi Y: 10-year clinical evaluation of a self-etching adhesive system. *Oper Dent* 32:3–10, 2007.

117. Clinician's preferences 2001. *CRA Newsletter* 25, 2001.

118. Tay FR, Sano H, Carvalho R, et al: An ultrastructural study of the influence of acidity of self-etching primers and smear layer thickness on bonding to intact dentin. *J Adhes Dent* 2:83–98, 2000.

119. Peumans M, De Munck J, Van Landuyt KL, et al: Eight-year clinical evaluation of a 2-step self-etch adhesive with and without selective enamel etching. *Dent Mater* 26:1176–1184, 2010.

120. Van Meerbeek B, Yoshihara K, Yoshida Y, et al: State of the art of self-etch adhesives. *Dent Mater* 27:17–28, 2011.

121. Christensen G: Preventing postoperative tooth sensitivity in Class I, II, and V restorations. *J Am Dent Assoc* 133:229–231, 2002.

122. Gordan VV, Mjör IA: Short- and long-term clinical evaluation of post-operative sensitivity of a new resin-based restorative material and self-etching primer. *Oper Dent* 27:543–548, 2002.

123. Akpata ES, Behbehani J: Effect of bonding systems on post-operative sensitivity from posterior composites. *Am J Dent* 19:151–154, 2006.

124. Browning WD, Blalock JS, Callan RS, et al: Postoperative sensitivity: a comparison of two bonding agents. *Oper Dent* 32:112–117, 2007.

125. Casselli DS, Martins LR: Postoperative sensitivity in Class I composite resin restorations in vivo. *J Adhes Dent* 8:53–58, 2006.

126. Wegehaupt F, Betke H, Solloch N, et al: Influence of cavity lining and remaining dentin thickness on the occurrence of postoperative hypersensitivity of composite restorations. *J Adhes Dent* 11:137–141, 2009.

127. Burrow MF, Banomyong D, Harnirattisai C, et al: Effect of glass-ionomer cement lining on postoperative sensitivity in occlusal cavities restored with resin composite—A randomized clinical trial. *Oper Dent* 34:648–655, 2009.

128. Perdigão J: Dentin bonding as a function of dentin structure. *Dent Clin North Am* 46:277–301, 2002.

129. Tay FR, Pashley DH, Peters MC: Adhesive permeability affects composite coupling to dentin treated with a self-etch adhesive. *Oper Dent* 28:610–621, 2003.

130. Tay FR, Pashley DH: Aggressiveness of contemporary self-etching adhesives: Part I. Depth of penetration beyond dentin smear layers. *Dent Mater* 17:296–308, 2001.

131. Ito S, Tay FR, Hashimoto M, et al: Effects of multiple coatings of two all-in-one adhesives on dentin bonding. *J Adhes Dent* 7:133–141, 2005.

132. Brackett WW, Covey DA, St Germain HA, Jr: One-year clinical performance of a self-etching adhesive in Class V resin composites cured by two methods. *Oper Dent* 27:218–222, 2002.

133. Kim S-Y, Lee KW, Seong SR, et al: Two-year clinical effectiveness of adhesives and retention form on resin composite restorations of non-carious cervical lesions. *Oper Dent* 34:507–515, 2009.

134. Loguercio AD, Bittencourt DD, Baratieri LN, et al: A 36-month evaluation of self-etch and etch-and-rinse adhesives in noncarious cervical lesions. *J Am Dent Assoc* 138:507–514, 2007.

135. Ritter AV, Heymann HO, Swift EJ, et al: Clinical evaluation of an all-in-one adhesive in non-carious cervical lesions with different degrees of dentin sclerosis. *Oper Dent* 33:370–378, 2008.

136. Loguercio AD, Amaral RC, Stanislawczuk R, et al: A 18-month randomized clinical trial of four bonding strategies. *J Dent Res* 84(Spec Iss A): abstract number 553, 2009.

137. Perdigão J, Dutra-Correa M, Anauate-Netto C, et al: Two-year clinical evaluation of elf-etch adhesives in posterior restorations. *J Adhes Dent* 11:149–159, 2009.

138. Reis A, Leite TM, Matte K, et al: Improving clinical retention of one-step self-etching adhesive systems with an additional hydrophobic adhesive layer. *J Am Dent Assoc* 140:877–885, 2009.

139. Reis A, Albuquerque M, Pegoraro M, et al: Can the durability of one-step self-etch adhesives be improved by double application or by an extra layer of hydrophobic resin? *J Dent* 36:309–315, 2008.

140. Van Landuyt KL, Peumans M, De Munck J, et al: Extension of a one-step self-etch adhesive into a multi-step adhesive. *Dent Mater* 22:533–544, 2006

141. Tay FR, Frankenberger R, Krejci I, et al: Single-bottle adhesives behave as permeable membranes after polymerization. I. In vivo evidence. *J Dent* 32:611–621, 2004.

142. Kanca J: Wet bonding: Effect of drying time and distance. *Am J Dent* 9:273–276, 1996.

143. Eick JD, Gwinnett AJ, Pashley DH, et al: Current concepts on adhesion to dentin. *Crit Rev Oral Biol Med* 8:306–335, 1997.

144. Maciel KT, Carvalho RM, Ringle RD, et al: The effect of acetone, ethanol, HEMA, and air on the stiffness of human decalcified dentin matrix. *J Dent Res* 75:1851–1858, 1996.

145. Perdigão J, Swift EJ, Cloe BC, et al: Effects of etchants, surface moisture, and resin composite on dentin bond strengths. *Am J Dent* 6:61–64, 1993.

146. Carvalho RM, Yoshiyama M, Pashley EL, et al: In vitro study on the dimensional changes of dentine after demineralization. *Arch Oral Biol* 41:369–377, 1996.

147. Perdigão J, Van Meerbeek B, Lopes MM, et al: The effect of a re-wetting agent on dentin bonding. *Dent Mater* 15:282–295, 1999.

148. Tay FR, Gwinnett AJ, Pang KM, et al: Resin permeation into acid-conditioned, moist, and dry dentin: a paradigm using water-free adhesive primers. *J Dent Res* 75:1034–1044, 1996.

149. Tay FR, Gwinnett AJ, Wei SH, et al: Micromorphological spectrum from over-drying to overwetting acid-conditioned dentin in water-free, acetone-based, single-bottle primer/adhesives. *Dent Mater* 12:236–244, 1996.

150. Swift EJ, Perdigao J, Heymann HO: Bonding to enamel and dentin: a brief history and state of the art, 1995. *Quintessence Int* 26:95–110, 1995.

151. Gwinnett AJ: Dentin bond strengths after air-drying and re-wetting. *Am J Dent* 7:144–148, 1994.

152. Van Meerbeek B, Yoshida Y, Lambrechts P, et al: A TEM study of two water-based adhesive systems bonded to dry and wet dentin. *J Dent Res* 77:50–59, 1998.

153. Sasaki N, Odajima S: Stress-strain curve and Young's modulus of a collagen molecule as determined by the x-ray diffraction technique. *J Biomech* 29:655–658, 1996.

154. Sasaki N, Shiwa S, Yagihara S, et al: X-ray diffraction studies on the structure of hydrated collagen. *Biopolymers* 22:2539–2547, 1983.

155. Van der Graaf ER, ten Bosch JJ: Changes in dimension and weight of human dentine after different drying procedures and during subsequent rehydration. *Arch Oral Biol* 38:97–99, 1993.

156. Eanes ED, Lundy DR, Martin GN: X-ray diffraction study of the mineralization of turkey leg tendon. *Calcif Tissue Res* 6:239–248, 1970.

157. Perdigão J, Frankenberger R: Effect of solvent and re-wetting time on dentin adhesion. *Quintessence Int* 32:385–390, 2001.

158. Tay FR, Pashley SH, Kapur RR, et al: Bonding BisGMA to dentin—a proof of concept for hydrophobic dentin bonding. *J Dent Res* 86:1034–1039, 2007.

159. Hosaka K, Nishitani Y, Tagami J, et al: Durability of resin-dentin bonds to water- vs. ethanol-saturated dentin. *J Dent Res* 88:146–151, 2009.

160. Spencer P, Swafford JR: Unprotected protein at the dentin-adhesive interface. *Quintessence Int* 30:501–507, 1999.

161. Finger WJ, Balkenhol M: Rewetting strategies for bonding to dry dentin with an acetone-based adhesive. *J Adhes Dent* 2:51–56, 2000.

162. Pilo R, Cardash HS, Oz-Ari B, et al: Effect of preliminary treatment of the dentin surface on the shear bond strength of resin composite to dentin. *Oper Dent* 26:569–575, 2001.

163. Goes MF, Pachane GC, García-Godoy F: Resin bond strength with different methods to remove excess water from the dentin. *Am J Dent* 10:298–301, 1997.

164. Magne P, Mahallati R, Bazos P, et al: Direct dentin bonding technique sensitivity when using air/suction drying steps. *J Esthet Restor Dent* 20:130–138, 2008.

165. Salz U, Zimmermann J, Zeuner F, et al: Hydrolytic stability of self-etching adhesive systems. *J Adhes Dent* 7:107–116, 2005.

166. Hiraishi N, Nishiyama N, Ikemura K, et al: Water concentration in self-etching primers affects their aggressiveness and bonding efficacy to dentin. *J Dent Res* 84:653–658, 2005.

167. Hosaka K, Nakajima M, Takahashi M, et al: Relationship between mechanical properties of one-step self-etch adhesives and water sorption. *Dent Mater* 26:360–367, 2010.

168. Ito S, Hoshino T, Iijima M, et al: Water sorption/solubility of self-etching dentin bonding agents. *Dent Mater* 26:617–626, 2010.

169. Clarkson BH, Feagin FF, McCurdy SP, et al: Effects of phosphoprotein moieties on the remineralization of human root caries. *Caries Res* 25:166–173, 1991.

170. Kato G, Nakabayashi N: Effect of phosphoric acid concentration on wet-bonding to etched dentin. *Dent Mater* 12:250–255, 1996.

171. Sano H, Shono T, Takatsu T, et al: Microporous dentin zone beneath resin-impregnated layer. *Oper Dent* 19:59–64, 1994.

172. Tatsumi T, Inokoshi S, Yamada T, et al: Remineralization of etched dentin. *J Prosthet Dent* 67:617–620, 1992.

173. Breschi L, Perdigão J, Gobbi P, et al: Immunolocalization of type I collagen in etched dentin. *J Biomed Mater Res* 66:764–769, 2003.

174. Mazzoni A, Pashley DH, Nishitani Y, et al: Reactivation of quenched endogenous proteolytic activities in hosphoric acid-etched dentine by etch-and-rinse adhesives. *Biomaterials*, 27:4470–4476, 2006.

175. Sulkala M, Larmas M, Sorsa T, et al: The localization of matrix metalloproteinase-20 (MMP-20, enamelysin) in mature human teeth. *J Dent Res* 81:603–638, 2002.

176. Martin-De Las Heras S, Valenzuela A, Overall CM: The matrix metalloproteinase gelatinase A in human dentine. *Arch Oral Biol* 45:757–765, 2000.

177. Gendron R, Grenier D, Sorsa T, et al: Inhibition of the activities of matrix metalloproteinases 2, 8, and 9 by chlorhexidine. *Clin Diagn Lab Immunol* 6:437–443, 1999.

178. Perdigao J, Denehy GE, Swift EJ, et al: Effects of chlorhexidine on dentin surfaces and shear bond strengths. *Am J Dent* 7:81–84, 1994.

179. Pashley DH, Tay FR, Yiu C, et al: Collagen degradation by host-derived enzyem during aging. *J Dent Res* 83:216–221, 2004.

180. Ricci HA, Sanabe ME, de Souza Costa CA, et al: Chlorhexidine increases the longevity of in vivo resin-dentin bonds. *Eur J Oral Sci* 118:411–416, 2010.

181. Carrilho MRO, Carvalho RM, de Goes MF, et al: Chlorhexidine preserves dentin bond in vitro. *J Dent Res* 86:90–94, 2007.

182. Hebling J, Pashley SH, Tjäderhane L, et al: Chlorhexidine arrests subclinical breakdown of dentin hybrid layers in vivo. *J Dent Res* 84:741–746, 2005.

183. Boushell LW, Kaku M, Mochida Y, et al: Immunohistochemical localization of matrixmetalloproteinase-2 in human coronal dentin. *Arch Oral Biol* 53:109–116, 2008.

184. De Munck J, Mine A, Van den Steen PE, et al: Enzymatic degradation of adhesive-dentin interfaces produced by mild self-etch adhesives. *Eur J Oral Sci* 118: 494–501, 2010.

185. Sadek FT, Castellan CS, Braga RR, et al: One-year stability of resin-dentin bonds created with a hydrophobic ethanol-wet bonding technique. *Dent Mater* 26:380–386, 2010.

186. Bergenholtz G, Cox CF, Loesche WJ, et al: Bacterial leakage around dental restorations its effect on the dental pulp. *J Oral Pathol* 11:439–450, 1982.

187. Brännström M, Nyborg H: Pulpal reaction to polycarboxylate and zinc phosphate cements used with inlays in deep cavity preparations. *J Am Dent Assoc* 94:308–310, 1977.

188. Brännström M, Vojinovic O, Nordenvall KJ, et al: Bacteria and pulpal reactions under silicate cement restorations. *J Prosthet Dent* 41:290–295, 1979.

189. Torstenson B, Nordenvall KJ, Brännström M: Pulpal reaction and microorganisms under Clearfil Composite Resin in deep cavities with acid etched dentin. *Swed Dent J* 6:167–176, 1982.

190. Pashley DH, Depew DD, Galloway SE, et al: Microleakage channels: Scanning electron microscopic observation. *Oper Dent* 14:68–72, 1989.

191. Brännström M, Nordenvall KJ: Bacterial penetration, pulpal reaction and the inner surface of Concise Enamel Bond: Composite fillings in etched and unetched cavities. *J Dent Res* 57:3–10, 1978.

192. Brännström M, Nyborg H: Cavity treatment with a microbicidal fluoride solution: Growth of bacteria and effect on the pulp. *J Prosthet Dent* 30:303–310, 1973.

193. Mejàre B, Mejàre I, Edwardsson S: Acid etching and composite resin restorations: a culturing and histologic study on bacterial penetration. *Acta Odontol Scand* 3:1–5, 1987.

194. Mejàre I, Mejàre B, Edwardsson S: Effect of a tight seal on survival of bacteria in saliva-contaminated cavities filled with composite resin. *Endod Dent Traumatol* 3:6–9, 1987.

195. Bergenholtz G: Effect of bacterial products on inflammatory reactions in dental pulp. *Scand J Dent Res* 85:122–129, 1977.

196. Bergenholtz G, Warfvinge J: Migration of leukocytes in dental pulp in response to plaque bacteria. *Scand J Dent Res* 90:354–362, 1982.

197. Brännström M: Communication between the oral cavity and the dental pulp associated with restorative treatment. *Oper Dent* 9:57–68, 1984.

198. Warfvinge J, Dahlén G, Bergenholtz G: Dental pulp response to bacterial cell wall material. *J Dent Res* 64:1046–1050, 1985.

199. Sano H, Takatsu T, Ciucchi B, et al: Nanoleakage: Leakage within the hybrid layer. *Oper Dent* 20:18–25, 1995.

200. Ruyter IE: The chemistry of adhesive agents. *Oper Dent* 5(Suppl):32–43, 1992.

201. Davidson CL, Abdalla AI: Effect of occlusal load cycling on the marginal integrity of adhesive Class V restorations. *Am J Dent* 7:111–114, 1994.

202. Gale MS, Darvell BW: Thermal cycling procedures for laboratory testing of dental restorations. *J Dent* 27:89–99, 1999.

203. Hashimoto M, Ohno H, Kaga M, et al: In vivo degradation of resin-dentin bonds in humans over 1 to 3 years. *J Dent Res* 79:1385–1391, 2000.

204. De Munck J, Van Landuyt K, Peumans M, et al: A critical review of the durability of adhesion to tooth tissue: Methods and results. *J Dent Res* 84:118–132, 2005.

205. Perdigão J, Lopes M: Dentin bonding—questions for the new millennium. *J Adhes Dent* 1:191–209, 1999.

206. Hashimoto M, Ohno H, Sano H, et al: Degradation patterns of different adhesives and bonding procedures. *J Biomed Mater Res* 66B:324–330, 2003.

207. Sano H, Yoshikawa T, Pereira PN, et al: Long-term durability of dentin bonds made with a self-etching primer, in vivo. *J Dent Res* 78:906–911, 1999.

208. De Munck J, Van Meerbeek B, Yoshida Y, et al: Four year water degradation of total-etch adhesives bonded to dentin. *J Dent Res* 82:136–140, 2003.

209. Malacarne J, Carvalho RM, de Goes MF, et al: Water sorption/solubility of dental adhesive resins. *Dent Mater* 22:973–980, 2006.

210. Sano H, Yoshiyama M, Ebisu S, et al: Comparative SEM and TEM observations of nanoleakage within the hybrid layer. *Oper Dent* 20:160–167, 1995.

211. Li HP, Burrow MF, Tyas MJ: The effect of long-term storage on nanoleakage. *Oper Dent* 26:609–616, 2001.

212. Tay FR, Pashley DH, Yoshiyama M, et al: Two modes of nanoleakage expression in single-step adhesives. *J Dent Res* 81:472–476, 2002.

213. Pashley DH, Ciucchi B, Sano H, et al: Permeability of dentin to adhesive agents. *Quintessence Int* 24:618–631, 1993.

214. Lee HL, Orlowski JA, Scheidt GC, et al: Effects of acid etchants on dentin. *J Dent Res* 52:1228–1233, 1973.

215. Marshall GW, Inai N, Wu-Magidi IC, et al: Dentin demineralization: Effects of dentin depth, pH and different acids. *Dent Mater* 13:338–343, 1997.

216. Selvig KA: Ultrastructural changes in human dentine exposed to a weak acid. *Arch Oral Biol* 13:719–734, 1968.

217. Wang J-D, Hume WR: Diffusion of hydrogen ion and hydroxyl ion from various sources through dentine. *Int Endod J* 21:17–26, 1988.

218. Uno S, Finger WJ: Effects of acidic conditioners on dentine demineralization and dimension of hybrid layers. *J Dent* 24:211–216, 1996.

219. Macko DJ, Rutberg M, Langeland K: Pulpal response to the application of phosphoric acid to dentin. *Oral Surg* 6:930–946, 1978.

220. Cox CF, Suzuki S: Re-evaluating pulp protection: Calcium hydroxide liners vs. cohesive hybridization. *J Am Dent Assoc* 125:823–831, 1994.

221. Cox CF, Keall CL, Keall HJ, et al: Biocompatibility of surface-sealed dental materials against exposed pulps. *J Prosthet Dent* 57:1–8, 1987.

222. Fuks AB, Funnell B, Cleaton-Jones P: Pulp response to a composite resin inserted in deep cavities with and without a surface seal. *J Prosthet Dent* 63:129–134, 1990.

223. Inokoshi S, Iwaku M, Fusayama T: Pulpal response to a new adhesive restorative resin. *J Dent Res* 61:1014–1019, 1982.

224. Qvist V, Stoltze K, Qvist J, et al: Human pulp reactions to resin restorations performed with different acid-etched restorative procedures. *Acta Odontol Scand* 47:253–263, 1989.

225. Snuggs HM, Cox CF, Powell CS, et al: Pulpal healing and dentinal bridge formation in an acidic environment. *Quintessence Int* 24:501–509, 1993.

226. Tsuneda Y, Hayakawa T, Yamamoto H, et al: A histopathological study of direct pulp capping with adhesive resins. *Oper Dent* 20:223–229, 1995.

227. White KS, Cox CF, Kanca J, 3rd, et al: Pulp response to adhesive resin systems applied to acid-etched vital dentin: damp versus dry primer application. *Quintessence Int* 25:259–268, 1994.

228. Heitman T, Unterbrink G: Direct pulp capping with a dentinal adhesive resin system: A pilot study. *Quintessence Int* 11:765–770, 1995.

229. Cox CF, Hafez AA, Akimoto N, et al: Biocompatibility of primer, adhesive and resin composite systems on non-exposed and exposed pulps of non-human primate teeth. *Am J Dent* 11:S55–S63, 1998.

230. Gwinnett AJ, Tay FR: Early and intermediate time response of the dental pulp to an acid etch technique in vivo. *Am J Dent* 11:S35–S44, 1998.

231. Hebling J, Giro EM, Costa CA, et al: Biocompatibility of an adhesive system applied to exposed human dental pulp. *J Endod* 25:676–682, 1999.

232. Pameijer CH, Stanley HR: The disastrous effects of the "total etch" technique in vital pulp capping in primates. *Am J Dent* 11:S45–S54, 1998.

233. Costa CA, Hebling J, Hanks CT: Current status of pulp capping with dentin adhesive systems: A review. *Dent Mater* 16:188–197, 2000.

234. Bergenholtz G: Iatrogenic injury to the pulp in dental procedures: Aspects of pathogenesis, management and preventive measures. *Int Dent J* 41:99–110, 1991.

235. Brännström M: The effect of dentin desiccation and aspirated odontoblasts on the pulp. *J Prosthet Dent* 20:165–171, 1968.

236. Hasegawa T, Retief DH: Laboratory evaluation of experimental restorative systems containing 4-META. *Am J Dent* 7:212–216, 1994.

237. Armstrong SR, Boyer DB, Keller JC: Microtensile bond strength testing and failure analysis of two dentin adhesives. *Dent Mater* 14:44–50, 1998.

238. Perinka L, Sano H, Hosoda H: Dentin thickness, hardness and Ca-concentration vs bond strength of dentin adhesives. *Dent Mater* 8:229–233, 1992.

239. Sano H, Ciucchi B, Matthews WG, et al: Tensile properties of mineralized and emineralized human and bovine dentin. *J Dent Res* 73:1205–1211, 1994.

240. Pashley DH, Carvalho RM, Sano H, et al: The microtensile test: A review. *J Adhes Dent* 1:299–309, 1999.

241. Finger WJ: Dentin bonding agents: relevance of in vitro investigations. *Am J Dent* 1:184–188, 1988.

242. Sudsangiam S, van Noort R: Do dentin bond strength tests serve a useful purpose? *J Adhes Dent* 1:57–67, 1999.

243. Øilo G: Bond strength testing—what does it mean? *Int Dent J* 43:492–498, 1993.

244. Versluis A, Tantbirojn D, Douglas WH: Why do shear bond tests pull out dentin? *J Dent Res* 76:1298–1307, 1997.

245. Van Meerbeek M, Peumans M, Poitevin A, et al: Relationship between bond-strength tests and clinical outcomes. *Dent Mater* 26:e100–e121, 2010.

246. Heintze SD, Bluck U, Göhring TN, et al: Marginal adaptation in vitro and clinical outcome of Class V restorations. *Dent Mater* 25:605–620, 2009.

247. Heintze SD, Thunpithayakul C, Armstrong SR, et al: Correlation between microtensile bond strength data and clinical outcome of Class V restoration. *Dent Mater* 27:114–125, 2011.

248. Paul SJ, Welter DA, Ghazi M, et al: Nanoleakage at the dentin adhesive interface vs microtensile bond strength. *Oper Dent* 24:181–188, 1999.

249. Yanagawa T, Finger WJ: Relationship between degree of polymerization of resin composite and bond strength of Gluma-treated dentin. *Am J Dent* 7:157–160, 1994.

250. Eick JD, Robinson SJ, Chappell RP, et al: The dentinal surface: Its influence on dentinal adhesion: Part III. *Quintessence Int* 24:571–582, 1993.

251. Tam LE, Pilliar RM: Fracture surface characterization of dentin-bonded interfacial fracture toughness specimens. *J Dent Res* 73:607–619, 1994.

252. Fortin D, Swift EJ, Jr, Denehy GE, et al: Bond strength and microleakage of current adhesive systems. *Dent Mater* 10:253–258, 1994.

253. Pashley DH: Dentin bonding: Overview of the substrate with respect to adhesive material. *J Esthet Dent* 3:46–50, 1991.

254. Pameijer CH, Louw NP: Significance of pulpal pressure during clinical bonding procedures. *Am J Dent* 10:214–218, 1997.

255. Sano H, Shono T, Sonoda H, et al: Relationship between surface area for adhesion and tensile bond strength: evaluation of a micro-tensile bond test. *Dent Mater* 10:236–240, 1994.

256. Nakajima M, Sano H, Burrow MF, et al: Tensile bond strength and SEM evaluation of caries-affected dentin using dentin adhesives. *J Dent Res* 74:1679–1688, 1995.

257. Phrukkanon S, Burrow MF, Tyas MJ: The influence of cross-sectional shape and surface area on the microtensile bond test. *Dent Mater* 14:212–221, 1998.

258. Shono Y, Ogawa T, Terashita M, et al: Regional measurement of resin-dentin bonding as an array. *J Dent Res* 78:699–705, 1999.

259. Yoshiyama M, Carvaho RM, Sano H, et al: Regional bond strengths of resins to human root dentine. *J Dent* 24:435–442, 1996.

260. Yoshiyama M, Sano H, Ebisu S, et al: Regional strengths of bonding agents to cervical sclerotic root dentin. *J Dent Res* 75:1404–1413, 1996.

261. Brännström M, Lindén LA, Aström A, et al: The hydrodynamics of the dental tubule and of pulp fluid: a discussion of its significance in relation to dentinal sensitivity. *Caries Res* 1:310–317, 1967.

262. Harnirattisai C, Inokoshi S, Shimada Y, et al: Adhesive interface between resin and etched dentin of cervical erosion/abrasion lesions. *Oper Dent* 18:138–143, 1993.

263. Kwong SM, Cheung GS, Kei LH, et al: Micro-tensile bond strengths to sclerotic dentin using a self-etching and a total-etching technique. *Dent Mater* 18:359–369, 2002.

264. Heymann HO, Sturdevant JR, Bayne SC, et al: Examining tooth flexure effects on cervical restorations: a two-year clinical study. *J Am Dent Assoc* 122:41–47, 1991.

265. Van Meerbeek B, Braem B, Lambrechts P, et al: Morphological characterization of the interface between resin and sclerotic dentine. *J Dent* 22:141–146, 1994.

266. van Dijken JWV: Clinical evaluation of three adhesive systems in Class V non-carious lesions. *Dent Mater* 16:285–291, 2000.

267. Braem M, Lambrechts P, Vanherle G, et al: Stiffness increase during the setting of dental composite resins. *J Dent Res* 66:1713–1716, 1987.

268. Heymann HO, Sturdevant JR, Brunson WD, et al: Twelve-month clinical study of dentinal adhesives in Class V cervical lesions. *J Am Dent Assoc* 116:179–183, 1988.

269. Reis A, Loguercio AD: A 36-month clinical evaluation of ethanol/water and acetone-based etch-and-rinse adhesives in non-carious cervical lesions. *Oper Dent* 34:384–391, 2009.

270. Gladys S, Van Meerbeek B, Braem M, et al: Comparative physico-mechanical characterization of new hybrid restorative materials with conventional glass-ionomer and resin composite restorative materials. *J Dent Res* 76:883–894, 1997.

271. Miyazaki M, Hinoura K, Onose H, et al: Effect of filler content of light-cured composites on bond strength to bovine dentine. *J Dent* 19:301–303, 1991.

272. Browning WD, Brackett WW, Gilpatrick RO: Two-year clinical comparison of a microfilled and a hybrid resin-based composite in non-carious Class V lesions. *Oper Dent* 25:46–50, 2000.

273. Peumans M, De Munck J, Van Landuyt KL, et al: Restoring cervical lesions with flexible composites. *Dent Mater* 23:749–754, 2007.

274. Kemp-Scholte CM, Davidson CL: Marginal integrity related to bond strength and strain capacity of composite resin restorative systems. *J Prosthet Dent* 64:658–664, 1990.

275. Kemp-Scholte CM, Davidson CL: Complete marginal seal of Class V resin composite restorations effected by increased flexibility. *J Dent Res* 69:1240–1243, 1990.

276. Lindberg A, van Dijken JW, Hörstedt P: In vivo interfacial adaptation of Class II resin composite restorations with and without a flowable resin composite liner. *Clin Oral Invest* 9:77–83, 2005.

277. Reis A, Loguercio AD: A 24-month follow-up of flowable resin composite as an intermediate layer in non-carious cervical lesions. *Oper Dent* 31:523–529, 2006.

278. Efes BG, Dörter C, Gömeç Y, et al: Two-year clinical evaluation of ormocer and nanofill composite with and without a flowable liner. *J Adhes Dent* 8:119–126, 2006.

279. Celik C, Ozgünaltay G, Attar N: Clinical evaluation of flowable resins in non-carious cervical lesions: Two-year results. *Oper Dent* 32:313–321, 2007.

280. van Dijken JWV, Pallesen U: Clinical performance of a hybrid resin composite with and without an intermediate layer of flowable resin composite: A 7-year evaluation. *Dent Mater* 27:150–156, 2011.

281. Morris MF, Davis RD, Richardson BW: Clinical efficacy of two dentin desensitizing agents. *Am J Dent* 12:72–76, 1999.

282. Sanares AME, Itthagarun A, King NM, et al: Adverse surface interactions between one-bottle light-cured adhesives and chemical-cured composites. *Dent Mater* 17:542–556, 2001.

283. Swift EJ, Perdigao J, Combe EC, et al: Effects of restorative and adhesive curing methods on dentin bond strengths. *Am J Dent* 14:137–140, 2001.

284. Tay FR, Pashley DH, Yiu CK, et al: Factors contributing to the incompatibility between simplified-step adhesives and chemically-cured or dual-cured composites: Part I. Single-step self-etching adhesive. *J Adhes Dent* 5:27–40, 2003.

285. Pashley DH, Matthews WG, Zhang Y, et al: Fluid shifts across human dentine in vitro in response to hydrodynamic stimuli. *Arch Oral Biol* 41:1065–1072, 1996.

286. Gray A, Ferguson MM, Wall JG: Wine tasting and dental erosion: Case report. *Aust Dent J* 43:32–34, 1988.

287. Grippo JO: Abfractions: A new classification of hard tissue lesions of teeth. *J Esthet Dent* 3:14–19, 1991.

288. Cuenin MF, Scheidt MJ, O'Neal RB, et al: An in vivo study of dentin sensitivity: the relation of dentin sensitivity and the patency of dentin tubules. *J Periodontol* 62:668–673, 1991.

289. Reinhardt JW, Stephens NH, Fortin D: Effect of Gluma desensitization on dentin bond strength. *Am J Dent* 8:170–172, 1995.

290. Kerns DG, Scheidt MJ, Pashley DH, et al: Dentinal tubule occlusion and root hypersensitivity. *J Periodontol* 62:421–428, 1991.

291. Camps J, Pizant S, Dejou J, et al: Effects of desensitizing agents on human dentin permeability. *Am J Dent* 11:286–290, 1998.

292. Gaffar A: Treating hypersensitivity with fluoride varnishes. *Comp Cont Educ Dent* 19:1088–1094, 1998.

293. Ide M, Morel AD, Wilson RF, et al: The role of a dentine-bonding agent in reducing cervical dentine sensitivity. *J Clin Periodontol* 25:286–290, 1998.

294. Moritz A, Schoop U, Goharkhay K, et al: Long-term effects of CO2 laser irradiation on treatment of hypersensitive dental necks: Results of an in vivo study. *J Clin Laser Med Surg* 16:211–215, 1998.

295. Quarnstrom F, Collier N, McDade E, et al: A randomized clinical trial of agents to reduce sensitivity after crown cementation. *Gen Dent* 46:68–74, 1988.

296. Touyz LZ, Stern J: Hypersensitive dentinal pain attenuation with potassium nitrate. *Gen Dent* 47:42–45, 1999.

297. West N, Addy M, Hughes J: Dentine hypersensitivity: The effects of brushing desensitizing toothpastes, their solid and liquid phases, and detergents on dentine and acrylic: Studies in vitro. *J Oral Rehabil* 25:885–895, 1998.

298. Yates R, West N, Addy M, et al: The effects of a potassium citrate, cetylpyridinium chloride, sodium fluoride mouthrinse on dentine hypersensitivity, plaque and gingivitis: A placebo-controlled study. *J Clin Periodontol* 25:813–820, 1998.

299. Zhang C, Matsumoto K, Kimura Y, et al: Effects of CO2 laser in treatment of cervical dentinal hypersensitivity. *J Endod* 24:595–597, 1998.

300. Schwartz RS, Conn LJ, Jr, Haveman CW: Clinical evaluation of two desensitizing agents for use under Class 5 silver amalgam restorations. *J Prosthet Dent* 80:269–273, 1998.

301. Cobb DS, Reinhardt JW, Vargas MA: Effect of HEMA-containing dentin desensitizers on shear bond strength of a resin cement. *Am J Dent* 10:62–65, 1997.

302. Swift EJ, Lloyd AH, Felton DA, et al: The effect of resin desensitizing agents on crown retention. *J Am Dent Assoc* 128:195–200, 1997.

303. Calamia JR, Styner DL, Rattet AH: Effect of Amalgambond on cervical sensitivity. *Am J Dent* 8:283–284, 1995.

304. Ferrari M, Cagidiaco MC, Kugel G, et al: Clinical evaluation of a one-bottle bonding system for desensitizing exposed roots. *Am J Dent* 12:243–249, 1999.

305. Nakabayashi N, Nakamura M, Yasuda N, et al: Hybrid layer as a dentin-bonding mechanism. *J Esthet Dent* 3:133–138, 1991.

306. Scherman A, Jacobsen PL: Managing dentin hypersensitivity: what treatment to recommend to patients. *J Am Dent Assoc* 123:57–61, 1992.

307. Nikaido T, Burrow MF, Tagami J, et al: Effect of pulpal pressure on adhesion of resin composite to dentin: Bovine serum versus saline. *Quintessence Int* 26:221–226, 1995.

308. Swift EJ, Hammel SA, Perdigao J, et al: Prevention of root surface caries using a dental adhesive. *J Am Dent Assoc* 125:571–576, 1994.

309. Felton DA, Bergenholtz G, Kanoy BE: Evaluation of the desensitizing effect of Gluma dentin bond on teeth prepared for complete coverage restorations. *Int J Prosthodont* 4:292–298, 1991.

310. Bowes JH, Cater CW: The reaction of glutaraldehyde with proteins and other biological materials. *J Royal Microsc Soc* 85:193–200, 1966.

311. Schüpbach P, Lutz F, Finger WJ: Closing of dentinal tubules by Gluma desensitizer. *Eur J Oral Sci* 105:414–421, 1997.

312. Duran I, Sengun A, Yildirim T, Ozturk B: In vitro dentine permeability evaluation of HEMA-based (desensitizing) products using split-chamber model following in vivo application in the dog. *J Oral Rehabil* 32:34–38, 2005.

313. Camps J, About I, Van Meerbeek B, et al: Efficiency and cytotoxicity of resin-based desensitizing agents. *Am J Dent* 15:300–304, 2002.

314. Ritter AV, Heymann HO, Swift EJ, et al: Effects of different re-wetting techniques on dentin shear bond strengths. *J Esthet Dent* 12:85–96, 2000.

315. Sobral MA, Garone-Netto N, Luz MA, et al: Prevention of postoperative tooth sensitivity: A preliminary clinical trial. *J Oral Rehabil* 32:661–668, 2005.

316. Barkmeier WW, Menis DL, Barnes DM, et al: Bond strength of a veneering porcelain using newer generation adhesive systems. *Pract Periodont Aesthet Dent* 5:50–55, 1993.

317. Kanca J: Dental adhesion and the All-Bond system. *J Esthet Dent* 3:129–132, 1991.

318. Watanabe F, Powers JM, Lorey RE: In vitro bonding of prosthodontic adhesives to dental alloys. *J Dent Res* 67:479–483, 1988.

319. Burke FJT, Watts DC: Fracture resistance of teeth restored with dentin-bonded crowns. *Quintessence Int* 25:335–340, 1994.

320. Suliman AA, Swift EJ, Jr, Perdigao J: Effects of surface treatment and bonding agents on bond strength of composite to porcelain. *J Prosthet Dent* 70:118–120, 1993.

321. Bjorksten J, Yaeger LL: Vinyl silane size for glass fabric, *Mod Plast* 29:124, 128, 1952.

322. Bowen RL, Rodriguez MS: Tensile strength and modulus of elasticity of tooth structure and several restorative materials. *J Am Dent Assoc* 64:378–387, 1962.

323. Diaz-Arnold AM, Schneider RL, Aquilino SA: Porcelain repairs: An evaluation of the shear strength of three porcelain repair systems (abstract 806). *J Dent Res* 66:207, 1987.

324. Newburg R, Pameijer CH: Composite resin bonded to porcelain with a silane solution. *J Am Dent Assoc* 96:288–291, 1978.

325. Sheth J, Jensen M, Tolliver D: Effect of surface treatment on etched porcelain and bond strength to enamel. *Dent Mater* 4:328–337, 1998.

326. Garvie RC, Hannink RH, Pascoe RT: Ceramic steel? *Nature* 258:703–704, 1975.

327. Hannink RHJ, Kelly PM, Muddle BC: Transformation toughening in zirconia-containing ceramics. *J Am Ceram Soc* 83:461–487, 2000.

328. Heuer AH: Transformation toughening in ZrO2-containing ceramics. *J Am Ceram Soc* 70:689–698, 1987.

329. Valandro LF, Ozcan M, Bottino MC, et al: Bond strength of a resin cement to high-alumina and zirconia-reinforced ceramics: The effect of surface conditioning. *J Adhes Dent* 8:175–181, 2006.

330. Magne P, Paranhos MP, Burnett LH, et al: New zirconia primer improves bond strength of resin-based cement. *Dent Mater* 26:345–352, 2010.

331. Kitayama S, Nikaido T, Takahashi R, et al: Effect of primer treatment on bonding of resin cements to zirconia ceramic. *Dent Mater* 26:426–432, 2010.

332. Darr AH, Jacobson PH: Conversion of dual-cure luting cements. *J Oral Rehabil* 22:43–47, 1995.

333. Hasegawa EA, Boyer DB, Chan DC: Hardening of dual-cured cements under composite resin inlays. *J Prosthet Dent* 66:187–192, 1991.

334. Peutzfeldt A: Dual-cure resin cements: In vitro wear and effect of quantity of remaining double-bonds, filler volume and light-curing. *Acta Odontol Scand* 53:29–34, 1995.

335. Gerth HU, Dammaschke T, Züchner H, et al: Chemical analysis and bonding reaction of RelyX Unicem and Bifix composites–a comparative study. *Dent Mater* 22:934–941, 2006.

336. Saskalauskaite E, Tam LE, McComb D: Flexural strength, elastic modulus, and pH profile of self-etch resin luting cements. *J Prosthodont* 17:262–268, 2008.

337. Vrochari AD, Eliades G, Hellwig E, et al: Curing efficiency of four self-etching, self-adhesive resin cements. *Dent Mater* 25:1104–1108, 2009.

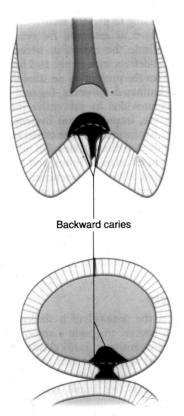

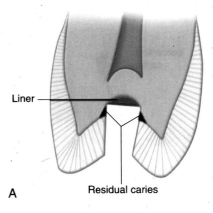

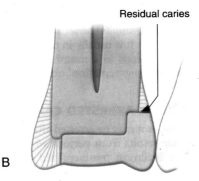

Fig. 5-2 Backward caries extends from the dentinoenamel junction (DEJ) into enamel.

Fig. 5-3 Unacceptable types of residual caries remaining after tooth preparation at the dentinoenamel junction (DEJ) (*A*) and on enamel wall of tooth preparation (*B*). In post-operative radiograph, *B* appears similar to secondary (recurrent) caries.

present and often are prevalent in older patients. Root caries is usually more rapid than other forms of caries and should be detected and treated early. Root caries is becoming more prevalent because a greater number of older individuals are retaining more of their teeth and experiencing gingival recession, both of which increase the likelihood of root caries development.

SECONDARY (RECURRENT) CARIES

Secondary caries occurs at the junction of a restoration and the tooth and may progress under the restoration. It is often termed *recurrent caries*. This condition usually indicates that microleakage is present, along with other conditions conducive to caries development (Fig. 5-5).

Extent of Caries
INCIPIENT CARIES (REVERSIBLE)

Incipient caries is the first evidence of caries activity in enamel. On smooth-surface enamel, the lesion appears opaque white when air-dried and seems to disappear when wet. This lesion of demineralized enamel has not extended to the DEJ, and the enamel surface is fairly hard, intact, and smooth to the touch. The lesion can be remineralized if immediate corrective measures alter the oral environment, including plaque removal and control. This lesion may be characterized as reversible. A remineralized lesion usually is either opaque white or a shade of brown-to-black from extrinsic coloration, has a hard surface, and appears the same whether wet or dry.

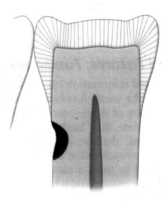

Fig. 5-4 Root-surface caries.

CAVITATED CARIES (IRREVERSIBLE)

In cavitated caries, the enamel surface is broken (not intact), and usually the lesion has advanced into dentin. Usually, remineralization is not possible, and treatment that includes tooth preparation and restoration is indicated.

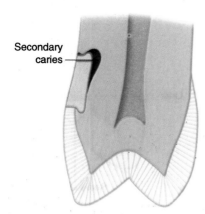

Secondary caries

Fig. 5-5 Secondary (recurrent) caries.

Rate (Speed) of Caries
ACUTE (RAMPANT) CARIES

Acute caries, often termed *rampant caries*, refers to disease that rapidly damages the tooth. It is usually in the form of numerous soft, light-colored lesions in a mouth and is infectious. Less time for extrinsic pigmentation explains the lighter coloration.

CHRONIC (SLOW) OR ARRESTED CARIES

Chronic caries is slow, or it may be arrested after several active phases. The slow rate results from periods when demineralized tooth structure is almost remineralized (the disease is episodic over time because of changes in the oral environment). The condition may be found in only a few locations in a mouth, and the lesion is discolored and fairly hard. The slow rate of caries allows time for extrinsic pigmentation. An arrested enamel lesion is brown-to-black in color and hard and as a result of fluoride may be more caries resistant than contiguous, unaffected enamel. An arrested, dentinal lesion typically is "open" (allowing debridement from toothbrushing), dark, and hard, and this dentin is termed *sclerotic* or *eburnated dentin*.

Grooves and Fissures; Fossae and Pits

Chapter 1 presented information on the development of the enamel surface of the tooth. Anatomic depressions mark the location of the union of developmental enamel lobes. Where such union is complete, this "landmark" is only slightly involuted, smooth, hard, shallow, accessible to cleansing, and termed *groove*. Where such union is incomplete, the landmark is sharply involuted to form a narrow, inaccessible canal of varying depths in the enamel and is termed *fissure*. The distinction made between a groove and a fissure also applies to an enamel surface *fossa*, which is nondefective enamel lobe union, and a *pit*, which is defective. A fissure (or pit) may be a trap for plaque and other oral elements that together can produce caries, unless the surface enamel of the fissure or pit walls is fluoride rich.

Extension for Prevention

Black noted that in tooth preparations for smooth-surface caries, the restoration should be extended to areas that are normally self-cleansing to prevent recurrence of caries.[1] This principle was known as *extension for prevention* and was broadened to include the extension necessary to remove remaining enamel defects such as pits and fissures. The practice of extension for the prevention on smooth surfaces virtually has been eliminated, however, because of the relative caries immunity provided by preventive measures such as fluoride application, improved oral hygiene, and a proper diet. This change has fostered a more conservative philosophy defining the factors that dictate extension on smooth surfaces to be (1) the extent of caries or injury and (2) the restorative material to be used. Likewise, extension for prevention to include the full length of enamel fissures has been reduced by treatments that conserve tooth structure. Tooth structure conservation ultimately leads to restored teeth that are stronger and more resistant to fracture. Such treatments are enameloplasty, application of pit-and-fissure sealant, and preventive resin or conservative composite restoration.[9]

Enameloplasty

Enameloplasty is the removal of a shallow developmental fissure or pit in enamel to create a smooth, saucer-shaped surface that is self-cleansing or easily cleaned. This prophylactic procedure can be applied not only to fissures and pits and deep supplemental grooves but also to some shallow, smooth-surface enamel defects (see Initial Tooth Preparation Stage later in the chapter).

Prophylactic Odontotomy

Prophylactic odontotomy is presented only as a historical concept.[10] The procedure involves minimal preparation and amalgam filling of the developmental, structural imperfections of enamel, such as pits and fissures, to prevent caries originating in these sites. Prophylactic odontotomy is no longer advocated as a preventive measure.

Affected and Infected Dentin

Fusayama reported that carious dentin consists of two distinct layers—an outer layer and an inner layer.[11] This textbook refers to the outer layer as *infected dentin* and the inner layer as *affected dentin*. In tooth preparation, it is desirable that only infected dentin be removed, leaving affected dentin, which may be remineralized in a vital tooth after the completion of restorative treatment. This principle for the removal of dentinal caries is supported by the observation by Fusayama et al. that the softening front of the lesion always precedes the discoloration front, which always precedes the bacterial front.[12]

Infected dentin has bacteria present, and collagen is irreversibly denatured. It is not remineralizable and must be removed. Affected dentin has no bacteria, and the collagen matrix is intact, is remineralizable, and should be preserved. To clinically distinguish these two layers, the operator traditionally observes the degree of discoloration (extrinsic staining) and tests the area for hardness by the feel of an explorer tine or a slowly revolving bur. Some difficulties occur with this approach because (1) the discoloration may be slight and gradually changeable in acute (rapid) caries, and (2) the hardness (softness) felt by the hand through an instrument may

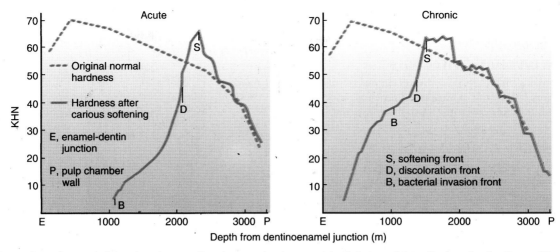

Fig. 5-6 Comparison of acute and chronic caries regarding closeness, hardness, and depth factors of the softening, discoloration, and bacterial invasion fronts.

be an inexact guide. To differentiate between remineralizable and non-remineralizable dentin, staining carious dentin was proposed by Fusayama.[11] Caries-detecting dyes are not specific for infected dentin and will stain the slightly demineralized protein matrix of affected dentin as well as normal DEJ.[13] Caries-detecting dyes should be used with caution and only as an adjunct to clinical evaluation.

In chronic caries, infected dentin usually is discolored, and because the bacterial front is close to the discoloration front, it is advisable, in caries removal, to remove all discolored dentin unless judged to be within 0.5 mm of the pulp (Fig. 5-6). Because the discoloration is slight in acute caries, and the bacterial front is well behind the discoloration front, some discolored dentin may be left, although any "clinically remarkable" discoloration should be removed.[12]

Non-carious Tooth Defects Terminology
Abrasion

Abrasion is abnormal tooth surface loss resulting from direct forces of friction between teeth and external objects or from frictional forces between contacting teeth components in the presence of an abrasive medium.[8] Abrasion may occur from (1) improper brushing techniques, (2) habits such as holding a pipe stem between teeth, (3) tobacco chewing, or (4) vigorous use of toothpicks between adjacent teeth. Toothbrush abrasion is the most common example and is usually seen as a sharp, V-shaped notch in the gingival portion of the facial aspect of a tooth.

Erosion

Erosion is the wear or loss of tooth surface by chemico-mechanical action. Regurgitation of stomach acid can cause this condition on the lingual surfaces of maxillary teeth (particularly anterior teeth). Other examples are the dissolution of the facial aspects of anterior teeth because of habitual sucking on lemons or the loss of tooth surface from ingestion of acidic beverages.

Attrition

Attrition is the mechanical wear of the incisal or occlusal surface as a result of functional or parafunctional movements of the mandible (tooth-to-tooth contacts). Attrition also includes proximal surface wear at the contact area because of physiologic tooth movement.

Abfraction

It has been proposed that the predominant causative factor of some cervical, wedge-shaped defects is a strong eccentric occlusal force (frequently manifested as an associated wear facet) resulting in microfractures or abfractures. Such microfractures occur as the cervical area of the tooth flexes under such loads. This defect is termed *idiopathic erosion* or *abfraction*.[14]

Fractures

Fractures are among the more difficult and challenging defects of teeth, in both diagnosis and treatment.

INCOMPLETE FRACTURE NOT DIRECTLY INVOLVING VITAL PULP

An incomplete fracture not directly involving vital pulp is often termed a "greenstick" fracture. This phenomenon is caused by excessive cyclic loading (or traumatic injury) from occlusal contact with resultant fracture development. The fracture begins in enamel, but becomes painful following propagation into dentin. This condition is very sensitive, and yet the patient may only be able to tell which side of the mouth is affected rather than the specific tooth. It is, therefore, sometimes challenging to diagnose and treat.

COMPLETE FRACTURE NOT INVOLVING VITAL PULP

This represents complete separation of a fragment of the tooth structure in such a way that the pulp is not involved. Usually, pain is not associated with this condition, unless the gingival border of the fractured segment is still held by periodontal tissue. Restorative treatment (sometimes along with periodontal treatment) is indicated.

FRACTURE INVOLVING VITAL PULP

Fracture involving vital pulp always results in pulpal infection and severe pain. If the tooth is restorable, immediate root canal therapy is indicated; otherwise the tooth must be extracted.

Non-hereditary Enamel Hypoplasia

Non-hereditary enamel hypoplasia occurs when ameloblasts are injured during enamel formation, resulting in defective enamel (diminished form, calcification, or both). It usually is seen on anterior teeth and the first molars in the form of opaque white or light brown areas with smooth, intact, hard surface or as pitted or grooved enamel, which is usually hard and discolored and caused by fluorosis or high fever. The reader should consult a textbook on oral pathology for additional information.

Amelogenesis Imperfecta

In *amelogenesis imperfecta* the enamel is defective in form or calcification as a result of heredity and has an appearance ranging from essentially normal to extremely unsightly.[15]

Dentinogenesis Imperfecta

Dentinogenesis imperfecta is a hereditary condition in which only dentin is defective. Normal enamel is weakly attached and lost early. The reader should consult a textbook on oral pathology for additional information.

Tooth Preparation Terminology
Simple, Compound, and Complex Tooth Preparations

A tooth preparation is termed *simple* if only one tooth surface is involved, *compound* if two surfaces are involved, and *complex* if a preparation involves three or more surfaces.

Abbreviated Descriptions of Tooth Preparations

For brevity in records and communication, the description of a tooth preparation is abbreviated by using the first letter, capitalized, of each tooth surface involved. Examples are as follows: (1) An occlusal tooth preparation is an "O"; (2) a preparation involving the mesial and occlusal surfaces is an "MO"; and (3) a preparation involving the mesial, occlusal, and distal surfaces is an "MOD".

Tooth Preparation Walls (Fig. 5-7)
INTERNAL WALL

The *internal wall* is the prepared surface that does not extend to the external tooth surface.

AXIAL WALL

The *axial wall* is the internal wall parallel to the long axis of the tooth.

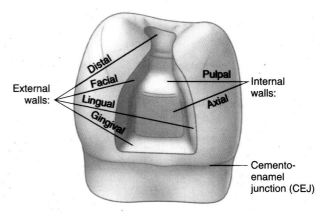

Fig. 5-7 The external and internal walls (floors) for an amalgam tooth preparation.

PULPAL WALL (FLOOR)

The *pulpal wall* is the internal wall that is perpendicular to the long axis of the tooth and occlusal of the pulp.

EXTERNAL WALL

The *external wall* is the prepared surface that extends to the external tooth surface. Such a wall takes the name of the tooth surface (or aspect) that the wall is adjacent to.

FLOOR (OR SEAT)

The *floor* (or seat) is the prepared wall that is reasonably horizontal and perpendicular to the occlusal forces that are directed occlusogingivally (generally parallel to the long axis of the tooth). Examples are pulpal and gingival floors. Such floors may be purposefully prepared to provide stabilizing seats for the restoration, distributing the stresses in the tooth structure rather than concentrating them. This preparation feature increases the resistance form of the restored tooth against post-restorative fracture.

ENAMEL WALL

The *enamel wall* is that portion of a prepared external wall consisting of enamel (see Fig. 5-1, *D*).

DENTINAL WALL

The *dentinal wall* is that portion of a prepared external wall consisting of dentin, in which mechanical retention features may be located (see Fig. 5-1, *D*).

Tooth Preparation Angles

Although the junction of two or more prepared surfaces is referred to as *angle*, the junction is almost always "softened" so as to present a slightly rounded configuration. Despite this rounding, these junctions are still referred to as *angles* for descriptive and communicative purposes.

LINE ANGLE

A *line angle* is the junction of two planar surfaces of different orientation along a line (Figs. 5-8 and 5-9). An *internal* line angle is the line angle whose apex points into the tooth. The

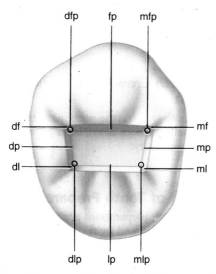

Fig. 5-8 Schematic representation (for descriptive purpose) illustrating tooth preparation line angles and point angles. Line angles are faciopulpal (*fp*), distofacial (*df*), distopulpal (*dp*), distolingual (*dl*), linguopulpal (*lp*), mesiolingual (*ml*), mesiopulpal (*mp*), and mesiofacial (*mf*). Point angles are distofaciopulpal (*dfp*), distolinguopulpal (*dlp*), mesiolinguopulpal (*mlp*), and mesiofaciopulpal (*mfp*).

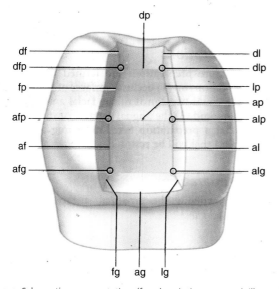

Fig. 5-9 Schematic representation (for descriptive purpose) illustrating tooth preparation line angles and point angles. Line angles are distofacial (*df*), faciopulpal (*fp*), axiofacial (*af*), faciogingival (*fg*), axiogingival (*ag*), linguogingival (*lg*), axiolingual (*al*), axiopulpal (*ap*), linguopulpal (*lp*), distolingual (*dl*), and distopulpal (*dp*). Point angles are distofaciopulpal (*dfp*), axiofaciopulpal (*afp*), axiofaciogingival (*afg*), axiolinguogingival (*alg*), axiolinguopulpal (*alp*), and distolinguopulpal (*dlp*).

external line angle is the line angle whose apex points away from the tooth.

POINT ANGLE

The *point angle* is the junction of three planal surfaces of different orientation (see Figs. 5-8 and 5-9).

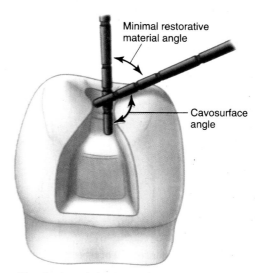

Fig. 5-10 Visualization of the cavosurface angle and the associated minimal restorative material angle for a typical amalgam tooth preparation.

CAVOSURFACE ANGLE AND CAVOSURFACE MARGIN

The *cavosurface angle* is the angle of tooth structure formed by the junction of a prepared wall and the external surface of the tooth. The actual junction is referred to as *cavosurface margin*. The cavosurface angle may differ with the location on the tooth, the direction of the enamel rods on the prepared wall, or the type of restorative material to be used. In Figure 5-1, *D*, the cavosurface angle (*cs*) is determined by projecting the prepared wall in an imaginary line (*w'*) and the unprepared enamel surface in an imaginary line (*us'*) and noting the angle (*cs'*) opposite to the cavosurface angle (*cs*). For better visualization, these imaginary projections can be formed by using two periodontal probes, one lying on the unprepared surface and the other on the prepared external tooth wall (Fig. 5-10).

Combination of Terms

When discussing or writing a term denoting a combination of two or more surfaces, the *-al* ending of the prefix word is changed to an *-o*. The angle formed by the lingual and incisal surfaces of an anterior tooth would be termed *linguoincisal line angle*. The tooth preparation involving the mesial and occlusal surfaces is termed *mesio-occlusal preparation*, or *MO preparation*. The preparation involving the mesial, occlusal, and distal surfaces is a *mesio-occluso-distal tooth preparation*, or *MOD preparation*.

Enamel Margin Strength

One of the important principles in tooth preparation is the concept of the *strongest enamel margin*. This margin has two significant features: (1) it is formed by full-length enamel rods whose inner ends are on sound dentin, and (2) these enamel rods are buttressed on the preparation side by progressively shorter rods whose outer ends have been cut off but whose

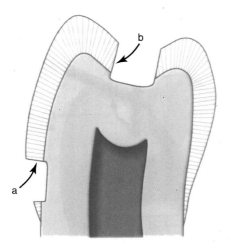

Fig. 5-11 All enamel walls must consist of either full-length enamel rods on sound dentin (*a*) or full-length enamel rods on sound dentin supported on preparation side by shortened rods also on sound dentin (*b*).

inner ends are on sound dentin (Fig. 5-11). Because enamel rods usually are perpendicular to the enamel surface, the strongest enamel margin results in a cavosurface angle greater than 90 degrees (see Fig. 5-1).

An enamel margin composed of full-length rods that are on sound dentin but are not buttressed tooth-side by shorter rods also on sound dentin is termed *strong*. Generally, this margin results in a 90-degree cavosurface angle. An enamel margin composed of rods that do not run uninterrupted from the surface to sound dentin is termed *unsupported*. Usually, this weak enamel margin either has a cavosurface angle less than 90 degrees or has no dentinal support.

Vertical (Longitudinal) and Horizontal (Transverse)

Tooth preparation features or sections that are parallel (or nearly so) to the long axis of the tooth crown are commonly described as *vertical*, such as vertical height of cusps, or vertical walls. Sometimes, the term *longitudinal* may be used in lieu of *vertical*. Tooth preparation features that are perpendicular (or nearly so) to the long axis of the tooth are termed *horizontal*, but sometimes referred to as *transverse*.

Intracoronal and Extracoronal Tooth Preparations

An intracoronal tooth preparation is usually "box-like," having internal and external preparation walls (see Figs. 5-7 to 5-9). With a conservative tooth preparation for the treatment of a small lesion, much of the tooth crown and crown surface is not involved. Nevertheless, the remaining tooth usually is weakened, and the restoration may or may not restore the tooth strength.

Conversely, the extracoronal preparation is usually "stump-like," having walls or surfaces that result from removal of most or all of the enamel. The extracoronal restoration, termed *crown*, envelops the remaining tooth crown and usually

restores some of its strength. This textbook does not include extracoronal tooth preparation for crown restorations.

Anatomic Tooth Crown and Clinical Tooth Crown

The anatomic tooth crown is the portion of the tooth covered by enamel. The clinical tooth crown is the portion of the tooth exposed to the oral cavity.

Classification of Tooth Preparations

Classification of tooth preparations according to the diseased anatomic areas involved and by the associated type of treatment was presented by Black.[1] These classifications were designated as Class I, Class II, Class III, Class IV, and Class V. Since Black's original classification, an additional class has been added, Class VI. Class I refers to pit-and-fissure lesions; the remaining classes are smooth-surface lesions. Classification originally was based on the observed frequency of carious lesions on certain aspects of the tooth. Although the relative frequency of caries locations may have changed over the years, the original classification is still used, and the various classes also are used to identify preparations and restorations (i.e., a Class I amalgam preparation or a Class I amalgam restoration).

Class I Preparations

All pit-and-fissure preparations are termed *Class I*. These include preparations on (1) occlusal surfaces of premolars and molars, (2) occlusal two-thirds of the facial and lingual surfaces of molars, and (3) the lingual surfaces of maxillary incisors. Note that a preparation takes the name of the tooth surface (aspect) that will be restored.

Class II Preparations

Preparations involving the proximal surfaces of posterior teeth are termed *Class II*.

Class III Preparations

Preparations involving the proximal surfaces of anterior teeth that do not include the incisal angle are termed *Class III*.

Class IV Preparations

Preparations involving the proximal surfaces of anterior teeth that include the incisal edge are termed *Class IV*.

Class V Preparations

Preparations on the gingival third of the facial or lingual surfaces of all teeth are termed *Class V*.

Class VI Preparations

Preparations on the incisal edges of anterior teeth or the occlusal cusp tips of posterior teeth are termed *Class VI*.

Box 5-1 Steps of Tooth Preparation

Initial tooth preparation stage
  Step 1: Outline form and initial depth
  Step 2: Primary resistance form
  Step 3: Primary retention form
  Step 4: Convenience form
Final tooth preparation stage
  Step 5: Removal of any remaining infected dentin or old restorative material (or both), if indicated
  Step 6: Pulp protection, if indicated
  Step 7: Secondary resistance and retention forms
  Step 8: Procedures for finishing external walls
  Step 9: Final procedures—cleaning, inspecting, desensitizing

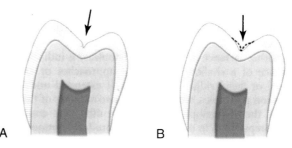

Fig. 5-12 **A,** Enameloplasty on area of imperfect coalescence of enamel. **B,** No more than one-third of the enamel thickness should be removed.

Initial and Final Stages of Tooth Preparation

The tooth preparation procedure is divided into two stages, each with several steps. Each stage should be thoroughly understood, and each step should be accomplished as perfectly as possible. The stages are presented in the sequence in which they should be followed if consistent, ideal results are to be obtained. The stages and steps in tooth preparation are listed in Box 5-1.

The sequence is changed under certain circumstances such as extensive caries that may involve the pulp. When this occurs, the sequence of these steps is altered to determine pulpal involvement and protect pulpal tissue as early in the procedure as possible. When necessary, it also is important to place the desired liner, base, or both in the preparation at this time, especially if a pulp capping procedure is necessary.

Before any restorative procedure can be undertaken, the environment in which the procedure will be done must be readied. Most restorative materials require a moisture-free environment; otherwise, the physical properties of the material are compromised. Chapter 7 presents methods of field isolation necessary to ensure the maximal effectiveness of the restorative material. In most cases, the use of the rubber dam best ensures correct isolation.

Treatment and management of the remainder of the oral environment also must be considered. Protecting the contiguous soft tissues in the operating site must be a primary objective. Oral mucosa, lips, cheek, and tongue should be protected against mechanical injury and the possible deleterious effects of substances placed in the mouth during the procedure and restoration.

The following sections present information regarding the initial and final stages of tooth preparation. The information presented is comprehensive and specific primarily for conventional (i.e., amalgam) tooth preparations. Major differences that exist for other types of tooth preparations (primarily for composite) are noted.

Initial Tooth Preparation Stage

Initial tooth preparation involves the extension of the external walls of the preparation at a specified, limited depth so as to provide access to the caries or defect and to reach the peripheral sound tooth structure. The placement and orientation of the preparation walls are designed to resist fracture of the tooth or restorative material from masticatory forces principally directed with the long axis of the tooth and to retain the restorative material in the tooth (except for a Class V preparation). In some situations, non-carious fissures or pits at the periphery of the anticipated external walls are best treated through minor modification of the enamel contours as part of the initial preparation. This procedure is referred to as *enameloplasty* (Fig. 5-12).

Enameloplasty involves the removal of a shallow, enamel developmental fissure or pit to create a smooth, saucer-shaped surface that is self-cleansing or easily cleaned. This prophylactic procedure can be applied not only to fissures and pits and deep supplemental grooves but also to some shallow, smooth-surface enamel defects. Sometimes, a groove or fossa (fissured or not) does not penetrate to any great depth into enamel but still does not allow proper preparation of tooth margins except by undesirable extension. This observation is always true of the end of a fissure. If such a shallow feature is removed, and the convolution of enamel is rounded or "saucered," the area becomes cleansable and finishable and allows conservative placement of preparation margins. Specific applications of this procedure are covered and illustrated in detail in other chapters pertaining to tooth preparations for gold and amalgam restorations. Enameloplasty does not extend the preparation outline form. The amalgam or gold restorative material is not placed into the recontoured area, and the only difference in the restoration is that the thickness of the restorative material at the enameloplastied margin (or pulpal depth of the external wall) is decreased. This approach differs from including adjacent faulty enamel areas in composite restorations because those areas are covered with the bonded composite material. Such inclusions may restore carious, decalcified, discolored, or poorly contoured areas.

Care is taken when choosing the area which will benefit from enameloplasty. Usually, a fissure should be removed by normal preparation procedures if it penetrates to more than one third the thickness of the enamel in the area. If one third or less of the enamel depth is involved, the fissure may be removed by enameloplasty without preparing or extending the tooth preparation. This procedure is applicable also to supplemental grooves (fissured or not) extending up cusp inclines. If the ends of these grooves were included in the tooth preparation, the cusp could be weakened to the extent that it would need to be capped. Provided that these areas are "saucered" by enameloplasty, the cusp strength can be retained and a smooth union effected between the restorative material and the enamel margin because the grooved enamel is eliminated.

Another instance in which enameloplasty is indicated is the presence of a shallow fissure that approaches or crosses a lingual or facial ridge. This fissure, if extended under tooth extension principles, would involve two surfaces of the tooth. Use of the enameloplasty procedure often can confine the tooth preparation to one surface and produce a smooth union of the tooth surface and restorative material. An example would be the lingual fissure of a mandibular first molar that terminates on the occlusolingual ridge. Conventional extension should terminate when approximately 2 mm of the tooth structure remains between the bur and the lingual surface, and the remainder of the fissure is then reshaped, provided that the terminal portion of the fissure is no more than one third of the enamel in depth. Otherwise, the tooth preparation must be extended onto the lingual surface.

Enameloplasty may be applied to teeth in which no preparation is anticipated. Extreme prudence must be exercised, however, in the selection of these areas and the depth of enamel removed. This procedure should not be used unless the fissure can be made into a groove with a saucer base by a minimal reduction of enamel, and unless centric contacts can be maintained. For composite preparations, it may be appropriate to seal shallow fissures with sealant or composite material, without any mechanical alteration to the fissure.[9] In the past, prophylactic odontotomy procedures were used, and these involved minimally preparing developmental or structural imperfections of the enamel, such as pits and fissures, and filling the preparation with amalgam to prevent caries from developing in these sites.[15] Prophylactic odontotomy is no longer advocated as a preventive measure.

Step 1: Outline Form and Initial Depth

The first step in initial tooth preparation is determining and developing the outline form while establishing the initial depth.

DEFINITION

Establishing the outline form means (1) placing the preparation margins in the positions they will occupy in the final preparation except for finishing enamel walls and margins and (2) preparing an initial depth of 0.2 to 0.5 mm pulpally of the DEJ position or 0.8 mm pulpally to normal root-surface position (no deeper initially whether in the tooth structure, air, old restorative material, or caries unless the occlusal enamel thickness is minimal, and greater dimension is necessary for the strength of the restorative material) (Fig. 5-13). The deeper dimension is necessary when placing secondary retention. The outline form must be visualized before any mechanical alteration to the tooth is begun.

PRINCIPLES

The three general principles on which outline form is established regardless of the type of tooth preparation being prepared are as follows: (1) all unsupported or weakened (friable) enamel usually should be removed, (2) all faults should be included, and (3) all margins should be placed in a position to allow finishing of the margins of the restoration. The third

principle has ramifications that differ for pit-and-fissure preparations compared with smooth-surface preparations.

FACTORS

In determining the outline form of a proposed tooth preparation, certain conditions or factors must first be assessed. These conditions affect the outline form and often dictate the extensions. The extent of the caries lesion, defect, or faulty old restoration affects the outline form of the proposed tooth preparation because the objective is to extend to sound tooth structure except in a pulpal direction. The one exception is that occasionally, a tooth preparation outline for a new restoration contacts or extends slightly into a sound, existing restoration (e.g., a new MO abutting a sound DO). This approach is sometimes an acceptable practice (i.e., to have a margin of a new restoration placed into an existing, sound restoration).

In addition to these factors, esthetic and occlusal conditions affect the proposed preparation. Esthetic considerations not only affect the choice of restorative material but also the design of the tooth preparation in an effort to maximize the esthetic result of the restoration. Correcting or improving occlusal relationships also may necessitate altering the tooth preparation to accommodate such changes, even when the involved tooth structure is not faulty (i.e., a cuspal form may need to be altered to effect better occlusal relationships). Likewise, the adjacent tooth contour may dictate specific preparation extensions that secure appropriate proximal relationships and provide the restored tooth with optimal form and strength. Lastly, the desired cavosurface marginal configuration of the proposed restoration affects the outline form. Restorative materials that need beveled margins require tooth preparation outline form extensions that must anticipate the final cavosurface position and form after the bevels have been placed.

FEATURES

Generally, the typical features of establishing proper outline form and initial depth are (1) preserving cuspal strength, (2) preserving marginal ridge strength, (3) minimizing faciolingual extensions, (4) connecting two close (<0.5 mm apart) defects or tooth preparations, and (5) restricting the depth of the preparation into dentin.

Step 2: Primary Resistance Form
DEFINITION

Primary resistance form may be defined as the shape and placement of the preparation walls that best enable the remaining tooth structure and the restoration to withstand, without fracture, masticatory forces delivered principally in the long axis of the tooth. The relatively horizontal pulpal and gingival floors prepared perpendicular to the tooth's long axis help resist forces in the long axis of the tooth and prevent tooth fracture from wedging effects caused by opposing cusps.

PRINCIPLES

The fundamental principles involved in obtaining primary resistance form include (1) using a box shape with a relatively horizontal floor, which helps the tooth resist occlusal loading by virtue of being at right angles to the forces of mastication that are directed in the long axis of the tooth; (2) restricting the extension of the external walls to allow strong cusp and

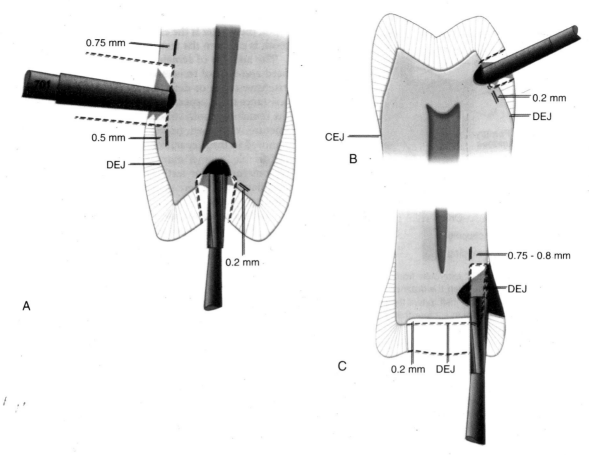

Fig. 5-13 Initial tooth preparation stage for conventional preparations. **A, B,** and **C,** Extensions in all directions are to sound tooth structure, while maintaining a specific limited pulpal or axial depth regardless of whether end (or side) of bur is in dentin, caries, old restorative material, or air. The dentinoenamel junction (DEJ) and the cementoenamel junction (CEJ) are indicated in *B*. In *A*, initial depth is approximately two-thirds of 3-mm bur head length, or 2 mm, as related to prepared facial and lingual walls, but is half the No. 245 bur head length, or 1.5 mm, as related to central fissure location.

ridge areas to remain with sufficient dentin support; (3) having a slight rounding of internal line angles to reduce stress concentrations in tooth structure; (4) reducing and covering (capping) weak cusps and enveloping or including enough of a weakened tooth within the restoration in extensive tooth preparations to prevent or resist fracture of the tooth by forces in the long axis and obliquely (laterally) directed forces (most resistance to oblique or lateral forces is attained later in the final tooth preparation stage); (5) providing enough thickness of restorative material to prevent its fracture under load; and (6) bonding the material to the tooth structure, when appropriate. Conventional and beveled preparation designs provide these resistance form principles. Modified tooth preparation designs are for small- to moderate-sized composite restorations and may not require uniform pulpal or axial depths or minimal thickness for the material.

When developing the outline form in conventional Class I and II preparations, the end of the cutting instrument prepares a relatively horizontal pulpal wall of uniform depth into the tooth (see Figs. 5-13, *A* and *C*). The pulpal wall follows the original occlusal surface contours and the DEJ (these roughly paralleling each other). Similarly, in the proximal portion of conventional Class II preparations, the end of the cutting

instrument prepares a gingival wall (floor) that is horizontal and relatively perpendicular to these forces.

Minimally extended faciolingual walls conserve dentin, supporting the cusps and faciolingual ridges, maintaining as much strength of the remaining tooth structure as possible. This resistance is against the obliquely delivered forces and the forces in the tooth's long axis.

Internal and external angles within the tooth preparation are slightly rounded so that stresses in the tooth and restoration from masticatory forces are not as concentrated at these line angles.[16,17] Rounding of internal line angles reduces the stress on the tooth, and resistance to fracture of the tooth is increased. Rounding of external angles within the tooth preparation (axiopulpal line angles) reduces the stress on some restorative materials (amalgam and ceramics), increasing resistance to fracture of the restorative material. A tooth weakened by extensive caries deserves consideration of the fourth principle [reducing and capping weakened cusps or extending to include cusps entirely] in obtaining the primary resistance form during tooth preparation. In extensive caries, facial or lingual extension of pulpal or gingival walls indicates (1) reduction of weak cusps for capping by the restorative material (Fig. 5-14) or (2) extension of the gingival floors around

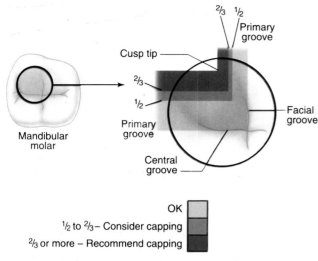

Fig. 5-14 Rule for cusp capping: If extension from a primary groove toward the cusp tip is no more than half the distance, no cusp capping should be done; if this extension is one half to two thirds of the distance, consider cusp capping; if the extension is more than two-thirds of the distance, usually cap the cusp.

axial tooth corners onto facial or lingual surfaces. Either of these features provides some resistance to forces in the long axis and to forces obliquely (laterally) directed. Reduction of cusps occurs as early as possible in the preparation to improve access and visibility. The decision to reduce a cusp is important and should be approached judiciously. The most important aspect in the evaluation of a suspicious cusp is the judgment of the amount of remaining dentin support. In addition, the cusp size and occlusal considerations may affect the decision. A basic general rule guides the reduction of cusps during initial tooth preparation: (1) cusp reduction should be considered when the outline form has extended half the distance from a primary groove to a cusp tip, and (2) cusp reduction usually is strongly recommended when the outline form has extended two-thirds the distance from a primary groove to a cusp tip. The exception to capping a cusp where extension has been two thirds from a primary groove toward the cusp tip is when the cusp is unusually large, when the operator judges that adequate cuspal strength (adequate dentin support) remains, or when a bonded restoration is being used and it is judged that bonding may provide for adequate remaining cuspal strength.[18]

In pulpless teeth, special consideration is applied in obtaining resistance form because of the weakened nature of the remaining structure.[19] The weakened cusps may need to be reduced, enveloped, and covered with restorative material to prevent the cracking or splitting of the remaining tooth structure in accord with the fourth principle mentioned previously.

FACTORS

The need to develop resistance form in a preparation is a result of several factors. Certain conditions must be assessed to reduce the potential for fracture of either the restoration or the tooth. Foremost is the assessment of the occlusal contact on the restoration and the remaining tooth structure. The greater the occlusal force and contacts, the greater is the

potential for future fracture (e.g., the further posterior the tooth, the greater is the effective masticatory force because the tooth is closer to the temporomandibular joint [TMJ]).

The amount of remaining tooth structure also affects the need and type of resistance form. Very large teeth, even with extensive caries or defects, may require less consideration of resistance form, especially in regard to capping cusps, because the remaining tooth structure still has sufficient bulk to resist fracture. Weakened, friable tooth structure always should be removed in the preparation, but sometimes unsupported, but not friable, enamel may be left. This is usually for esthetic reasons in anterior teeth, especially on the facial surfaces of maxillary teeth where stresses are minimal and a bonded restoration typically is used.

The type of restorative material also dictates resistance form needs. The minimal occlusal thickness for amalgam for appropriate resistance to fracture is 1.5 mm; cast metal, 1 to 2 mm (depending on the region); and ceramics, 2 mm. The dimensional needs of composite depend more on the occlusal wear potential of the restored area. The thickness requirement is greater for posterior teeth than for anterior teeth. Composite can be used in thinner applications such as veneers or minor esthetic enhancements as long as the wear potential is considered.

The last factor relates to the enhancement of resistance form simply by bonding a restoration to the tooth. Bonding amalgam, composite, or ceramic to prepared tooth structure may increase the strength of the remaining unprepared tooth, reducing the potential for fracture.[18] The benefits of the bonding procedures may permit the operator to leave a portion of the tooth in a more weakened state than usual or not to cap a cusp.

FEATURES

The design features of tooth preparation that enhance primary resistance form are as follows:

1. Relatively horizontal floors
2. Box-like shape
3. Inclusion of weakened tooth structure
4. Preservation of cusps and marginal ridges
5. Rounded internal line angles
6. Adequate thickness of restorative material
7. Reduction of cusps for capping, when indicated

Step 3: Primary Retention Form
DEFINITION

Primary retention form is the shape or form of the conventional preparation that prevents displacement or removal of the restoration by tipping or lifting forces for nonbonded restorations. In many respects, retention form and resistance form are accomplished at the same time (Fig. 5-15). The retention form developed during initial tooth preparation may be adequate to retain the restorative material in the tooth. Sometimes, however, additional retention features must be incorporated in the final stage of tooth preparation. Often, features that enhance the retention form of a preparation also enhance the resistance form (e.g., pins placed in a manner so that one portion of a tooth supports another portion of the tooth).

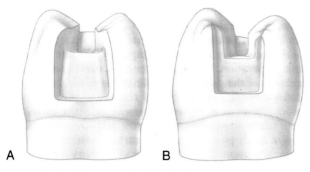

Fig. 5-15 Basic primary retention form in Class II tooth preparations for amalgam (A) with vertical external walls of proximal and occlusal portions converging occlusally and for inlay (B) with similar walls slightly diverging occlusally.

PRINCIPLES

Because retention needs are related to the restorative material used, the principles of primary retention form vary, depending on the material. For amalgam restorations in most Class I and all Class II conventional preparations, the material is retained in the tooth by developing external tooth walls that converge occlusally (see Fig. 5-15, A). In this way, when the amalgam is placed in the preparation and hardens, it cannot be dislodged without some type of fracture occurring. The occlusal convergence should not be excessive which would result in unsupported enamel rods at the cavosurface margin. In other conventional preparations for amalgam (e.g., Class III and V), the external walls diverge outwardly to provide strong enamel margins, and retention coves or grooves are prepared in the dentinal walls to provide the retention form (see Step 7: Secondary Resistance and Retention Forms).

Adhesive systems provide some retention by micromechanically bonding amalgam to tooth structure and reducing or eliminating microleakage.[20,21] However, these effects appear to have little clinical value for tooth reinforcement. Studies show that bonded amalgams do not result in long-term reinforcement of teeth or improved resistance to fracture.[22] Therefore, this book does not promote the use of bonded amalgam restorations.[23,24]

Composite restorations primarily are retained in the tooth by a micromechanical bond that develops between the material and the etched and primed tooth structure. In such restorations, enamel and dentin are etched by an acid (when using an etch-and-rinse adhesive), and dentin is primed with an adhesive before placement of the composite. Additional retention may be accomplished when the surface area of the enamel available for bonding is increased by a beveled or flared (>90 degrees) enamel marginal configuration. Sometimes, tooth preparation for a composite restoration also requires the use of the mechanical retention form used in preparations for nonbonded restoration, which is considered part of the final stage of preparation.

Cast metal (usually a gold alloy) intracoronal restorations rely primarily on almost parallel vertical walls to provide retention of the casting in the tooth. During the initial tooth preparation, the preparation walls must be designed not only to provide for draw (for the casting to be placed into the tooth) but also to provide for an appropriate small angle of divergence (2-5 degrees per wall) from the line of draw that would enhance retention form. The degree of divergence needed primarily depends on the length of the prepared walls: The greater the vertical height of the walls, the more divergence is permitted and recommended, but within the range described.

In inlay and onlay preparations for cast-metal restorations, the opposing vertical walls diverge outwardly by only a few degrees to each other and to a draw path that is usually perpendicular to the floor of the preparation (see Fig. 5-15, B). Close parallelism of prepared vertical walls is a principal retention form for cast-metal restorations, another being the use of a luting agent that bonds to tooth structure.

Step 4: Convenience Form

Convenience form is the shape or form of the preparation that provides for adequate observation, accessibility, and ease of operation in preparing and restoring the tooth. Occasionally, obtaining this form may necessitate the extension of distal, mesial, facial, or lingual walls to gain adequate access to the deeper portion of the preparation. The arbitrary extension of facial margins on anterior teeth usually is contraindicated, however, for esthetic reasons.

The occlusal divergence of vertical walls of tooth preparations for Class II cast restorations also may be considered convenience form. Extending proximal preparations beyond proximal contacts is another convenience form procedure. Although exceptions may be made to such an extension, preparing the proximal walls to obtain clearance with an adjacent proximal surface affords better access to finish the preparation walls and the restorative material and to place a matrix. For cast gold restorations, clearance with the adjacent proximal surface is mandatory to finish the preparation walls, make an accurate impression of the prepared tooth, and try-in the casting.

Final Tooth Preparation Stage

When the extensions and wall designs have fulfilled the objectives of initial tooth preparation, the preparation should be inspected carefully for other needs. With very conservative amalgam or composite restorations, the preparation may be complete after initial tooth preparation except for (1) desensitizing the prepared dentin walls for amalgam or (2) etching and priming the prepared walls for the adhesive for amalgam or composite. More involved lesions require additional steps (see steps 5 through 9 below) in the final tooth preparation stage.

Step 5: Removal of Any Remaining Enamel Pit or Fissure, Infected Dentin, or Old Restorative Material, If Indicated
DEFINITION

Removal of any remaining enamel pit or fissure, infected dentin, or old restorative material is the elimination of any infected carious tooth structure or faulty restorative material left in the tooth after initial tooth preparation. In preparations that remain in enamel, removal of any remaining enamel pit or fissure typically occurs as small, minimally extended excavations on isolated faulty areas of the pulpal floor.

In dentin, as caries progresses, an area of decalcification precedes the penetration of microorganisms. This area of decalcification often appears discolored compared with undisturbed dentin, and yet it does not exhibit the soft texture of caries. This dentin condition may be termed *affected dentin* and differs from *infected dentin* in that it has not lost structural integrity to the point which allows ready invasion by microorganisms. It is accepted and appropriate practice to allow affected dentin to remain in a prepared tooth.

The use of color alone to determine how much dentin to remove is unreliable. Often, soft, acute (rapid) caries manifests itself entirely within the normal range of color for dentin; the eye may not differentiate among infected, affected, or unaffected (normal) dentin. Distinctly discolored dentin, certainly affected, may simply be stained or sclerotic and is often comparable in hardness with surrounding unaffected (normal) dentin. A clinical description of exactly where infected dentin stops and affected dentin begins is practically impossible. It is an empiric decision made possible by practical knowledge and experience. The decision does not require exactness, for it is not necessary that all dentin invaded by microorganisms be removed. In shallow or moderately deep lesions, the removal of the masses of microorganisms and the subsequent sealing of the preparation by a restoration at best destroy those comparatively few remaining microorganisms and at worst reduce them to inactivity or dormancy.[25] Even in deep caries in which actual invasion of the pulp may have occurred, the recovery of the pulp requires only that a favorable balance be established for the pulp between the virulence of the organisms and the resistance of the host. This balance is often accomplished by removing all soft caries with its numerous organisms.[26] See Chapter 2 for caries detection and treatment modalities. However, leaving carious dentin at the DEJ area is unacceptable primarily because enamel requires an uncompromised attachment to dentin to be able to withstand the rigors of the oral environment (see Fig. 5-3).

After initial tooth preparation, the initial depths may result in old restorative material remaining on the pulpal or axial walls. Any remaining old restorative material should be removed if any of the following conditions are present: (1) the old material may affect negatively the esthetic result of the new restoration (i.e., old amalgam material left under a new composite restoration), (2) the old material may compromise the amount of needed retention (i.e., old glass ionomer material having a weaker bond to the tooth than the new composite restoration using enamel and dentin bonding), (3) radiographic evidence indicates caries is under the old material, (4) the tooth pulp was symptomatic pre-operatively, or (5) the periphery of the remaining old restorative material is not intact (i.e., some breach has occurred in the junction of the material with the adjacent tooth structure that may indicate caries under the old material). If none of these conditions is present, it is acceptable to leave the remaining old restorative material to serve as a base, rather than risk unnecessary excavation nearer to the pulp, which may result in pulpal irritation or exposure.

TECHNIQUES

When a pulpal or axial wall has been established at the proper initial tooth preparation position, and a small amount of infected carious material remains, only this material should be removed, leaving a rounded, concave area in the wall. The level or position of the wall peripheral to the caries removal depression should not be altered.

In large preparations with extensive soft caries, the removal of infected dentin may be accomplished early in the initial tooth preparation. When the extensive caries is removed, the condition of the pulp and the remaining tooth structure has a definite bearing on the type of restoration placed. For this reason, it is more expedient to remove extensive caries early in the tooth preparation before time and effort are spent in doing a tooth preparation for a certain restorative material that is then deemed inadequate for satisfactory restoration of the tooth.

Another instance in which the removal of caries is indicated early in tooth preparation is when a patient has numerous teeth with extensive caries. In one appointment, infected dentin is removed from several teeth, and temporary restorations are placed. After all the teeth containing extensive caries are so treated, individual teeth are restored definitively. This procedure stops the progression of caries and is often referred to as a *caries-control procedure* (see Chapter 2).

With regard to the removal of the harder, heavily discolored dentin, opinions vary among the use of spoon excavators, round steel burs at very low speed, and round carbide burs rotating at high speeds. Several factors must be taken into consideration in the removal of this type of caries in deep-seated lesions, although basically the primary concern is for the pulp. Pulpal damage may result from the creation of frictional heat with the use of a bur. The pulp may become infected by forcing microorganisms into the dentinal tubules through excessive pressure with a spoon excavator, or it may be exposed when either instrument is used. The ideal method of removing this material would be one in which minimal pressure is exerted, frictional heat is minimized, and complete control of the instrument is maintained. Consideration of these factors usually favors the use of a round carbide bur, in a slow- or high-speed handpiece, with air coolant and slow speed. This technique gives the operator complete control of the instrument, minimizes pressure and heat generation, and permits adequate vision of the area being operated on. Examination of the area with an explorer after the removal of infected dentin is advisable, but this should be done judiciously to avoid perforation into the pulp. Caries that rapidly develops sometimes is relatively unstained, and unless the sense of touch is relied on to detect softness, the operator unintentionally may leave infected dentin. Ideally, removal of infected dentin should continue until the remaining dentin hardness approaches that of normal dentin. Heavy pressure should not be applied with an explorer, however, or any other instrument, on what is believed to be a thin layer of reasonably firm dentin next to a healthy pulp, to avoid creating unnecessary pulpal exposure.

Removal of remaining old restorative material, when indicated, also is accomplished with use of a round carbide bur, at slow speed (just above stall-out) with air or air-water coolant. The water spray (along with high-volume evacuation) is used when removing old amalgam material to reduce the amount of mercury vapor.

Step 6: Pulp Protection, If Indicated

Although the placement of liners and bases is not a step in tooth preparation, in the strict sense of the term, it is a step in adapting the preparation for receiving the final restorative material. The reason for using liners or bases is to protect the pulp or to aid pulpal recovery or both. Pulpal irritation that occurs during or after operative procedures may result from (1) heat generated by rotary instruments, (2) some ingredients of various materials, (3) thermal changes conducted through restorative materials, (4) forces transmitted through materials to the dentin, (5) galvanic shock, and (6) the ingress of noxious products and bacteria through microleakage.[27]

Because the ingress of bacteria is most commonly associated with various pulpal responses, more emphasis should be given to the complete sealing of the prepared dentinal tubules. Effective tubular sealing may prevent penetration of bacteria into the tubules and limit the retrograde diffusion of bacterial toxins toward the pulp.

Certain physical, chemical, and biologic factors should be considered in the selection of a liner or base. The material used should be one that, under the circumstances, more nearly satisfies the needs of the individual tooth and is based on an assessment of the anatomic, physiologic, and biologic response characteristics of the pulp and the physical and chemical properties of the considered material.

In the following discussion of liners and bases, the use of the term *liners* may include suspensions or dispersions of zinc oxide, calcium hydroxide, or resin-modified glass ionomer (RMGI) that can be applied to a tooth surface in a relatively thin film.[20] Liners also may provide (1) a barrier that protects the dentin from noxious agents from either the restorative material or oral fluids, (2) initial electrical insulation, or (3) some thermal protection.[28] *Bases* are materials, most commonly cements, that are used in thicker dimensions beneath permanent restorations to provide for mechanical, chemical, and thermal protection of the pulp. Examples of bases include zinc phosphate, zinc oxide–eugenol, polycarboxylate, and the most common, some type of glass ionomer (usually an RMGI).

A liner is used to medicate the pulp when suspected trauma has occurred. The desired pulpal effects include sedation and stimulation, the latter resulting in reparative dentin formation. The specific pulpal response desired dictates the choice of liner. If the removal of infected dentin does not extend deeper than 1 to 2 mm from the initially prepared pulpal or axial wall, usually no liner is indicated. If the excavation extends into or within 0.5 mm of the pulp, a calcium hydroxide liner usually is selected to stimulate reparative dentin (indirect pulp cap procedure).[29]

Zinc oxide–eugenol and calcium hydroxide liners (chemosetting types that harden) in thicknesses of approximately 0.5 mm or greater have adequate strength to resist condensation forces of amalgam and provide protection against short-term thermal changes.[30] *Calcium hydroxide liners must always be covered with an RMGI to prevent dissolution of the liner over time when used under amalgam restorations.* Generally, it is desirable to have approximately a 2-mm dimension of bulk between the pulp and a metallic restorative material. This bulk may include remaining dentin, liner, or base. Base materials offer pulpal protection from mechanical, thermal, and chemical irritants. For composite restorative materials, which are thermal insulators, the calcium hydroxide should be covered by an RMGI to protect the liner from dissolution from the etchant used for the composite placement.[27,31] Very deep excavations may contain microscopic pulpal exposures that are not visible to the naked eye. Hemorrhage is the usual evidence of a vital pulp exposure, but with microscopic exposures, such evidence may be lacking. Nevertheless, these exposures are large enough to allow direct pulpal access for bacteria and fluids. The ability of hard-setting calcium hydroxide materials to stimulate the formation of reparative dentin when it is in contact with pulpal tissue makes it the usual material of choice for application to very deep excavations and known pulpal exposures (direct pulp cap procedures).[29] Liners and bases in exposure areas should be applied without pressure.

Usually, an RMGI is used for "base" needs. These materials effectively bond to tooth structure, release fluoride, and have sufficient strength. They are easily placed and contoured, when necessary. Because of their chemical and micromechanical bond to tooth structure, retentive preparation features are not typically required. These materials are excellent for use under amalgam, gold, ceramic, and composite restorations.

The protective qualities of zinc phosphate, polycarboxylate, and glass ionomer cements are in proportion to the bulk of material used. A thin layer does not afford the protection of a thicker layer. The level to which a base is built should never compromise the desired tooth preparation depth, resulting in inadequate restorative material thickness.

Step 7: Secondary Resistance and Retention Forms

After any remaining enamel pit or fissure, infected dentin, or old restorative material (if indicated) has been removed, and pulpal protection has been provided by appropriate liners and bases, additional resistance and retention features may be deemed necessary for the preparation. Many compound and complex preparations require these additional features. When a tooth preparation includes occlusal and proximal surfaces, each of those areas should have independent retention and resistance features.

Because many preparation features that improve retention form also improve resistance form, and the reverse is true, they are presented together. The *secondary retention and resistance forms* are of two types: (1) mechanical preparation features and (2) treatments of the preparation walls with etching, priming, and adhesive materials. The second type is not really considered a part of tooth preparation but, rather, the first step for the insertion of the restorative material. Regardless, some general comments are presented about such treatments.

MECHANICAL FEATURES

A variety of mechanical alterations to the preparation enhance retention form, and these alterations require additional removal of tooth structure.

Retention Grooves and Coves

Vertically oriented retention grooves are used to provide additional retention for the proximal portions of some conventional tooth preparations. Horizontally oriented retention grooves are prepared in most Class III and Class V preparations for amalgam and in some root-surface tooth preparations for composite. Retention coves are placed for the incisal retention of Class III amalgams.

Historically, retention grooves in Class II preparations for amalgam restorations were recommended to increase retention of the proximal portion against movement proximally secondary to creep. Also, it was thought that they may increase the resistance form of the restoration against fracture at the junction of the proximal and occlusal portions. In vivo studies do not substantiate the necessity of these grooves in proximo-occlusal preparations with occlusal dovetail outline forms or in MOD preparations.[4,32] They are recommended, however, for extensive tooth preparations for amalgam involving wide faciolingual proximal boxes, cusp capping, or both. Therefore, mastery of the techniques of optimal groove design and placement is indicated.

Preparation Extensions

Additional retention of the restorative material may be obtained by arbitrarily extending the preparation for molars onto the facial or lingual surface to include a facial or lingual groove. Such an extension, when performed for cast metal restorations, results in additional vertical, almost-parallel walls for retention. This feature also enhances resistance for the remaining tooth owing to envelopment.

Skirts

Skirts are preparation features used in cast gold restorations that extend the preparation around some, if not all, of the line angles of the tooth. When properly prepared, skirts provide additional, opposed vertical walls for added retention. The placement of skirts also significantly increases resistance form by enveloping the tooth, resisting fracture of the remaining tooth from occlusal forces.

Beveled Enamel Margins

Cast metal and some composite restorations include beveled marginal configurations. The bevels for cast metal may improve retention form slightly when opposing bevels are present but are used primarily to afford a better junctional relationship between the metal and the tooth. Enamel margins of some composite restorations may have a beveled or flared configuration to increase the surface area of etchable enamel and to maximize the effectiveness of the bond by etching more enamel rod ends.

Pins, Slots, Steps, and Amalgam Pins

When the need for increased retention form is unusually great, especially for amalgam restorations, several other features may be incorporated into the preparation. Pins and slots increase retention and resistance forms. Amalgam pins and properly positioned steps also improve retention form, but not to the extent of pins or slots.

PLACEMENT OF ETCHANT, PRIMER, OR ADHESIVE ON PREPARED WALLS

In addition to mechanical alterations to the tooth preparation, certain alterations to the preparation walls by actions of various materials also afford increased retention and resistance to fracture. Enamel and dentin surfaces may be treated with etchants or primers or both for certain restorative procedures.

Enamel Wall Etching

Enamel walls are etched for bonded restorations that use ceramic, composite, and amalgam materials. This procedure consists of etching the enamel with an appropriate acid, resulting in a microscopically roughened surface to which the bonding material is mechanically bound.

Dentin Treatment

Dentinal surfaces may require etching and priming when using bonded ceramic, composite, or amalgam restorations. The actual treatment varies with the restorative material used, but for most composite restorations, a dentin bonding agent is recommended. Retention of indirect restorations may be enhanced by the luting agent used. Although not considered part of the tooth preparation, the cementation procedure does affect the retention of these restorations, and some cementing materials require pretreatment of the dentin, resulting in varying degrees of micromechanical bonding.

Step 8: Procedures for Finishing the External Walls of the Tooth Preparation

Finishing the external walls of the preparation entails consideration of degree of smoothness and cavosurface design because each restorative material has its maximal effectiveness when the appropriate conditions are developed for that specific material. Not all preparations require special finishing of the external walls at this stage because the walls already may have been finished during earlier steps in the preparation. This is particularly true for many composite preparations and most amalgam preparations.

Because most preparations have external walls in enamel, most of the following discussion relates to the appropriate finishing of enamel walls. Nevertheless, when a preparation has extended onto the root surface (no enamel present), the root-surface cavosurface angle should be either 90 degrees (for amalgam, composite, or ceramic restorations) or beveled (for intracoronal cast metal restorations). The 90-degree, root-surface margin provides a butt joint relationship between the restorative material and the cementum or dentin preparation wall, a configuration that provides appropriate strength to both.

DEFINITION

Finishing the preparation walls is the further development, when indicated, of a specific cavosurface design and degree of smoothness or roughness that produces the maximum effectiveness of the restorative material being used.

OBJECTIVES

The objectives of finishing the prepared walls are to (1) create an optimal marginal junction between the restorative material and the tooth structure, (2) afford a smooth marginal junction, and (3) provide maximal strength of the tooth and the restorative material at and near the margin. The following factors must be considered in the finishing of enamel walls and margins: (1) the direction of the enamel rods, (2) the support of the enamel rods at the DEJ and laterally (preparation side), (3) the type of restorative material to be placed in the preparation, (4) the location of the margin, and (5) the degree of smoothness or roughness desired.

Theoretically, the enamel rods radiate from the DEJ to the external surface of the enamel and are perpendicular to the tooth surface. All rods extend full length from dentin to the enamel surface. The rods converge from the DEJ toward

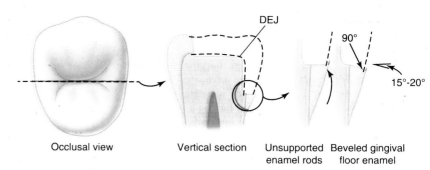

Fig. 5-16 Vertical section of Class II tooth preparation. Gingival floor enamel (and margin) is unsupported on dentin and friable unless removed.

Occlusal view　Vertical section　Unsupported enamel rods　Beveled gingival floor enamel

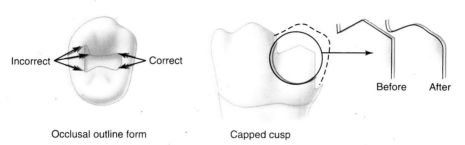

Occlusal outline form　Capped cusp

Fig. 5-17 The junctions of enamel walls (and respective margins) should be slightly rounded, whether obtuse or acute.

concave enamel surfaces and diverge outwardly toward convex surfaces. In general, the rods converge toward the center of developmental grooves and diverge toward the height of cusps and ridges (see Figs. 5-1, *B* and *C*). In the gingival third of enamel of the smooth surfaces in the permanent dentition, the rods incline slightly apically (Fig. 5-16).

In some instances, the rods of occlusal enamel seem to be harder than those of axial (mesial, facial, distal, lingual) enamel. This difference can be attributed to the amount of interlacing or twisting of the rods in the former compared with the straight rods of the latter. Enamel with such interlacing of the rods is termed *gnarled enamel.*

Enamel walls should be oriented such that all rods forming the prepared enamel wall have their inner ends resting on sound dentin. Enamel rods that do not run uninterrupted from the preparation margin to dentin tend to split off, leaving a V-shaped ditch along the cavosurface margin area of the restoration. This should not be interpreted to mean that all enamel walls should consist of full-length rods. The strongest enamel margin is one that is composed of full-length enamel rods supported on the preparation side by shorter enamel rods, all of which extend to sound dentin (see Fig. 5-11). The shorter enamel rods buttress the full-length enamel rods that form the margin, increasing the strength of the enamel margin.

An acute, abrupt change in an enamel wall outline form results in fracture potential, even though the enamel may have dentin support. The preparation outline and walls should have smooth curves or straight lines. When two enamel walls join, the resulting line angle may be "sharp." If so, it should be slightly curved ("softened"). This slight rounding usually results in a similar curve at the margin. In other words, line angles formed by the junction of enamel walls should be slightly rounded whether they are obtuse or acute (Fig. 5-17).

FEATURES

Finishing of external walls has two primary features: (1) the design of the cavosurface angle and (2) the degree of smoothness or roughness of the wall. The design of the cavosurface angle depends on the restorative material being used. Because of the low edge strength of amalgam and ceramic, a 90-degree cavosurface angle produces maximal strength for these materials and the tooth. No bevels are placed at the cavosurface margin. On occlusal surfaces for Class I and Class II amalgam restorations, the incline planes of the cusp and the converging walls (for retentive purposes) of the preparation approximate the desirable 90 degree butt joint junction, even though the actual occlusal enamel margin may be greater than 90 degrees.

Beveling the external walls is a preparation technique used for some materials, such as intracoronal cast-gold or cast-metal and composite restorations.

Beveling can serve four useful purposes in the tooth preparation for a casting: (1) it produces a stronger enamel margin, (2) it permits a marginal seal in slightly undersized castings, (3) it provides marginal metal that is more easily burnished and adapted, and (4) it assists in adaptation of gingival margins of castings that fail to seat by a slight amount.

When amalgam is used, beveling is contraindicated except on the gingival floor of a Class II preparation when enamel is still present. In these instances, it is usually necessary to place a slight bevel (approximately 15-20 degrees) only on the enamel portion of the wall to remove unsupported enamel rods. This is necessary because of the gingival orientation of enamel rods in the cervical area of the tooth crown. This minimal bevel may be placed with an appropriate gingival margin trimmer hand instrument and, when placed, still results in a 90 degree amalgam marginal angle (see Fig. 5-16).

Sometimes, the unsupported enamel rods are removed simply by an explorer tip pulled along the margin.

Beveling enamel margins in composite preparations is indicated primarily for larger restorations that have increased retention needs. The use of a beveled marginal form with a composite tooth preparation may be advocated because the potential for retention is increased by increasing the surface area of enamel available for etch and having a more effective area of etch obtained by etching the cut ends of the enamel rods. Other advantages of beveling composites are as follows: (1) adjacent, minor defects can be included with a bevel, (2) esthetic quality may be enhanced by a bevel creating an area of gradual increase in composite thickness from the margin to the bulk of the restoration, and (3) the marginal seal may be enhanced.

The degree of desired smoothness or roughness is the second consideration in finishing the external walls. The advent of high-speed cutting procedures has produced two pertinent factors related to finishing the enamel walls: (1) the lessening of tactile sense and (2) the rapid removal of tooth structure. High speed can lead to over-extension of margins, grooved walls, or rounded cavosurface angles, especially on proximal margins. If this method is used, plain-cut fissure burs produce the finest surface.[33] These burs produce a smoother surface than crosscut burs, diamonds, or carborundum stones.[34] An excellent finish is achieved with this type of bur at lower rotational speeds.

In instances when proximal margins are left at minimal extension for esthetic reasons, rotating instruments (burs, stones, wheels, or disks) may not be usable because of lack of proper access. In such locations, hand instruments may need to be used. The planing action of a sharp hand instrument can result in a smooth enamel wall, although it may not be as smooth as that achieved with other instruments.[35] Hand instruments such as enamel hatchets and margin trimmers may be used in planing enamel walls, cleaving enamel, and establishing enamel bevels.

The restorative material used is the primary factor dictating the desired smoothness or roughness of an enamel wall. The prepared walls of inlay or onlay preparations require a smooth surface to permit undistorted impressions and close adaptation of the casting to the enamel margins.[36] In areas of sufficient access, fine sandpaper disks can create a smooth surface; however, proper use of hand instruments, plain fissure burs, finishing carbide burs, or fine diamond stones also creates satisfactory enamel margins. Prepared walls and margins of composite restorations can be roughened, usually by a coarse diamond rotary instrument, to provide increased surface area for bonding. Likewise when using amalgam restorative materials, a smooth preparation wall is not as desirable as for cast restorations. When amalgam materials are used, it has been shown that a rougher prepared wall markedly improves resistance to marginal leakage.[37] This observation does not mean, however, that finishing of the enamel wall should be ignored, but it does indicate that no strict rule for the selection of the finishing instrument can be applied in all instances.

Step 9: Final Procedures: Cleaning, Inspecting, and Desensitizing

The usual procedure in cleaning is to free the preparation of visible debris with water from the syringe and then to remove

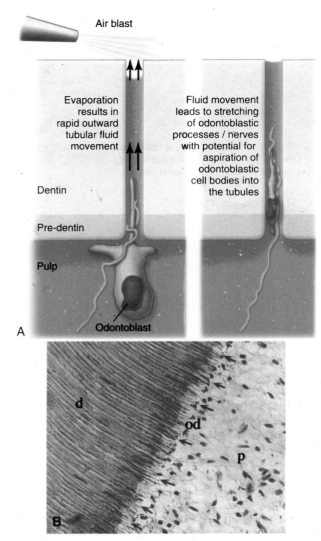

Fig. 5-18 **A,** Excessive drying of tooth preparations can cause odontoblasts to be aspirated into dentinal tubules. **B,** Nuclei are seen as dark rods in dentinal tubules. Red arrows indicate the nuclei of the aspirated odontoblasts. Green arrows indicate location of the odontoblasts prior to them being sucked into the tubules. *d,* dentin; *od,* odontoblasts; *p,* pulp. (**B,** *From Mitsiadis TA, De Bari C, About I: Apoptosis in development and repair-related human tooth remodeling: A view from the inside.* Exp Cell Res *314(4):869–877, 2008.*)

the visible moisture with a few light bursts of air from the air syringe. In some instances, debris clings to walls and angles despite the aforementioned efforts, and it may be necessary to loosen this material with an explorer or small cotton pellet. After all of the visible debris has been removed, the excess moisture is removed. It is important not to dehydrate the tooth by overuse of air as this may damage the odontoblasts associated with the desiccated tubules (Fig. 5-18). When the preparation has been cleaned adequately, it is visually inspected to confirm complete debridement.

Composite restorations require some treatment of the preparation before insertion of the restorative material. This treatment usually includes etching enamel and dentin and placing a resin-based adhesive. The smear layer usually is either altered or removed, and a hybrid layer is formed, which is characterized by an intermingling of the resin adhesive with collagen fibrils of the intertubular dentin. This creates a strong mechanical bond between the composite and dentin. It has been identified that the bond to dentin deteriorates over time as a result of hydrolysis of the adhesive resin component of the hybrid layer and proteolytic degradation of the collagen component of the hybrid layer.[38] Ongoing dental research has sought to optimize the long-term stability of the hybrid layer. For example, *in vivo* studies have shown that chlorhexidine (2 weight percent [wt%] solution) application to etched dentin is able to limit the activity of local collagenolytic enzymes (matrix metalloproteinases [MMPs]), which are able to degrade the exposed collagen matrix, and thus may help stabilize the hybrid layer, at least in Class I preparations for the short-term.[39] Long-term hybrid layer stability as a result of chlorhexidine use has not been demonstrated. These findings, as well as the decision to incorporate chlorhexidine or other dentin protease inhibitors as a final preparation step for hybrid layer stabilization, are to be considered in light of clinical studies that reveal that the clinical performance of composite resin systems that did not use chlorhexidine is comparable with that of amalgam.[40] In addition to the dentin bond, strong mechanical bonding occurs between the composite and the etched enamel, when enamel is present.

In accomplishing the final procedures before insertion of the restorative material, disinfection of the preparation may be considered. Although in the past, the term *sterilization* was used in the discussion of this topic, *disinfection* is a more accurate term to describe the objective. Chlorhexidine (2 wt%) solutions may be used in preparations for disinfection purposes in addition to the enzyme inhibition step mentioned above. The dentin tubule lumen, varying from 1 to 4 μm in diameter at varying distances between the DEJ and the pulp, presents a pathway for the entrance of microorganisms. Investigators have verified the presence of microorganisms in the dentin tubules beneath preparation walls. This fact in no way indicates, however, that caries is progressing or that failures will automatically result. It has been contended that caries in dentin stops or gradually ceases as soon as the caries lesion is closed to the oral environment, even if microorganisms remain in dentin.[41] Investigators have noted that the number of bacteria in the dentin tubules is relatively small compared with the numerous microorganisms found in the superficial carious lesion. The question is whether these remaining organisms are capable of extending caries under the environmental circumstances of a restored tooth.[26]

The possible infection of the pulp is always a consideration when bacteria remain in a channel that terminates in the pulp chamber. In this respect, the resistance of vital tissue to the ingress of bacteria must be considered. The precipitation of mineral in the dentinal tubules beneath a caries lesion (giving it a transparent appearance) creates a physical barrier to bacterial ingress. In addition to this host defense mechanism, the presence of reparative dentin deposited as a result of pulpal insult constitutes a significant deterrent to bacterial progress. Bacteria may be in a dormant condition as the result of the more sealed environment of a restored tooth.

Assuming that a surface disinfectant is successful, it is doubtful that the disinfection can exist for any appreciable length of time because of the difference between the thermal coefficients of expansion of the tooth and filling materials.[42,43] Although differing in amounts, marginal leakage has been shown for most restorative materials.[32,44,45] A large percentage of non-disinfected restorations exhibit no caries on the internal wall as a result of this oral fluid penetration; it is possible that the natural defense mechanism of the tooth or the germicidal action of the restorative material destroys any invading bacteria. Some protection from further carious action is afforded by some restorative materials.[46] The germicidal or protective effect ranges from the fluoride content of some materials to the deposition of corrosive products at the interface of the preparation wall in an amalgam. Zinc oxide-eugenol cement has significant germicidal properties over an extended period. The use of desensitizers (for non-bonded restorations) and dentin bonding agents (for bonded restorations) to limit post-operative sensitivity has been recognized.

Occlusion of the dentinal tubules limits the potential for tubular fluid movement and resultant sensitivity. Desensitizers are effective disinfectants, provide crosslinking of any exposed dentin matrix and occlude ("plug") the dentinal tubules by crosslinking tubular proteins.[47] Preparations designed for amalgam restoration should be desensitized with a solution that contains 5% glutaraldehyde and 35% 2-hydroxyethyl methacrylate (HEMA) before amalgam placement.[47,48] Desensitizers may be used before cementing restorations with nonbonding luting agents. Desensitizers may be used immediately after etching and before priming of the dentin, if desired. All bonded restorations (composites, amalgams, glass ionomer materials, and bonded indirect restorations) use various adhesive systems that not only bond the material to the tooth but also seal the prepared tooth structure.

Additional Concepts in Tooth Preparation

Any new techniques which are advocated for the restoration of teeth should be assessed on the basis of the fundamentals of tooth preparation presented in this chapter. Understanding these fundamental principles makes the assessment of new approaches easier and wiser. Because amalgam and composite restorations are done more often than other operative procedures, most of the proposed new ways to restore teeth relate to these types of restorations.

Preparations for Amalgam Restorations

Several other restorative techniques have been advocated for use with amalgam restorations. These preparation techniques should be evaluated in light of the following pre-requisites for amalgam success: (1) 90-degree junctions of amalgam with tooth structure, (2) mechanical retention form, and (3) adequate thickness for the amalgam material.

Amalgam Box-Only Tooth Preparations

Box-only tooth preparations for amalgam may be advocated for some posterior teeth in which a proximal surface requires restoration, but the occlusal surface is not faulty. A proximal box is prepared and specific retention form is provided, but no occlusal step is included. Such restorations are more conservative in that less tooth structure is removed. That conservation of tooth structure must be weighed against possible loss of retention form provided by the occlusal step of a typical Class II amalgam preparation. Proximal retention grooves may be indicated as part of this preparation design.

Amalgam Tunnel Tooth Preparations

In an effort to be conservative of tooth structure removal, other investigators advocate a tunnel tooth preparation. This preparation joins an occlusal lesion with a proximal lesion by means of a prepared tunnel under the involved marginal ridge. In this way, the marginal ridge remains essentially intact. In assessing this technique, the adequacy of preparation access may be controversial. Developing appropriately formed preparation walls and excavating caries may be compromised by lack of access and visibility. Whether or not the marginal ridge is preserved in a strong state also is controversial, especially since the dentinal support (essential for enamel longevity) of the marginal ridge is no longer present. This technique is controversial and is not supported in this textbook.

Adhesive Amalgam Restorations

Other techniques advocated for amalgam restorations use adhesive systems.[21,49,50] Some of these materials mechanically bond the amalgam material to tooth structure. Others seal the prepared tooth structure with an adhesive resin before amalgam placement.[51] The technique for the adhesive resin liner is different in that the adhesive is placed and polymerized before the amalgam placement. Although the proposed bonding techniques vary for bonded amalgams, the essential procedure is to prepare the tooth in a fashion similar to typical amalgam preparations except that more weakened, remaining tooth structure may be retained. Next, the preparation walls are treated or covered with specific adhesive lining materials that mechanically bond to the tooth and the amalgam. The amalgam is condensed into this adhesive material before polymerization, and a bond develops between the amalgam and adhesive. Because studies demonstrate no long-term benefit with regards to tooth reinforcement, this book does not promote the use of bonded amalgams.[22-24]

Preparations for Composite Restorations

Other concepts relate to the use of composite to restore teeth. Some newer concepts relating to preparations for composite restorations are presented in Chapters 8 to 12. In these chapters, more conservative preparations and preparations relating to expanded uses of composite, such as for esthetic enhancements, the conservative composite restoration of posterior occlusal surfaces, preventive resin restoration, veneers, and ceramic inlays cemented with composite materials, are presented.

Understanding the requirements of successful composite restorations is essential when assessing any proposed modifications. For a composite restoration to be successful, (1) marginal enamel may be beveled or have a flared form, and all should be etched; (2) dentin bonding systems should be used; and (3) non-enamel (root surface) external walls should provide butt-joint shapes, when necessary, and have

appropriately placed mechanical retention form, when indicated (see Table 5-1).

Composite Box-Only Tooth Preparations

The box-only preparations for composite restorations are similar to the preparations for amalgam restorations except that the box form is less distinct, having "roughed-out" marginal configurations rather than refined, 90-degree butt joints. The prepared tooth structure (enamel and dentin) is etched, primed, or both, which provides the retention form of the material in the tooth.

Composite Tunnel Tooth Preparations

The tunnel preparation, as described earlier, also has been advocated for composite restorations. Usually, it also is advocated to use an RMGI liner under the composite, and some investigators suggest that this preparation design be partially or completely restored with a glass ionomer restorative material. The same disadvantages exist as with amalgam tunnel restorations, and this technique is not recommended in this textbook.

Summary

This chapter has addressed the principles of tooth preparation. What should be apparent at this time is that a tooth preparation is determined by many factors, and each time a tooth is to be restored, each of these factors must be assessed. Tooth preparation for composite restorations is simpler and more conservative than for amalgam restorations because of the physical requirements necessary for amalgam (see Table 5-1). If the principles of tooth preparation are followed, the success of any restoration is greatly increased. No two tooth preparations are the same.

Numerous factors may need to be considered before initiating a tooth preparation. Box 5-2 lists many of these factors, but it is not an all-inclusive list. The increasing bond strengths of enamel and dentin bonding materials are likely to result in significant emphasis on adhesive restorations. Likewise, the improved ability to bond to tooth structure is likely to

---

Box 5-2 Factors to Consider before Tooth Preparation

Extent of Caries	Extent of Defect
Occlusion	Pulpal protection
Pulpal involvement	Contours
Esthetics	Economics
Patient's age	Patient's risk status
Patient's home care	Bur design
Gingival status	Radiographic assessment
Anesthesia	Other treatment factors
Bone support	Patient cooperation
Patient's desires	Fracture lines
Material limitations	Tooth anatomy
Operator skill	Ability to isolate area
Enamel rod direction	
Extent of old restorative material	

continue to alter the entire tooth preparation procedure. When materials can be bonded effectively to a tooth while restoring the inherent strength of the tooth, the need for refined tooth preparations is reduced.

References

1. Black GV: *Operative dentistry*, ed 8, Woodstock, Ill, 1947–1948, Medico-Dental.
2. Bronner FJ: Mechanical, physiological, and pathological aspects of operative procedures. *Dent Cosmos* 73:577, 1931.
3. Markley MR: Restorations of silver amalgam. *J Am Dent Assoc* 43:133, 1951.
4. Sturdevant JR, Wilder AD, Roberson TM, et al: Clinical study of conservative designs for Class II amalgams (abstract 1549). *J Dent Res* 67:306, 1988.
5. Sockwell CL: Dental handpieces and rotary cutting instruments. *Dent Clin North Am* 15:219, 1971.
6. Sturdevant CM: *The art and science of operative dentistry*, ed 1, New York, 1968, McGraw-Hill.
7. Charbeneau GT, Peyton FA: Some effects of cavity instrumentation on the adaptation of gold castings and amalgam. *J Prosthet Dent* 8:514, 1958.
8. Marzouk MA: *Operative dentistry*, St Louis, 1985, Ishiyaku EuroAmerica.
9. Simonsen RJ: Preventive resin restoration. *Quintessence Int* 9:69–76, 1978.
10. Hyatt TP: Prophylactic odontotomy: The ideal procedure in dentistry for children. *Dent Cosmos* 78:353, 1936.
11. Fusayama T: Two layers of carious dentin: Diagnosis and treatment. *Oper Dent* 4:63–70, 1979.
12. Fusayama T, Okuse K, Hosoda H: Relationship between hardness, discoloration, and microbial invasion in carious dentin. *J Dent Res* 45:1033–1046, 1966.
13. McComb D: Caries-detector dyes—how accurate and useful are they? *J Can Dent Assoc* 66(4):195–198, 2000.
14. Lee WC, Eakle WS: Possible role of tensile stress in the etiology of cervical erosive lesions of teeth. *J Prosthet Dent* 52:374–380, 1984.
15. Shafer WG, Hine MK, Levy BM: *Textbook of oral pathology*, ed 4, Philadelphia, 1983, WB Saunders.
16. Guard WF, Haack DC, Ireland RL: Photoelastic stress analysis of buccolingual sections of Class II cavity restorations. *J Am Dent Assoc* 57:631, 1958.
17. Massler M, Barber TK: Action of amalgam on dentin. *J Am Dent Assoc* 47:415, 1953.
18. Boyer DB, Roth L: Fracture resistance of teeth with bonded amalgams. *Am J Dent* 7:91–94, 1994.
19. Frank AL: Protective coronal coverage of the pulpless tooth. *J Am Dent Assoc* 59:895, 1959.
20. Going RE: Status report on cement bases, cavity liners, varnishes, primers, and cleaners. *J Am Dent Assoc* 85:654, 1972.
21. Mach Z, Regent J, Staninec M, et al: The integrity of bonded amalgam restorations: A clinical evaluation after five years. *J Am Dent Assoc* 133:460–467, 2002.
22. Smales RJ, Wetherell JD: Review of bonded amalgam restorations, and assessment in a general practice over five years. *Oper Dent* 25:374–381, 2000.
23. Baratieri LN, Machado A, Van Noort R, et al: Effect of pulp protection technique on the clinical performance of amalgam restorations: Three-year results. *Oper Dent* 29:319–324, 2002.
24. Summitt JB, Burgess JO, Berry TG, et al: Six-year clinical evaluation of bonded and pin-retained complex amalgam restorations. *Oper Dent* 29:261–268, 2004.
25. Reeves R, Stanley HR: The relationship of bacterial penetration and pulpal pathosis in carious teeth. *Oral Surg* 22:59, 1966.
26. Stanley HR: *Human pulp response to operative dental procedures*, Gainesville, FL, 1976, Storter Printing.
27. Ritter AV, Swift EJ: Current restorative concepts of pulp protection. *Endod Topics* 5:41–48, 2003.
28. Murray PE, Hafez AA, Smith AJ, et al: Bacterial microleakage and pulp inflammation associated with various restorative materials. *Dent Mater* 18:470–478, 2002.
29. Swift EJ, Trope M, Ritter AV: Vital pulp therapy for the mature tooth—can it work? *Endod Topics* 5: 49–56, 2003.
30. Chong WF, Swartz ML, Phillips RW: Displacement of cement bases by amalgam condensation. *J Am Dent Assoc* 74:97, 1967.
31. Goracci G, Giovani M: Scanning electron microscopic evaluation of resin-dentin and calcium hydroxide-dentin interface with resin composite restorations. *Quintessence Int* 27:129–135, 1996.
32. Swartz ML, Phillips RW: In vitro studies on the marginal leakage of restorative materials. *J Am Dent Assoc* 62:141, 1961.
33. Hartley JL, Hudson DC: *Clinical evaluation of devices and techniques for the removal of tooth structure*, Randolph Air Force Base, Texas, 1959, Air University.
34. Cantwell KR, Aplin AW, Mahler DB: Cavity finish with high-speed handpieces. *Dent Prog* 1:42, 1960.
35. Street EV: Effects of various instruments on enamel walls. *J Am Dent Assoc* 46:274, 1953.
36. Charbeneau GT, Peyton FA: Some effects of cavity instrumentation on the adaptation of gold castings and amalgam. *J Prosthet Dent* 8:514, 1958.
37. Menegale CM, Swartz ML, Phillips RW: Adaptation of restorative materials as influenced by the roughness of cavity walls. *J Dent Res* 39:825, 1960.
38. Pashley DH, Tay FR, Breschi L, et al: State of the art etch-and-rinse adhesives. *Dent Mater* 27:1–16, 2011.
39. Carrilho MRO, Geraldeli S, Tay F, et al: *J Dent Res* 86:529–533, 2007.
40. Opdam NJ, Bronkhorst EM, Loomans BAC, et al: 12-year survival of composite vs. amalgam restorations. *J Dent Res* 89:1063–1067, 2010.
41. Besic FC: The fate of bacteria sealed in dental cavities. *J Dent Res* 22:349, 1943.
42. Going RE, Massler M, Dute HL: Marginal penetration of dental restorations by different radioactive isotopes. *J Dent Res* 39:273, 1960.
43. Going RE, Massler M: Influence of cavity liners under amalgam restorations on penetration by radioactive isotopes. *J Dent Res* 11:298, 1961.
44. Nelson RJ, Wolcott RB, Paffenbarger GC: Fluid exchange at the margins of dental restorations. *J Am Dent Assoc* 44:288, 1962.
45. Swartz ML, Phillips RW, Norman RD, et al: Role of cavity varnishes and bases in the penetration of cement constituents through tooth structure. *J Prosthet Dent* 16:963, 1966.
46. Shay DE, Allen TJ, Mantz RF: Antibacterial effects of some dental restorative materials. *J Dent Res* 35:25, 1956.
47. Schüpbach P, Lutz F, Finger WJ: Closing of dentinal tubules by Gluma Desensitizer. *Eur J Oral Sci* 105:414–421, 1997.
48. Reinhardt JW, Stephens NH, Fortin D: Effect of Gluma desensitization on dentin bond strength. *Am J Dent* 8:170–172, 1995.
49. Staninec M, Setcos JC: Bonded amalgam restorations: current research and clinical procedure. *Dent Update* 30:430–434, 2003.
50. Zidan O, Abdel-Keriem U: The effect of amalgam bonding on the stiffness of teeth weakened by cavity preparation. *Dent Mater* 19:680–685, 2003.
51. Ben-Amar A: Reduction of microleakage around new amalgam restorations. *J Am Dent Assoc* 119:725, 1989.

Chapter 6

Instruments and Equipment for Tooth Preparation

Terrence E. Donovan, R. Scott Eidson

Hand Instruments for Cutting

Removal and shaping of tooth structure are essential aspects of restorative dentistry. Initially, this was a difficult process accomplished entirely by the use of hand instruments. The introduction of rotary, powered cutting equipment was a truly major advance in dentistry. From the time of the first hand-powered dental drill to the present-day electric and air-driven handpiece, tremendous strides have been made in the mechanical alteration of tooth structure and in the ease with which teeth can be restored. Modern high-speed equipment has eliminated the need for many hand instruments for tooth preparation. Nevertheless, hand instruments remain an essential part of the armamentarium for restorative dentistry.

The early hand-operated instruments—with their large, heavy handles (Fig. 6-1) and inferior (by present standards) metal alloys in the blades—were cumbersome, awkward to use, and ineffective in many situations. As the commercial manufacture of hand instruments increased, and dentists began to express ideas about tooth preparation, it became apparent that some scheme for identifying these instruments was necessary. Among his many contributions to modern dentistry, Black is credited with the first acceptable nomenclature for and classification of hand instruments.[1] His classification system enabled dentists and manufacturers to communicate more clearly and effectively about instrument design and function.

Modern hand instruments, when properly used, produce beneficial results for the operator and the patient. Some of these results can be satisfactorily achieved only with hand instruments and not with rotary instruments. Preparation form dictates some circumstances in which hand instruments are to be used, whereas accessibility dictates others.

Terminology and Classification
Categories

The hand instruments used in the dental operatory may be categorized as (1) cutting (excavators, chisels, and others) or (2) non-cutting (amalgam condensers, mirrors, explorers, probes).[1] Excavators may be subdivided further into ordinary hatchets, hoes, angle formers, and spoons. Chisels are primarily used for cutting enamel and may be subdivided further into straight chisels, curved chisels, bin-angle chisels, enamel hatchets, and gingival margin trimmers. Other cutting instruments may be subdivided as knives, files, scalers, and carvers. In addition to the cutting instruments, a large group of noncutting instruments (see Fig. 14-21, *D* and *E*) is also in use.

Design

Most hand instruments, regardless of use, are composed of three parts: handle, shank, and blade (Fig. 6-2). For many non-cutting instruments, the part corresponding to the blade is termed *nib*. The end of the nib, or working surface, is known as *face*. The blade or nib is the working end of the instrument and is connected to the handle by the shank. Some instruments have a blade on both ends of the handle and are known as double-ended instruments. The blades are of many designs and sizes, depending on their functions.

Handles are available in various sizes and shapes. Early hand instruments had handles of quite large diameter and were grasped in the palm of the hand. A large, heavy handle is not always conducive to delicate manipulation. In North America, most instrument handles are small in diameter (5.5 mm) and light. They are commonly eight-sided and knurled to facilitate control. In Europe, the handles are often larger in diameter and tapered.

Shanks, which serve to connect the handles to the working ends of the instruments, are normally smooth, round, and tapered. They often have one or more bends to overcome the tendency of the instrument to twist while in use when force is applied.

Enamel and dentin are difficult substances to cut and require the generation of substantial forces at the tip of the instrument. Hand instruments must be balanced and sharp. Balance allows for the concentration of force onto the blade without causing rotation of the instrument in the operator's

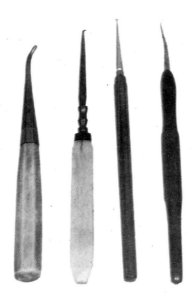

Fig. 6-1 Designs of some early hand instruments. These instruments were individually handmade, variable in design, and cumbersome to use. Because of the nature of the handles, effective sterilization was a problem.

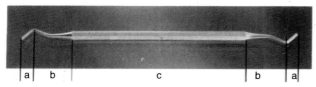

Fig. 6-2 Double-ended instrument illustrating three component parts of hand instruments: blade (*a*), shank (*b*), and handle (*c*). *(Modified from Boyd LRB: Dental instruments: A pocket guide, ed 4, St. Louis, 2012, Saunders.)*

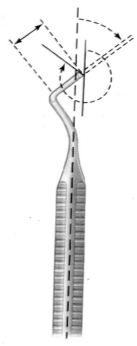

Fig. 6-3 Instrument shank and blade design (with primary cutting edge positioned close to handle axis to produce balance). The complete instrument formula (four numbers) is expressed as the blade width (1) in 0.1-mm increments, cutting edge angle (2) in centigrades, blade length (3) in millimeters, and blade angle (4) in degrees.

grasp. Sharpness concentrates the force onto a small area of the edge, producing a high stress.

Balance is accomplished by designing the angles of the shank so that the cutting edge of the blade lies within the projected diameter of the handle and nearly coincides with the projected axis of the handle (Fig. 6-3; see also Fig. 6-2). For optimal anti-rotational design, the blade edge must not be off-axis by more than 1 to 2 mm. All dental instruments and equipment need to satisfy this principle of balance.

Shank Angles

The functional orientation and length of the blade determine the number of angles in the shank necessary to balance the instrument. Black classified instruments on the basis of the number of shank angles as mon-angle (one), bin-angle (two), or triple-angle (three).[2] Instruments with small, short blades may be easily designed in mon-angle form while confining the cutting edge within the required limit. Instruments with longer blades or more complex orientations may require two or three angles in the shank to bring the cutting edge close to the long axis of the handle. Such shanks are termed *contra-angled*.

Names

Black classified all of the instruments by name.[2] In addition, for hand-cutting instruments, he developed a numeric formula to characterize the dimensions and angles of the working end (see the next section for details of the formula). Black's classification system by instrument name categorized instruments by (1) function (e.g., scaler, excavator), (2) manner of use (e.g., hand condenser), (3) design of the working end (e.g., spoon excavator, sickle scaler), or (4) shape of the shank (e.g., mon-angle, bin-angle, contra-angle).[2] These names were combined to form the complete description of the instrument (e.g., bin-angle spoon excavator).

Formulas

Cutting instruments have formulas describing the dimensions and angles of the working end. These are placed on the handle using a code of three or four numbers separated by dashes or spaces (e.g., 10–8.5–8–14) (see Fig. 6-3). The first number indicates the width of the blade or primary cutting edge in tenths of a millimeter (0.1 mm) (e.g., 10 = 1 mm). The second number of a four-number code indicates the primary cutting edge angle, measured from a line parallel to the long axis of the instrument handle in clockwise centigrades. The angle is expressed as a percent of 360 degrees (e.g., 85 = 85% × 360 degrees = 306 degrees). The instrument is positioned so that this number always exceeds 50. If the edge is locally perpendicular to the blade, this number is normally omitted, resulting in a three-number code. The third number (second number of a three-number code) indicates the blade length in

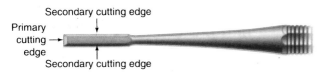

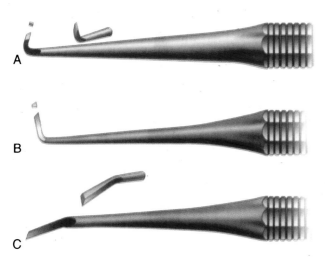

Fig. 6-4 Chisel blade design showing primary and secondary cutting edges.

Fig. 6-5 Examples of hand instruments called excavators (with corresponding instrument formulas). **A,** Bi-beveled ordinary hatchet (3–2–28). **B,** Hoe (4½–1½—22). **C,** Angle former (12–85–5–8).

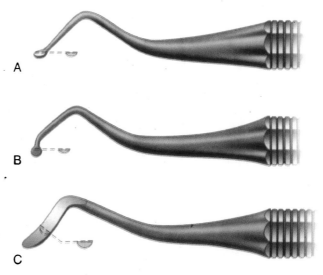

Fig. 6-6 Examples of hand instruments called spoon excavators (with corresponding instrument formulas). **A,** Bin-angle spoon (13–7–14). **B,** Triple-angle spoon (13–7–14). **C,** Spoon (15–7–14).

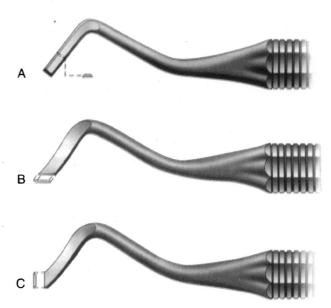

Fig. 6-7 Examples of hand instruments called chisels (with corresponding instrument formulas). **A,** Enamel hatchet (10–7–14). **B,** Gingival margin trimmer (12½—100–7–14). **C,** Gingival margin trimmer (12½—100–7–14).

millimeters (e.g., 8 = 8 mm). The fourth number (third number of a three-number code) indicates the blade angle, relative to the long axis of the handle in clockwise centigrade (e.g., 14 = 50 degrees). For these measurements, the instrument is positioned such that this number is always 50 or less. The most commonly used hand instruments, including those specified in this text, are shown in Figures 6-5 through 6-9 with their formulas indicated.

In some instances, an additional number on the handle is the manufacturer's identification number. It should not be confused with the formula number. This identification number is included simply to assist the specific manufacturer in cataloging and ordering.

Bevels

Most hand cutting instruments have on the end of the blade a single bevel that forms the primary cutting edge. Two additional edges, called *secondary cutting edges*, extend from the primary edge for the length of the blade (Fig. 6-4). Bi-beveled instruments such as ordinary hatchets have two bevels that form the cutting edge (Fig. 6-5, *A*).

Certain single-beveled instruments such as spoon excavators (Fig. 6-6) and gingival margin trimmers (Fig. 6-7, *B* and *C*) are used with a scraping or lateral cutting motion. Others such as enamel hatchets (see Fig. 6-7, *A*) may be used with a planing or direct cutting motion and a lateral cutting motion. For such single-beveled designs, the instruments must be made in pairs, with the bevels on opposite sides of the blade. Such instruments are designated as right beveled or left beveled and are indicated by appending the letter R or L to

the instrument formula. To determine whether the instrument has a right or left bevel, the primary cutting edge is held down and pointing away, and if the bevel appears on the right side of the blade, it is the right instrument of the pair. This instrument, when used in a scraping motion, is moved from right to left. The opposite holds true for the left instrument of the pair. One instrument is suited for work on one side of the preparation, and the other is suited for the opposite side of the preparation.

Most instruments are available with blades and shanks on both ends of the handle. Such instruments are termed

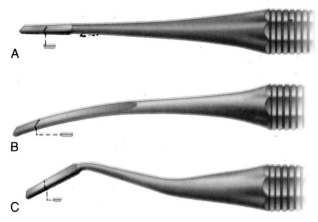

Fig. 6-8 Examples of hand instruments called chisels (with corresponding instrument formulas). **A,** Straight (12–7–0). **B,** Wedelstaedt (11½—15–3). **C,** Bin-angle (10–7–8).

double-ended. In many cases, the right instrument of the pair is on one end of the handle, and the left instrument is on the other end. Sometimes, similar blades of different widths are placed on double-ended instruments. Single-ended instruments may be safer to use, but double-ended instruments are more efficient because they reduce instrument exchange.

Instruments having the cutting edge perpendicular to the axis of the handle (Fig. 6-8), such as bin-angle chisels (see Fig. 6-8, *C*), instruments with a slight blade curvature (Wedelstaedt chisels) (see Fig. 6-8, *B*), and hoes (see Fig. 6-5, *B*), are single-beveled and not designated as rights or lefts but as having a mesial bevel or a distal bevel. If when one observes the inside of the blade curvature (or the inside of the angle at the junction of the blade and shank) the primary bevel is not visible, the instrument has a distal bevel. Conversely, if the primary bevel can be seen (from the same viewpoint), the instrument has a mesial or reverse bevel (see Fig. 6-8).

As previously described, instruments such as chisels and hatchets have three cutting edges, one primary and two secondary. These allow cutting in three directions, as the need presents. The secondary edges permit more effective cutting than the primary edge in several instances. They are particularly effective in work on the facial and lingual walls of the proximal portion of a proximo-occlusal tooth preparation. The operator should not forget the usefulness of these secondary cutting edges because they enhance the use of the instrument.

Applications

The cutting instruments are used to cut the hard or soft tissues of the mouth. Excavators are used for removal of caries and refinement of the internal parts of the preparation. Chisels are used primarily for cutting enamel.

Excavators

The four subdivisions of excavators are (1) ordinary hatchets, (2) hoes, (3) angle-formers, and (4) spoons. An ordinary hatchet excavator has the cutting edge of the blade directed in the same plane as that of the long axis of the handle and is bi-beveled (see Fig. 6-5, *A*). These instruments are used primarily on anterior teeth for preparing retentive areas and sharpening internal line angles, particularly in preparations for direct gold restorations.

The hoe excavator has the primary cutting edge of the blade perpendicular to the axis of the handle (see Fig. 6-5, *B*). This type of instrument is used for planing tooth preparation walls and for forming line angles. It is commonly used in Class III and V preparations for direct gold restorations. Some sets of cutting instruments contain hoes with longer and heavier blades, with the shanks contra-angled. These are intended for use on enamel or posterior teeth.

A special type of excavator is the angle-former (see Fig. 6-5, *C*). It is used primarily for sharpening line angles and creating retentive features in dentin in preparation for gold restorations. It also may be used in placing a bevel on enamel margins. It is mon-angled and has the primary cutting edge at an angle (other than 90 degrees) to the blade. It may be described as a combination of a chisel and a gingival margin trimmer. It is available in pairs (right and left).

Spoon excavators (see Fig. 6-6) are used for removing caries and carving amalgam or direct wax patterns. The blades are slightly curved, and the cutting edges are either circular or claw-like. The circular edge is known as a discoid, whereas the claw-like blade is termed *cleoid* (Fig. 6-9, *C* and *D*). The shanks may be bin-angled or triple-angled to facilitate accessibility.

Chisels

Chisels are intended primarily for cutting enamel and may be grouped as (1) straight, slightly curved, or bin-angle; (2) enamel hatchets; and (3) gingival margin trimmers. The straight chisel has a straight shank and blade, with the bevel on only one side. Its primary edge is perpendicular to the axis of the handle. It is similar in design to a carpenter's chisel (see Fig. 6-8, *A*). The shank and blade of the chisel also may be slightly curved (Wedelstaedt design) (see Fig. 6-8, *B*) or may be bin-angled (see Fig. 6-8, *C*). The force used with all these chisels is essentially a straight thrust. A right or left type is not needed in a straight chisel because a 180-degree turn of the instrument allows for its use on either side of the preparation. The bin-angle and Wedelstaedt chisels have the primary cutting edges in a plane perpendicular to the axis of the handle and may have either a distal bevel or a mesial (reverse) bevel. The blade with a distal bevel is designed to plane a wall that faces the blade's inside surface (see Fig. 6-5, *A* and *B*). The blade with a mesial bevel is designed to plane a wall that faces the blade's outside surface (see Fig. 6-8, *B* and *C*).

The enamel hatchet is a chisel similar in design to the ordinary hatchet except that the blade is larger, heavier, and beveled on only one side (see Fig. 6-7, *A*). It has its cutting edges in a plane that is parallel with the axis of the handle. It is used for cutting enamel and comes as right or left types for use on opposite sides of the preparation.

The gingival margin trimmer is designed to produce a proper bevel on gingival enamel margins of proximo-occlusal preparations. It is similar in design to the enamel hatchet except the blade is curved (similar to a spoon excavator), and the primary cutting edge is at an angle (other than perpendicular) to the axis of the blade (see Fig. 6-7, *B* and *C*). It is made as right and left types. It also is made so that a right and left pair is either a mesial pair or a distal pair. When the second number in the formula is 90 to 100, the pair is used

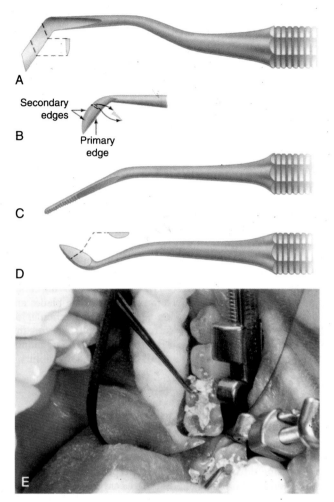

Fig. 6-9 Examples of other hand instruments for cutting. **A,** Finishing knife. **B,** Alternative finishing knife design emphasizing secondary cutting edges. **C,** Dental file. **D,** Cleoid blade. **E,** Discoid blade carving amalgam.

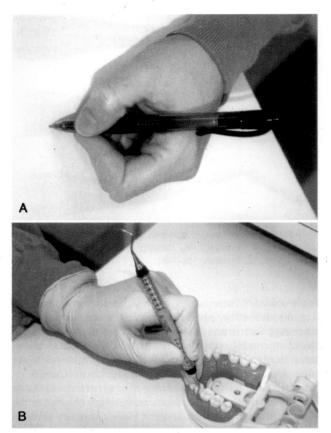

Fig. 6-10 Pen grasps. **A,** Conventional pen grasp. Side of middle finger is on writing instrument. **B,** Modified pen grasp. Correct position of middle finger is near the "topside" of the instrument for good control and cutting pressure. The rest is tip (or tips) of ring finger (or ring and little fingers) on tooth (or teeth) of same arch.

on the distal gingival margin. When this number is 75 to 85, the pair is used to bevel the mesial margin. The 100 and 75 pairs are for inlay–onlay preparations with steep gingival bevels. The 90 and 85 pairs are for amalgam preparations with gingival enamel bevels that decline gingivally only slightly. Among other uses for these instruments is the rounding or beveling of the axiopulpal line angle of two-surface preparations.

Other Cutting Instruments

Other hand cutting instruments such as the knife, file, and discoid–cleoid instrument are used for trimming restorative material rather than for cutting tooth structure. Knives, known as *finishing knives, amalgam knives,* or *gold knives,* are designed with a thin, knife-like blade that is made in various sizes and shapes (see Fig. 6-9, *A* and *B*). Knives are used for trimming excess restorative material on the gingival, facial, or lingual margins of a proximal restoration or trimming and contouring the surface of a Class V restoration. Sharp secondary edges on the heel aspect of the blade are useful in a scrape–pull mode.

Files (see Fig. 6-9, *C*) also can be used to trim excess restorative material. They are particularly useful at gingival margins. The blades of the file are extremely thin, and the teeth of the instrument on the cutting surfaces are short and designed to make the file a push instrument or a pull instrument. Files are manufactured in various shapes and angles to allow access to restorations.

The discoid-cleoid (see Fig. 6-9, *D* and *E*) instrument is used principally for carving occlusal anatomy in unset amalgam restorations. It also may be used to trim or burnish inlay–onlay margins. The working ends of this instrument are larger than the discoid or cleoid end of an excavator.

Hand Instrument Techniques

Four grasps are used with hand instruments: (1) modified pen, (2) inverted pen, (3) palm-and-thumb, and (4) modified palm-and-thumb. The conventional pen grasp is not an acceptable instrument grasp (Fig. 6-10, *A*).

Modified Pen Grasp

The grasp that permits the greatest delicacy of touch is the modified pen grasp (see Fig. 6-10, *B*). As the name implies, it is similar, but not identical, to that used in holding a pen. The

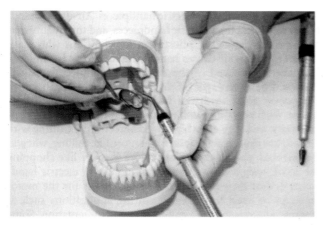

Fig. 6-11 Inverted pen grasp. Palm faces more toward operator. The rest is similar to that shown for modified pen grasp (see Fig. 6-10, *B*).

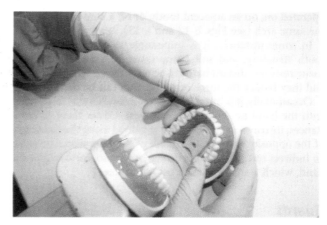

Fig. 6-12 Palm-and-thumb grasp. This grasp has limited use, such as preparing incisal retention in a Class III preparation on a maxillary incisor. The rest is tip of thumb on tooth in same arch.

pads of the thumb and of the index and middle fingers contact the instrument, while the tip of the ring finger (or tips of the ring and little fingers) is placed on a nearby tooth surface of the same arch as a rest. The palm of the hand generally is facing away from the operator. The pad of the middle finger is placed near the topside of the instrument; by this finger working with the wrist and the forearm, cutting or cleaving pressure is generated on the blade. The instrument should not be allowed to rest on or near the first joint of the middle finger as in the conventional pen grasp (see Fig. 6-10, *A*). Although this latter position may appear to be more comfortable, it limits the application of pressure. A balanced instrument design allows the application of suitable force without the instrument tending to rotate in the fingers (see Fig. 6-3).

Inverted Pen Grasp

The finger positions of the inverted pen grasp are the same as for the modified pen grasp. The hand is rotated, however, so that the palm faces more toward the operator (Fig. 6-11). This grasp is used mostly for tooth preparations employing the lingual approach on anterior teeth.

Palm-and-Thumb Grasp

The palm-and-thumb grasp is similar to that used for holding a knife while paring an apple. The handle is placed in the palm of the hand and grasped by all the fingers, while the thumb is free of the instrument, and the rest is provided by supporting the tip of the thumb on a nearby tooth of the same arch or on a firm, stable structure. For suitable control, this grasp requires careful use during cutting. An example of an appropriate use is holding a handpiece for cutting incisal retention for a Class III preparation on a maxillary incisor (Fig. 6-12).

Modified Palm-and-Thumb Grasp

The modified palm-and-thumb grasp may be used when it is feasible to rest the thumb on the tooth being prepared or the adjacent tooth (Fig. 6-13). The handle of the instrument is held by all four fingers, whose pads press the handle against the distal area of the palm and the pad and first joint of the thumb. Grasping the handle under the first joints of the ring

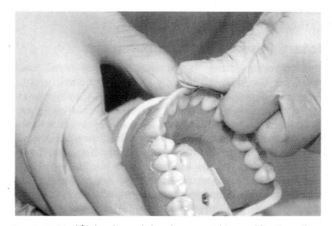

Fig. 6-13 Modified palm-and-thumb grasp. This modification allows greater ease of instrument movement and more control against slippage during thrust stroke compared with palm-and-thumb grasp. The rest is tip of thumb on tooth being prepared or adjacent tooth. Note how the instrument is braced against pad and end joint of thumb.

finger and little finger provides stabilization. This grip fosters control against slippage.

The modified pen grasp and the inverted pen grasp are used practically universally. The modified palm-and-thumb grasp usually is employed in the area of the maxillary arch and is best adopted when the dentist is operating from a rear-chair position.

Rests

A proper instrument grasp must include a firm rest to steady the hand during operating procedures. When the modified pen grasp and the inverted pen grasp are used, rests are established by placing the ring finger (or both ring and little fingers) on a tooth (or teeth) of the same arch and as close to the operating site as possible (see Figs. 6-10 and 6-11). The closer the rest areas are to the operating area, the more reliable they are. When the palm-and-thumb grasps are used, rests are created by placing the tip of the thumb on the tooth being operated on, on an adjacent tooth, or on a convenient area of the same arch (see Figs. 6-12 and 6-13).

In some instances, it is impossible to establish a rest on tooth structure, and soft tissue must be used. Neither soft tissue rests nor distant hard tissue rests afford reliable control, and they reduce the force or power that can be used safely.

Occasionally, it is impossible to establish normal finger rests with the hand holding the instrument. Under these circumstances, instrument control may be gained using the forefinger of the opposite hand on the shank of the instrument or using an indirect rest (i.e., the operating hand rests on the opposite hand, which rests on a stable oral structure).

Guards

Guards are hand instruments or other items, such as interproximal wedges, used to protect soft tissue from contact with sharp cutting or abrasive instruments (see Fig. 6-10, *B*).

Contemporary Powered Cutting Equipment

Rotary Power Cutting Equipment

Powered rotary cutting instruments, known as *dental handpieces*, are the most commonly used instruments in contemporary dentistry. Dentistry as practiced today would not be possible without the use of powered cutting instruments. Current dental handpieces are now highly efficient and sophisticated instruments that have evolved from their beginnings in the early 1950s. Many evolutionary changes to handpieces have dramatically improved their use and efficiency over the years. Changes in ergonomic design, weight, and balance have made handpieces more comfortable to use for longer periods. This improved design can minimize arm and shoulder fatigue in the clinician. Better visibility with incorporation of durable fiberoptics greatly improves the clinician's ability to see more detail with less eye strain. Development of LED (light-emitting diode) technology has improved the quality of light to be more akin to daylight and has vastly enhanced bulb life. Noise levels, which have a considerable impact on the long-term hearing health of clinicians and their staff, have been reduced. The durability of the handpiece that undergoes frequent sterilization has been improved significantly over the years, thus avoiding material degradation. New bearing materials and cartridges have been developed to enhance their service longevity and to contribute to noise level reductions. Chucking mechanisms have evolved such that pushbuttons, instead of bur tools, are used to release and change burs.

Two technologies are used today for dental handpieces, and each has unique characteristics and benefits. The air-driven handpiece was, for many years, the mainstay for cutting teeth in dentistry. The electric motor-driven handpiece is now becoming increasingly popular for use in all cutting applications in dentistry. The technologies for both air-driven and electric systems continue to evolve, and both systems remain very popular for everyday use in operative dentistry procedures.

Electric and air-driven systems have both advantages and disadvantages. Air-driven systems are less costly on initial startup and are less expensive with regard to replacing

turbines compared with electric handpieces. Air-driven handpieces weigh less than electric handpieces, and this quality may be the most significant adjustment for clinicians who make the change from air-driven handpieces to electric handpieces. The size of the head of the air-driven handpiece is usually smaller. The advantages of electric handpieces are that they are quieter than air-driven handpieces, they cut with high torque with very little stalling, they maintain high bur concentricity, and they offer high-precision cutting. Cutting with electric handpieces is smoother and more like milling, whereas cutting with the air-driven handpiece is more like chopping the tooth with the bur. Another advantage of electric handpieces is that they offer multiple attachments for the motor that can be used for different cutting applications such as denture adjustments and endodontic instrumentation. Some disadvantages of air-driven handpieces are that they create a loud, high-pitched noise that can affect the hearing of the operator and the staff over years. The torque and concentricity of the air turbines degrade in a relatively short period. Air-driven handpieces need turbine replacement and repairs more frequently. More vibration and bur chatter are associated with air-driven handpieces. Some disadvantages of electric handpieces are the initial setup expense and weight and balance issues for some clinicians.

Rotary Speed Ranges for Different Cutting Applications

The rotational speed of an instrument is measured in revolutions per minute (rpm). Three speed ranges are generally recognized: low or slow speeds (<12,000 rpm), medium or intermediate speeds (12,000–200,000 rpm), and high or ultra-high speeds (>200,000 rpm). The terms *low-speed*, *medium-speed*, and *high-speed* are used preferentially in this textbook. Most useful instruments are rotated at either low speed or high speed. Electric handpiece motors generate up to 200,000 rpm of rotation. This speed is significantly less than the 400,000 rpm generated by air-driven handpieces. However, the electric handpiece motor has attachments with speed increase multipliers that can increase rotation in ratios of 5:1 or 4:1, which makes them effective in the same range as air-driven handpieces. The difference in the amount of cutting power is substantial in electric handpieces. Electric handpieces can produce up to 60 watts of cutting power versus less than 20 watts by air-driven handpieces. The extra cutting power in electric handpieces allow the constant torque necessary to cut various restorative materials and tooth structure regardless of the load. Unlike in the air-driven handpiece, the bur in the electric handpiece can resist slowing down or stopping as the load is increased.

The crucial factor for some purposes is the surface speed of the instrument, that is, the velocity at which the edges of the cutting instrument pass across the surface being cut. This speed is proportional to the rotational speed and the diameter of the instrument, with large instruments having higher surface speeds at any given rate of rotation.

Although intact tooth structure can be removed by an instrument rotating at low speeds, it is a traumatic experience for the patient and the dentist. Low-speed cutting is ineffective, is time-consuming, and requires a relatively heavy force application; this results in heat production at the operating site and produces vibrations of low frequency and high amplitude. Heat and vibration are the main sources of patient discomfort.[3] At low speeds, burs have a tendency to roll out of the tooth preparation and mar the proximal margin or tooth surface. In addition, carbide burs do not last long because their brittle blades are easily broken at low speeds. Many of these disadvantages of low-speed operation do not apply when the objective is some procedure other than cutting tooth structure. The low-speed range is used for cleaning teeth, caries excavation, and finishing and polishing procedures. At low speeds, tactile sensation is better, and generally, overheating of cut surfaces is less likely. The availability of a low-speed option provides a valuable adjunct for many dental procedures.

At high speed, the surface speed needed for efficient cutting can be attained with smaller and more versatile cutting instruments. This speed is used for tooth preparation and removing old restorations. Other advantages are the following: (1) diamond and carbide cutting instruments remove tooth structure faster and with less pressure, vibration, and heat generation; (2) the number of rotary cutting instruments needed is reduced because smaller sizes are more universal in application; (3) the operator has better control and greater ease of operation; (4) instruments last longer; (5) patients are generally less apprehensive because annoying vibrations and operating time are decreased; and (6) several teeth in the same arch can be treated at the same appointment (as they should be).

Variable control to regulate the speed makes the handpiece more versatile. This feature allows the operator to obtain easily the optimal speed for the size and type of rotating instrument at any stage of a specific operation. All electric handpieces have an adjustable rheostat that can easily set the maximum rpms to specific situations for different operative procedures. Air-driven handpieces can be controlled, but usually the control is more difficult and less precise, since the operator's pressure on the foot-operated rheostat controls the speed of the handpiece.

For infection control, all dental handpieces are now sterilized, but the process is associated with some challenges. Continual sterilization can produce degradation in clinical performance (longevity, power, turbine speed, fiberoptic transmission, eccentricity, noise, chuck performance, visibility angle, interocclusal clearance, water spray pattern).[4] Most handpieces require re-oiling after sterilization, and excess oil may be sprayed during the start-up operation. Several companies offer automated equipment to precisely clean and lubricate the handpiece after each use. It is recommended to run the handpiece for a few seconds before initiating dental procedures in which the deposition of oil spray onto tooth structure might interfere with processes such as dental adhesion.

Laser Equipment

Lasers are devices that produce beams of coherent and very-high-intensity light. Numerous current and potential uses of lasers in dentistry have been identified that involve the treatment of soft tissues and the modification of hard tooth structures.[5,6] The word *laser* is an acronym for "light amplification by stimulated emission of radiation." A crystal or gas is excited to emit photons of a characteristic wavelength that are amplified and filtered to make a coherent light beam. The effects of the laser depend on the power of the beam and the extent to which the beam is absorbed.

Current laser units are relatively expensive compared with air-driven and electric motor cutting instruments and must be used frequently in a dental practice to justify the expense. At the moment, lasers are used primarily for either soft tissue applications or hard tissue surface modification. They can be used for tooth preparations, however, it is more difficult to generate a defined margin or tooth preparation surface than with conventional rotary instruments. Lasers are inefficient and awkward for removing large amounts of enamel or dentin, and that process with a laser has the potential to generate unwanted amounts of heat. They cannot be used to remove existing amalgam or ceramic dental restorations. No single laser type is suitable for all potential laser applications. Lasers may never replace a high-speed dental handpiece. For several years, the use of lasers to prepare teeth held great promise; however, that promise has failed to materialize. Currently, available laser instruments have proven to be relatively inefficient and impractical for tooth preparation and have not achieved widespread popularity. Although lasers can be extremely useful for soft tissue surgery, current versions are of limited value for tooth preparation.

Other Equipment

Alternative methods of cutting enamel and dentin have been assessed periodically. In the mid-1950s, air-abrasive cutting was tested, but several clinical problems precluded general acceptance. Most importantly, no tactile sense was associated with air-abrasive cutting of tooth structure. This made it difficult for the operator to determine the cutting progress within the tooth preparation. Additionally, the abrasive dust interfered with visibility of the cutting site and tended to mechanically etch the surface of the dental mirror. Preventing the patient or office personnel from inhaling abrasive dust posed an additional difficulty.

Contemporary air abrasion equipment (Fig. 6-14) is helpful for stain removal, debriding pits and fissures before sealing, and micromechanical roughening of surfaces to be bonded (enamel, cast metal alloys, or porcelain).[7] This approach works well when organic material is being removed and when only

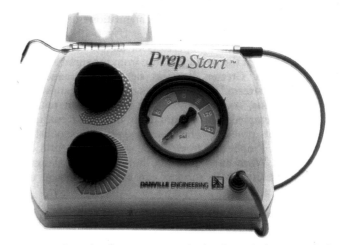

Fig. 6-14 Example of contemporary air abrasion unit for removal of superficial enamel defects or stains, debriding pits and fissures for sealant application, or roughening surfaces to be bonded or luted. *(Courtesy Danville Materials, Inc., San Ramon, CA.)*

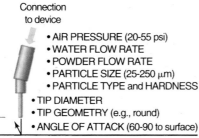

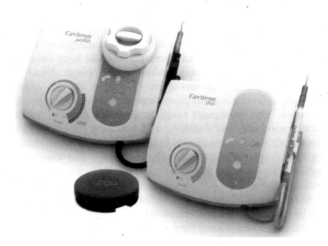

Fig. 6-15 Schematic representation of range of variables associated with any type of air abrasion equipment. The cleaning or cutting action is a function of kinetic energy imparted to the actual surface, and this is affected by variables concerning the particle size, air pressure, angulation with surface, type of substrate, and method of clearance. (*Courtesy of B. Kunselman [Master's thesis, 1999], School of Dentistry, University of North Carolina, Chapel Hill, NC.*)

Fig. 6-16 Example of air abrasion equipment used for tooth cleaning showing the Prophy tip and handle attached by a flexible cord to the control unit with the reservoir of powder and source of water (*left*). (*Courtesy of DENTSPLY International, York, PA.*)

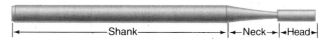

Fig. 6-17 Normal designation of three parts of rotary cutting instruments.

a limited amount of enamel or dentin is involved. Although promoted for caries excavation, air abrasion cannot produce well-defined preparation wall and margin details that are possible with conventional rotary cutting techniques. Generally, the finest stream of abrading particles still generates an effective cutting width that is far greater than the width of luted cement margins or the errors tolerable in most caries excavations. Roughening of surfaces to be bonded, luted, or repaired is an advantage and can occur intraorally or extraorally, depending on the situation. Roughening by air abrasion by itself is not a substitute for acid-etching techniques. Roughening improves bonding. Acid-etching alone or after roughening, however, always produces a better bond than air abrasion alone.[8]

Air abrasion techniques rely on the transfer of kinetic energy from a stream of powder particles on the surface of tooth structure or a restoration to produce a fractured surface layer, resulting in roughness for bonding or disruption for cutting. The energy transfer event is affected by many things, including powder particle, pressure, angulation, surface composition, and clearance angle variables (Fig. 6-15). The most common error made by operators of air abrasion units is holding the tip at the wrong distance from the surface for the desired action. Greater distances significantly reduce the energy of the stream.[9] Short distances may produce unwanted cutting actions, such as when only surface stain removal is being attempted. The potential for unwanted cutting is a significant problem when employing an air-polishing device (e.g., Prophy Jet) to clean the surfaces of dentin and enamel.[10-13] When used properly, however, units designed for air polishing tooth surfaces can be quite efficient and effective (Fig. 6-16).

Rotary Cutting Instruments

The individual instruments intended for use with dental handpieces are manufactured in hundreds of sizes, shapes, and types. This variation is, in part, a result of the need for specialized designs for particular clinical applications or to fit particular handpieces, but much of the variation also results from individual preferences on the part of dentists. Since the introduction of high-speed techniques in clinical practice, a rapid evolution of technique and an accompanying proliferation of new instrument designs have occurred. Nevertheless, the number of instruments essential for use with any one type of handpiece is comparatively small, especially in the case of high-speed turbine handpieces.

Common Design Characteristics

Despite the great variation among rotary cutting instruments, they share certain design features. Each instrument consists of three parts: (1) shank, (2) neck, and (3) head (Fig. 6-17). Each has its own function, influencing its design and the materials used for its construction. The term *shank* has different meanings as applied to rotary instruments and to hand instruments.

Shank Design

The *shank* is the part that fits into the handpiece, accepts the rotary motion from the handpiece, and provides a bearing surface to control the alignment and concentricity of the instrument. The shank design and dimensions vary with the handpiece for which it is intended. The American Dental Association (ADA) Specification No. 23 for dental excavating burs includes five classes of instrument shanks.[14] Three of these (Fig. 6-18)—the straight handpiece shank, the latch-type angle handpiece shank, and the friction-grip angle handpiece shank—are commonly encountered. The shank portion of the straight handpiece instrument is a simple cylinder. It is

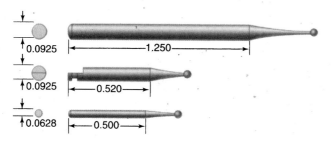

Fig. 6-18 Characteristics and typical dimensions (in inches) of three common instrument shank designs for straight handpiece (*A*), latch-angle handpiece (*B*), and friction-grip angle handpiece type (*C*).

held in the handpiece by a metal chuck that accepts a range of shank diameters. Precise control of the shank diameter is not as crucial as for other shank designs. Straight handpiece instruments are now rarely used for preparing teeth except for caries excavation. They are commonly used, however, for finishing and polishing completed restorations.

The more complicated shape of the latch-type shank reflects the different mechanisms by which these instruments are held in the handpiece. Their shorter overall length permits substantially improved access to posterior regions of the mouth compared with straight handpiece instruments. Handpieces that use latch-type burs normally have a metal bur tube within which the instruments fit as closely as possible, while still permitting easy interchange. The posterior portion of the shank is flattened on one side so that the end of the instrument fits into a D-shaped socket at the bottom of the bur tube, causing the instrument to be rotated. Latch-type instruments are not retained in the handpiece by a chuck but, rather, by a retaining latch that slides into the groove found at the shank end of the instrument. This type of instrument is used predominantly at low and medium speed ranges for finishing procedures. At these speeds, the small amount of potential wobble inherent in the clearance between the instrument and the handpiece bur tube is controlled by the lateral pressure exerted during cutting procedures. At higher speeds, the latch-type shank design is inadequate to provide a true-running instrument head, and as a result, an improved shank design is required for these speeds.

The friction-grip shank design was developed for use with high-speed handpieces. This design is smaller in overall length than the latch-type instruments, providing a further improvement in access to the posterior regions of the mouth. The shank is a simple cylinder manufactured to close dimensional tolerances. As the name implies, friction-grip instruments originally were designed to be held in the handpiece by friction between the shank and a plastic or metal chuck. Newer handpiece designs have metal chucks that close to make a positive contact with the bur shank. Careful dimensional control on the shanks of these instruments is important because for high-speed use, even minor variations in shank diameter can cause substantial variation in instrument performance and problems with insertion, retention, and removal.

Neck Design

As shown in Fig. 6-17, the *neck* is the intermediate portion of an instrument that connects the head to the shank. It corresponds to the part of a hand instrument that is referred to as *shank*. Except in the case of the larger, more massive instruments, the neck normally tapers from the shank diameter to a smaller size immediately adjacent to the head. The main function of the neck is to transmit rotational and translational forces to the head. At the same time, it is desirable for the operator to have the greatest possible visibility of the cutting head and the greatest manipulative freedom. For this reason, the neck dimensions represent a compromise between the need for a large cross-section to provide strength and a small cross-section to improve access and visibility.

Head Design

The *head* is the working part of the instrument, the cutting edges or points that perform the desired shaping of tooth structure. The shape of the head and the material used to construct it are closely related to its intended application and technique of use. The heads of instruments show greater variation in design and construction than either of the other main portions. For this reason, the characteristics of the head form the basis on which rotary instruments are usually classified.

Many characteristics of the heads of rotary instruments could be used for classification. Most important among these is the division into bladed instruments and abrasive instruments. Material of construction, head size, and head shape are additional characteristics that are useful for further subdivision. Bladed and abrasive instruments exhibit substantially different clinical performances, even when operated under nearly identical conditions. This appears to result from differences in the mechanism of cutting that are inherent in their designs.

Dental Burs

The term *bur* is applied to all rotary cutting instruments that have bladed cutting heads. This includes instruments intended for finishing metal restorations and surgical removal of bone and instruments primarily intended for tooth preparation.

Historical Development of Dental Burs

The earliest burs were hand-made. They were not only expensive but also variable in dimension and performance. The shapes, dimensions, and nomenclature of modern burs are directly related to those of the first machine-made burs introduced in 1891.[15] Early burs were made of steel. Steel burs perform well, cutting human dentin at low speeds, but dull rapidly at higher speeds or when cutting enamel. When burs are dulled, the reduced effectiveness in cutting creates increased heat and vibration.

Carbide burs, which were introduced in 1947, have largely replaced steel burs for tooth preparation. Steel burs now are used mainly for finishing procedures. Carbide burs perform better than steel burs at all speeds, and their superiority is greatest at high speeds. All carbide burs have heads of cemented carbide in which microscopic carbide particles, usually tungsten carbide, are held together in a matrix of cobalt or nickel. Carbide is much harder than steel and less prone to dulling during cutting.

In most burs, the carbide head is attached to a steel shank and neck by welding or brazing. The substitution of steel for carbide in the portions of the bur where greater wear resistance is not required has several advantages. It permits the manufacturer more freedom of design in attaining the characteristics desired in the instrument and allows economy in the cost of materials of construction.

Although most carbide burs have the joint located in the posterior part of the head, others are sold that have the joint located within the shank and have carbide necks and heads. Carbide is stiffer and stronger than steel, but it is also more brittle. A carbide neck subjected to a sudden blow or shock fractures, whereas a steel neck bends. A bur that is even slightly bent produces increased vibration and overcutting as a result of increased runout. Although steel necks reduce the risk of fracture during use, they may cause severe problems if bent. Either type can be satisfactory, and other design factors are varied to take maximal advantage of the properties of the material used.

Bur Classification Systems

To facilitate the description, selection, and manufacture of burs, it is highly desirable to have some agreed-on shorthand designation, which represents all variables of a particular head design by some simple code. In the United States, dental burs traditionally have been described in terms of an arbitrary numerical code for head size and shape (e.g., 2 = 1-mm diameter round bur; 57 = 1-mm diameter straight fissure bur; 34 = 0.8-mm diameter inverted cone bur).[16] Despite the complexity of the system, it is still in common use. Other countries developed and used similarly arbitrary systems. Newer classification systems such as those developed by the International Dental Federation (Federation Dentaire Internationale) and International Standards Organization (ISO) tend to use separate designations for shape (usually a shape name) and size (usually a number giving the head diameter in tenths of a millimeter) (e.g., round 010; straight fissure plain 010; inverted cone 008).[17,18]

Shapes

The term *bur shape* refers to the contour or silhouette of the head. The basic head shapes are round, inverted cone, pear, straight fissure, and tapered fissure (Fig. 6-19). A *round bur* is spherical. This shape customarily has been used for initial entry into the tooth, extension of the preparation, preparation of retention features, and caries removal.

An *inverted cone bur* is a portion of a rapidly tapered cone with the apex of the cone directed toward the bur shank. Head length is approximately the same as the diameter. This shape is particularly suitable for providing undercuts in tooth preparations.

A *pear-shaped bur* is a portion of a slightly tapered cone with the small end of the cone directed toward the bur shank. The end of the head either is continuously curved or is flat with rounded corners where the sides and flat end intersect. An elongated pear bur (length three times the width) is advocated for tooth preparations for amalgam.

A *straight fissure bur* is an elongated cylinder. Some dentists advocate this shape for amalgam tooth preparation. Modified burs of this design with slightly curved tip angles are available. A tapered fissure bur is a portion of a slightly tapered cone with the small end of the cone directed away from the bur shank. This shape is used for tooth preparations for indirect restorations, for which freedom from undercuts is essential for successful withdrawal of patterns and final seating of the restorations. Tapered fissure burs can have a flat end with the tip corners slightly rounded.

Among these basic shapes, variations are possible. Fissure and inverted cone burs may have half-round or domed ends. Taper and cone angles may vary. The ratio of head length to diameter may be varied. In addition to shape, other features may be varied, such as the number of blades, spiral versus axial patterns for blades, and continuous versus crosscut blade edges.

Sizes

In the United States, the number designating bur size also traditionally has served as a code for head design. This numbering system for burs was originated by the S.S. White Dental Manufacturing Company in 1891 for their first machine-made burs. It was extensive and logical, so other domestic manufacturers found it convenient to adopt it for their burs as well. As a result, for more than 60 years, a general uniformity existed for bur numbers in the United States. Table 6-1 shows the correlation of bur head sizes with dimensions and shapes. The table includes not only many bur sizes that are still in common use but also others that have become obsolete.

The original numbering system grouped burs by 9 shapes and 11 sizes. The $\frac{1}{2}$ and $\frac{1}{4}$ designations (both very small round burs) were added later when smaller instruments were included in the system. All original bur designs had continuous blade edges. Later, when crosscut burs were found to be more effective for cutting dentin at low speeds, crosscut versions of many bur sizes were introduced. This modification was indicated by adding 500 to the number of the equivalent noncrosscut size. A No. 57 with crosscut was designated No. 557. Similarly, a 900 prefix was used to indicate a head design intended for end cutting only. Except for differences in blade design, a No. 957, No. 557, and No. 57 bur all had the same head dimensions. These changes occurred gradually over time without disrupting the system. The sizes in common use in 1955 are shown in Table 6-2. The system changed rapidly thereafter, but where the numbers are still used, the designs and dimensions remain the same.

Modifications in Bur Design

As available handpiece speeds increased after 1950, particularly after the high-speed turbine handpieces were introduced,

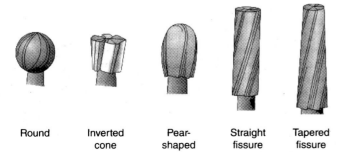

| Round | Inverted cone | Pear-shaped | Straight fissure | Tapered fissure |

Fig. 6-19 Basic bur head shapes. *(From Finkbeiner BL, Johnson CS: Mosby's comprehensive dental assisting, St. Louis, 1995, Mosby.)*

Table 6-1 Original Bur Head Sizes (1891–1954)

Head Shapes	Head Diameters in Inches (mm*)												
	0.020	0.025	0.032	0.039	0.047	0.055	0.063	0.072	0.081	0.090	0.099	0.109	0.119
	(0.5)	(0.6)	(0.8)	(1.0)	(1.2)	(1.4)	(1.6)	(1.8)	(2.1)	(2.3)	(2.5)	(2.8)	(3.0)
Round	¼	½	1	2	3	4	5	6	7	8	9	10	11
Wheel	—	11½	12	13	14	15	16	17	18	19	20	21	22
Cone	—	22½	23	24	25	26	27	28	29	30	31	32	33
Inverted cone	—	33½	34	35	36	37	38	39	40	41	42	43	44
Bud	—	44½	45	46	47	48	49	50	51	—	—	—	—
Straight fissure (flat end)	55¼	55½	56	57	58	59	60	61	62	—	—	—	—
Straight fissure (pointed end)	.	66½	67	68	69	70	71	72	73	—	—	—	—
Pear		77½	78	79	80	81	82	83	84	85	86	87	88
Oval		88½	89	90	91	92	93	94	95	—	—	—	—

*Millimeter values rounded to the nearest 0.1 mm.
Courtesy of H.M. Moylan, S.S. White Dental Manufacturing Company, Lakewood, NJ.

Table 6-2 Standard Bur Head Sizes—Carbide and Steel (1955–Present)

Head Shapes	Head Diameters in Inches (mm*)													
	0.020	0.025	0.032	0.040	0.048	0.056	0.064	0.073	0.082	0.091	0.100	0.110	0.120	0.130
	(0.5)	(0.6)	(0.8)	(1.0)	(1.2)	(1.4)	(1.6)	(1.9)	(2.1)	(2.3)	(2.5)	(2.8)	(3.0)	(3.3)
Round	¼	½	1	2	3	4	5	6	7	8	9	10	11	—
Wheel	—	11½	12	—	14	—	16	—	—	—	—	—	—	—
Inverted cone	—	33½	34	35	36	37	38	39	40	—	—	—	—	—
Plain fissure	—	55½	56	57	58	59	60	61	62	—	—	—	—	—
Round crosscut	—	—	—	502	503	504	505	506	—	—	—	—	—	—
Straight fissure crosscut	—	—	556	557	558	559	560	561	562	563	—	—	—	—
Tapered fissure crosscut	—	—	—	700	701	—	702	—	703	—	—	—	—	—
End cutting fissure	—	—	—	957	958	959	—	—	—	—	—	—	—	—

*Millimeter values rounded to the nearest 0.1 mm.
Note: Non-standard burs are not shown in this table.

a new cycle of modification of bur sizes and shapes occurred. Numerous other categories have arisen as new variations in blade number or design have been created. Some of the numbers assigned to the burs were selected arbitrarily. With the introduction of new bur sizes and elimination of older sizes, much of the logic in the system has no longer been maintained, and many dentists and manufacturers no longer recognize the original significance of the numbers used for burs. The number of standard sizes that have continued in use has been reduced. This has been most obvious in the decreased popularity of large-diameter burs. The cutting effectiveness of carbide burs is greatly increased at high speeds.[19] This is particularly true of the small-diameter sizes, which did not have sufficient peripheral speed for efficient cutting when used at lower rates of rotation. As the effectiveness of small burs has increased, they have replaced larger burs in many procedures. Three other major trends in bur design are discernible: (1)

reduced use of crosscuts, (2) extended heads on fissure burs, and (3) rounding of sharp tip angles.

Crosscuts are needed on fissure burs to obtain adequate cutting effectiveness at low speeds, but they are not needed at high speeds. Because crosscut burs used at high speeds tend to produce unduly rough surfaces, many of the crosscut sizes originally developed for low-speed use have been replaced by non-crosscut instruments of the same dimension for high-speed use.[20] In many instances, the non-crosscut equivalents were available; a No. 57 bur might be used at high speed, whereas a No. 557 bur was preferred for low-speed use. Non-crosscut versions of the 700 series burs have become popular, but their introduction precipitated a crisis in the bur numbering system because no number traditionally had been assigned to burs of this type.

Carbide fissure burs with extended head lengths two to three times those of the normal tapered fissure burs of similar

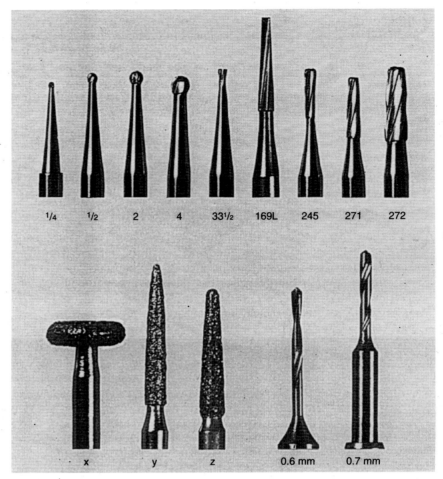

Fig. 6-20 Burs used in recommended procedures. Bur sizes ¼, ½–, 2, 4, 33½–, and 169L are standard carbide burs available from various sources. The 245, 271, and 272 burs are non-standard carbide burs that do not conform to the current American Dental Association (ADA) standard numbering system. They are designed to combine rounded corners with flat ends and are available from several manufacturers. The diamond instruments shown are wheel (Star No. 110) (*x*), flame (Star No. 265-8F) (*y*), and tapered cylinder (R & R No. 770 × 7) (*z*). Two sizes of twist drill are illustrated. Particular drills often are provided as specified by manufacturers of pin-retention systems.

diameter have been introduced. Such a design would never have been practical using a brittle material such as carbide if the bur were to be used at low speed. The applied force required to make a bur cut at speeds of 5000 to 6000 rpm would normally be sufficient to fracture such an attenuated head. The extremely light applied pressures needed for cutting at high speed permit many modifications of burs, however, that would have been impractical at low speed.

The third major trend in bur design has been toward rounding of the sharp tip corners. Early contributions to this trend were made by Markley and also Sockwell.[8] Because teeth are relatively brittle, the sharp angles produced by conventional burs can result in high stress concentrations and increase the tendency of the tooth to fracture. Bur heads with rounded corners result in lower stresses in restored teeth, enhance the strength of the tooth by preserving vital dentin, and facilitate the adaptation of restorative materials. Carbide burs and diamond instruments of these designs last longer because no sharp corners to chip and wear are present. Such burs facilitate tooth preparation with desired features of a flat preparation floor and rounded internal line angles.

Many of these new and modified bur designs simplify the techniques and reduce the effort needed for optimal results. Although the development of new bur sizes and shapes has increased greatly the number of different types in current use, the number actually required for clinical effectiveness has

been reduced. Most instruments recommended in this text for the preparation of teeth are illustrated in Fig. 6-20. The selection includes standard head designs and modified designs of the types just discussed. Table 6-3 lists the significant head dimensions of these standard and modified burs.

A problem related to the dimensions and designations of rotary dental instruments worldwide arose because each country developed its own system of classification. Dentists in the United States often were not aware of the problem because they predominantly used domestic products, and all U.S. manufacturers used the same system. The rapid rate at which new bur designs were introduced during the transition to high-speed techniques threatened to cause a complete breakdown in the numbering system. As different manufacturers developed and marketed new burs of similar design almost simultaneously, the risk of similar burs being given different numbers or different burs being given the same number increased. Combined with the growing use of foreign products in the United States, this situation has led to more interest in the establishment of international standards for dimensions, nomenclature, and other characteristics.

Progress toward the development of an international numbering system for basic bur shapes and sizes under the auspices of the ISO (International Standards Organization) has been slow. For other design features, the trend instead seems to be toward the use of individual manufacturer's code

Table 6-3 Names and Key Dimensions of Recommended Burs

Manufacturer's Size Number	ADA Size Number	ISO Size Number	Head Diameter (mm)	Head Length (mm)	Taper Angle (degrees)	Shape
¼	¼	005	0.50	0.40	—	Round
½	½	006	0.60	0.48	—	Round
2	2	010	1.00	0.80	—	Round
4	4	014	1.40	1.10	—	Round
33½	33½	006	0.60	0.45	12	Inverted cone
169	169	009	0.90	4.30	6	Tapered fissure
169L*	169L	009	0.90	5.60	4	Elongated tapered fissure
329	329	007	0.70	0.85	8	Pear, normal length
330	330	008	0.80	1.00	8	Pear, normal length
245†‡	330L	008	0.80	3.00	4	Pear, elongated
271†	171	012	1.20	4.00	6	Tapered fissure
272†	172	016	1.60	5.00	6	Tapered fissure

*Similar to the No. 169 bur except for greater head length.
†These burs differ from the equivalent ADA size by being flat ended with rounded corners. The manufacturer's number has been changed to indicate this difference.
‡Similar to the No. 330 bur except for greater head length.
ADA, American Dental Association; *ISO*, International Standard Organization.

numbers. Throughout the remaining text, the traditional U.S. numbers are used, where possible. The few exceptions are shown in Fig. 6-20 and Table 6-3.

Additional Features in Head Design

Numerous factors other than head size and shape are involved in determining the clinical effectiveness of a bur design.[21,22] Figure 6-21 shows a lateral view and a cross-sectional view of a No. 701 crosscut tapered fissure bur in which several of these factors are illustrated. The lateral view (see Fig. 6-21, *A*) shows neck diameter, head diameter, head length, taper angle, blade spiral angle, and crosscut size and spacing as they apply to this bur size. Of these features, head length and taper angle are primarily descriptive and may be varied within limits consistent with the intended use of the bur. This bur originally was designed for use at low speeds in preparing teeth for cast restorations. The taper angle is intended to approximate the desired occlusal divergence of the lateral walls of the preparations, and the head length must be long enough to reach the full depth of the normal preparation. These factors do not otherwise affect the performance of the bur.

Neck diameter is important functionally because a neck that is too small results in a weak instrument unable to resist lateral forces. Too large a neck diameter may interfere with visibility and the use of the part of the bur head next to the neck and may restrict access for coolants. As the head of a bur increases in length or diameter, the moment arm exerted by lateral forces increases, and the neck needs to be larger.

Compared with these factors, two other design variables, the spiral angle and crosscutting, have considerably greater influence on bur performance. There is a tendency toward reduced spiral angles on burs intended exclusively for high-speed operation in which a large spiral is not needed to produce a smoother preparation and a smaller angle, which produces more efficient cutting.

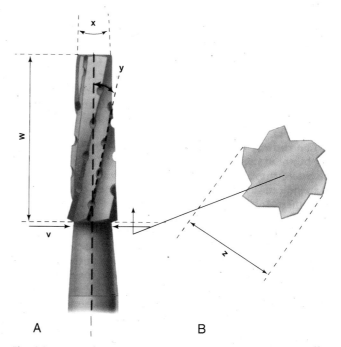

Fig. 6-21 Design features of bur heads (illustrated using No. 701 bur). **A,** Lateral view—neck diameter (*v*), head length (*w*), taper angle (*x*), and spiral angle (*y*). **B,** End view—head diameter (*z*).

As noted previously, crosscut bur designs have notches in the blade edges to increase cutting effectiveness at low and medium speeds. A certain amount of perpendicular force is required to make a blade grasp the surface and start cutting as it passes across the surface. The harder the surface, the duller the blade, and the greater its length, the more is the force required to initiate cutting. By reducing the total length of bur blade that is actively cutting at any one time, the crosscuts effectively increase the cutting pressure resulting from rotation of the bur and the perpendicular pressure holding the blade edge against the tooth.

As each crosscut blade cuts, it leaves small ridges of tooth structure standing behind the notches. Because the notches in two succeeding blades do not line up with each other, the ridges left by one blade are removed by the following one at low or medium speeds. At the high speed attained with air-driven handpieces, however, the contact of the bur with the tooth is not continuous, and usually only one blade cuts effectively.[23] Under these circumstances, although the high cutting rate of crosscut burs is maintained, the ridges are not removed, and a much rougher cut surface results.[20]

A cross-sectional view of the same No. 701 bur is shown in Figure 6-21, *B*. This cross-section is made at the point of largest head diameter and is drawn as seen from the shank end. The bur has six blades uniformly spaced with depressed areas between them. These depressed areas are properly known as *flutes*. The number of blades on a bur is always even because even numbers are easier to produce in the manufacturing process, and instruments with odd numbers of blades cut no better than those with even numbers. The number of blades on an excavating bur may vary from 6 to 8 to 10. Burs intended mainly for finishing procedures usually have 12 to 40 blades. The greater the number of blades, the smoother is the cutting action at low speeds. Most burs are made with at least 6 blades because they may need to be used in this speed range. In the high-speed range, no more than one blade seems to cut effectively at any one time, and the remaining blades are, in effect, spares. The tendency for the bur to cut on a single blade is often a result of factors other than the bur itself. Nevertheless, it is important that the bur head be as symmetrical as possible. Two terms are in common use to measure this characteristic of bur heads: *concentricity* and *runout*.

Concentricity is a direct measurement of the symmetry of the bur head itself. It measures how closely a single circle can be passed through the tips of all of the blades. Concentricity is an indication of whether one blade is longer or shorter than the others. It is a static measurement not directly related to function. *Runout* is a dynamic test measuring the accuracy with which all blade tips pass through a single point when the instrument is rotated. It measures not only the concentricity of the head but also the accuracy with which the center of rotation passes through the center of the head. Even a perfectly concentric head exhibits substantial runout if the head is off center on the axis of the bur, the bur neck is bent, the bur is not held straight in the handpiece chuck, or the chuck is eccentric relative to the handpiece bearings. The runout can never be less than the concentricity, and it is usually substantially greater. *Runout* is the more significant term clinically because it is the primary cause of vibration during cutting and is the factor that determines the minimum diameter of the hole that can be prepared by a given bur. Because of runout errors, burs normally cut holes measurably larger than the head diameter.

Bur Blade Design

The actual cutting action of a bur (or a diamond) occurs in a very small region at the edge of the blade (or at the point of a diamond chip). In the high-speed range, this effective

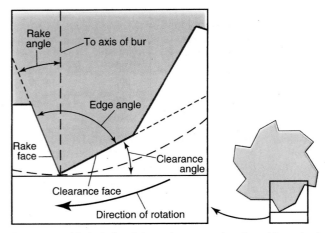

Fig. 6-22 Bur blade design. Schematic cross-section viewed from shank end of head to show rake angle, edge angle, and clearance angle.

portion of the individual blade is limited to no more than a few thousandths of a centimeter adjacent to the blade edge. Figure 6-22 is an enlarged schematic view of this portion of a bur blade. Several terms used in the discussion of blade design are illustrated.

Each blade has two sides—the *rake face* (toward the direction of cutting) and the *clearance face*—and three important angles—the *rake angle*, the *edge angle*, and the *clearance angle*. The optimal angles depend on such factors as the mechanical properties of the blade material, the mechanical properties of the material being cut, the rotational speed and diameter of the bur, and the lateral force applied by the operator to the handpiece and to the bur.

The rake angle is the most important design characteristic of a bur blade. For cutting hard, brittle materials, a negative rake angle minimizes fractures of the cutting edge, increasing the tool life. A rake angle is said to be negative when the rake face is ahead of the radius (from cutting edge to axis of bur), as illustrated in Figure 6-22. Increasing the edge angle reinforces the cutting edge and reduces the likelihood for the edge of the blade to fracture. Carbide bur blades have higher hardness and are more wear-resistant, but they are more brittle than steel blades and require greater edge angles to minimize fractures. The three angles cannot be varied independently of each other. An increase in the clearance angle causes a decrease in the edge angle. The clearance angle eliminates rubbing friction of the clearance face, provides a stop to prevent the bur edge from digging into the tooth structure excessively, and reduces the radius of the blade back of the cutting edge to provide adequate flute space or clearance space for the chips formed ahead of the following blade.

Carbide burs normally have blades with slight negative rake angles and edge angles of approximately 90 degrees. Their clearance faces either are curved or have two surfaces to provide a low clearance angle near the edge and a greater clearance space ahead of the following blade.

Diamond Abrasive Instruments

The second major category of rotary dental cutting instruments involves abrasive cutting rather than blade cutting. Abrasive instruments are based on small, angular particles of a hard substance held in a matrix of softer material. Cutting occurs at numerous points where individual hard particles protrude from the matrix, rather than along a continuous blade edge. This difference in design causes definite differences in the mechanisms by which the two types of instruments cut and in the applications for which they are best suited.

Abrasive instruments are generally grouped as diamond or other instruments. Diamond instruments have had great clinical impact because of their long life and great effectiveness in cutting enamel and dentin. Diamond instruments for dental use were introduced in the United States in 1942 at a time before carbide burs were available and at a time when interest in increased rotational speeds was beginning to expose the limitations of steel burs. The earliest diamond instruments were substitutes for previously used abrasive points of other types used for grinding and finishing.[24] Their vastly superior performance in these applications led to their immediate acceptance. The shortage of burs as a result of wartime demands emphasized the relative durability of diamond instruments for cutting enamel and promoted the development of operative techniques employing them.

Terminology

Diamond instruments consist of three parts: (1) a metal blank, (2) the powdered diamond abrasive, and (3) a metallic bonding material that holds the diamond powder onto the blank (Fig. 6-23). The blank in many ways resembles a bur without blades. It has the same essential parts: head, neck, and shank.

The shank dimensions, similar to those for bur shanks, depend on the intended handpiece. The neck is normally a tapered section of reduced diameter that connects the shank to the head, but for large disk-shaped or wheel-shaped instruments, it may not be reduced below the shank diameter. The head of the blank is undersized compared with the desired final dimensions of the instrument, but its size and shape determine the size and shape of the finished instrument. Dimensions of the head make allowance for a fairly uniform thickness of diamonds and bonding material on all sides. Some abrasive instruments are designed as a mandrel and a detachable head. This is much more practical for abrasive disks that have very short lifetimes.

The diamonds employed are industrial diamonds, either natural or synthetic, that have been crushed to powder, then carefully graded for size and quality. The shape of the individual particle is important because of its effect on the cutting efficiency and durability of the instrument, but the careful control of particle size is probably of greater importance. The diamonds generally are attached to the blank by electroplating a layer of metal on the blank while holding the diamonds in place against it. Although the electroplating holds the diamonds in place, it also tends to cover much of the diamond surfaces. Some proprietary techniques do allow greater diamond exposure and more effective cutting.

Classification

Diamond instruments currently are marketed in myriad head shapes and sizes (Table 6-4) and in all of the standard shank designs. Most of the diamond shapes parallel those for burs (Fig. 6-24). This great diversity arose, in part, as a result of the relative simplicity of the manufacturing process. Because it is possible to make diamond instruments in almost any shape for which a blank can be manufactured, they are produced in many highly specialized shapes, on which it would be impractical to place cutting blades. This has been a major factor in establishing clinical uses for these points, which are not in direct competition with burs.

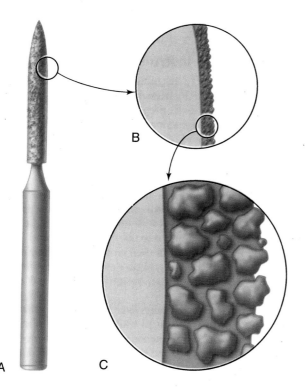

Fig. 6-23 Diamond instrument construction. **A,** Overall view. **B,** Detail of abrasive layer. **C,** Detail of particle bonding.

Table 6-4 Standard Categories of Shapes and Sizes for Diamond Cutting Instruments

Head Shapes	Profile Variations
Round	—
Football	Pointed
Barrel	—
Cylinder	Flat-, bevel-, round- or, safe-end
Inverted cone	—
Taper	Flat-, round-, or safe-end
Flame	—
Curettage	—
Pear	—
Needle	"Christmas tree"
Interproximal	Occlusal anatomy
Donut	—
Wheel	—

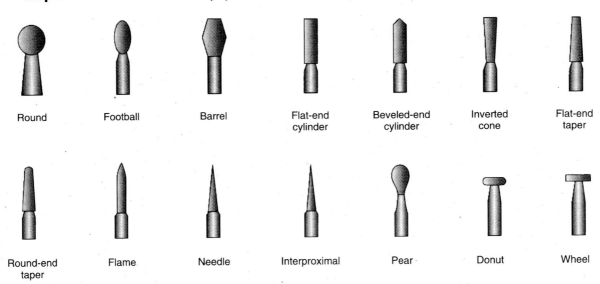

| Round | Football | Barrel | Flat-end cylinder | Beveled-end cylinder | Inverted cone | Flat-end taper |

| Round-end taper | Flame | Needle | Interproximal | Pear | Donut | Wheel |

Fig. 6-24 Characteristic shapes and designs for a range of diamond cutting instruments.

Head Shapes and Sizes

Diamond instruments are available in a wide variety of shapes and in sizes that correspond to all except the smallest-diameter burs. The greatest difference lies in the diversity of other sizes and shapes in which diamond instruments are produced. Even with many subdivisions, the size range within each group is large compared with that found among the burs. More than 200 shapes and sizes of diamonds are currently marketed.

Because of their design with an abrasive layer over an underlying blank, the smallest diamond instruments cannot be as small in diameter as the smallest burs, but a wide range of sizes is available for each shape. No one manufacturer produces all sizes, but each usually offers an assortment of instruments, including the popular sizes and shapes. Because of the lack of uniform nomenclature for diamond instruments, it is often necessary to select them by inspection to obtain the desired size and shape. It is essential to indicate the manufacturer when attempting to describe diamond instruments by catalogue number.

Diamond Particle Factors

The clinical performance of diamond abrasive instruments depends on the size, spacing, uniformity, exposure, and bonding of the diamond particles. Increased pressure causes the particles to dig into the surface more deeply, leaving deeper scratches and removing more tooth structure.

Diamond particle size is commonly categorized as coarse (125–150 μm), medium (88–125 μm), fine (60–74 μm), and very fine (38–44 μm) for diamond preparation instruments.[24] These ranges correspond to standard sieve sizes for separating particle sizes. When using large particle sizes, the number of abrasive particles that can be placed on a given area of the head is decreased. For any given force that the operator applies, the pressure on each particle tip is greater. The resulting pressure also is increased if diamond particles are more widely spaced so that fewer are in contact with the surface at any one time. The final clinical performance of diamond instruments is strongly affected by the technique used to take advantage of the design factors for each instrument.

Diamond finishing instruments use even finer diamonds (10–38 μm) to produce relatively smooth surfaces for final finishing with diamond polishing pastes. Surface finishes of less than 1 μm are considered clinically smooth (see the section on composites in online Chapter 18) and can be routinely attained by using a series of progressively finer polishing steps.

Proper diamond instrument speed and pressure are the major factors in determining service life.[25] Properly used diamond instruments last almost indefinitely. Almost the only cause of failure of diamond instruments is loss of the diamonds from critical areas. This loss results from the use of excess pressure in an attempt to increase the cutting rate at inadequate speeds.[26]

Other Abrasive Instruments

Many types of abrasive instruments are used in dentistry in addition to diamond instruments. At one time, they were extensively used for tooth preparation, but their use is now primarily restricted to shaping, finishing, and polishing restorations in the clinic and in the laboratory.

Classification

In these instruments, as in the diamond instruments, the cutting surfaces of the head are composed of abrasive particles held in a continuous matrix of softer material. Other than this and their use of standard shank designs, diamond instruments have little similarity in their construction. They may be divided into two distinct groups—*molded instruments* and *coated instruments*. Each uses various abrasives and matrix materials.

Molded abrasive instruments have heads that are manufactured by molding or pressing a uniform mixture of abrasive and matrix around the roughened end of the shank or cementing a premolded head to the shank. In contrast to diamond instruments, molded instruments have a much softer matrix and wear during use. The abrasive is distributed throughout the matrix so that new particles are exposed by the wear. These instruments are made in a full range of shapes and sizes. The mounted heads are often termed *points* and *stones*. Hard and rigid molded instrument heads use rigid polymer or ceramic materials for their matrix and commonly are used for grinding and shaping procedures. Other molded instrument heads use flexible matrix materials, such as rubber, to hold the abrasive particles. These are used predominantly for finishing and polishing procedures. Molded unmounted disks or wheelstones are attached by a screw to a mandrel of suitable size for a given handpiece that has a threaded hole in the end. This design permits the instruments to be changed easily and discarded economically.

The coated abrasive instruments are mostly disks that have a thin layer of abrasive cemented to a flexible backing. This construction allows the instrument to conform to the surface contour of a tooth or restoration. Most flexible disks are designed for reversible attachment to a mandrel. Coated abrasive instruments may be used in the finishing and smoothing procedures of certain enamel walls (and margins) of tooth preparations for indirect restorations but most often in finishing procedures for restorations.

The abrasives are softer and are less wear resistant than diamond powder, and as a result, they tend to lose their sharp edges and their cutting efficiency with use. When this happens to coated instruments, they are discarded. In contrast, molded instruments are intended to partially regenerate through the gradual loss of their worn outer layers but may require that the operator reshape them to improve their concentricity. This is accomplished by applying a truing or shaping stone against the rotating instrument.

Materials

The matrix materials usually are phenolic resins or rubber. Some molded points may be sintered, but most are resin bonded. A rubber matrix is used primarily to obtain a flexible head on instruments to be used for polishing. A harder, nonflexible rubber matrix is often used for molded silicon carbide (SiC) disks. The matrix of coated instruments is usually one of the phenolic resins.

Synthetic or natural abrasives may be used, including silicon carbide, aluminum oxide, garnet, quartz, pumice, and cuttlebone. The hardness of the abrasive has a major effect on the cutting efficiency. The Mohs hardness values for important dental abrasives are shown in Table 6-5. SiC usually is used in molded rounds, tree or bud shapes, wheels, and cylinders of various sizes. These points are normally gray-green, available in various textures, and usually fast cutting (except on enamel) and produce a moderately smooth surface. Molded unmounted disks are black or a dark color, have a soft matrix, wear more rapidly than stones, and produce a moderately rough surface texture. These disks are termed *carborundum disks* or *separating disks*. Aluminum oxide is used for the same instrument designs as those for silicon carbide disks. Points are usually white, rigid, fine textured, and less porous and produce a smoother surface than SiC.

Garnet (reddish) and quartz (white) are used for coated disks that are available in a series of particle sizes and range from coarse to medium-fine for use in initial finishing. These abrasives are hard enough to cut tooth structure and all restorative materials, with the exception of some porcelains. Pumice is a powdered abrasive produced by crushing foamed volcanic glass into thin glass flakes. The flakes cut effectively, but they

Table 6-5 Hardness Values of Restorative Materials, Tooth Structure, and Abrasives

	Knoop Hardness	Brinell Hardness	Mohs Hardness
Dentin	68	48	3–4
Enamel	343	300	5
Dental composite	41–80	60–80	5–7
Dental amalgam	110	—	4–5
Gold alloy (type III)	—	110	—
Feldspathic porcelain	460	—	6–7
Pumice	—	—	6
Cuttlebone	—	—	7
Garnet	—	—	6.5–7
Quartz	800	600	7
Aluminum oxide	1500	1200	9
Silicon carbide	2500	—	9.5
Diamond	>7000	>5000	10

break down rapidly. Pumice is used with rubber disks and wheels, usually for initial polishing procedures. Cuttlebone is derived from the cuttlefish, a relative of squid and octopus. It is becoming scarce and gradually is being replaced by synthetic substitutes. It is a soft white abrasive, used only in coated disks for final finishing and polishing. It is soft enough that it reduces the risk of unintentional damage to tooth structure during the final stages of finishing.

Cutting Mechanisms

For cutting, it is necessary to apply sufficient pressure to make the cutting edge of a blade or abrasive particle dig into the surface. Local fracture occurs more easily if the strain rate is high (high rotary instrument surface speed) because the surface that is being cut responds in a brittle fashion. The process by which rotary instruments cut tooth structure is complex and not fully understood. The following discussion of cutting addresses cutting evaluations, cutting instrument design, proposed cutting mechanisms, and clinical recommendations for cutting.

Evaluation of Cutting

Cutting can be measured in terms of effectiveness and efficiency. Certain factors may influence one, but not the other.[27] Cutting effectiveness is the rate of tooth structure removal (mm/min or mg/s). Effectiveness does not consider potential side effects such as heat or noise. Cutting efficiency is the percentage of energy actually producing cutting. Cutting efficiency is reduced when energy is wasted as heat or noise. It is possible to increase effectiveness while decreasing efficiency. A dull bur may be made to cut faster than a sharp bur by applying a greater pressure, but experience indicates that this results in a great increase in heat production and reduced efficiency.[28]

It is generally agreed that increased rotational speed results in increased effectiveness and efficiency. Adverse effects associated with increased speeds are heat, vibration, and noise. Heat has been identified as a primary cause of pulpal injury. Air-water sprays do not prevent the production of heat, but do serve to remove it before it causes a damaging increase in temperature within the tooth.

Bladed Cutting

The following discussion focuses on rotary bladed instruments but also is applicable to bladed hand instruments. Tooth structure, similar to other materials, undergoes brittle and ductile fracture. Brittle fracture is associated with crack production, usually by tensile loading. Ductile fracture involves plastic deformation of material, usually proceeding by shear. Extensive plastic deformation also may produce local work hardening and encourage brittle fracture. Low-speed cutting tends to proceed by plastic deformation before tooth structure fracture. High-speed cutting, especially of enamel, proceeds by brittle fracture.

The rate of stress application (or strain rate) affects the resultant properties of materials. In general, the faster the rate of loading, the greater are the strength, hardness, modulus of elasticity, and brittleness of a material. A cutting instrument with a large diameter and high rotational speed produces a high surface speed and a high stress (or strain) rate.

Many factors interact to determine which cutting mechanism is active in a particular situation. The mechanical properties of tooth structure, the design of the cutting edge or point, the linear speed of the instrument's surface, the contact force applied, and the power output characteristics of the handpiece influence the cutting process in various ways.[19,29]

For the blade to initiate the cutting action, it must be sharp, must have a higher hardness and modulus of elasticity than the material being cut, and must be pressed against the surface with sufficient force. The high hardness and modulus of elasticity are essential to concentrate the applied force on a small enough area to exceed the shear strength of the material being cut. As shown in Figure 6-25, sheared segments accumulate in a distorted layer that slides up along the rake face of the blade until it breaks or until the blade disengages from the surface as it rotates. These chips accumulate in the clearance space between blades until washed out or thrown out by centrifugal force.

Mechanical distortion of tooth structure ahead of the blade produces heat. Frictional heat is produced by the rubbing action of the cut chips against the rake face of the blade and the blade tip against the cut surface of the tooth immediately behind the edge. This can produce extreme temperature increases in the tooth and the bur in the absence of adequate cooling. The transfer of heat is not instantaneous, and the reduced temperature increase observed in teeth cut at very high speeds may be caused, in part, by the removal of the heated surface layer of the tooth structure by a following blade before the heat can be conducted into the tooth.

Abrasive Cutting

The following discussion is pertinent to all abrasive cutting situations, but diamond instruments are used as the primary example.[12] The cutting action of diamond abrasive instruments is similar in many ways to that of bladed instruments, but key differences result from the properties, size, and distribution of the abrasive. The very high hardness of diamonds provides superior resistance to wear. A diamond instrument that is not abused has little or no tendency to dull with use. Individual diamond particles have very sharp edges, are randomly oriented on the surface, and tend to have large negative rake angles.

When diamond instruments are used to cut ductile materials, some material is removed as chips, but much material flows laterally around the cutting point and is left as a ridge of deformed material on the surface (Fig. 6-26). Repeated deformation work hardens the distorted material until irregular portions become brittle, break off, and are removed. This type of cutting is less efficient than that by a blade; burs are generally preferred for cutting ductile materials such as dentin.

Diamonds cut brittle materials by a different mechanism. Most cutting results from tensile fractures that produce a series of subsurface cracks (Fig. 6-27). Diamonds are most efficient when used to cut brittle materials and are superior to burs for the removal of dental enamel. Diamond abrasives are commonly used for milling in computer-aided design/computer-assisted manufacturing (CAD/CAM) or copy-milling applications (see section on machined restorations in Online Chapter 18).

Cutting Recommendations

Overall, the requirements for effective and efficient cutting include using a contra-angle handpiece, air-water spray for cooling, high operating speed (> 200,000 rpm), light pressure,

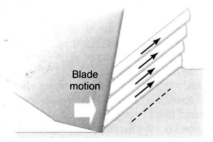

Fig. 6-25 Schematic representation of bur blade (*end view*) cutting a ductile material by shearing mechanism. Energy is required to deform the material removed and produce new surface.

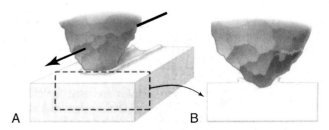

Fig. 6-26 Schematic representation of an abrasive particle cutting ductile material. **A,** Lateral view. **B,** Cross-sectional view. Material is displaced laterally by passage of an abrasive particle, work hardened, and subsequently removed by other particles.

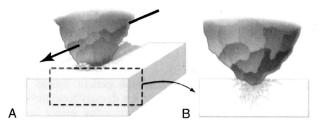

Fig. 6-27 Schematic representation of abrasive particle cutting brittle material. **A,** Lateral view. **B,** Cross-sectional view. Subsurface cracks caused by the passage of abrasive particles intersect, undermining small pieces of material, which are removed easily by following abrasive particles.

and a carbide bur or diamond instrument. Carbide burs are better for end cutting, produce lower heat, and have more blade edges per diameter for cutting. They are used effectively for punch cuts to enter tooth structure, intracoronal tooth preparation, amalgam removal, small preparations, and secondary retention features. Diamond instruments have higher hardness, and coarse diamonds have high cutting effectiveness. Diamonds are more effective than burs for intracoronal and extracoronal tooth preparations, beveling enamel margins on tooth preparations, and enameloplasty.

Hazards with Cutting Instruments

Almost everything done in a dental office involves some risk to the patient, the dentist, or the auxiliaries. For the patient, pulpal dangers arise from tooth preparation and restoration procedures. Soft tissue dangers are also present. Everyone is potentially susceptible to eye, ear, and inhalation dangers. Careful adherence to normal precautions can, however, eliminate or minimize most risks associated with the use of cutting instruments.

Pulpal Precautions

The use of cutting instruments can harm the pulp by exposure to mechanical vibration, heat generation, desiccation and loss of dentinal tubule fluid, or transection of odontoblastic processes. As the thickness of remaining dentin decreases, the pulpal insult (and response) from heat or desiccation increases. Slight to moderate injury produces a localized, protective pulpal response in the region of the cut tubules. In severe injury, destruction extends beyond the cut tubules, often resulting in pulpal abscess and death of the pulp. These pulpal sequelae (recovery or necrosis) take 2 weeks to 6 months or longer, depending on the extent and degree of the trauma. Although a young pulp is more prone to injury, it also recovers more effectively compared with an older pulp, in which the recuperative powers are slower and less effective.

Enamel and dentin are good thermal insulators and protect the pulp if the quantity of heat is not too great and the remaining thickness of tissue is adequate. The longer the time of cutting and the higher the local temperature produced, the greater is the threat of thermal trauma. The remaining tissue is effective in protecting the pulp in proportion to the square of its thickness. Steel burs produce more heat than carbide

burs because of inefficient cutting. Burs and diamond instruments that are dull or plugged with debris do not cut efficiently, resulting in heat production. When used without coolants, diamond instruments generate more damaging heat compared with carbide burs.

The most common instrument coolants are air and air-water sprays. Air alone as a coolant is not effective in preventing pulpal damage because it needlessly desiccates dentin and damages odontoblasts. Air has a much lower heat capacity than water and is much less efficient in absorbing unwanted heat. An air coolant alone should be used only when visibility is a problem, such as during the finishing procedures of tooth preparations. At such times, air coolant combined with lower speed and light, intermittent application should be used to enhance vision and minimize trauma. Air-water spray is universally used to cool, moisten, and clear the operating site during normal cutting procedures. In addition, the spray lubricates, cleans, and cools the cutting instrument, increasing its efficiency and service life. A well-designed and properly directed air-water spray also helps keep the gingival crevice open for better visualization when gingival extension is necessary. The use of a water spray and its removal by an effective high-volume evacuator are especially important when old amalgam restorations are removed because they decrease mercury vapor release and increase visibility.

During normal cutting procedures, a layer of debris, described as a smear layer, is created that covers the cut surfaces of the enamel and dentin. The smear layer on dentin is moderately protective because it occludes the dentinal tubules and inhibits the outward flow of tubular fluid and the inward penetration of microleakage contaminants. The smear layer is, however, still porous. When air alone is applied to dentin, local desiccation may produce fluid flow and affect the physiologic status of the odontoblastic processes in the underlying dentin. Air is applied only to the extent of removing excess moisture, leaving a glistening surface.

Soft Tissue Precautions

The lips, tongue, and cheeks of the patient are the most frequent areas of soft tissue injury. The handpiece should never be operated unless good access to and visualization of the cutting site are available. A rubber dam is helpful in isolating the operating site. When the dam is not used, the dental assistant can retract the soft tissue on one side with a mouth mirror, cotton roll, or evacuator tip. The dentist usually can manage the other side with a mirror or cotton roll or both. If the dentist must work alone, the patient can help by holding a retraction-type saliva ejector evacuator tip, after it is positioned in the mouth.

With air-driven handpieces, the rotating instrument does not stop immediately when the foot control is released. The operator must wait for the instrument to stop or be extremely careful when removing the handpiece from the mouth so as not to lacerate soft tissues. The large disk is one of the most dangerous instruments used in the mouth. Such disks are seldom indicated intraorally. They should be used with light, intermittent application and with extreme caution.

With electric handpieces, patients have been severely burned when these handpieces have overheated during dental procedures (Fig. 6-28). Some patients suffered third-degree burns that required reconstructive surgery. Burns may not be

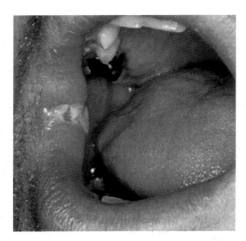

Fig. 6-28 This patient suffered burn from the overheated bearing of an electric handpiece. Because the patient was anesthetized, he was unaware of the burn as it occurred from the overheated handpiece.

apparent to the operator or the patient until after the tissue damage has occurred because the anesthetized patient cannot feel the tissue burning and the handpiece housing insulates the operator from the heated attachment. Although the reported burns have occurred during cutting of tooth and bone, tooth extraction and other dental surgical procedures, overheating could occur during any dental procedure.

With high-speed and low-speed air-driven handpieces, sluggish handpiece performance will alert the dental practitioner to maintenance issues such as a dull bur or worn or clogged gears or bearings. A poorly maintained electric handpiece does not provide a similar warning that maintenance is needed. Instead, if an electric handpiece is worn out, damaged, or clogged, the electric motor sends increased power to the handpiece head or attachment in order to maintain handpiece performance. This increased power can rapidly generate heat at the head of the handpiece attachment. Because the heat buildup is so rapid and is efficiently conducted through the metal handpiece, a burn occurring in the patient may be the first indication of handpiece problems. Adhering to strict maintenance guidelines recommended by the manufacturers is critical to prevent overheating in electric handpieces. The clinician must be aware that improperly maintained, damaged, or worn-out devices have the potential to overheat without warning.

The dentist and the assistant always must be aware of the patient's response during the cutting procedures. A sudden reflex movement by the patient such as gagging, swallowing, or coughing could result in serious injury. If an accident does occur and soft tissue is damaged, the operator should remain calm and control any hemorrhage with a pressure pack. The patient should be told what has happened, and medical assistance should be obtained, if needed.

The chance of mechanical pulpal involvement may be greater if a hand excavator is used to remove the last portions of soft caries in a deep preparation. When the remaining dentinal wall is thin, the pressure exerted on the excavator may be sufficient to break into the pulp chamber. A round bur may be used at a low speed with light, intermittent pressure for caries removal. Air-driven handpieces should be operated just above stall-out speed to improve tactile sense for caries

removal. The dentist should proceed with caution and inspect the area frequently.

Eye Precautions

The operator, the assistant, and the patient should wear glasses with side shields to prevent eye damage from airborne particles during operative procedures using rotary instrumentation. When high speeds are used, particles of old restorations, tooth structure, bacteria, and other debris are discharged at high speeds from the patient's mouth. Sufficiently strong high-volume evacuation applied by the dental assistant near the operating site helps alleviate this problem. Protective glasses are always indicated when rotary instrumentation is being used. The dentist, being in the direct path of such particles, is more likely to receive injury than the assistant or the patient. If an eye is injured, it should be covered by a clean gauze pad until medical attention can be obtained.

In addition to routine airborne debris, airborne particles may be produced occasionally by matrix failure of molded abrasive cutting instruments. Hard matrix wheels may crack or shatter into relatively large pieces. Soft abrasive wheels or points may increase in temperature during use, causing the rubber matrix to debond explosively from the abrasive into fine particles.

Precautions must be taken to prevent eye injury from unusual light sources such as visible light–curing units and laser equipment. Dental personnel and patients should be protected from high-intensity visible light with the use of colored plastic shields (attached to the fiberoptic tip). Laser light can be inadvertently reflected from many surfaces in the dental operatory; the operatory should be closed, and everyone should wear protective goggles (see the earlier section on laser equipment).

Ear Precautions

Various sounds are known to affect people in different ways. Soft music or random sounds such as rainfall usually have a relaxing or sedative effect. Loud noises are generally annoying and may contribute to mental and physical distress. A noisy environment decreases the ability to concentrate, increases proneness to accidents, and reduces overall efficiency. Extremely loud noises such as explosions or continuous exposure to high noise levels can cause permanent damage to the hearing mechanism.

An objectionable high-pitched whine is produced by some air-driven handpieces at high speeds. Aside from the annoying aspect of this noise, hearing loss could result from continued exposure. Potential damage to hearing from noise depends on (1) the intensity or loudness (decibels [db]), (2) frequency (cycles per second [cps]) of the noise, (3) duration (time) of the noise, and (4) susceptibility of the individual. Older age, existing ear damage, disease, and medications are other factors that can accelerate hearing loss.

Normal ears require that the intensity of sound reach a certain minimal level before the ear can detect it. This is known as *auditory threshold*. It can vary with the frequency and exposure to other sounds. When subjected to a loud noise of short duration, a protective mechanism of the ear causes it to lose some sensitivity temporarily. This is described as *temporary threshold shift.* If sufficient time is allowed between exposures, complete recovery occurs. Extended or continuous exposure is much more likely to result in a permanent threshold shift, with persistent hearing loss. The loss may be caused by all frequencies, but often high-frequency sounds affect hearing more severely. A certain amount of unnoticed noise (ambient noise level) is present even in a quiet room (20–40 db). An ordinary conversation averages 50 to 70 db in a frequency range of 500 to 2500 cps.

Air-driven handpieces with ball bearings, free running at 30-lb air pressure, may have noise levels of 70 to 94 db at high frequencies. Noise levels greater than 75 db in frequency ranges of 1000 to 8000 cps may cause hearing damage. Noise levels vary among handpieces produced by the same manufacturer. Handpiece wear and eccentric rotating instruments can cause increased noise. Protective measures are recommended when the noise level reaches 85 db with frequency ranges of 300 to 4800 cps. Protection is mandatory in areas where the level transiently reaches 95 db. The effect of excessive noise levels depends on exposure times. Normal use of a dental handpiece is one of intermittent application that generally is less than 30 minutes per day. Earplugs can be used to reduce the level of exposure, but these have several drawbacks. Room soundproofing helps and can be accomplished with absorbing materials used on walls and floors. Anti-noise devices also can be used to cancel unwanted sounds.

Inhalation Precautions

Aerosols and vapors are created by cutting tooth structure and restorative materials. Aerosols and vapors are a health hazard to all present. The aerosols are fine dispersions in air of water, tooth debris, microorganisms, or restorative materials. Cutting amalgams or composites produce submicron particles and vapor. The particles that may be inadvertently inhaled have the potential to produce alveolar irritation and tissue reactions. Vapor from cutting amalgams is predominantly mercury and should be eliminated, as much as possible, by careful evacuation near the tooth being operated on. The vapors generated during cutting or polishing by thermal decomposition of polymeric restorative materials (sealants, acrylic resin, composites) are predominantly monomers. They may be eliminated efficiently by careful intraoral evacuation during the cutting or polishing procedures.

A rubber dam protects the patient against oral inhalation of aerosols or vapors, but nasal inhalation of vapor and finer aerosol still may occur. Disposable masks worn by dental office personnel filter out bacteria and all but the finest particulate matter. Masks do not, however, filter out mercury or monomer vapors. The biologic effects of mercury hazards and appropriate office hygiene measures are discussed in online Chapter 18 on Biomaterials.

References

1. Black GV: *The technical procedures in filling teeth*, 1899, Henry O. Shepard.
2. Black GV: *Operative dentistry*, ed 8, Woodstock, IL, 1947, Medico-Dental.
3. Peyton FA: Temperature rise in teeth developed by rotating instruments. *J Am Dent Assoc* 50:629–630, 1955.
4. Leonard DL, Charlton DG: Performance of high-speed dental handpieces. *J Am Dent Assoc* 130:1301–1311, 1999.
5. Myers TD: Lasers in dentistry. *J Am Dent Assoc* 122:46–50, 1991.
6. Zakariasen KL, MacDonald R, Boran T: Spotlight on lasers—a look at potential benefits. *J Am Dent Assoc* 122:58–62, 1991.
7. Berry EA, III, Eakle WS, Summitt JB: Air abrasion: an old technology reborn. *Compend Cont Educ Dent* 20:751–759, 1999.
8. Sockwell CL: Dental handpieces and rotary cutting instruments. *Dent Clin North Am* 15:219–244, 1971.
9. Kunselman B: *Effect of air-polishing shield on the abrasion of PMMA and dentin* [thesis], Chapel Hill, NC, 1999, University of North Carolina.
10. Atkinson DR, Cobb CM, Killoy WJ: The effect of an air-powder abrasive system on in vitro root surfaces. *J Periodontol* 55:13–18, 1984.
11. Boyde A: Airpolishing effects on enamel, dentin and cement. *Br Dent J* 156:287–291, 1984.
12. Galloway SE, Pashley DH: Rate of removal of root structure by use of the Prophy-Jet device. *J Periodontol* 58:464–469, 1987.
13. Peterson LG, Hellden L, Jongebloed W, et al: The effect of a jet abrasive instrument (Prophy Jet) on root surfaces. *Swed Dent J* 9:193–199, 1985.
14. American Dental Association: Council on Dental Research adopts standards for shapes and dimensions of excavating burs and diamond instruments. *J Am Dent Assoc* 67:943, 1963.
15. SS White Dental Manufacturing Company: *A century of service to dentistry*, Philadelphia, 1944, SS White Dental Manufacturing.
16. American National Standards Institute: American Dental Association Specification No. 23 for dental excavating burs. *J Am Dent Assoc* 104:887, 1982.
17. International Standards Organization: *Standard ISO 2157: Head and neck dimensions of designated shapes of burs*, Geneva, 1972, International Standards Organization.
18. Morrant GA: Burs and rotary instruments: Introduction of a new standard numbering system. *Br Dent J* 147:97–98, 1979.
19. Eames WB, Nale JL: A comparison of cutting efficiency of air-driven fissure burs. *J Am Dent Assoc* 86:412–415, 1973.
20. Cantwell KR, Rotella M, Funkenbusch PD, et al: Surface characteristics of tooth structure after cutting with rotary instruments. *Dent Progr* 1:42–46, 1960.
21. Henry EE, Peyton FA: The relationship between design and cutting efficiency of dental burs. *J Dent Res* 33:281–292, 1954.
22. Henry EE: Influences of design factors on performance of the inverted cone bur. *J Dent Res* 35:704–713, 1956.
23. Hartley JL, Hudson DC: Modern rotating instruments: burs and diamond points. *Dent Clin North Am* 737–745, 1958.
24. Grajower R, Zeitchick A, Rajstein J: The grinding efficiency of diamond burs. *J Prosthet Dent* 42:422–428, 1979
25. Eames WB, Reder BS, Smith GA: Cutting efficiency of diamond stones: effect of technique variables. *Oper Dent* 2:156–164, 1977.
26. Hartley JL, Hudson DC, Richardson WP, et al: Cutting characteristics of dental burs as shown by high speed photomicrography. *Armed Forces Med J* 8:209, 1957.
27 Koblitz FF, Tateosian LH, Roemer FD, et al: An overview of cutting and wear related phenomena in dentistry. In Pearlman S, editor: *The cutting edge (DHEW Publication No. [NIH] 76-670)*, Washington, D.C., 1976, US Government Printing Office.
28. Westland IN: The energy requirement of the dental cutting process. *J Oral Rehabil* 7:51, 1980.
29. Lindhe J: Orthogonal cutting of dentine. *Odontol Revy (Malma)* 15(Suppl 8):11–100, 1964.

Chapter 7

Preliminary Considerations for Operative Dentistry

Lee W. Boushell, Ricardo Walter, Aldridge D. Wilder, Jr.

This chapter addresses routine chairside pre-operative procedures (before actual tooth preparation). Primarily, these procedures include patient and operator positions and isolation of the operating field.

Preoperative Patient and Dental Team Considerations

In preparation for a clinical procedure, it is important to ensure that patient and operator positions are properly selected, that instrument exchange between the dentist and the assistant is efficient, that proper illumination is present, and that magnification is used, if needed.

Patient and Operator Positions

Efficient patient and operator positions are beneficial for the welfare of both individuals. A patient who is in a comfortable position is more relaxed, has less muscle tension, and is more capable of cooperating with the dentist.

The practice of dentistry is demanding and stressful. Physical problems may arise if appropriate operating positions are neglected.[1] Most restorative dental procedures can be accomplished with the dentist seated. Positions that create unnecessary curvature of the spine or slumping of the shoulders should be avoided. Proper balance and weight distribution on both feet is essential when operating from a standing position. Generally, any uncomfortable or unnatural position that places undue strain on the body should be used only rarely.

Chair and Patient Positions

Chair and patient positions are important considerations. Dental chairs are designed to provide total body support in any chair position. An available chair accessory is an adjustable headrest cushion or an articulating headrest attached to the chair back. A contoured or lounge-type chair provides complete patient support and comfort. Most chairs also are equipped with programmable operating positions.

The most common patient positions for operative dentistry are almost supine or reclined 45 degrees (Fig. 7-1). The choice of patient position varies with the operator, the type of procedure, and the area of the mouth involved in the operation. In the almost supine position, the patient's head, knees, and feet are approximately the same level. The patient's head should not be lower than the feet; the head should be positioned lower than the feet only in an emergency, as when the patient is in syncope.

Operating Positions

Operating positions can be described by the location of the operator or by the location of the operator's arms in relation to patient position. A right-handed operator uses essentially three positions—right front, right, and right rear. These are sometimes referred to as the *7-o'clock, 9-o'clock,* and *11-o'clock positions* (Fig. 7-2, *A*). For a left-handed operator, the three positions are the *left front, left,* and *left rear positions,* or the *5-o'clock, 3-o'clock,* and *1-o'clock* positions. A fourth position, *direct rear position,* or *12-o'clock position,* has application for certain areas of the mouth. As a rule, the teeth being treated should be at the same level as the operator's elbow. The operating positions described here are for the right-handed operator; the left-handed operator should substitute left for right.

RIGHT FRONT POSITION

The right front position facilitates examination and treatment of mandibular anterior teeth (see Fig. 7-2, *B*), mandibular posterior teeth (especially on the right side), and maxillary anterior teeth. It is often advantageous to have the patient's head rotated slightly toward the operator.

RIGHT POSITION

In the right position, the operator is directly to the right of the patient (see Fig. 7-2, *C*). This position is convenient for operating on the facial surfaces of maxillary and mandibular right posterior teeth and the occlusal surfaces of mandibular right posterior teeth.

RIGHT REAR POSITION

The right rear position is the position of choice for most operations. The operator is behind and slightly to the right of

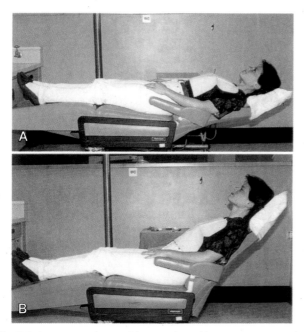

Fig. 7-1 Common patient positions. Both positions are recommended for sit-down dentistry. Use depends on the arch being treated. **A,** Supine. **B,** Reclined 45 degrees. *(From Darby ML, Walsh MM: Dental hygiene: Theory and practice, ed 3, St. Louis, 2010, Saunders.)*

the patient. The left arm is positioned around the patient's head (see Fig. 7-2, *D*). When operating from this position, the lingual and incisal (occlusal) surfaces of maxillary teeth are viewed in the mouth mirror. Direct vision may be used on mandibular teeth, particularly on the left side, but the use of a mouth mirror is advocated for visibility, light reflection, and retraction.

DIRECT REAR POSITION

The direct rear position is used primarily for operating on the lingual surfaces of mandibular anterior teeth. The operator is located directly behind the patient and looks down over the patient's head (see Fig. 7-2, *E*).

General Considerations

Several general considerations regarding chair and patient positions are important. The operator should not hesitate to rotate the patient's head backward or forward or from side to side to accommodate the demands of access and visibility of the operating field. Minor rotation of the patient's head is not uncomfortable to the patient and allows the operator to maintain his or her basic body position. As a rule, when operating in the maxillary arch, the maxillary occlusal surfaces should be oriented approximately perpendicular to the floor. When operating in the mandibular arch, the mandibular occlusal surfaces should be oriented approximately 45 degrees to the floor.

The operator's face should not come too close to the patient's face. The ideal distance, similar to that for reading a book, should be maintained. Another important aspect of proper operating position is to minimize body contact with the patient. A proper operator does not rest the forearms on

the patient's shoulders or the hands on the patient's face or forehead. The patient's chest should not be used as an instrument tray. From most positions, the left hand should be free to hold the mouth mirror to reflect light onto the operating field, to view the tooth preparation indirectly, or to retract the cheek or tongue. In certain instances, it is more appropriate to retract the cheek with one or two fingers of the left hand than to use a mouth mirror. It is often possible, however, to retract the cheek and reflect light with the mouth mirror at the same time.

When operating for an extended period, the operator can obtain a certain amount of rest and muscle relaxation by changing operating positions. Operating from a single position through the day, especially if standing, produces unnecessary fatigue. Changing positions, if only for a short time, reduces muscle strain and lessens fatigue.[1]

Operating Stools

A variety of operating stools are available for the dentist and the dental assistant. The seat should be well padded with smooth cushion edges and should be adjustable up and down. The backrest should be adjustable forward and backward as well as up and down.

Some advantages of the seated work position are lost if the operator uses the stool improperly. The operator should sit back on the cushion, using the entire seat and not just the front edge. The upper body should be positioned so that the spinal column is straight or bent slightly forward and supported by the backrest of the stool. The thighs should be parallel to the floor, and the lower legs should be perpendicular to the floor. If the seat is too high, its front edge cuts off circulation to the user's legs. Feet should be flat on the floor.

The seated work position for the assistant is essentially the same as for the operator except that the stool is 4 to 6 inches higher for maximal visual access. It is important that the stool for the assistant have an adequate footrest so that a parallel thigh position can be maintained with good foot support. When properly seated, the operator and the assistant are capable of providing dental service throughout the day without an unnecessary decline in efficiency and productivity because of muscle tension and fatigue (Fig. 7-3).

Instrument Exchange

All instrument exchanges between the operator and the assistant should occur in the exchange zone below the patient's chin and a few inches above the patient's chest. Instruments should not be exchanged over the patient's face. During the procedure, the operator should anticipate the next instrument required, and inform the assistant accordingly; this allows the instrument to be brought into the exchange zone for a timely exchange.

During proper instrument exchange, the operator should not need to remove his or her eyes from the operating field. The operator should rotate the instrument handle forward to cue the assistant to exchange instruments. Any sharp instrument should be exchanged with appropriate deliberation. The assistant should take the instrument from the operator, rather than the operator dropping it into the assistant's hand, and vice versa. Each person should be sure that the other has a firm grasp on the instrument before it is released.

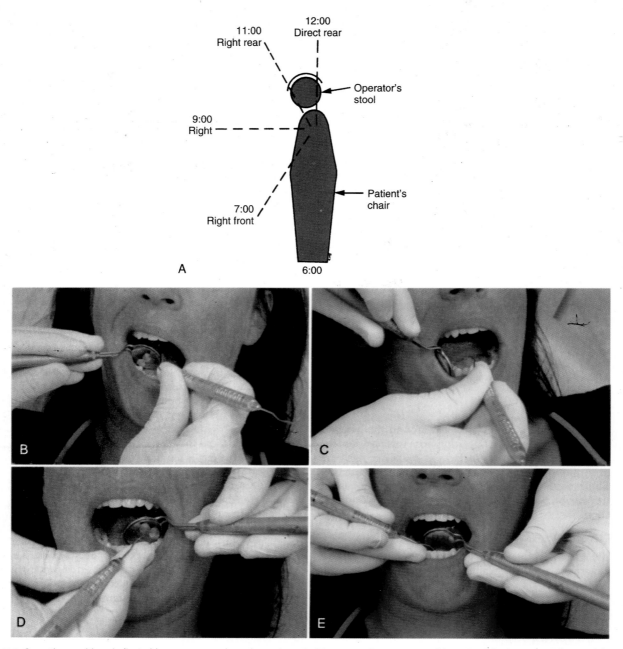

Fig. 7-2 Operating positions indicated by arm approach to the patient. **A,** Diagrammatic operator positions. **B,** Right front. **C,** Right. **D,** Right rear. **E,** Direct rear.

Magnification and Headlamp Illumination

Another key to the success of clinical operative dentistry is visual acuity. The operator must be able to see clearly to attend to the details of each procedure. The use of magnification facilitates attention to detail and does not adversely affect vision. Magnifying lenses have a fixed focal length that often requires the operator to maintain a proper working distance, which ensures good posture. Several types of magnification devices are available, including bifocal eyeglasses, loupes, and surgical telescopes (Fig. 7-4). The use of such magnification devices also provides some protection from eye injury. To further improve visual acuity, headlamps are recommended in operative dentistry. Their greatest advantage is the light source being parallel to the clinician's vision, eliminating shadows at the operating field. Current headlamps use light-emitting diode (LED) technology and produce whiter light than conventional tungsten halogen light sources.

Isolation of the Operating Field

The goals of operating field isolation are moisture control, retraction, and harm prevention.

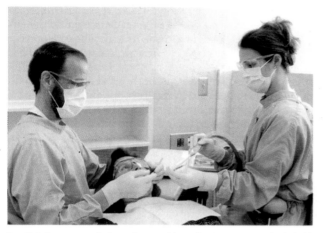

Fig. 7-3 Recommended seating positions for operator and chairside assistant, with the height of the operating field approximately at elbow level of the operator. *(From Robinson DS, Bird DL: Essentials of dental assisting, ed 4, St. Louis, 2007, Saunders.)*

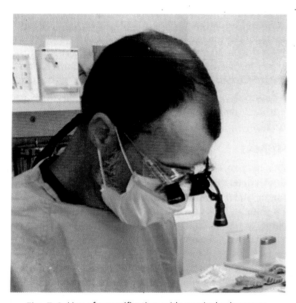

Fig. 7-4 Use of magnification with surgical telescopes.

Goals of Isolation
Moisture Control

Operative dentistry cannot be executed properly unless the moisture in the mouth is controlled. Moisture control refers to excluding sulcular fluid, saliva, and gingival bleeding from the operating field. It also involves preventing the spray from the handpiece and restorative debris from being swallowed or aspirated by the patient. The rubber dam, suction devices, and absorbents are variously effective in moisture control. Generally, the rubber dam is the recommended technique for moisture control. Raskin et al. and Fusayama have reported, however, that achieving effective isolation is more important than the specific technique used.[2,3]

Retraction and Access

The details of a restorative procedure cannot be managed without proper retraction and access. Retraction and access provides maximal exposure of the operating site and usually involves having the patient maintain an open mouth and depressing or retracting the gingival tissue, tongue, lips, and cheek. The rubber dam, high-volume evacuator, absorbents, retraction cord, mouth prop, and other isolation devices such as the Isolite (Isolite Systems, Santa Barbara, CA) are used for retraction and access.

Harm Prevention

An important consideration of isolating the operating field is preventing harm to the patient during the operation.[4,5] Excessive saliva and handpiece spray can alarm the patient. Small instruments and restorative debris can be aspirated or swallowed. Soft tissue can be damaged accidentally. The same devices used for moisture control and retraction contribute not only to harm prevention but also to patient comfort and operator efficiency. Harm prevention is achieved as much by the manner in which the devices are used as by the devices themselves.

Local Anesthesia

Local anesthetics play a role in eliminating the discomfort of dental treatment and controlling moisture by reducing salivary flow. Local anesthetics incorporating a vasoconstrictor also reduce blood flow, which helps control hemorrhage at the operating site.

Rubber Dam Isolation

In 1864, S.C. Barnum, a New York City dentist, introduced the rubber dam into dentistry. Use of the rubber dam ensures appropriate dryness of the teeth and improves the quality of clinical restorative dentistry.[6,7] The rubber dam is used to define the operating field by isolating one or more teeth from the oral environment. The dam eliminates saliva from the operating site and retracts the soft tissue.

Advantages

The advantages of rubber dam isolation of the operating field are (1) a dry, clean operating field; (2) improved access and visibility; (3) potentially improved properties of dental materials; (4) protection of the patient and the operator; and (5) operating efficiency.

DRY, CLEAN OPERATING FIELD

For most procedures, rubber dam isolation is the preferred method of obtaining a dry, clean field. The operator can best perform procedures such as caries removal, proper tooth preparation, and insertion of restorative materials in a dry field. The time saved by operating in a clean field with good visibility may more than compensate for the time spent applying the rubber dam.[8] When excavating a deep caries lesion and risking pulpal exposure, use of the rubber dam is strongly recommended to prevent pulpal contamination from oral fluids.

ACCESS AND VISIBILITY

→ Non-reflective background

The rubber dam provides maximal access and visibility. It controls moisture and retracts soft tissue. Gingival tissue is retracted mildly to enhance access to and visibility of the gingival aspects of the tooth preparation. The dam also retracts the lips, cheeks, and tongue. A dark-colored rubber dam provides a non-reflective background in contrast to the operating site. Because the dam remains in place throughout the operative procedure, access and visibility are maintained without interruption.

IMPROVED PROPERTIES OF DENTAL MATERIALS

The rubber dam prevents moisture contamination of restorative materials during insertion and promotes improved properties of dental materials. Amalgam restorative material does not achieve its optimum physical properties if used in a wet field.[6] Bonding to enamel and dentin is unpredictable if the tooth substrate is contaminated with saliva, blood, or other oral fluids.[9,10] Some studies have concluded that no difference exists between the use of the rubber dam and cotton roll isolation as long as control of sources of contamination is maintained during the restorative procedures.[2,11-13]

PROTECTION OF THE PATIENT AND THE OPERATOR

The rubber dam protects the patient and the operator. It protects the patient from aspirating or swallowing small instruments or debris associated with operative procedures.[14] A properly applied rubber dam protects soft tissue from irritating or distasteful medicaments (e.g., etching agents). The dam also offers some soft tissue protection from rotating burs and stones. Authors disagree on whether the rubber dam protects the patient from mercury exposure during amalgam removal.[15,16] However, it is generally agreed that the rubber dam is an effective infection control barrier for the dental office.[17-19]

OPERATING EFFICIENCY

Use of the rubber dam allows for operating efficiency and increased productivity. Excessive conversation with the patient is discouraged. The rubber dam retainer (discussed later) helps provide a moderate amount of mouth opening during the procedure. (For additional mouth-opening aids, see the section on Mouth Props.) Quadrant restorative procedures are facilitated. Many state dental practice acts permit the assistant to place the rubber dam, thus saving time for the dentist. Christensen reported that use of a rubber dam increases the quality and quantity of restorative services.[8]

Disadvantages

Rubber dam use is low among private practitioners.[20-22] Time consumption and patient objection are the most frequently quoted disadvantages of the rubber dam. However, the rubber dam usually can be placed in less than 5 minutes. The advantages previously mentioned certainly outweigh the time spent with placement.

Certain situations may preclude the use of the rubber dam, including (1) teeth that have not erupted sufficiently to support a retainer, (2) some third molars, and (3) extremely malpositioned teeth. In addition, patients may not tolerate the rubber dam if breathing through the nose is difficult. In rare

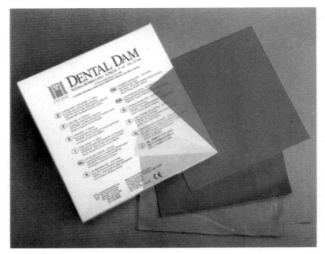

Fig. 7-5 Rubber dam material as supplied in sheets. *(From Boyd LRB: Dental instruments: A pocket guide, ed 4, St. Louis, 2012, Saunders.)*

instances, the patient cannot tolerate a rubber dam because of psychological reasons or latex allergy.[12,23] Latex-free rubber dam material is, however, currently available (Fig. 7-5). Jones and Reid reported that use of the rubber dam was well accepted by patients and operators.[24]

Materials and Instruments

The materials and instruments necessary for the use of the rubber dam are available from most dental supply companies.

MATERIAL

thicker dam → Class V

Rubber dam material (latex and nonlatex), as with all rubber products, deteriorates over time, resulting in low tear strength. The dam material is available in 5 × 5 inch (12.5 × 12.5 cm) or 6 × 6 inch (15 × 15 cm) sheets. The thicknesses or weights available are thin (0.006 inch [0.15 mm]), medium (0.008 inch [0.2 mm]), heavy (0.010 inch [0.25 mm]), and extra heavy (0.012 inch [0.30 mm]). Light and dark dam materials are available, and darker colors are generally preferred for contrast. The rubber dam material has a shiny side and a dull side. Because the dull side is less light reflective, it is generally placed facing the occlusal side of the isolated teeth. A thicker dam is more effective in retracting tissue and more resistant to tearing; it is especially recommended for isolating Class V lesions in conjunction with a cervical retainer. The thinner material has the advantage of passing through the contacts easier, which is particularly helpful when contacts are tight.

FRAME

The rubber dam holder (frame) maintains the borders of the rubber dam in position. The Young holder is a U-shaped metal frame (Fig. 7-6) with small metal projections for securing the borders of the rubber dam.

RETAINER

The rubber dam retainer consists of four prongs and two jaws connected by a bow (Fig. 7-7). The retainer is used to anchor the dam to the most posterior tooth to be isolated. Retainers also are used to retract gingival tissue. Many different sizes and

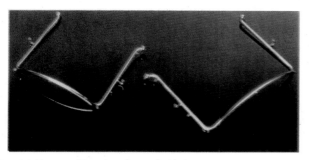

Fig. 7-6 Young rubber dam frame (holder). *(From Hargreaves KM, Cohen S: Cohen's pathways of the pulp, ed 10, St. Louis, 2011, Mosby.)*

shapes are available, with specific retainers designed for certain teeth (Fig. 7-8). Table 7-1 lists suggested retainer applications. When positioned on a tooth, a properly selected retainer should contact the tooth in its four line angles (see Fig. 7-7). This four-point contact prevents rocking or tilting of the retainer. Movement of the retainer on the anchor tooth can injure the gingiva and the tooth, resulting in postoperative soreness or sensitivity.[25] The prongs of some retainers are gingivally directed (inverted) and are helpful when the anchor tooth is only partially erupted or when additional soft tissue retraction is indicated (Fig. 7-9). The jaws of the retainer should not extend beyond the mesial and distal line angles of the tooth because (1) they may interfere with matrix and wedge placement, (2) gingival trauma is more likely to occur, and (3) a complete seal around the anchor tooth is more difficult to achieve.

Wingless and winged retainers are available (see Fig. 7-8). The winged retainer has anterior and lateral wings (Fig. 7-10).

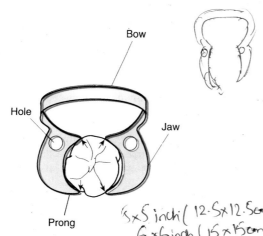

Fig. 7-7 Rubber dam retainer. Note four-point prong contact *(arrows)* with tooth. *(From Daniel SJ, Harfst SA, Wilder RS: Mosby's dental hygiene: Concepts, cases, and competencies, ed 2, St. Louis, 2008, Mosby.)*

Table 7-1 **Suggested Retainers for Various Anchor Tooth Applications**	
Retainer	**Application**
W56	Most molar anchor teeth
W7	Mandibular molar anchor teeth
W8	Maxillary molar anchor teeth
W4	Most premolar anchor teeth
W2	Small premolar anchor teeth
W27	Terminal mandibular molar anchor teeth requiring preparations involving the distal surface

FIESTA® Color Coded Matte Finish Winged and Wingless Clamps

ANTERIOR

MOLAR

Small lower   Lower   Lower

PREMOLAR

Upper   Small upper   Upper and lower

Large bicuspids   Bicuspids

MOLAR - SPECIAL USE
For irregularly shaped, structurally compromised or partially erupted molars

SERRATED JAWS
Serrations for improved retention

Lower right molars/   Lower left molars/
Upper left molars   Upper right molars

Small   Large

Fig. 7-8 Selection of rubber dam retainers. Note retainers with wings. *(Pictured:* Color Coded Matte Finish Winged and Wingless Clamps.) *(Courtesy Coltène/Whaledent Inc., Cuyahoga Falls, OH.)*

The wings are designed to provide extra retraction of the rubber dam from the operating field and to allow attachment of the dam to the retainer before conveying the retainer (with dam) to the anchor tooth, after which the dam is removed from the lateral wings. As seen in Figure 7-10, the anterior wings can be cut away if they are not wanted.

The bow of the retainer (except the No. 212, which is applied after the rubber dam is in place) should be tied with dental floss (Fig. 7-11) approximately 12 inches (30 cm) in length before the retainer is placed in the mouth. For maximal protection, the tie may be threaded through both holes in the jaws of the retainer because the bow of the retainer could break. The floss allows retrieval of the retainer or its broken parts if they are accidentally swallowed or aspirated. It is sometimes necessary to re-contour the jaws of the retainer to the shape of the tooth by grinding with a mounted stone

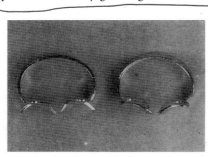

Fig. 7-9 Retainers with prongs directed gingivally are helpful when the anchor tooth is only partially erupted.

(Fig. 7-12). A retainer usually is not required when the dam is applied for treatment of the anterior teeth except for the cervical retainer for Class V restorations.

PUNCH

The rubber dam punch is a precision instrument having a rotating metal table (disk) with holes of varying sizes and a tapered, sharp-pointed plunger (Fig. 7-13). Care should be exercised when changing from one hole to another. The plunger should be centered in the cutting hole so that the edges of the holes are not at risk of being chipped by the plunger tip when the plunger is closed. Otherwise, the cutting quality of the punch is ruined, as evidenced by incompletely cut holes. These holes tear easily when stretched during application over the retainer or tooth.

RETAINER FORCEPS

The rubber dam retainer forceps is used for placement and removal of the retainer from the tooth (Fig. 7-14).

NAPKIN

The rubber dam napkin, placed between the rubber dam and the patient's skin, has the following benefits:

1. It improves patient comfort by reducing direct contact of the rubber material with the skin.
2. It absorbs any saliva seeping at the corners of the mouth.
3. It acts as a cushion.

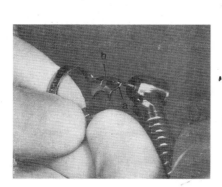

Fig. 7-10 Removing anterior wings (*a*) on molar retainer. Lateral wings (*b*) are for holding lip of stretched rubber dam hole.

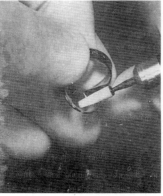

Fig. 7-12 Re-contouring jaws of retainer with mounted stone.

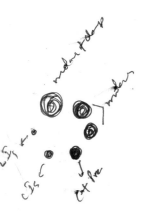

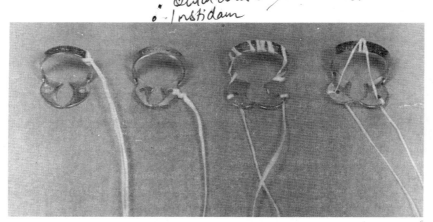

Fig. 7-11 Methods of tying retainers with dental floss.

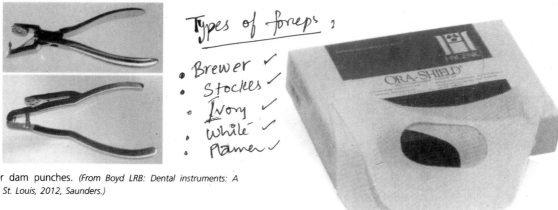

Fig. 7-13 Rubber dam punches. (*From Boyd LRB: Dental instruments: A pocket guide, ed 4, St. Louis, 2012, Saunders.*)

Types of forceps :
- *Brewer* ✓
- *Stockes* ✓
- *Ivory* ✓
- *White* ✓
- *Flamer* ✓

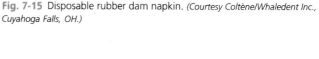

Fig. 7-15 Disposable rubber dam napkin. (*Courtesy Coltène/Whaledent Inc., Cuyahoga Falls, OH.*)

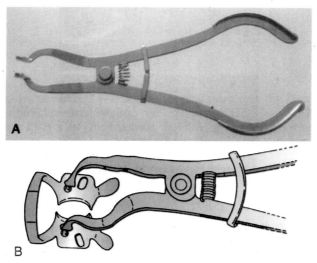

Fig. 7-14 Rubber dam forceps (*A*) engaging retainer (*B*). (**A,** *From Boyd LRB: Dental instruments: A pocket guide, ed 4, St. Louis, 2012, Saunders.* **B,** *From Baum L, Phillips RW, Lund MR: Textbook of operative dentistry, ed 3, Philadelphia, 1995, Saunders.*)

4. It provides a convenient method of wiping the patient's lips on removal of the dam.
5. The rubber dam napkin adds to the comfort of the patient, particularly when the dam must be used for long appointments (Fig. 7-15).

LUBRICANT

A water-soluble lubricant applied in the area of the punched holes facilitates the passing of the dam septa through the proximal contacts. A rubber dam lubricant is commercially available, but other lubricants such as shaving cream also are satisfactory. Applying the lubricant to both sides of the dam in the area of the punched holes aids in passing the dam through the contacts. Cocoa butter or petroleum jelly may be applied at the corners of the patient's mouth to prevent irritation. These two materials are not satisfactory rubber dam lubricants, however, because both are oil-based and not easily rinsed from the dam when the dam is placed.

ANCHORS (OTHER THAN RETAINERS)

Besides retainers, other anchors may also be used. The proximal contact may be sufficient to anchor the dam on the tooth

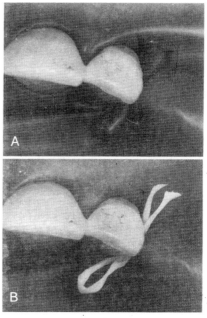

Fig. 7-16 **A,** Anchor formed from dental tape. **B,** Anchor formed from rubber dam material.

farthest from the posterior retainer (in the isolated field), eliminating the need for a second retainer (see Step 13 of Procedure 7-1). To secure the dam further anteriorly or to anchor the dam on any tooth where a retainer is contraindicated, waxed dental tape (or floss) or a small piece of rubber dam material (cut from a sheet of dam) or a rubber Wedjet (Hygenic, Akron, OH) may be passed through the proximal contact. When dental tape is used, it should be passed through the contact, looped, and passed through a second time (Fig. 7-16, *A*). The cut piece of dam material is first stretched, passed through the contact, and then released (see Fig. 7-16, *B*). When the anchor is in place, the tape, floss, dam material, or Wedjet should be trimmed to prevent interference with the operating site.

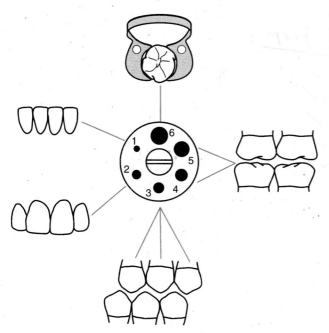

Fig. 7-17 Cutting table on rubber dam punch, illustrating use of hole size. *(From Daniel SJ, Harfst SA, Wilder RS: Mosby's dental hygiene: Concepts, cases, and competencies, ed 2, St. Louis, 2008, Mosby.)*

Hole Size and Position

Successful isolation of teeth and maintenance of a dry, clean operating field largely depend on hole size and position in the rubber dam.[26] Holes should be punched by following the arch form, making adjustments for malpositioned or missing teeth. Most rubber dam punches have either five or six holes in the cutting table. The smaller holes are used for the incisors, canines, and premolars and the larger holes for the molars. The largest hole generally is reserved for the posterior anchor tooth (Fig. 7-17). The following guidelines and suggestions can be helpful when positioning the holes:

- (Optional) Punch an identification hole in the upper left (i.e., the patient's left) corner of the rubber dam for ease of location of that corner when applying the dam to the holder.
- When operating on the incisors and mesial surfaces of canines, isolate from first premolar to first premolar. Metal retainers usually are not required for this isolation (Fig. 7-18, *A*). If additional access is necessary after isolating teeth, as described, a retainer can be positioned over the dam to engage the adjacent nonisolated tooth, but care must be exercised not to pinch the gingiva beneath the dam (see Fig. 7-18, *B* and *C*).
- When operating on a canine, it is preferable to isolate from the first molar to the opposite lateral incisor. To treat a Class V lesion on a canine, isolate posteriorly to include the first molar to provide access for placement of the cervical retainer on the canine.
- When operating on posterior teeth, isolate anteriorly to include the lateral incisor on the opposite side of the arch from the operating site. In this case, the hole for the lateral incisor is the most remote from the hole for the posterior anchor tooth. Anterior teeth included in the isolation

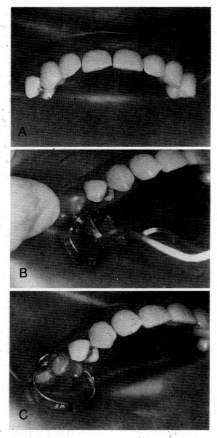

Fig. 7-18 A, Isolation for operating on incisors and mesial surface of canines. **B** and **C,** Increasing access by application of metal retainer over dam and adjacent nonisolated tooth.

provide finger rests on dry teeth and better access and visibility for the operator and the assistant.

- When operating on premolars, punch holes to include one to two teeth distally, and extend anteriorly to include the opposite lateral incisor.
- When operating on molars, punch holes as far distally as possible, and extend anteriorly to include the opposite lateral incisor.
- Isolation of a minimum of three teeth is recommended except when endodontic therapy is indicated, and in that case, only the tooth to be treated is isolated. The number of teeth to be treated and the tooth surface influence the pattern of isolation.
- The distance between holes is equal to the distance from the center of one tooth to the center of the adjacent tooth, measured at the level of the gingival tissue. When the distance between holes is excessive, the dam material is excessive and wrinkles between teeth. Conversely, too little distance between holes causes the dam to stretch, resulting in space around the teeth and leakage. When the distance is correct, the dam intimately adapts to the teeth and covers and slightly retracts the interdental tissue.
- When the rubber dam is applied to maxillary teeth, the first holes punched (after the optional identification hole) are for the central incisors. These holes are positioned approximately 1 inch (25 mm) from the superior border of the dam (Fig. 7-19, *A*), providing sufficient material to

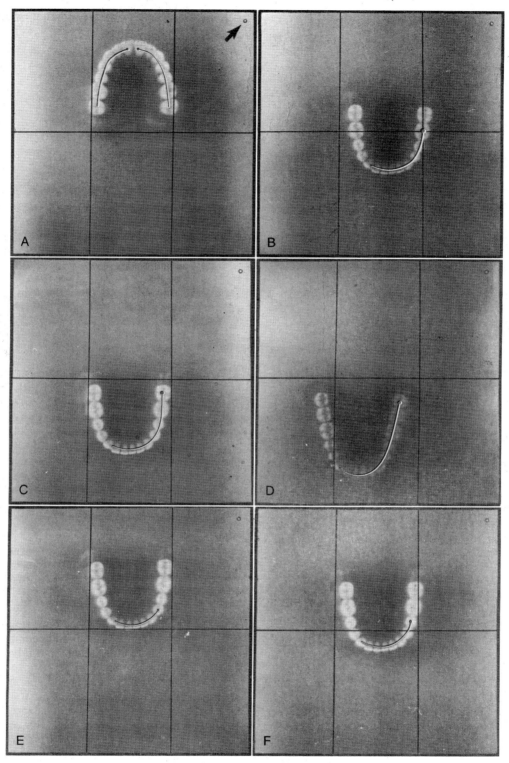

Fig. 7-19 Hole position. **A,** When maxillary teeth are to be isolated, the first holes punched are for central incisors, approximately 1 inch (2.5 cm) from superior border. **B,** Hole position when the anchor tooth is the mandibular first molar. **C,** Hole position when the anchor tooth is the mandibular second molar. **D,** Hole position when the anchor tooth is the mandibular third molar. **E,** Hole position when the anchor tooth is the mandibular first premolar. **F,** Hole position when the anchor tooth is the mandibular second premolar. Note the hole punched in each of these six representative rubber dam sheets for identification of the upper left corner (*arrow in A*).

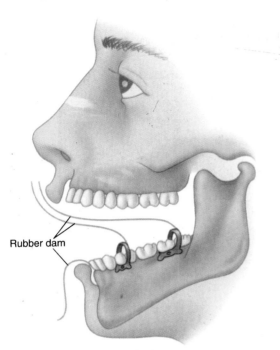

Fig. 7-20 The more posterior the mandibular anchor tooth, the more dam material is required to come from behind retainer over the upper lip.

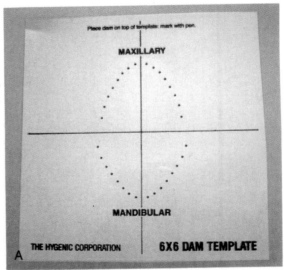

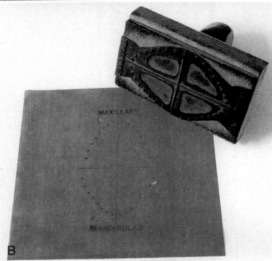

Fig. 7-21 Commercial products to aid in locating hole position. **A,** Dental dam template. **B,** Dental dam stamp. *(From Boyd LRB: Dental instruments: A pocket guide, ed 4, St. Louis, 2012, Saunders.)*

cover the patient's upper lip. For a patient with a large upper lip or mustache, position the holes more than 1 inch from the edge. Conversely, for a child or an adult with a small upper lip, the holes should be positioned less than 1 inch from the edge. When the holes for the incisors are located, the remaining holes are punched.

- When the rubber dam is applied to mandibular teeth, the first hole punched (after the optional identification hole) is for the posterior anchor tooth that is to receive the retainer. To determine the proper location, mentally divide the rubber dam into three vertical sections: left, middle, and right. If the anchor tooth is the mandibular first molar, punch the hole for this tooth at a point halfway from the superior edge to the inferior edge and at the junction of the right (or left) and middle thirds (see Fig. 7-19, *B*). If the anchor tooth is the second or third molar, the position for the hole moves toward the inferior border and slightly toward the center of the rubber dam compared with the first molar hole just described (see Fig. 7-19, *C* and *D*). If the anchor tooth is the first premolar, the hole is placed toward the superior border compared with the hole for the first molar and toward the center of the dam (see Fig. 7-19, *E*). The farther posterior the mandibular anchor tooth, the more dam material is required to come from behind the retainer over the upper lip. Figure 7-20 illustrates the difference in the amount of dam required, comparing the first premolar and the second molar as anchor teeth. The distances also may be compared by noting the length of dam between the superior edge of the dam and the position of the hole for the posterior anchor tooth (see Fig. 7-19, *B* to *F*).
- When a thinner rubber dam is used, smaller holes must be punched to achieve an adequate seal around the teeth because the thin dam has greater elasticity.

Until these guidelines and suggestions related to hole position are mastered, an inexperienced operator may choose to use commercial products to aid in locating hole position (Fig. 7-21). A rubber stamp that imprints permanent and primary arch forms on the rubber dam is available, and several sheets of dam material can be stamped in advance. A plastic template also can be used to mark hole position. Experienced operators and assistants may not require these aids, and accurate hole location is best achieved by noting the patient's arch form and tooth position.

Placement

Usually, administering the anesthetic precedes application of the rubber dam. This approach allows for the beginning of profound anesthesia and more comfortable retainer placement on the anchor tooth. Occasionally, the posterior anchor tooth in the maxillary arch may need to be anesthetized if it is remote from the anesthetized operating site.

The technique for the application of the rubber dam is presented by numerous authors.[7,27,28] The step-by-step application and removal of the rubber dam using the maxillary left first molar for the posterior retainer and including the maxillary right lateral incisor as the anterior anchor is described and illustrated here. The procedure is described as if the operator and the assistant are working together.

Compared with the alternative procedures discussed in a later section, Procedures 7-1 and 7-2 allow the retainer and the dam to be placed sequentially. This approach provides for maximal visibility when placing the retainer, which reduces the risk of impinging on gingival tissue. Isolating a greater number of teeth, as illustrated in Procedure 7-1, is indicated for quadrant operative procedures. For limited operative procedures, it is often acceptable to isolate fewer teeth. Appropriate seal of each tooth is accomplished by inversion of the rubber material in a gingival direction. Interproximal inversion is accomplished first by using dental floss. Inversion of the dam on the facial and lingual surfaces is accomplished by air-drying the surfaces and use of a blunt instrument (see Procedure 7-1, step 18).

Alternative and Additional Methods and Factors

The procedure detailed in Procedure 7-1 describes the method of sequentially placing the retainer and rubber dam on the anchor tooth.

APPLYING THE DAM AND RETAINER SIMULTANEOUSLY

The retainer and dam may be placed simultaneously to reduce the risk of the retainer being swallowed or aspirated before the dam is placed. This approach also solves the occasional difficulty of trying to pass the dam over a previously placed retainer, the bow of which is pressing against oral soft tissues.

In this method, the posterior retainer is applied first to verify a stable fit. The operator removes the retainer and, still holding the retainer with forceps, passes the bow through the proper hole from the underside of the dam (the lubricated rubber dam is held by the assistant) (Fig. 7-22, A). The free end of the floss tie should be threaded through the anchor hole before the retainer bow is inserted. When using a retainer with lateral wings, place the retainer in the hole punched for the anchor tooth by stretching the dam to engage these wings (Fig. 7-23).

The operator grasps the handle of the forceps in the right hand and gathers the dam with the left hand to clearly visualize the jaws of the retainer and facilitate its placement (see Fig. 7-22, B). The operator conveys the retainer (with the dam) into the mouth and positions it on the anchor tooth. Care is needed when applying the retainer to prevent the jaws of the retainer from sliding gingivally and impinging on the soft tissue (see Fig. 7-22, C).

Text continued on p. 204.

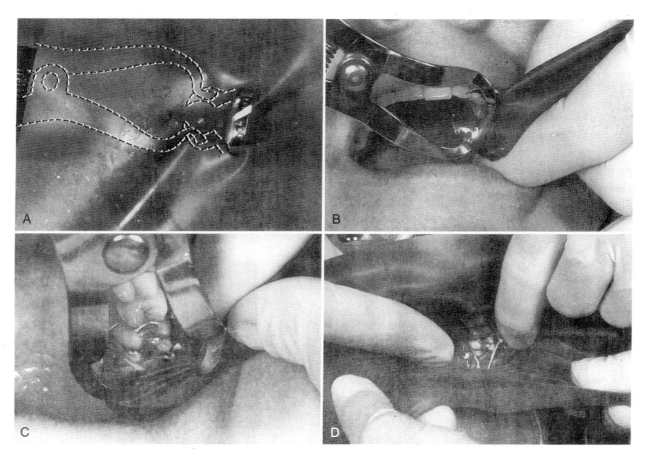

Fig. 7-22 A, Bow being passed through the posterior anchor hole from the underside of the dam. **B,** Gathering the dam to facilitate placement of the retainer. **C,** Positioning the retainer on the anchor tooth. **D,** Stretching the anchor hole borders over and under the jaws of the retainer.

Procedure 7-1 Application of Rubber Dam Isolation

The application procedure is described for right-handed operators. Left-handed users should change right to left. Each step number has a corresponding illustration.

Step 1: Testing and Lubricating the Proximal Contacts

The operator receives the dental floss from the assistant to test the interproximal contacts and remove debris from the teeth to be isolated. Passing (or attempting to pass) the floss through the contacts identifies any sharp edges of restorations or enamel that must be smoothed or removed to prevent tearing the dam. Using waxed dental tape may lubricate tight contacts to facilitate dam placement. Tight contacts that are difficult to floss but do not cut or fray the floss may be wedged apart slightly to permit placement of the rubber dam. A blunt hand instrument may be used for separation. For some clinical situations, the proximal portion of the tooth to be restored may need to be partially prepared to eliminate a sharp or difficult contact before the dam is placed.

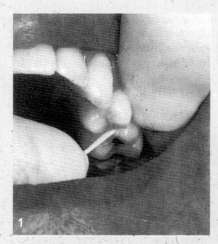

Step 1: Testing and lubricating the proximal contacts.

Step 2: Punching Holes

It is recommended that the assistant punch the holes after assessing the arch form and tooth alignment. Some operators prefer to have the assistant pre-punch the dam, however, using holes marked by a template or a rubber dam stamp.

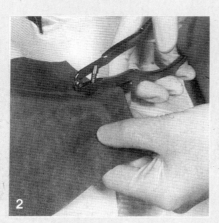

Step 2: Punching the holes.

Step 3: Lubricating the Dam

The assistant lubricates both sides of the rubber dam in the area of the punched holes using a cotton roll or gloved fingertip to apply the lubricant. This facilitates passing the rubber dam through the contacts. The lips and especially the corners of the mouth may be lubricated with petroleum jelly or cocoa butter to prevent irritation.

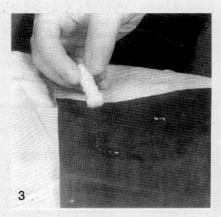

Step 3: Lubricating the dam.

Step 4: Selecting the Retainer

The operator receives (from the assistant) the rubber dam retainer forceps with the selected retainer and floss tie in position (A). The free end of the tie should exit from the cheek side of the retainer. Try the retainer on the tooth to verify retainer stability. If the retainer fits poorly, it is removed either for adjustment or for selection of a different size.[24] (Retainer adjustment, if needed to provide stability, is discussed in the previous section on rubber dam retainer.) Whenever the forceps is holding the retainer, care should be taken not to open the retainer more than necessary to secure it in the forceps. Stretching the retainer open for extended periods causes it to lose its elastic recovery. Retainers that have been deformed ("sprung"), such as the one shown in B, should be discarded.

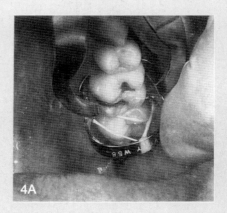

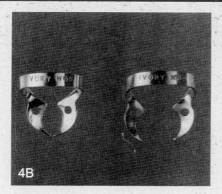

Step 4: Selecting the retainer. *(From Peterson JE, Nation WA, Matsson L: Effect of a rubber dam clamp (retainer) on cementum and junctional epithelium, Oper Dent 11:42-45, 1986.)*

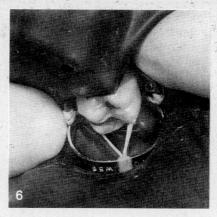

Step 6: Positioning the dam over the retainer.

Step 5: Testing the Retainer's Stability and Retention

If during trial placement the retainer seems acceptable, remove the forceps. Test the retainer's stability and retention by lifting gently in an occlusal direction with a fingertip under the bow of the retainer. An improperly fitting retainer rocks or is easily dislodged.

Step 7: Applying the Napkin

The operator now gathers the rubber dam in the left hand, while the assistant inserts the fingers and thumb of the right (or left) hand through the napkin's opening and grasps the bunched dam held by the operator.

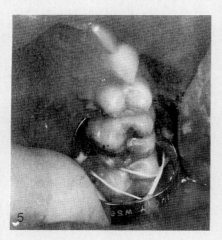

Step 5: Testing the retainer's stability and retention.

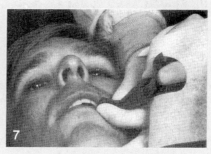

Step 7: Applying the napkin.

Step 8: Positioning the Napkin

The assistant pulls the bunched dam through the napkin and positions it on the patient's face. The operator helps by positioning the napkin on the patient's right side. The napkin reduces skin contact with the dam.

Step 6: Positioning the Dam over the Retainer

Before applying the dam, the floss tie may be threaded through the anchor hole, or it may be left on the underside of the dam. With the forefingers, stretch the anchor hole of the dam over the retainer (bow first) and then under the retainer jaws. The lip of the hole must pass completely under the retainer jaws. The forefingers may thin out, to a single thickness, the septal dam for the mesial contact of the retainer tooth and attempt to pass it through the contact, lip of the hole first. The septal dam always must pass through its respective contact in single thickness. If it does not pass through readily, it should be passed through with dental tape later in the procedure.

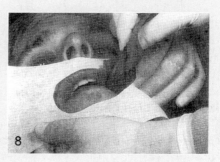

Step 8: Positioning the napkin.

Continued

Procedure 7-1 Application of Rubber Dam Isolation—cont'd

Step 9: Attaching the Frame

The operator unfolds the dam. (If an identification hole was punched, it is used to identify the upper left corner.) The assistant aids in unfolding the dam and, while holding the frame in place, attaches the dam to the metal projections on the left side of the frame. Simultaneously, the operator stretches and attaches the dam on the right side. The frame is positioned outside the dam. The curvature of the frame should be concentric with the patient's face. The dam lies between the frame and napkin. Either the operator or the assistant attaches the dam along the inferior border of the frame. Attaching the dam to the frame at this time controls the dam to provide access and visibility. The free ends of the floss tie are secured to the frame.

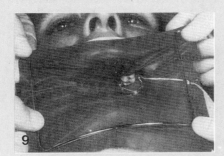

Step 9: Attaching the frame.

Step 10 (Optional): Attaching the Neck Strap

The assistant attaches the neck strap to the left side of the frame and passes it behind the patient's neck. The operator attaches it to the right side of the frame. Neck strap tension is adjusted to stabilize the frame and hold the frame (and periphery of the dam) gently against the face and away from the operating field. If desired, using soft tissue paper between the neck and strap may prevent contact of the patient's neck against the strap.

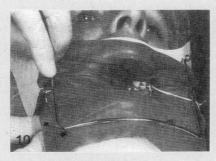

Step 10 (optional): Attaching the neck strap.

Step 11: Passing the Dam through the Posterior Contact

If a tooth is present distal to the retainer, the distal edge of the posterior anchor hole should be passed through the contact (single thickness, with no folds) to ensure a seal around the anchor tooth.

If necessary, use waxed dental tape to assist in this procedure (see step 15 for the use of dental tape). If the retainer comes off unintentionally as this is done or during subsequent procedures, passage of the dam through the distal contact anchors the dam sufficiently to allow easier reapplication of the retainer or placement of an adjusted or different retainer.

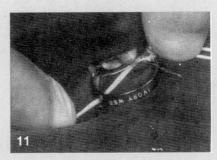

Step 11: Passing the dam through the posterior contact.

Step 12 (Optional): Applying a Rigid Supporting Material

If the stability of the retainer is questionable, a rigid supporting material such as low-fusing modeling compound may be applied.

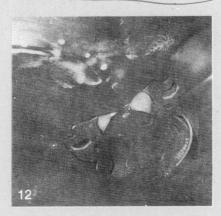

Step 12 (optional): Applying the rigid material.

Step 13: Applying the Anterior Anchor (If Needed)

The operator passes the dam over the anterior anchor tooth, anchoring the anterior portion of the rubber dam. Usually, the dam passes easily through the mesial and distal contacts of the anchor tooth if it is passed in single thickness starting with the lip of the hole. Stretching the lip of the hole and sliding it back and forth aids in positioning the septum. When the contact farthest from the retainer is minimal ("light"), an anchor may be required in the form of a double thickness of dental tape or a narrow strip of dam material or Wedjet that is stretched, inserted, and released. If the contact is open, a rolled piece of dam material may be used.

Procedure 7-1 Application of Rubber Dam Isolation—cont'd

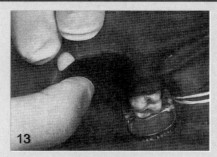

Step 13: Applying the anterior anchor (if needed).

Step 14: Passing the Septa through the Contacts without Dental Tape

The operator passes the septa through as many contacts as possible without the use of dental tape by stretching the septal dam faciogingivally and linguogingivally with the forefingers. Each septum must not be allowed to bunch or fold. Rather, its passage through the contact should be started with a single edge and continued with a single thickness. Passing the dam through as many contacts as possible without using dental tape is urged because the use of dental tape always increases the risk of tearing holes in the septa. Slight separation (wedging) of the teeth is sometimes an aid when the contacts are extremely tight. Pressure from a blunt hand instrument (e.g., beaver-tail burnisher) applied in the facial embrasure gingival to the contact usually is sufficient to obtain enough separation to permit the septum to pass through the contact.

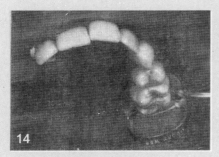

Step 14: Passing the septa through the contacts without dental tape.

Step 15: Passing the Septa through the Contacts with Tape

Use waxed dental tape to pass the dam through the remaining contacts. Dental tape is preferred over floss because its wider dimension more effectively carries the rubber septa through the contacts. Also, dental tape is not as likely to cut the septa. The waxed variety makes passage easier and decreases the chances for cutting holes in the septa or tearing the edges of the holes. The leading edge of the septum should be over the contact, ready to be drawn into and through the contact with dental tape. As before, the septal rubber should be kept in single thickness with no folds. Dental tape should be placed at the contact on a slight angle. With a good finger rest on the tooth, dental tape should be controlled

so that it slides (not snaps) through the proximal contact, preventing damage to the interdental tissues. When the leading edge of the septum has passed the contact, the remaining interseptal dam can be carried through more easily.

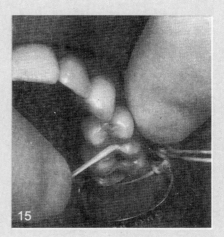

Step 15: Passing the septa through the contacts with dental tape.

Step 16 (Optional): Technique for Using Dental Tape

Often, several passes with dental tape are required to carry a reluctant septum through a tight contact. When this happens, previously passed tape should be left in the gingival embrasure until the entire septum has been placed successfully with subsequent passage of dental tape. This prevents a partially passed septum from being removed or torn. The double strand of the tape is removed from the facial embrasure.

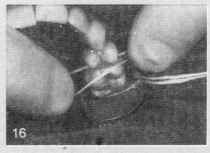

Step 16 (optional): Technique for using dental tape.

Step 17: Inverting the Dam Interproximally

Invert the dam into the gingival sulcus to complete the seal around the tooth and prevent leakage. Often, the dam inverts itself as the septa are passed through the contacts as a result of the dam being stretched gingivally. The operator should verify that the dam is inverted interproximally. Inversion in this region is best accomplished with dental tape.

Continued

Procedure 7-1 Application of Rubber Dam Isolation—cont'd

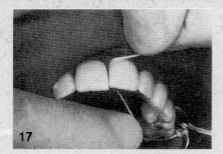

Step 17: Inverting the dam interproximally.

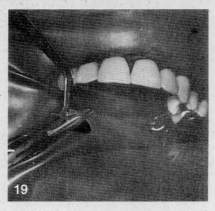

Step 19 (optional): Using a saliva ejector.

Step 18: Inverting the Dam Faciolingually

With the edges of the dam inverted interproximally, complete the inversion facially and lingually using an explorer or a beaver-tail burnisher while the assistant directs a stream of air onto the tooth. Move the explorer around the neck of the tooth facially and lingually with the tip perpendicular to the tooth surface or directed slightly gingivally. A dry surface prevents the dam from sliding out of the crevice. Alternatively, the dam can be inverted facially and lingually by drying the tooth while stretching the dam gingivally and releasing it slowly.

Step 20: Confirming Proper Application of the Rubber Dam

The properly applied rubber dam is securely positioned and comfortable to the patient. The patient should be assured that the rubber dam does not prevent swallowing or mouth closing (about halfway) during a pause in the procedure.

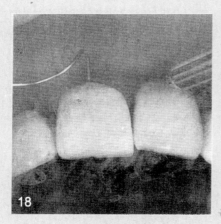

Step 18: Inverting the dam faciolingually.

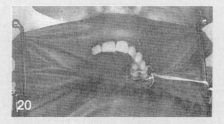

Step 20: Confirming proper application of the rubber dam.

Step 21: Checking for Access and Visibility

Check to see that the completed rubber dam provides maximal access and visibility for the operative procedure.

Step 19 (Optional): Using a Saliva Ejector

The use of a saliva ejector is optional because most patients are able, and usually prefer, to swallow excess saliva. Salivation is greatly reduced when profound anesthesia is obtained. If salivation is a problem, the operator or assistant uses cotton pliers to pick up the dam lingual to mandibular incisors and cuts a small hole through which the saliva ejector is inserted. The hole should be positioned so that the rubber dam helps support the weight of the ejector, preventing pressure on the delicate tissues in the floor of the mouth.

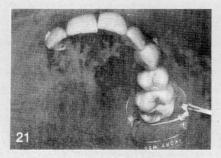

Step 21: Checking for access and visibility.

Procedure 7-1 Application of Rubber Dam Isolation—cont'd

Step 22: Inserting the Wedges

For proximal surface preparations (Classes II, III, and IV), many operators consider the insertion of interproximal wedges as the final step in rubber dam application. Wedges are generally round toothpick ends about ½ inch (12 mm) in length that are snugly inserted into the gingival embrasures from the facial or lingual embrasure, whichever is greater, using No. 110 pliers.

To facilitate wedge insertion, first stretch the dam slightly by fingertip pressure in the direction opposite wedge insertion (*A*), then insert the wedge while slowly releasing the dam. This results in a passive dam under the wedge (i.e., the dam does not rebound the wedge) and prevents bunching or tearing of the septal dam during wedge insertion. The inserted wedges appear in *B*.

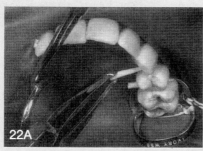
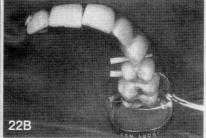

Step 22: Inserting the wedges.

Procedure 7-2 Removal of Rubber Dam Isolation

Before the removal of the rubber dam, rinse and suction away any debris that may have collected to prevent it from falling into the floor of the mouth during the removal procedure. If a saliva ejector was used, remove it at this time. Each numbered step has a corresponding illustration.

Step 1: Cutting the Septa

Stretch the dam facially, pulling the septal rubber away from gingival tissue and the tooth. Protect the underlying soft tissue by placing a fingertip beneath the septum. Clip each septum with blunt-tipped scissors, freeing the dam from the interproximal spaces, but leave the dam over the anterior and posterior anchor teeth. To prevent inadvertent soft tissue damage, curved nose scissors are preferred.

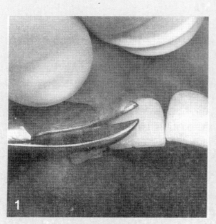

Step 1: Cutting the septa.

Step 2: Removing the Retainer

Engage the retainer with retainer forceps. It is unnecessary to remove any compound, if used, because it will break free as the retainer is spread and lifted from the tooth. While the operator removes the retainer, the assistant releases the neck strap, if used, from the left side of the frame.

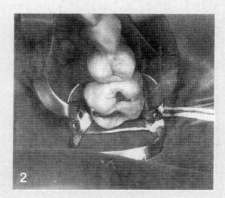

Step 2: Removing the retainer.

Step 3: Removing the Dam

After the retainer is removed, release the dam from the anterior anchor tooth, and remove the dam and frame simultaneously. While doing this, caution the patient not to bite on newly inserted amalgam restorations until the occlusion can be evaluated.

Continued

Procedure 7-2 Removal of Rubber Dam Isolation—cont'd

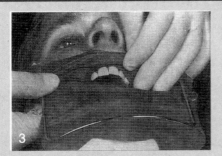

Step 3: Removing the dam.

Step 4: Wiping the Lips

Wipe the patient's lips with the napkin immediately after the dam and frame are removed. This helps prevent saliva from getting on the patient's face and is comforting to the patient.

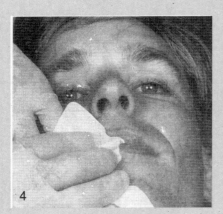

Step 4: Wiping the lips.

Step 5: Rinsing the Mouth and Massaging the Tissue

Rinse teeth and the mouth using the air-water spray and the high-volume evacuator. To enhance circulation, particularly around anchor teeth, massage the tissue around the teeth that were isolated.

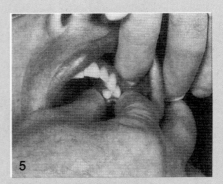

Step 5: Rinsing the mouth and massaging the tissue.

Step 6: Examining the Dam

Lay the sheet of rubber dam over a light-colored flat surface, or hold it up to the operating light to determine that no portion of the rubber dam has remained between or around the teeth. Such a remnant would cause gingival inflammation.

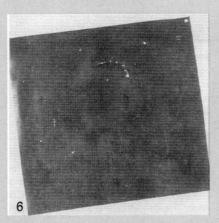

Step 6: Examining the dam.

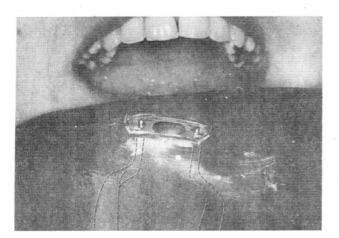

Fig. 7-23 The lip of hole for the anchor tooth is stretched to engage the lateral wings of the retainer.

The assistant gently pulls the inferior border of the dam toward the patient's chin, while the operator positions the superior border over the upper lip. As the assistant holds the borders of the dam, the operator uses the second or middle finger of both hands, one finger facial and the other finger lingual to the bow, to pass the anchor hole borders over and under the jaws of the retainer (see Fig. 7-22, *D*). At this point, the application procedure continues as was previously described, beginning with step 7 in Procedure 7-1.

APPLYING THE DAM BEFORE THE RETAINER

The dam may be stretched over the anchor tooth before the retainer is placed. The advantage of this method is that it is not necessary to manipulate the dam over the retainer. The operator places the retainer, while the dental assistant stretches and holds the dam over the anchor tooth (Fig. 7-24). The

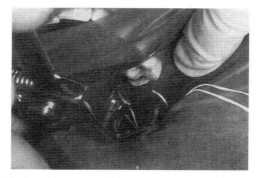

Fig. 7-24 The retainer is applied after the dam is stretched over the posterior anchor tooth.

disadvantage is the reduced visibility of underlying gingival tissue, which may become impinged on by the retainer.

CERVICAL RETAINER PLACEMENT

The use of a No. 212 cervical retainer for restoration of Class V tooth preparations was recommended by Markley.[29] When punching holes in the rubber dam, the hole for the tooth to receive this retainer for a facial cervical restoration should be positioned slightly facial to the arch form to compensate for the extension of the dam to the cervical area (Fig. 7-25, *A*). The farther gingivally the lesion extends, the farther the hole must be positioned from the arch form. In addition, the hole should be slightly larger, and the distance between it and the adjacent holes should be slightly increased (Fig. 7-26). If the cervical retainer is to be placed on an incisor, isolation should be extended to include the first premolars, and metal retainers usually are not needed to anchor the dam (see Fig. 7-25, *B*). If the cervical retainer is to be placed on a canine or a posterior

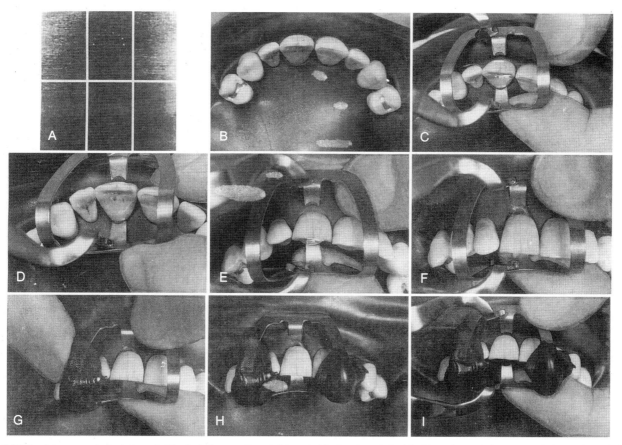

Fig. 7-25 Applying a cervical retainer. **A,** The hole for maxillary right central incisor is punched facial to the arch form. **B,** Isolation is extended to include the first premolars; metal posterior retainers are unnecessary. **C,** First, position the lingual jaw touching the height of contour, while keeping the facial jaw from touching the tooth; steady the retainer with the fingers of the left hand using the index finger under the lingual bow and the thumb under the facial bow. **D,** Note the final position of the lingual jaw after gently moving it apical of height of contour, with fingers continually supporting and guiding the retainer and with the facial jaw away from the tooth. **E,** Stretch the facial rubber apically by the thumb to expose the lesion and soft tissue, with the forefinger maintaining the position of the lingual jaw and with the facial jaw not touching. **F,** Note the facial jaw having apically retracted the tissue and the dam and in position against the tooth 0.5 to 1 mm apical of lesion. The thumb has now moved from under the facial bow to apply holding pressure, while the index finger continues to maintain the lingual jaw position. **G,** Apply stabilizing material over and under the bow and into the gingival embrasures, while the fingers of left hand hold the retainer's position. **H,** Application of the retainer is completed by the addition of a stabilizing material to the other bow and into the gingival embrasures. The retainer holes are accessible to the forceps for removal. **I,** Note the removal of the retainer by ample spreading of the retainer jaws before lifting the retainer from the site of the operation.

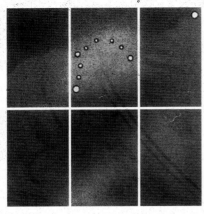

Fig. 7-26 The hole position for the tooth (maxillary right canine) to receive the cervical retainer is positioned facially to the arch form.

tooth, the anchor tooth retainer is positioned sufficiently posterior so as to not interfere with placement of the cervical retainer. If this is not possible, the anchor tooth retainer should be removed before positioning the cervical retainer. A heavier rubber dam usually is recommended for better tissue retraction in such restorations.

The operator engages the jaws of the cervical retainer with the forceps, spreads the retainer sufficiently, and positions its lingual jaw against the tooth at the height of contour (see Fig. 7-25, C). The operator gently moves the retainer jaw gingivally, depressing the dam and soft tissue, until the jaw of the retainer is positioned slightly apical of the height of contour (see Fig. 7-25, D). Care should be exercised in not allowing the lingual jaw to pinch the lingual gingiva or injure the gingival attachment. While positioning the lingual jaw, the index finger of the left hand should help in supporting and guiding the retainer jaw gingivally to the proper location.

While stabilizing the lingual jaw with the index finger, the operator uses the thumb of the left hand to pull the dam apically to expose the facial lesion and gingival crest (see Fig. 7-25, E). The operator positions the facial jaw gingival to the lesion and releases the dam held by the thumb. Next, the operator moves the thumb onto the facial jaw to secure it (see Fig. 7-25, F). Care should be exercised while positioning the facial jaw so as to not scar enamel or cementum. The tip of each retainer jaw should not be sharp and should conform to the contour of the engaged tooth surface. The retainer jaw should not be positioned too close to the lesion because of the danger of collapsing carious or weak tooth structure. Such proximity also would limit access and visibility to the operating site. As a rule, the facial jaw should be at least 0.5 mm gingival to the anticipated location of the gingival margin of the completed tooth preparation. While maintaining the retainer's position with the fingers of the left hand, the operator removes the forceps.

At times, the No. 212 retainer needs to be stabilized on the tooth with a fast-setting rigid material (e.g., polyvinyl siloxane bite registration material or stick compound) (see Figure 7-25). To remove the cervical retainer, the operator engages it with the forceps, spreads the retainer jaws to free the compound support, and lifts the retainer incisally (occlusally), being careful to spread the retainer sufficiently to prevent its jaws from scraping the tooth or damaging the newly inserted

restoration (see Fig. 7-25, I). The embrasures are freed of any remaining compound before removing the rubber dam.

A modified No. 212 retainer is recommended, especially for treatment of cervical lesions with greatly extended gingival margins. The modified No. 212 retainer can be ordered, if specified, or the operator can modify an existing No. 212 retainer. The modification technique involves heating each jaw of the retainer in an open flame, then bending it with No. 110 pliers from its oblique orientation to a more horizontal one. Allowing the modified retainer to bench-cool returns it to its original hardened state.

FIXED BRIDGE ISOLATION

It is sometimes necessary to isolate one or more abutment teeth of a fixed bridge. Indications for fixed bridge isolation include restoration of an adjacent proximal surface and cervical restoration of an abutment tooth.

The technique suggested for this procedure is as follows.[30] The rubber dam is punched as usual, except for providing one large hole for each unit in the bridge. Fixed bridge isolation is accomplished after the remainder of the dam is applied (Fig. 7-27, A). A blunted, curved suture needle with dental floss attached is threaded from the facial aspect through the hole for the anterior abutment and then under the anterior connector and back through the same hole on the lingual side (see Fig. 7-27, B). The needle's direction is reversed as it is passed from the lingual side through the hole for the second bridge unit, then under the same anterior connector, and through the hole of the second bridge unit on the facial side (see Fig. 7-27, C). A square knot is tied with the two ends of the floss, pulling the dam material snugly around the connector and into the gingival embrasure. The free ends of the floss should be cut closely so that they neither interfere with access and visibility nor become entangled in a rotating instrument. Each terminal abutment of the bridge is isolated by this method (see Fig. 7-27, D). If the floss knot on the facial aspect interferes with cervical restoration of an abutment tooth, the operator can tie the septum from the lingual aspect. Removal of the rubber dam isolating a fixed bridge is accomplished by cutting the interseptal rubber over the connectors with scissors and removing the floss ties (see Fig. 7-27, E). As always, after dam removal, the operator needs to verify that no dam segments are missing and massage the adjacent gingival tissue.

SUBSTITUTION OF A RETAINER WITH A MATRIX

When a matrix band must be applied to the posterior anchor tooth, the jaws of the retainer often prevent proper positioning and wedging of the matrix (Fig. 7-28, A). Successful application of the matrix can be accomplished by substituting the retainer with the matrix. Figure 7-28, B through D, illustrates this exchange on a mandibular right molar, as the index finger of the operator depresses gingivally and distally the rubber dam adjacent to the facial jaw, while the assistant similarly depresses the dam on the lingual side. After the matrix band is placed, the tension is released on the dam, allowing it to invert around the band. The matrix, in contrast to the retainer, has neither jaws nor a bow, so the dam tends to slip occlusally and over the matrix unless dryness is maintained.

The operator obtains access and visibility for insertion of the restorative material by reflecting the dam distally and occlusally with the mirror. Care must be exercised, however, not to stretch the dam so much that it is pulled away from the

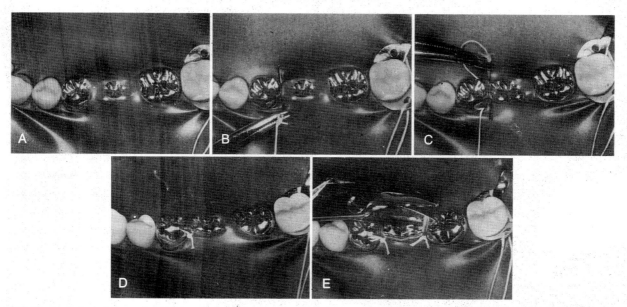

Fig. 7-27 Procedure for isolating a fixed bridge. **A,** Apply the dam except in the area of the fixed bridge. **B,** Thread the blunted suture needle from the facial to the lingual aspect through the anterior abutment hole, then under the anterior connector and back through the same hole on the lingual surface. **C,** Pass the needle facially through the hole for the second bridge unit, then under the same connector and through the hole for the second unit. **D,** Tie off the first septum. **E,** Cut the posterior septum to initiate removal of the dam.

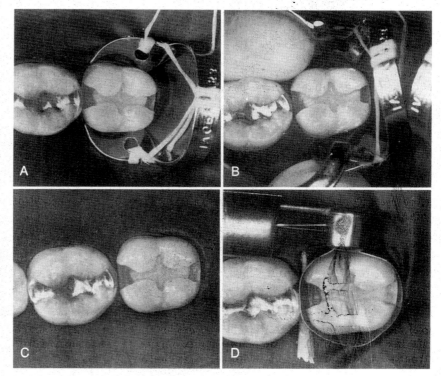

Fig. 7-28 Substituting the retainer with matrix on the terminal tooth. **A,** Completed preparation of the terminal tooth with the retainer in place. **B,** The dentist and the assistant stretch the dam distally and gingivally as the retainer is being removed. **C,** The retainer is removed before placement of the matrix. **D,** Completed matrix is in place. To maximize access and visibility during insertion, the mouth mirror is used to reflect the dam distally and occlusally.

matrix, permitting leakage around the tooth or slippage over the matrix. After insertion, the occlusal portion is contoured before removing the matrix. To complete the procedure, the operator has the choice of removing the matrix, replacing the retainer, and completing the contouring or removing the matrix and rubber dam and completing the contouring.

VARIATIONS WITH PATIENT AGE

The age of a patient often dictates changes in the procedures of rubber dam application. A few variations are described here. Because young patients have smaller dental arches compared with adult patients, holes should be punched in the dam accordingly. For primary teeth, isolation is usually from the most posterior tooth to the canine on the same side. The sheet of rubber dam may be smaller for young patients so that the rubber material does not cover the nose. The unpunched rubber dam is attached to the frame, the holes are punched, the dam with the frame is applied over the anchor tooth, and the retainer applied (Fig. 7-29). Because the dam is generally

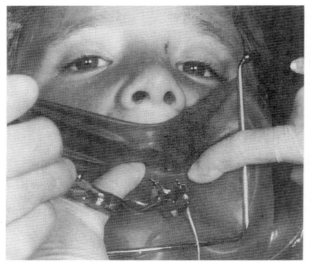

Fig. 7-29 On a child, the rubber dam often is attached to a frame before holes are punched. The dam is positioned over the anchor tooth before a retainer is applied (as in Fig. 7-24).

in place for shorter intervals than in an adult patient, the napkin might not be used.

The jaws of the retainers used on primary and young permanent teeth need to be directed more gingivally because of short clinical crowns or because the anchor tooth's height of contour is below the crest of the gingival tissue. The S.S. White No. 27 retainer is recommended for primary teeth. The Ivory No. W14 retainer is recommended for young permanent teeth.

Isolated teeth with short clinical crowns (other than the anchor tooth) may require ligation to hold the dam in position. Generally, ligation is unnecessary if enough teeth are isolated by the rubber dam. When ligatures are indicated, however, a surgeon's knot is used to secure the ligature (Fig. 7-30). The knot is tightened as the ligature is moved gingivally and then secured. Ligatures may be removed by teasing them occlusally with an explorer or by cutting them with a hand instrument or scissors. Ligatures should be removed first during rubber dam removal.

ERRORS IN APPLICATION AND REMOVAL

Certain errors in application and removal can prevent adequate moisture control, reduce access and visibility, or cause injury to the patient.

Off-Center Arch Form

A rubber dam punched off-center (off-center arch form) may not shield the patient's oral cavity adequately, allowing foreign matter to escape down the patient's throat. An off-center dam can result in an excess of dam material superiorly that may

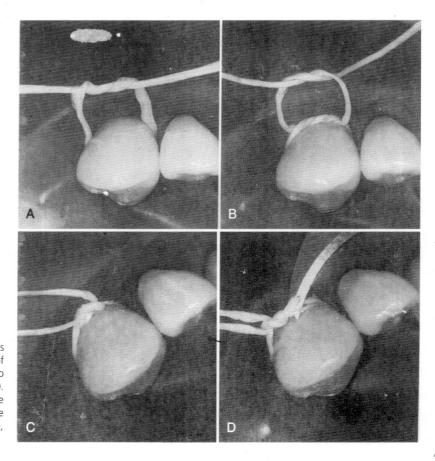

Fig. 7-30 Surgeon's knot. **A** and **B,** Dental tape is placed around the tooth gingival to the height of contour (A), and a knot is tied by first making two loops with the free ends, followed by a single loop (B). **C,** The free ends are not cut but tied to frame to serve as a reminder that ligature is in place. **D,** To remove the ligature, simply cut the tape with a scalpel blade, amalgam knife, or scissors.

occlude the patient's nasal airway (Fig. 7-31, *A*). If this happens, the superior border of the dam can be folded under or cut from around the patient's nose (see Fig. 7-31, *B* and *C*). It is important to verify that the rubber dam frame has been applied properly so that its ends are not dangerously close to the patient's eyes.

Inappropriate Distance between the Holes

Too little distance between holes precludes adequate isolation because the hole margins in the rubber dam are stretched and do not fit snugly around the necks of the teeth. Conversely, too much distance results in excess septal width, causing the

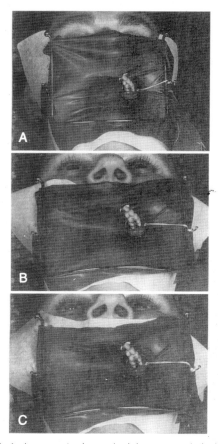

Fig. 7-31 A, An inappropriately punched dam may occlude the patient's nasal airway. **B,** Excess dam material along the superior border is folded under to the proper position. **C,** Excess dam material is cut from around the patient's nose.

dam to wrinkle between the teeth, interfere with proximal access, and provide inadequate tissue retraction.

Incorrect Arch Form of Holes

If the punched arch form is too small (incorrect arch form), the holes are stretched open around the teeth, permitting leakage. If the punched arch form is too large, the dam wrinkles around the teeth and may interfere with access.

Inappropriate Retainer

An inappropriate retainer may (1) be too small, resulting in occasional breakage when the retainer jaws are overspread; (2) be unstable on the anchor tooth; (3) impinge on soft tissue; or (4) impede wedge placement. An appropriate retainer should maintain a stable four-point contact with the anchor tooth and not interfere with wedge placement.

Retainer-Pinched Tissue

The jaws and prongs of the rubber dam retainer usually slightly depress the tissue, but they should not pinch or impinge on it.

Shredded or Torn Dam

Care should be exercised to prevent shredding or tearing the dam, especially during hole punching or passing the septa through the contacts.

Sharp Tips on No. 212 Retainer

Sharp tips on a No. 212 retainer should be sufficiently dulled to prevent damaging cementum.

Incorrect Technique for Cutting Septa

During removal of the rubber dam, an incorrect technique for cutting the septa may result in cut tissue or torn septa. Stretching the septa away from the gingiva, protecting the lip and cheek with an index finger, and using curve-beaked scissors decreases the risk of cutting soft tissue or tearing the septa with the scissors as the septa are cut.

Cotton Roll Isolation and Cellulose Wafers

Absorbents, such as cotton rolls (Fig. 7-32), also can provide isolation. Absorbents are isolation alternatives when rubber dam application is impractical or impossible. In selected situations, cotton roll isolation can be as effective as rubber dam isolation.[2,31] In conjunction with profound anesthesia, absorbents provide acceptable moisture control for most clinical procedures. Using a saliva ejector in conjunction with

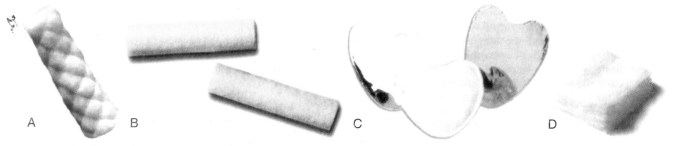

Fig. 7-32 Absorbents such as cotton rolls (*A* and *B*), reflective shields (*C*), and gauze sponges (*D*) provide satisfactory dryness for short periods. *(Courtesy Richmond Dental, Charlotte, NC.)*

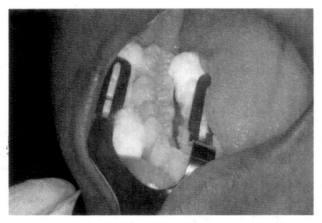

Fig. 7-33 A cotton roll holder in position. *(Courtesy R. Scott Eidson, DDS.)*

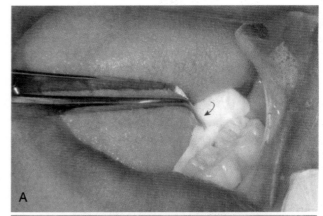

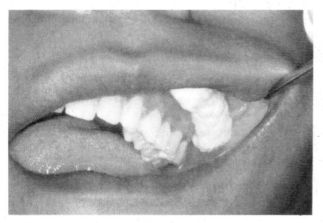

Fig. 7-34 Isolate maxillary posterior teeth by placing the cotton roll in the vestibule adjacent to teeth. *(Courtesy R. Scott Eidson, DDS.)*

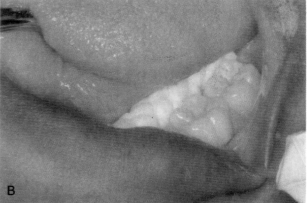

Fig. 7-35 **A,** Position a large cotton roll between the tongue and teeth by "rolling" the cotton to place it in the direction of the arrow. **B,** Properly positioned facial and lingual cotton rolls improve access and visibility. *(Courtesy R. Scott Eidson, DDS.)*

absorbents may abate salivary flow further. Cotton rolls should be replaced, as needed. It is sometimes permissible to suction the free moisture from a saturated cotton roll in place in the mouth; this is done by placing the evacuator tip next to the end of the cotton roll while the operator secures the roll.

Several commercial devices for holding cotton rolls in position are available (Fig. 7-33). It is generally necessary to remove the holding appliance from the mouth to change the cotton rolls. An advantage of cotton roll holders is that they may slightly retract the cheeks and tongue from teeth, which enhances access and visibility.

Placing a cotton roll in the facial vestibule (Fig. 7-34) isolates maxillary teeth. Placing a cotton roll in the vestibule and another between teeth and the tongue (Fig. 7-35) isolates mandibular teeth. Although placement of a cotton roll in the facial vestibule is simple, placement on the lingual of mandibular teeth is more difficult. Lingual placement is facilitated by holding the mesial end of the cotton roll with operative pliers and positioning the cotton roll over the desired location. The index finger of the other hand is used to push the cotton roll gingivally while twisting the cotton roll with the operative pliers toward the lingual aspect of teeth. Cellulose wafers may be used to retract the cheek and provide additional

absorbency. After the cotton rolls, cellulose wafers, or both are in place, the saliva ejector may be positioned. When removing cotton rolls or cellulose wafers, it may be necessary to moisten them using the air-water syringe to prevent inadvertent removal of the epithelium from the cheeks, floor of the mouth, or lips.

Other Isolation Techniques
Throat shields

When the rubber dam is not being used, throat shields are indicated when the risk of aspirating or swallowing small objects is present. Throat shields are particularly important when treating teeth in the maxillary arch. A gauze sponge (2 × 2 inch [5 × 5cm]), unfolded and spread over the tongue and the posterior part of the mouth, is helpful in recovering a small object, for example, an indirect restoration, should it be dropped (Fig. 7-36). Without a throat shield, it is possible for a small object to be aspirated or swallowed (Fig. 7-37).[32]

High-Volume Evacuators and Saliva Ejectors

Air-water spray is supplied through the head of the high-speed handpiece to wash the operating site and act as a coolant for the bur and the tooth. High-volume evacuators are preferred for suctioning water and debris from the mouth (Fig. 7-38)

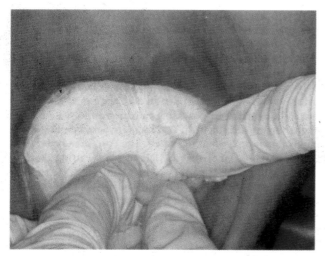

Fig. 7-36 A throat screen is used during try-in and removal of indirect restorations. *(Courtesy R. Scott Eidson, DDS.)*

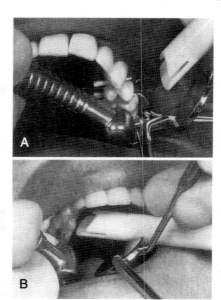

Fig. 7-38 Position of evacuator tip for maximal removal of water and debris in operating area. **A,** With rubber dam applied. **B,** With cotton roll isolation.

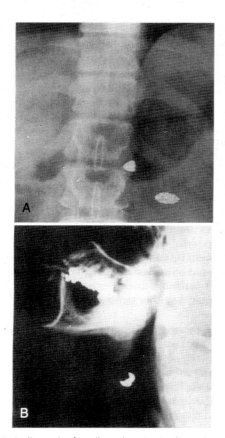

Fig. 7-37 A, Radiograph of swallowed casting in the patient's stomach. **B,** Radiograph of casting lodged in the patient's throat.

because saliva ejectors remove water slowly and have little capacity for picking up solids. A practical test for the adequacy of a high-volume evacuator is to submerge the evacuator tip in a 5-oz (150-mL) cup of water. The water should disappear in approximately 1 second. The combined use of water spray or air-water spray and a high-volume evacuator during cutting procedures has the following advantages:

1. Cuttings of tooth and restorative material and other debris are removed from the operating site.
2. A clean operating field improves access and visibility.
3. Dehydration of oral tissues does not occur.
4. Precious metals can be more readily salvaged if desired.

The assistant places the evacuator tip as close as possible to the tooth being prepared. It should not, however, obstruct the operator's access or vision. Also, the evacuator tip should not be so close to the handpiece head that the air-water spray is diverted from the rotary instrument (i.e., bur or diamond). The assistant should place the evacuator tip in the mouth before the operator positions the handpiece and the mirror. The assistant usually places the tip of the evacuator just distal to the tooth to be prepared. For maximal efficiency, the orifice of the evacuator tip should be positioned such that it is parallel to the facial (lingual) surface of the tooth being prepared. The assistant's right hand holds the evacuator tip; the left hand manipulates the air-water syringe. (Hand positions are reversed if the operator is left-handed.) When the operator needs to examine the progress of tooth preparation, the assistant rinses and dries the tooth using air from the syringe in conjunction with the evacuator.

In most patients, the use of saliva ejectors is not required for removal of saliva because salivary flow is greatly reduced when the operating site is profoundly anesthetized. The dentist or assistant positions the saliva ejector if needed. The saliva ejector removes saliva that collects on the floor of the mouth. It may be used in conjunction with sponges, cotton rolls, and the rubber dam. It should be placed in an area least likely to interfere with the operator's movements.

The tip of the ejector must be smooth and made of a nonirritating material. Disposable plastic ejectors that may be shaped by bending with the fingers are preferable because of improved infection control (Fig. 7-39). The ejector should be placed to prevent occluding its tip with tissue from the floor of the mouth. Some ejectors are designed to prevent

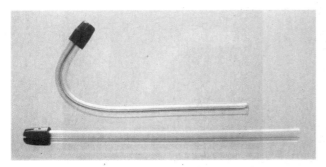

Fig. 7-39 Saliva ejectors. *(From Boyd LRB: Dental instruments: A pocket guide, ed 4, St. Louis, 2012, Saunders.)*

suctioning of tissue. It also may be necessary to adjust the suction for each patient to prevent this occurrence. Svedopter (saliva ejector with tongue retractor) moisture control systems, which aid in providing suction, retraction, illumination, and jaw opening support, are available (Isolite Systems, Santa Barbara, CA). When using the Isolite, a reduction in operating time when placing sealants has been reported. The same study reported that the majority of patients were indifferent with regard to isolation with Isolite and cotton rolls, considering both techniques confortable.[33]

Retraction Cord

When properly applied, retraction cord often can be used for isolation and retraction in direct procedures involving accessible subgingival areas and in indirect procedures involving gingival margins. When the rubber dam is not used, is impractical, or is inappropriate, retraction cord, usually moistened with a noncaustic hemostatic agent, may be placed in the gingival sulcus to control sulcular seepage, hemorrhage, or both. To achieve adequate moisture control, retraction cord isolation should be used in conjunction with salivation control. A properly applied retraction cord improves access and visibility and helps prevent abrasion of gingival tissue during tooth preparation. Retraction cord may help restrict excess restorative material from entering the gingival sulcus and provide better access for contouring and finishing the restorative material. When the proper cord is correctly inserted, its mild physical and chemical (hemostatic) effects achieve isolation from fluids (along with cotton roll use), it provides access and visibility, and it does not cause harm. Anesthesia of the operating site may or may not be needed for patient comfort.

The operator chooses a diameter of cord that can be inserted gently into the gingival sulcus and that produces lateral displacement of the free gingiva ("opening" the sulcus) without blanching it (caused by ischemia secondary to pressure). The length of the cord should be sufficient to extend approximately 1 mm beyond the gingival width of the tooth preparation. A thin, blunt-edged instrument blade or the side of an explorer is used to insert the cord progressively. To prevent displacement of a previously inserted cord, the placement instrument should be moved slightly backward at each step as it is stepped along the cord (Fig. 7-40). Cord placement should not harm gingival tissue or damage the epithelial attachment. If ischemia of gingival tissue is observed, the cord may need to be replaced with a smaller-diameter cord. The objective is to obtain minimal, yet sufficient, lateral displacement of the free gingiva and not to force it apically. Cord insertion results in adequate apical retraction of the gingival crest in a short time. Occasionally, it may be helpful to insert a second, usually larger, cord over the initially inserted cord.

In procedures for an indirect restoration, inserting the cord before removal of infected dentin and placement of any necessary liner assists in providing maximum moisture control. It also opens the sulcus in readiness for any beveling of the gingival margins, when indicated. The cord may be removed before beveling, or it may be left in place during beveling. Inserting the cord as early as possible in tooth preparation helps prevent abrasion of the gingival tissue, thus reducing the potential for bleeding and allowing only minimal absorption of any medicament from the cord into the circulatory system.

Mirror and Evacuator Tip Retraction

A secondary function of the mirror and the evacuator tip is to retract the cheek, lip, and tongue (Fig. 7-41). This retraction is particularly important when a rubber dam is not used.

Mouth Props

A potential aid to restorative procedures on posterior teeth (for a lengthy appointment) is a mouth prop (Fig. 7-42, *A*). A prop should establish and maintain suitable mouth opening, relieving the patient's muscles of this task, which often produces fatigue and sometimes pain. The ideal characteristics of a mouth prop are as follows:

1. It should be adaptable to all mouths.
2. It should be easily positionable, without causing discomfort to the patient.
3. It should be easily adjusted, if necessary, to provide the proper mouth opening or improve its position in the mouth.
4. It should be stable once applied.
5. It should be easily and readily removable by the operator or patient in case of emergency.
6. It should be either sterilizable or disposable.

Mouth props are generally available as either a block type or a ratchet type (see Fig. 7-42, *B* and *C*). Although the ratchet type is adjustable, its size and cost are disadvantages.

The use of a mouth prop may be beneficial to the operator and the patient. The most outstanding benefits to the patient are relief of responsibility of maintaining adequate mouth opening and relief of muscle fatigue and muscle pain. For the dentist, the prop ensures constant and adequate mouth opening and permits extended or multiple operations, if desired.

Drugs

The use of drugs to control salivation is rarely indicated in restorative dentistry and is generally limited to atropine. As with any drug, the operator should be familiar with its indications, contraindications, and adverse effects. Atropine is contraindicated for nursing mothers and patients with glaucoma.[34]

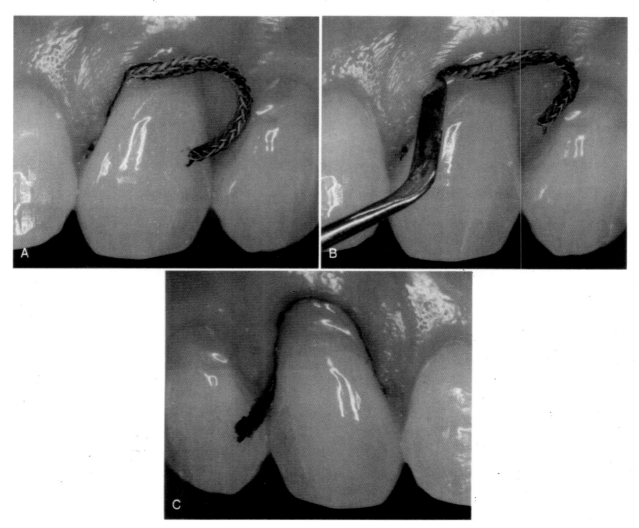

Fig. 7-40 Retraction cord placed in the gingival crevice. **A,** Cord placement initiated. **B,** A thin, flat-bladed instrument is used for cord placement. **C,** Cord placed.

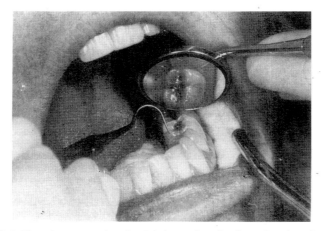

Fig. 7-41 Chairside assistant uses air syringe to dry teeth and to keep the mirror free of debris.

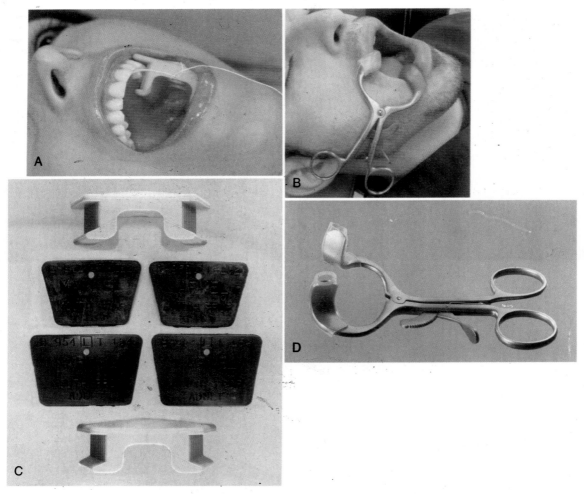

Fig. 7-42 Mouth props. **A,** Block-type prop maintaining mouth opening. **B,** Ratchet-type prop maintaining mouth opening. **C,** Block-type prop. **D,** Ratchet-type prop. (**A** and **B,** From Malamed SF: Sedation: A guide to patient management, ed 5, St. Louis, 2010, Mosby. **C** and **D,** From Hupp JR, Ellis E, Tucker MR: Contemporary oral and maxillofacial surgery, ed 5, St. Louis, 2008, Mosby.)

Summary

A thorough knowledge of the preliminary procedures addressed in this chapter reduces the physical strain on the dental team associated with daily dental practice. Maintaining optimal moisture control is a necessary component in the delivery of high-quality operative dentistry.

References

1. Shugars DA, Williams D, Cline SJ, et al: Musculoskeletal back pain among dentists. *Gen Dent* 32:481–485, 1984.
2. Raskin A, Setcos JC, Vreven J, et al: Influence of the isolation method on the 10-year clinical behaviour of posterior resin composite restorations. *Clin Oral Invest* 25:148–152, 2000.
3. Fusayama T: Total etch technique and cavity isolation. *J Esthet Dent* 4:105–109, 1992.
4. Heling I, Sommer M, Kot I: Rubber dam—an essential safeguard. *Quintessence Int* 19:377–378, 1988.
5. Huggins DR: The rubber dam—an insurance policy against litigation. *J Indiana Dent Assoc* 65:23–24, 1986.
6. Anusavice KJ, editor: *Phillips' science of dental materials*, ed 11, St. Louis, 2003, Saunders.
7. Medina JE: The rubber dam—an incentive for excellence. *Dent Clin North Am* 255–264, 1967.
8. Christensen GJ: Using rubber dams to boost quality, quantity of restorative services. *J Am Dent Assoc* 125:81–82, 1994.
9. American Dental Association Council on Scientific Affairs; ADA Council on Dental Benefit Programs: Statement on posterior resin-based composites. *J Am Dent Assoc* 129:1627–1628, 1998.
10. Barghi N, Knight GT, Berry TG: Comparing two methods of moisture control in bonding to enamel: A clinical study. *Oper Dent* 16:130–135, 1991.
11. Smales RJ: Rubber dam usage related to restoration quality and survival. *Br Dent J* 174:330–333, 1993.
12. Roy A, Epstein J, Onno E: Latex allergies in dentistry: Recognition and recommendations. *J Can Dent Assoc* 63:297–300, 1997.
13. Albani F, Ballesio I, Campanella V, et al: Pit and fissure sealants: Results at five and ten years. *Eur J Paediatr Dent* 6:61–65, 2005.
14. Nimmo A, Werley MS, Martin JS, et al: Particulate inhalation during the removal of amalgam restorations. *J Prosthet Dent* 63:228–233, 1990.
15. Berglund A, Molin M: Mercury levels in plasma and urine after removal of all amalgam restorations: The effect of using rubber dams. *Dent Mater* 13:297–304, 1997.
16. Kremers L, Halbach S, Willruth H, et al: Effect of rubber dam on mercury exposure during amalgam removal. *Eur J Oral Sci* 107:202–207, 1999.
17. Cochran MA, Miller CH, Sheldrake MA: The efficacy of the rubber dam as a barrier to the spread of microorganisms during dental treatment. *J Am Dent Assoc* 119:141–144, 1989.
18. Samaranayake LP, Reid J, Evans D: The efficacy of rubber dam isolation in reducing atmospheric bacterial contamination. *ASDC J Dent Child* 56:442–444, 1989.

19. Harrel SK, Molinari J: Aerosols and splatter in dentistry: A brief review of the literature and infection control implications. *J Am Dent Assoc* 135: 429–437, 2004.

20. Joynt RB, Davis EL, Schreier PH: Rubber dam usage among practicing dentists. *Oper Dent* 14:176–181, 1989.

21. Marshall K, Page J: The use of rubber dam in the UK: A survey. *Br Dent J* 169:286–291, 1990.

22. Gilbert GH, Litaker MS, Pihlstrom DJ, et al: DPBRN Collaborative Group: Rubber dam use during routine operative dentistry procedures: Findings from the dental PBRN. *Oper Dent* 35:491–499, 2010.

23. de Andrade ED, Ranali J, Volpato MC, et al: Allergic reaction after rubber dam placement. *J Endod* 26:182–183, 2000.

24. Jones CM, Reid JS: Patient and operator attitudes toward rubber dam. *ASDC J Dent Child* 55:452–454, 1988.

25. Peterson JE, Nation WA, Matsson L: Effect of a rubber dam clamp (retainer) on cementum and junctional epithelium. *Oper Dent* 11:42–45, 1986.

26. Ingraham R, Koser JR: *An atlas of gold foil and rubber dam procedures*, Buena Park, CA, 1961, Uni-Tro College Press.

27. Brinker HA: Access—the key to success. *J Prosthet Dent* 28:391–401, 1972.

28. Cunningham PR, Ferguson GW: The instruction of rubber dam technique. *J Am Acad Gold Foil Oper* 13:5–12, 1970.

29. Markley MR: Amalgam restorations for Class V cavities. *J Am Dent Assoc* 50:301–309, 1955.

30. Baum L, Phillips RW, Lund MR: *Textbook of operative dentistry*, ed 3, Philadelphia, 1995, Saunders.

31. Brunthaler A, König F, Lucas T, et al: Longevity of direct resin composite restorations in posterior teeth. *Clin Oral Invest* 7:63–70, 2003.

32. Nelson JF: Ingesting an onlay: A case report. *J Am Dent Assoc* 123:73–74, 1992.

33. Collette J, Wilson S, Sullivan D: A study of the Isolite system during sealant placement: Efficacy and patient acceptance. *Pediatr Dent* 32:146–150, 2010.

34. Ciancio SG, editor: *ADA/PDR dental therapeutics*, ed 5, 2009, PDR Network.

Chapter 8

Introduction to Composite Restorations

Harald O. Heymann, André V. Ritter, Theodore M. Roberson

The search for an ideal esthetic material for restoring teeth has resulted in significant improvements in esthetic materials and in the techniques for using these materials. Composites and the acid-etch technique represent two major advances in restorative dentistry.[1-4] Adhesive materials that have strong bonds to enamel and dentin further simplify restorative techniques.[5-10] The possibilities for innovative uses of esthetic materials are exciting and almost unlimited. Many of the specific applications of these materials are presented in Chapters 9 through 12; this chapter provides a general introduction to composites, the predominant direct esthetic restorative materials (Fig. 8-1).

Although these materials are referred to as *resin-based composites, composite resins,* and by other terms, this book refers to most direct esthetic restorations as *composites.* Some information also is presented about various types of composites, including macrofill, microfill, hybrid, nanofill, nanohybrid, flowable, and packable types, as well as other direct tooth-colored restorative materials such as glass ionomers and resin-modified glass ionomers. A brief historical perspective of other tooth-colored materials that may still be encountered clinically is also provided.

The choice of a material to restore caries lesions and other defects in teeth is not always simple. Tooth-colored materials such as composites are used in almost all types and sizes of restorations. Such restorations are accomplished with minimal loss of tooth structure, little or no discomfort, relatively short operating time, and modest expense to the patient compared with indirect restorations. When a tooth is significantly weakened by extensive defects (especially in areas of heavy occlusal function), however, and esthetics is of primary concern, the best treatment usually is a ceramic onlay or crown or a porcelain-fused-to-metal crown.

It is the dentist's responsibility to present all logical restorative alternatives to a patient, but the patient should be given the opportunity to make the final decision regarding which alternative will be selected. Explaining the procedure and showing the patient color photographs and models of teeth that have been restored by various methods are helpful. Simulation of possible treatment outcomes, using computer imaging technology, also is helpful.

The lifespan of an esthetic restoration depends on many factors, including the nature and extent of the initial caries lesion or defect; the treatment procedure; the restorative material and technique used; the operator's skill; and patient factors such as oral hygiene, occlusion, caries risk, and adverse habits. Because all direct esthetic restorations are bonded to tooth structure, the effectiveness of generating the bond is paramount for the success and longevity of such restorations. Failures can result from numerous causes, including trauma, improper tooth preparation, inferior materials, and misuse of dental materials. The dentist is responsible for performing or accomplishing each operative procedure with meticulous care and attention to detail. Patient cooperation is crucial, however, in maintaining the clinical appearance and influencing the longevity of any restoration. Long-term clinical success requires that a patient be knowledgeable about the causes of dental disease and be motivated to practice preventive measures, including a proper diet, good oral hygiene, and maintenance recall visits to the dentist.

This chapter primarily presents the properties and clinical uses of composite materials. Composites can be used in almost any tooth surface for any kind of restorative procedure. Naturally, certain factors must be considered for each specific application. The reasons for such expanded usage of these materials relate to the improvements in their ability to bond to tooth structure (enamel and dentin) and in their physical properties. The ability to bond a relatively strong material (composite) to tooth structure (enamel and dentin) results in a restored tooth that is well sealed and possibly regains a portion of its strength.[11,12]

Types of Esthetic Restorative Materials

Many esthetic restorative materials are available. To gain a full historical appreciation of the types of conservative esthetic materials that might be encountered, a representative list of tooth-colored materials is briefly reviewed. These materials are presented in greater detail in online Chapter 18, Biomaterials.

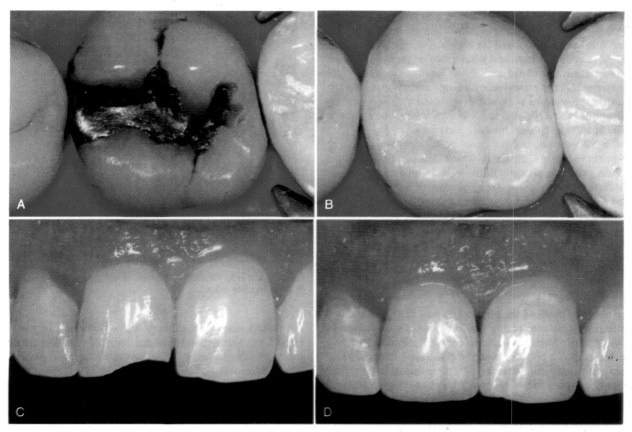

Fig. 8-1 Composite restorations. **A** and **B,** Class II composite restoration, before and after. **C** and **D,** Class IV composite restoration, before and after.

Ceramic Inlays and Onlays

The fused (baked) feldspathic porcelain inlay, an indirect ceramic restoration, dates from 1908, when Byram described several designs of tooth preparations for its use.[13,14] Since the development of adhesive resin cements, interest in using feldspathic porcelain for inlays and onlays in posterior teeth (see examples in Chapter 11) and veneers in anterior teeth (see examples in Chapter 12) has been renewed.[15-19] Many of these restorations are fabricated in a dental laboratory with materials and equipment similar to those used for other types of fused porcelain. Newer versions of ceramics, from which indirect restorations are either pressed or cast, also are available whose physical properties and ease of fabrication are much improved from classic feldspathic porcelain materials (see online Chapter 18). Sophisticated computer-aided design/computer-assisted machining (CAD/CAM) systems enable fabrication of ceramic restorations chairside, thus eliminating the need for impressions, temporary restorations, laboratory procedures and costs, and additional appointments (see Chapter 11 and online Chapter 18).[20-22]

Silicate Cement

Silicate cement, the first translucent restorative material, was introduced in 1878 in England by Fletcher.[14] For more than 60 years, silicate cement was used extensively to restore caries lesions in anterior teeth. Silicate cement powder is composed of acid-soluble glasses, and the liquid contains phosphoric

acid, water, and buffering agents. Although silicate cement is not used as a restorative material today, a practitioner still might encounter silicate restorations in older patients. Of particular interest is that glass ionomer materials are basically contemporary versions of silicate cements. The primary difference relates to the use of polyacrylic acid as opposed to phosphoric acid, rendering glass ionomers less soluble.

Silicate cement was recommended for small restorations in the anterior teeth of patients with high caries activity.[23] By virtue of the high fluoride content and solubility of this restorative material, the adjacent enamel was thought to be rendered more resistant to recurrent caries. Although the average life of a silicate cement restoration was approximately four years, some of these restorations were reported to last for 10 years and longer in some patients.[24,25]

The failures of silicate cement are easy to detect because of the discoloration and loss of contour of the restoration. When examined with an explorer tip, silicate cement is rough and has the feel of ground glass. Old composite restorations may exhibit a similar surface texture and discoloration, but they are less subject to extensive ditching or loss of contour.

Acrylic Resin

Self-curing (chemically activated) acrylic resin for anterior restorations was developed in Germany in the 1930s.[26] Early acrylic materials were disappointing because of their inherent weaknesses such as poor activator systems, high polymerization shrinkage, high coefficient of thermal expansion, and lack of wear resistance, all of which resulted in marginal leakage, pulp injury, recurrent caries, color changes, and excessive wear.[26,27] It was not indicated for high-stress areas because the material had low strength and would flow under load. Its high polymerization shrinkage and linear coefficient of thermal expansion (LCTEs) caused microleakage and eventual discoloration at the margins as a result of percolation.[26] Acrylic resin restorations are rarely used today but, as with silicate cement restorations, may be seen in older patients.

As a restoration, acrylic resin was most successful in the protected areas of teeth where temperature change, abrasion, and stress were minimal.[28] It also was used as an esthetic veneer on the facial surface of Class II and IV metal restorations and for facings in crowns and bridges. A current, although limited, use of acrylic resin is for making temporary restorations in operative and fixed prosthodontic indirect restoration procedures requiring two or more appointments.

Composite

In an effort to improve the physical characteristics of unfilled acrylic resins, Bowen, of the National Bureau of Standards (now called the National Institute of Standards and Technology), developed a polymeric dental restorative material reinforced with inorganic particles.[1,29] The introduction in 1962 of this filled resin material became the basis for the restorations that are generically termed *composites*. Basically, composite restorative materials consist of a continuous polymeric or resin matrix in which an inorganic filler is dispersed. This inorganic filler phase significantly enhances the physical properties of the composite (compared with previous tooth-colored materials) by increasing the strength of the restorative material and reducing thermal expansion.[30] Composites possess LCTEs that are one-half to one-third the value typically found for unfilled acrylic resins and nearer to that of tooth structure. (See online Chapter 18 for details on composite components and properties.)

For a composite to have good mechanical properties, a strong bond must exist between the organic resin matrix and the inorganic filler. This bond is achieved by coating the filler particles with a silane coupling agent, which not only increases the strength of the composite but also reduces its solubility and water absorption.[30,31]

Composites are usually classified primarily on the basis of the size, amount, and composition of the inorganic filler. Different types of composite used since its introduction include macrofill composites (also called *conventional composites*), microfill composites, hybrid composites (including traditional hybrid, microhybrid, and nanohybrid composites), and nanofill composites. Composites also have been classified on the basis of their handling characteristics, for example, as flowable and packable composites.

Macrofill (or Conventional) Composites

Macrofill composites were the first type of composites introduced in the early 1960s. Although these types of composite restorations are sometimes found in some older patients, they are no longer used in clinical practice. Macrofill composites generally contained approximately 75% to 80% inorganic filler by weight. The average particle size of conventional

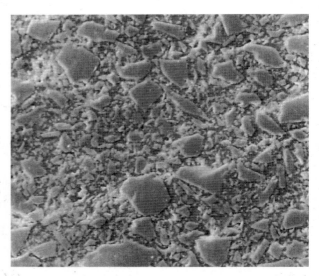

Fig. 8-2 Scanning electron micrograph of polished surface of a conventional composite (×300).

composites was approximately 8 μm.[29] Because of the relatively large size and extreme hardness of the filler particles, macrofill composites typically exhibit a rough surface texture. (This characteristic can be seen in the scanning electron micrograph in Fig. 8-2.) The resin matrix wears at a faster rate than do the filler particles, further roughening the surface. This type of surface texture causes the restoration to be more susceptible to discoloration from extrinsic staining. Macrofill composites have a higher amount of initial wear at occlusal contact areas than do the microfill or hybrid types.

Most conventional composites currently have been supplanted by hybrid composites (see later) but may still be encountered in older patients.

Microfill Composites

Microfill composites were introduced in the late 1970s. These materials were designed to replace the rough surface characteristic of conventional composites with a smooth, lustrous surface similar to tooth enamel. Instead of containing the large filler particles typical of the conventional composites, microfill composites contain colloidal silica particles whose average diameter is 0.01 to 0.04 μm. As illustrated in the scanning electron micrograph in Figure 8-3, this small particle size results in a smooth, polished surface in the finished restoration that is less receptive to plaque or extrinsic staining. Because of the greater surface area per unit volume of these microfine particles, however, microfill composites cannot be as heavily filled because of the significant surface area per unit of volume.[31] Typically, microfill composites have an inorganic filler content of approximately 35% to 60% by weight. Because these materials contain considerably less filler than do conventional or hybrid composites, some of their physical and mechanical characteristics are inferior. Nonetheless, microfill composites are clinically highly wear resistant. Also, their low modulus of elasticity may allow microfill composite restorations to flex during tooth flexure, better protecting the bonding interface. This feature may not have any effect on material selection for Class V restorations in general, but it might make microfill composites an appropriate choice for restoring

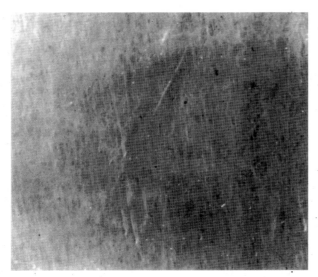

Fig. 8-3 Scanning electron micrograph of polished surface of a microfill composite (×300).

Class V cervical lesions or defects in which cervical flexure can be significant (e.g., bruxism, clenching, stressful occlusion).[32]

Hybrid Composites

Hybrid composites were developed in an effort to combine the favorable physical and mechanical properties characteristic of macrofill composites with the smooth surface typical of the microfill composites. These materials generally have an inorganic filler content of approximately 75% to 85% by weight. Classically, the filler has been a mixture of microfiller and small filler particles that results in a considerably smaller average particle size (0.4–1 μm) than that of conventional composites. Because of the relatively high content of inorganic fillers, the physical and mechanical characteristics are generally superior to those of conventional composites. Classic versions of hybrid materials exhibit a smooth "patina-like" surface texture in the finished restoration.

Current versions of hybrid composites also contain ultrasmall nanofillers, resulting in superior characteristics. These newer versions of hybrid composites are called *nanohybrid composites*.

Nanofill

Nanofill composites contain filler particles that are extremely small (0.005–0.01 μm). Because these small primary particles can be easily agglomerated, a full range of filler sizes is possible, and optimal particle packing is facilitated. Alternatively, many classic hybrid composites have simply incorporated nanofillers into the existing filler composition, thereby optimizing the material further. Consequently, high filler levels can be generated in the restorative material, which results in good physical properties and improved esthetics. The small primary particle size also makes nanofills highly polishable. Because of these qualities, nanofill and nanohybrid composites are the most popular composite restorative materials in use. These composites have almost universal clinical applicability and are the primary materials referred to as *composites* throughout this book.

Packable Composites

Packable composites are designed to be inherently more viscous to afford a "feel" on insertion, similar to that of amalgam. Because of increased viscosity and resistance to packing, some lateral displacement of the matrix band is possible. Their development is an attempt to accomplish two goals: (1) easier restoration of a proximal contact and (2) similarity to the handling properties of amalgam. Packable composites do not completely accomplish either of these goals. Because of the increased viscosity, it is typically more difficult to attain optimal marginal adaptation, prompting some clinicians to first apply a small amount of flowable composite along proximal marginal areas to enhance adaptation.

Flowable Composites

Flowable composites generally have lower filler content and consequently inferior physical properties such as lower wear resistance and lower strength compared with the more heavily filled composites. They also exhibit much higher polymerization shrinkage. Although manufacturers promote widespread use of these products, they seem to be more appropriate for use in some small Class I restorations, as pit-and-fissure sealants, as marginal repair materials, or, more infrequently, as the first increment placed as a stress-breaking liner under posterior composites. Additionally, flowable composites are being used as first small increments in the proximal box of a Class II restoration in an effort to improve marginal adaptation. This approach is somewhat controversial but may be indicated in conjunction with the use of thicker, packable composites, where optimal marginal adaptation is more difficult to achieve.

Some manufacturers also are currently marketing flowable composites as bulk-fill materials, to be used to restore most, if not all, of a tooth preparation in posterior teeth. The manufacturers claim reduced polymerization shrinkage stress, which may occur because of the low elastic modulus of the flowable materials. However, the physical properties of flowable composites are generally poor, and the long-term performance of such restorations is not yet proven. Whether or not flowable composites are used for bulk-filling, they should never be placed in areas of high proximal or occlusal stress because of their comparatively poor wear resistance. More heavily filled composites are far superior for restorations involving occlusal or proximal contact areas.

Glass Ionomer
Conventional Glass Ionomers

Glass ionomers were developed first by Wilson and Kent in 1972.[33] Similar to silicate cements, their predecessors, the original glass ionomer restorative materials were powder/liquid systems. Glass ionomers have the same favorable characteristics of silicate cements—they release fluoride into the surrounding tooth structure, yielding a potential anticariogenic effect, and possess a favorable coefficient of thermal expansion.[34,35] In contrast to silicate cements, which have phosphoric acid liquid, glass ionomers use polyacrylic acid, which renders the final restorative material less soluble.

Although conventional glass ionomers are relatively technique-sensitive with regard to mixing and insertion procedures, they may be good materials for restoration of teeth with root-surface caries because of their inherent potential anti-cariogenic quality and adhesion to dentin. Similarly, because of the potential for sustained fluoride release, glass ionomers may be indicated for other restorations in patients exhibiting high caries activity.[36] Because of their low resistance to wear and relatively low strength compared with composite or amalgam, glass ionomers are not recommended for the restoration of the occlusal areas of posterior teeth. Glass ionomer cements also have been widely advocated for permanent cementation of crowns.

Today, most glass ionomers also are available in encapsulated forms that are mixed by trituration. The capsule containing the mixed material subsequently is placed in an injection syringe for easy insertion into the tooth preparation.

Resin-Modified Glass Ionomers

In an effort to improve the physical properties and esthetic qualities of conventional glass ionomer cements, resin-modified glass ionomer (RMGI) materials have been developed (Table 8-1). RMGIs are probably best described as glass ionomers to which resin has been added. An acid-base setting reaction, similar to that of conventional glass ionomer cements, is present. This is the primary feature that distinguishes these materials from compomers (see the next section). Additionally, the resin component affords the potential for light-curing, autocuring, or both. RMGIs are easier to use and possess better strength, wear resistance, and esthetics than do conventional glass ionomers. Their physical properties are generally inferior to those of composites, however, and their indications for clinical use are limited. Because they have the potential advantage of sustained fluoride release, they may be best indicated for Class V restorations in adults who are at high risk for caries and for Class I and II restorations in primary teeth that would not require long-term service.[37]

Compomers (Polyacid-Modified Composites)

Compomers probably are best described as composites to which some glass ionomer components have been added. Primarily light-cured, they are easy to use and gained popularity because of their superb handling properties. Overall, their physical properties are superior to traditional glass ionomers and RMGIs, but inferior to those of composites. Their indications for clinical use are limited. Although compomers are capable of releasing fluoride, the release is not sustained at a constant rate, and anti-cariogenicity is questionable.

Table 8-1 Tooth-Colored Materials

Conventional Glass Ionomer	Resin-Modified Glass Ionomer Compomer	Composite
High fluoride release	←	Low fluoride release
Low strength		High strength
Poor esthetics		Excellent esthetics
Low wear resistance		High wear resistance

Important Properties of Composites

The various properties of composites should be understood for achieving a successful composite restoration. These properties generally require that specific techniques be incorporated into the restorative procedure, either in tooth preparation or in the application of the material. The various property factors are presented here, with additional information provided primarily in online Chapter 18 but also in Chapters 9 through 12.

Linear Coefficient of Thermal Expansion

The *LCTE* is the rate of dimensional change of a material per unit change in temperature. The closer the LCTE of the material is to the LCTE of enamel, the lower the chance for creating voids or openings at the junction of the material and the tooth when temperature changes occur. The LCTE of modern composites is approximately three times that of tooth structure.[38] Bonding a composite to etched tooth structure reduces the potential negative effects as a result of the difference between the LCTE of the tooth structure and that of the material.

Water Sorption

Water sorption is the amount of water that a material absorbs over time per unit of surface area or volume. When a restorative material absorbs water, its properties change, and its effectiveness is usually diminished. All of the available tooth-colored materials exhibit some water absorption. Materials with higher filler contents exhibit lower water absorption values than materials with lower filler content.

Wear Resistance

Wear resistance refers to a material's ability to resist surface loss as a result of abrasive contact with opposing tooth structure, restorative material, food boli, and such items as toothbrush bristles and toothpicks. The filler particle size, shape, and content affect the potential wear of composites and other tooth-colored restorative materials. The location of the restoration in the dental arch and occlusal contact relationships also affect the potential wear of these materials.

Wear resistance of contemporary composite materials is generally good. Although not yet as resistant as amalgam, the difference is becoming smaller.[39,40] A composite restoration offers stable occlusal relationship potential in most clinical conditions, particularly if the occlusal contacts are shared with the contacts on natural tooth structure.

Surface Texture

Surface texture is the smoothness of the surface of the restorative material. Restorations in close approximation to gingival tissues require surface smoothness for optimal gingival health. The size and composition of the filler particles primarily determine the smoothness of a restoration, as does the material's ability to be finished and polished. Although microfill composites historically have offered the smoothest restorative surface, nanohybrid and nanofill composites also provide surface textures that are polishable, esthetically satisfying, and compatible with soft tissues.

Radiopacity

Esthetic restorative materials must be sufficiently *radiopaque* so that the radiolucent image of recurrent caries around or under a restoration can be seen more easily in a radiograph. Most composites contain radiopaque fillers such as barium glass to make the material radiopaque.

Modulus of Elasticity

Modulus of elasticity is the stiffness of a material. A material having a higher modulus is more rigid; conversely, a material with a lower modulus is more flexible. A microfill composite material with greater flexibility may perform better in certain Class V restorations than a more rigid hybrid composite.[32,41] This is particularly true for Class V restorations in teeth experiencing heavy occlusal forces, where stress concentrations exist in the cervical area. Such stress can cause tooth flexure that can disrupt the bonding interface.[42] Using a more flexible material such as a microfill composite allows the restorations to bend with the tooth, better protecting the bonding interface. The elastic modulus of the material may be less significant, however, with current bonding systems unless significant occlusal stress from bruxism, clenching, or other forms of stressful occlusion are present. Stress-breaking liners that possess a lower elastic modulus also can be used to potentially protect the bonding interface from polymerization shrinkage effects.

Solubility

Solubility is the loss in weight per unit surface area or volume secondary to dissolution or disintegration of a material in oral fluids, over time, at a given temperature. Composite materials do not show any clinically relevant solubility.

Polymerization of Composite

Polymerization Shrinkage

Composite materials shrink while polymerizing. This is referred to as *polymerization shrinkage*. This phenomenon cannot be avoided, and important clinical procedural techniques must be incorporated to help offset the potential problems associated with a material pulling away from the preparation walls as it polymerizes. Careful control of the amount and insertion point of the material and appropriate use of an adhesive on the prepared tooth structure to improve bonding reduce these problems.

Polymerization shrinkage usually does not cause significant problems with restorations cured in preparations having all-enamel margins. When a tooth preparation has extended onto the root surface, however, polymerization shrinkage can (and usually does) cause a gap formation at the junction of the composite and root surface.[43,44] This problem can be minimized by using the appropriate technique but probably cannot be eliminated. The clinical significance of the gap is not fully known. The gap occurs because the force of the polymerization of the composite is greater than the initial bond strength of the composite to the dentin of the root. The gap is probably composed of composite on the restoration side and hybridized dentin on the root side. If extending onto the root surface, it may be beneficial to place an RMGI first in the gingival portion of the preparation on the root followed by the composite. This approach may reduce the potential for microleakage and gap formation and render the surrounding tooth structure more resistant to recurrent caries.[45-51]

Another important clinical consideration regarding the effects of polymerization shrinkage is the configuration factor (C-factor). The C-factor is the ratio of bonded surfaces to the unbonded, or free, surfaces in a tooth preparation. The higher the C-factor, the greater is the potential for bond disruption from polymerization effects. A Class IV restoration (one bonded surface and four unbonded surfaces) with a C-factor of 0.25 is at low risk for adverse polymerization shrinkage effects. A Class I restoration with a C-factor of 5 (five bonded surfaces, one unbonded surface) is at much higher risk of bond disruption associated with polymerization shrinkage, particularly along the pulpal floor (Fig. 8-4).[52] Internal stresses can be reduced in restorations subject to potentially high disruptive contraction forces (e.g., Class I preparations with a high C-factor) by using (1) "soft-start" polymerization instead of high-intensity light-curing; (2) incremental additions to reduce the effects of polymerization shrinkage; and (3) a stress-breaking liner such as a filled dentinal adhesive, flowable composite, or RMGI.

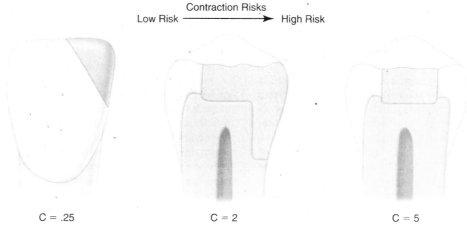

Contraction Risks

Low Risk ——————→ High Risk

C = .25   C = 2   C = 5

Fig. 8-4 Configuration factor (C-factor) (bonded surfaces/unbonded surfaces).

Another approach to reducing polymerization shrinkage stress with composites is to use a different polymer as the matrix. Typical hybrid composites using BIS-GMA or UDMA as the matrix shrink approximately 2.4% to 2.8%. Microfilled and flowable composites shrink considerably more because they are less highly filled. One product, Filtek LS (3M ESPE, St. Paul, MN) uses a silorane polymer matrix and the linear shrinkage of this composite is approximately 0.7%. These materials have very different chemistry compared with conventional composites and require dedicated bonding systems. The efficacy of such materials will be determined by ongoing clinical trials.

Method of Polymerization

The method of polymerization of a composite may affect the technique of insertion, direction of polymerization shrinkage, finishing procedure, color stability, and amount of internal porosity in the material. The two polymerization methods are (1) the self-cured method and (2) the light-cured method using visible light. Self-cured materials require mixing two components, a catalyst and a base, which then react to cause the material to polymerize. Because the components are mixed, the risk for air inclusion in the mixture and internal porosity is greater. Also, the working time to insert the self-cured material is restricted by the speed of chemical reaction and can result in the need for increased finishing time because limited contouring can be done before setting occurs. The color stability of self-cured materials also is lower because of the eventual breakdown of tertiary amines, the polymerization-initiating chemical ingredients. The direction of polymerization shrinkage for self-cured materials is generally centralized (toward the center of the mass). It is theorized that this may help maintain marginal adaptation to prevent microleakage.

Light-cured materials require the use of light-curing units or generators. The use of light sources may cause retinal damage unless appropriate precautions are taken to avoid direct, prolonged exposure to the light source. Light-cured materials do provide increased working time during insertion of the material, however, and may require less finishing time. They also exhibit greater color stability and less internal porosity. Effects of polymerization shrinkage can be partially compensated for by an incremental insertion (and curing) technique. In some clinical situations, however, positioning the light source close enough to the material is difficult or compromised. Despite these disadvantages, almost all contemporary composites are of the light-cured type.

Interest in improving the light-curing methods continues to grow. In addition to the classic quartz, tungsten, or halogen light-curing systems, plasma arc curing systems have been available for rapid polymerization of light-cured materials. These provide high-intensity and high-speed curing compared with the quartz, tungsten, or halogen systems. However, they also significantly increase the stresses from heat generation and polymerization shrinkage. Light-curing systems using blue light-emitting diodes (LEDs) are predominantly used today. Blue LED light-curing units are more efficient, more portable, and more durable than the systems noted previously. All of these efforts have been made to develop a light-curing system that is consistent and faster and produces a stress-free cured material. These features, along with the development of composites with less volumetric polymerization shrinkage, are expected to make light-curing more successful and more economical and to possibly result in restorations with better bonding and improved properties.

General Considerations for Composite Restorations

A composite restoration is placed as follows: (1) The defect is removed from the tooth; (2) the prepared tooth structure is treated with an appropriate enamel and dentin adhesive; and (3) a filled restorative material (composite) is inserted, contoured, and polished. A successful composite restoration requires careful attention to technique detail, resulting in gaining the maximum benefit of the material's properties and appropriate bonding of the material to the tooth (the main advantage of composite is its ability to be bonded to the tooth). The fundamental concepts of adhesion of a restorative material to tooth structure are presented in Chapter 4.

This section summarizes general considerations about all composite restorations. Information for specific clinical applications is presented in Chapters 9 through 12. In selecting a direct restorative material, practitioners usually choose between composite and amalgam. Consequently, some of the following information provides comparative analyses between those two materials.

Indications

Directly placed composite can be used for most clinical applications. Limiting factors for a specific clinical use are identified in later chapters. Generally, the indications for use are as follows:

1. Class I, II, III, IV, V, and VI restorations
2. Foundations or core buildups
3. Sealants and preventive resin restorations (conservative composite restorations)
4. Esthetic enhancement procedures:
   Partial veneers
   Full veneers
   Tooth contour modifications
   Diastema closures
5. Cements (for indirect restorations)
6. Temporary restorations
7. Periodontal splinting

Isolation Factors

For a composite restoration to be successful (i.e., to restore function, to be harmonious with adjacent tissues, and to be retained within the tooth), it must be bonded appropriately to the tooth structure (enamel and dentin). Bonding to the tooth structure requires an environment isolated from contamination by oral fluids or other contaminants; such contamination prohibits bond development. The ability to isolate the operating area (usually by using a rubber dam or cotton rolls) is a major factor in selecting a composite material for a restoration. If the operating area can be isolated, a bonding procedure can be done successfully. This would include the use of a composite or an RMGI restoration and the bonding of an indirect restoration with an appropriate cementing agent. If the operating area cannot be totally protected from contamination, an amalgam restoration may be the material of choice because the presence of some oral fluids may not cause significant clinical problems with amalgam.

Occlusal Factors

Composite materials exhibit less wear resistance than amalgam; however, studies indicate that with contemporary composites, the wear resistance is not substantially different from that of amalgam.[39,40] For patients with heavy occlusion, bruxism, or restorations that provide all of a tooth's occlusal contacts, usually the material of choice is amalgam, rather than composite. Nevertheless, for most teeth experiencing normal occlusal loading and having occlusal contacts that are at least shared with the tooth structure, composite restorations perform well.

Operator Factors

Compared with an amalgam restoration, tooth preparation for a composite restoration is relatively easier and less complex, but tooth isolation; placement of adhesive on the tooth structure; and insertion, finishing, and polishing of the composite are more difficult. The operator must pay greater attention to detail to accomplish a composite restoration successfully. Technical ability and knowledge of the material's use and limitations are required.

Contraindications

The primary contraindications for the use of composite as a restorative material relate to the factors presented above—isolation, occlusion, and operator factors. If the operating site cannot be isolated from contamination by oral fluids, composite (or any other bonded material) should not be used. If all of the occlusion is on the restorative material, composite may not be the right choice. The need to strengthen the remaining weakened, unprepared tooth structure with an economical composite restoration procedure (compared with an indirect restoration) and the commitment to recall the patient routinely and in a timely manner may override any concern about excessive wear potential. Also, as discussed previously, composite restoration extensions on the root surface may exhibit gap formation at the junction of the composite and the root. The use of an RMGI liner beneath the composite in the root-surface area may reduce the potential for microleakage, gap formation, and recurrent caries.[45-51] Any restoration that extends onto the root surface may result in less than ideal marginal integrity. An amalgam exhibits a slight space at the margin until corrosion products seal the area better. Lastly, the operator must be committed to pursuing procedures, such as tooth isolation, that make bonded restorations successful. These additional procedures may make the procedures associated with successful bonded restorations more difficult and time consuming.

Advantages

Some advantages of composite restorations have been stated already, but the following list provides the reasons composite restorations have become so popular, especially compared with amalgam restorations. Composite restorations are:

1. Esthetic.
2. Conservative in tooth structure removal (less extension, uniform depth not necessary, mechanical retention usually not necessary).
3. Less complex when preparing the tooth.
4. Insulating; having low thermal conductivity.
5. Used almost universally.
6. Bonded to tooth structure, resulting in good retention, relatively low microleakage, minimal interfacial staining, and increased strength of remaining tooth structure.
7. Repairable.

Disadvantages

The primary disadvantages of composite restorations relate to potential gap formation and procedural difficulties. Composite restorations:

1. May have a gap formation, usually occurring on root surfaces as a result of the forces of polymerization shrinkage of the composite material being greater than the initial early bond strength of the material to dentin. A gap also can result from improper insertion of the composite by the clinician.
2. Are more difficult, time-consuming, and costly (compared with amalgam restorations) because bonding usually requires multiple steps; insertion is more difficult; establishing proximal contacts, axial contours, embrasures, and occlusal contacts may be more difficult; and finishing and polishing procedures are more difficult.
3. Are more technique-sensitive because the operating site must be appropriately isolated, and proper technique is mandatory in the placement of etchant, primer, and adhesive on the tooth structure (enamel and dentin).
4. May exhibit greater occlusal wear in areas of high occlusal stress or when all of the tooth's occlusal contacts are on the composite material.
5. Have a higher LCTE, resulting in potential marginal percolation if an inadequate bonding technique is used.

Clinical Technique

Initial Clinical Procedures

A complete examination, diagnosis, and treatment plan should be finalized before the patient is scheduled for operative appointments (emergencies excepted). A brief review of the chart (including medical factors), treatment plan, and radiographs should precede each restorative procedure (see Chapter 3).

Local Anesthesia

Local anesthesia usually is required for many operative procedures. Profound anesthesia contributes to a more comfortable

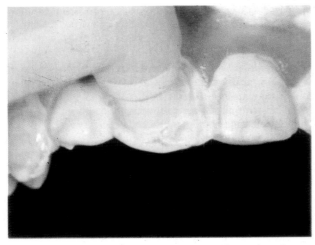

Fig. 8-5 Cleaning operating site with slurry of flour of pumice.

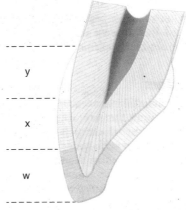

Fig. 8-6 Cross-section of anterior tooth showing three color zones. Incisal third (w) is a lighter shade and more translucent than cervical third (y), whereas middle third (x) represents blending of incisal and cervical thirds.

and uninterrupted procedure and usually results in a marked reduction in salivation. These effects of local anesthesia contribute to better operative dentistry, especially when placing bonded restorations.

Preparation of the Operating Site

Prior to beginning any composite restoration, it may be necessary to clean the operating site with a slurry of pumice to remove plaque, pellicle, and superficial stains (Fig. 8-5). Calculus removal with appropriate instruments also may be needed. These steps create a site more receptive to bonding. Prophy pastes containing flavoring agents, glycerin, or fluorides may act as contaminants and should be avoided to prevent a possible conflict with the acid-etch technique.

Shade Selection

Special attention should be given to matching the color of the natural tooth with the composite material. The shade of the tooth should be determined before teeth are subjected to any prolonged drying because dehydrated teeth become lighter in shade as a result of a decrease in translucency. Normally, teeth are predominantly white, with varying degrees of yellow, gray, or orange tints. The color also varies with the translucency, thickness, and distribution of enamel and dentin and the age of the patient. Other factors such as fluorosis, tetracycline staining, and endodontic treatment also affect tooth color. Because of so many variables, it is necessary to match the individual surface of the tooth to be restored. A cross-section of an anterior tooth (Fig. 8-6) illustrates why color zones exist. The incisal third (w) (mostly enamel) is lighter and more translucent than the cervical third (y) (mostly dentin), whereas the middle third (x) is a blend of the incisal and cervical colors.

Most manufacturers provide shade guides for their specific materials, which usually are not interchangeable with materials from other manufacturers. Different manufacturers vary in the numbers of shades available. Most manufacturers also cross-reference their shades with those of the Vita Classical shade guide (Vident, Brea, CA), a universally adopted shade guide. Also, most composite materials are available in enamel and dentin shades and translucent and opaque shades. The

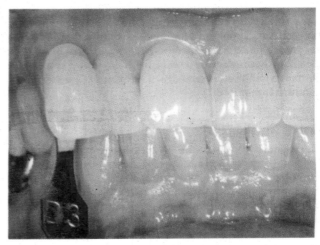

Fig. 8-7 Shade selection. Shade tab is held near the area to be restored.

translucency of the composite material selected depends on the translucency of the tooth structure in the area of the tooth to be restored. Enamel shades are more translucent and typically are indicated for restoration of translucent areas such as incisal edges. Because of the current popularity of bleaching, many manufacturers also offer composites in very light shades.

Good lighting is necessary for effective color selection. Natural light is preferred for selection of shades. If no windows are present in the operatory to provide natural daylight, color-corrected operating lights or ceiling lights should be available to facilitate accurate shade selection. If the dental operating light is used, it should be moved away to decrease the intensity, allowing the effect of shadows to be seen.

In choosing the appropriate shade, the entire shade guide should be held near the patient's teeth to determine the general color. A specific shade tab is selected and held beside the area of the tooth to be restored (Fig. 8-7). The cervical area of the tooth is usually darker than the incisal area. The selection should be made as rapidly as possible because physiologic limitations of the color receptors in the eye make it increasingly difficult to distinguish between similar colors after approximately 30 seconds. If more time is needed, the operator should rest the eyes by looking at a blue or violet object for a few seconds.[53,54] These are the complementary colors of orange and yellow, which are the predominant colors in teeth. By looking at complementary colors, the color receptors in the operator's eye are revitalized and resensitized to perceiving minor variations in yellow and orange. Some dentists request that their assistants make or assist in the shade selection. This practice saves time not only for the dentist but also for the assistant, who, when adequately trained to select shades, may feel a greater sense of responsibility and involvement. Final shade selection can be verified by the patient with the use of a hand mirror.

Most teeth can be matched from manufacturers' basic shades, although some composites from different manufacturers do not match a Vita shade guide the same way. Layering of various shades or opacities also may be required to achieve the desired result.

The shade is recorded in the patient's chart. Because teeth darken with age, a different shade or material may be required if a replacement becomes necessary later. If bleaching (whitening) of teeth is contemplated, it should be done before any restorations are placed (see Chapter 12).

To be more certain of the proper shade selection, a small amount of material of the selected shade can be placed directly on the tooth, close to the area to be restored, and cured. This step may provide a more accurate assessment of the selected shade. If the shade is correct, an explorer is used to remove the cured material from the tooth surface. (A more comprehensive review of factors affecting the esthetic considerations of tooth restoration is presented in Chapter 12.)

Isolation of the Operating Site

Complete instructions for the control of moisture are given in Chapter 7. Isolation for tooth-colored restorations can be accomplished with a rubber dam or cotton rolls, with or without a retraction cord. Regardless of the method, isolation of the area is imperative if the desired bond is to be obtained. Contamination of etched enamel or dentin by saliva results in a significantly decreased bond; likewise, contamination of the composite material during insertion results in degradation of physical properties.

RUBBER DAM

The rubber dam is an excellent means of acquiring access, vision, and moisture control. For proximal surface restorations, the dam should attempt to isolate several teeth mesial and distal to the operating site; this provides adequate access for tooth preparation, application of the matrix, and insertion and finishing of the material. If a lingual approach is indicated for an anterior tooth restoration, it is better to isolate all anterior teeth and include the first premolars to provide more access to the lingual area. For some Class V carious lesions and other facial or lingual defects, it may be necessary to apply a No. 212 retainer (clamp).

If a proximal restoration involves all of the contact area or extends subgingivally, a wedge should be inserted in the gingival embrasure after dam application and before tooth preparation. The wedge (1) depresses interproximal soft tissue, (2) shields the dam and soft tissue from injury during the operative procedure, and (3) produces separation of teeth to help compensate for the thickness of the matrix that will be used later. Adequate preoperative wedging assists the eventual proximal contact restoration. Wedge insertion should occur whether or not a rubber dam is being used. Usually, the wedge is inserted into the larger facial or lingual embrasure, but this is at the discretion of the operator.

COTTON ROLLS (WITH OR WITHOUT A RETRACTION CORD)

An alternative method of obtaining a dry operating field is the use of cotton roll isolation. When the dentist and the dental assistant are experienced and careful, cotton roll isolation results in an operating site conducive to accomplishing a successful composite (or any other) restoration. A cotton roll is placed in the facial vestibule directly adjacent to the tooth being restored. When restoring a mandibular tooth, a second, preferably larger, cotton roll should be placed adjacent to the tooth in the lingual vestibule.

When the gingival extension of a tooth preparation is to be positioned subgingivally, or near the gingiva, a retraction cord can be used to retract the tissue temporarily and reduce seepage of tissue fluids into the operating site. If hemorrhage control is needed, the cord can be saturated first with a liquid astringent material.

Other Pre-operative Considerations

When restoring posterior proximal surfaces, a wedge should be placed firmly into the gingival embrasure pre-operatively. This wedge causes separation of the operated tooth from the adjacent tooth and creates some space to compensate for the thickness of the matrix used later in the procedure. Pre-operative wedging assists in re-establishing a proximal contact with a composite restoration. A complement for pre-wedging is the use of sectional matrix systems with bitine separating rings (see Chapter 10 for specifics related to sectional matrix systems).

Also, a pre-operative assessment of the occlusion should be made. This assessment should occur before rubber dam placement and should identify not only the occlusal contacts of the tooth or teeth to be restored but also the occlusal contacts on adjacent teeth. Knowing the pre-operative location of occlusal contacts is important in planning the restoration outline form and establishing the proper occlusal contact on the restoration. Remembering where the contacts are located on adjacent teeth provides guidance in knowing when the restoration contacts are correctly adjusted.

Tooth Preparation and Restoration for Composite Restorations

Detailed descriptions of specific composite tooth preparations and restorations are presented in Chapters 5, 9, 10, and 12. The reader is referred to these chapters for specific clinical procedures involved in the preparation for all classes of composite restorations.

Reparing Composite Restorations

If a patient presents with a composite restoration that has a localized defect, a repair usually can be made. Easily accessible areas may be roughened with a diamond stone; the area is etched; an appropriate enamel/dentin adhesive is applied; and finally the composite is inserted, contoured, and polished. If the defect is not easily accessible, a tooth preparation must be created that exposes the defective area, and a matrix may be necessary; the adhesive and the composite are then placed.

If a void is detected immediately after insertion of a composite restoration, but before contouring is initiated, more composite can be added directly to the void area. These materials bond because the void area has an oxygen-inhibited surface layer that permits composite additions. If any contouring has occurred, however, the oxygen-inhibited layer may have been removed or altered, and the area must be re-etched and the adhesive placed before adding more composite.

Common Problems: Causes and Potential Solutions

This section lists the causes of common problems associated with some composite restorations and potential solutions to those problems. The subsequent chapters on techniques refer back to these because they describe specific composite procedures.

Poor Isolation of the Operating Area

Causes of poor isolation of the operating area include the following:

- No rubber dam or leaking rubber dam
- Inadequate cotton roll isolation
- Careless technique
- Preparation so deep gingivally that the operating area cannot be isolated

Potential solutions for poor isolation of the operating area include the following:

- Use of better technique
- Use of a matrix to help isolation
- Use of a restorative material other than composite that does not require bonding
- Repeating bonding procedures (if the area is contaminated)

White Line or Halo Adjacent to the Enamel Margin

The following factors cause micro-fracture of marginal enamel:

- Traumatic contouring or finishing techniques
- Inadequate etching and bonding of that area
- High-intensity light-curing, resulting in excessive polymerization stresses

Potential solutions are as follows:

- Re-etching, priming, and bonding the area
- Conservatively removing the defect and re-restoring

- Using atraumatic finishing techniques (e.g., light intermittent pressure)
- Using soft-start polymerization techniques
- Leaving as is and monitoring for leakage

Voids

Causes of voids include the following:

- Mixing of self-cured composites (however, self-cured materials are rarely used today)
- Spaces left between increments during insertion
- Tacky composite pulling away from the preparation during insertion

Potential solutions are as follows:

- Using a more careful technique
- Repairing marginal voids by preparing the area and re-restoring

Weak or Missing Proximal Contacts (Class II, III, and IV)

Causes of weak and missing proximal contacts are as follows:

- Inadequately contoured matrix band
- Inadequate wedging, preoperatively and during the composite insertion
- Matrix band movement during composite insertion or matrix band not in direct contact with the adjacent proximal surface
- A circumferential matrix being used when restoring only one contact
- Tacky composite pulling away from matrix contact area during insertion
- Matrix band too thick

Potential solutions include the following:

- Properly contouring the matrix band
- Having the matrix in contact with the adjacent tooth
- Using a firm preoperative and insertion wedging technique
- Using a matrix system that places the matrix only around the proximal surface to be restored
- Using specially designed, triangular light-curing tips to hold the matrix against the adjacent tooth while curing
- Using a hand instrument to hold the matrix against the adjacent tooth while curing the incremental placements of composite
- Being careful with insertion technique

Inaccurate Shade

Causes of an incorrect shade include the following:

- Inappropriate operator lighting while selecting the shade
- Selection of shade after the tooth is dried
- Shade tab not matching the actual composite shade
- Wrong shade selected

Potential solutions are as follows:

- Using natural light when selecting shade, if possible
- Selecting the shade before isolating the tooth
- Pre-operatively placing some of the selected shade on the tooth and curing (then removing)
- Not shining the operating light directly on the area during shade selection
- Understanding the typical zones of different shades for natural teeth

Poor Retention

Causes of poor retention include the following:

- Inadequate preparation form
- Contamination of the operating area
- Poor bonding technique
- Use of incompatible bonding materials

Potential solutions include the following:

- Preparing the tooth with appropriate bevels or flares and secondary retention feature, when necessary
- Keeping the area isolated while bonding
- Following the manufacturer's directions strictly

Contouring and Finishing Problems

Causes of contouring or finishing problems are as follows:

- Injuring adjacent unprepared tooth structure
- Over-contouring the restoration
- Under-contouring the restoration
- Ditching cementum
- Creating inadequate anatomic tooth form
- Dealing with difficult-to-see margins

Potential solutions include the following:

- Being careful with the use of rotary instruments to avoid adversely affecting the structure of the adjacent tooth or teeth
- Having a proper matrix with appropriate axial and line angle contours
- Creating embrasures to match the adjacent tooth embrasure form
- Not using rotary instruments that leave roughened surfaces
- Using a properly shaped contouring instrument for the area being contoured
- Remembering the outline form of the preparation
- Viewing the restoration from all angles as it is contoured

Controversial Issues

Because of the dynamic nature of the practice of operative dentistry, changes are occurring constantly. As new products and techniques are developed, their effectiveness cannot be assessed until they have been tested by appropriately designed research protocols. Many such developments are taking place at any time, and many of these developments do not have the necessary documentation to prove their effectiveness, even though they receive positive publicity.

Liners and Bases Under Composite Restorations

Various materials have been promoted for routine use as liners or bases under composite restorations. These include RMGIs and flowable composites. Proponents of this approach do not promote these materials for pulp protection in the traditional sense but as materials that provide a better seal for composite restorations when extended onto the root surface. RMGI materials may improve the seal in root-surface areas, which would protect the pulp and render surrounding tooth structure more resistant to recurrent caries and act as stress breakers, which may resist polymerization or flexural stresses placed on the composite restoration.[45-51,55,56]

Retention in Class V Root-Surface Preparations

This book recommends the use of retention grooves in composite tooth preparations when the operator believes that an additional retention form is necessary. It is likely, however, that with the bonding systems available, retention groove placement is usually not necessary.

Wear Problems

This book recommends that occlusal factors be considered when selecting composite as a restorative material, especially in clinical situations when heavy occlusal forces are anticipated or when all of the occlusal contacts will be on the restoration only. The wear resistance of some composites is similar to that of amalgam, however, and composite restorations should be successful for most occlusal patterns where occlusal contacts are shared with the tooth structure.

Significance of Gap Formation

As discussed previously, the gap formation that usually occurs when the composite restoration is extended onto the root surface may not have any long-term clinical effects. With the two vectors of the defect being primarily resin or composite, recurrent caries may not be a problem. How long the exposed hybridized resin layer on the root stays intact is unknown, however, and if it deteriorates in a short time, the area is exposed to risk for caries. Use of an RMGI liner material may reduce the effect of gap formation by rendering the surrounding tooth structure more resistant to recurrent caries.[45-51]

Summary

The use of composite restorations is increasing because of the benefits accrued from adhesive bonding to tooth structure, esthetic qualities, and almost universal clinical use. When done properly, a composite restoration can provide excellent service for many years. When used in posterior teeth, however, composite restorations are more difficult and sensitive to the operator's technique and ability than are amalgam restorations. To achieve the bond that provides the desired benefits, the operating site must be free from contamination, and the material and bonding technique must be used properly. Subsequent chapters provide additional information about the specific uses of composite as restorative material.

References

1. Bowen RL: *Dental filling material comprising vinyl-silane treated fused silica and a binder consisting of the reaction product of bis-phenol and glycidyl acrylate*, U.S. Patent No. 3,06,112, November 27, 1962.

2. Buonocore M, Buonocore M, Wileman W: A report on a resin composition capable of bonding to human dentin surfaces. *J Dent Res* 35:846, 1956.

3. Buonocore MG: A simple method of increasing the adhesion of acrylic filling materials to enamel surfaces. *J Dent Res* 34:849, 1955.

4. Silverstone LM, Dogan IL, editors: *Proceedings of the international symposium on the acid etch technique*, St Paul, MN, 1975, North Central Publishing.

5. Bowen RL: Adhesive bonding of various materials to hard tooth tissues: The effect of a surface active comonomer on adhesion to diverse substrates V. *J Dent Res* 44:1369, 1965.

6. Reinhardt JW, Chan DC, Boyer DB: Shear strengths of ten commercial dentin bonding agents. *Dent Mater* 3:43–45, 1987.

7. Retief DH, Gross JD, Bradley EL, et al: Tensile bond strengths of dentin bonding agents to dentin. *Dent Mater* 2:72–77, 1986.

8. Tagami J, Hosoda H, Fusayama T: Optimal technique of etching enamel. *Oper Dent* 13:181–184, 1988.

9. Ritter AV, Swift EJ, Heymann HO, et al: An eight-year clinical evaluation of filled and unfilled one-bottle dental adhesives. *J Am Dent Assoc* 140:28–37, 2009.

10. Wilder AD, Swift EJ, Heymann HO, et al: A 12-year clinical evaluation of a three-step dentin adhesive in noncarious cervical lesions. *J Am Dent Assoc* 140:526–535, 2009.

11. Ausiello P, De Gee AJ, Rengo S, et al: Fracture resistance of endodontically-treated premolars adhesively restored. *Am J Dent* 10:237–241, 1997.

12. Liberman R, Ben-Amar A, Gontar G, et al: The effect of posterior composite restorations on the resistance of cavity walls to vertically applied loads. *J Oral Rehabil* 17:99–105, 1990.

13. Byram JQ: *Principles and practice of filling teeth with porcelain*, New York, 1908, Consolidated Dental Manufacturing Co.

14. Charbeneau GT: *Principles and practice of operative dentistry*, ed 1, Philadelphia, 1975, Lea & Febiger.

15. Calamia JR: High-strength porcelain bonded restorations: Anterior and posterior. *Quintessence Int* 20:717–726, 1989.

16. Friedman MJ: The enamel ceramic alternative: Porcelain veneers vs metal ceramic crowns. *CDA J* 20:27–32, 1992.

17. Qualtrough AJE, Wilson NH, Smith GA: The porcelain inlay: A historical view. *Oper Dent* 15:61–70, 1990.

18. Taleghani M, Leinfelder KF, Lane J: Posterior porcelain bonded inlays. *Compend Cont Educ Dent* 8:410–415, 1987.

19. Friedman MJ: A 15-year review of porcelain veneer failure: A clinician's observation. *Compend Cont Ed Dent* 19:625–636, 1998.

20. Leinfelder KF, Isenberg BP, Essig ME: A new method for generating ceramic restorations: A CAD-CAM system. *J Am Dent Assoc* 118:703–707, 1989.

21. Mörmann WH, Brandestini M, Lutz F, et al: Chairside computer-aided direct ceramic inlays. *Quintessence Int* 20:329–339, 1989.

22. Mörmann WH, Brandestini M, Lutz F, et al: CAD-CAM ceramic inlays and onlays: A case report after 3 years in place. *J Am Dent Assoc* 120:517–520, 1990.

23. Volker J, et al: Some observations on the relationship between plastic filling materials and dental caries. *Tufts Dent Outlook* 18:4, 1944.

24. Paffenbarger GC: Silicate cement: an investigation by a group of practicing dentists under the direction of the ADA research fellowship at the National Bureau of Standards. *J Am Dent Assoc* 27:1611, 1940.

25. Davis WC: *Operative dentistry*, ed 5, St. Louis, 1945, Mosby.

26. Nelson RJ, Wolcott RB, Paffenbarger GC: Fluid exchange at the margins of dental restorations. *J Am Dent Assoc* 44:288, 1952.

27. Seltzer S: The penetration of microorganisms between the tooth and direct resin fillings. *J Am Dent Assoc* 51:560, 1955.

28. Sockwell CL: Clinical evaluation of anterior restorative materials. *Dent Clin North Am* 20:403, 1976.

29. Craig RG, editor: *Restorative dental materials*, ed 11, St. Louis, 2001, Mosby.

30. Bowen RL: Properties of a silica-reinforced polymer for dental restorations. *J Am Dent Assoc* 66:57, 1963.

31. Craig RG: Chemistry, composition, and properties of composite resins. *Dent Clin North Am* 25:219, 1981.

32. Heymann HO, Sturdevant JR, Bayne S, et al: Examining tooth flexure effects on cervical restorations: A two-year clinical study. *J Am Dent Assoc* 122: 41–47, 1991.

33. Wilson AD, Kent BE: A new translucent cement for dentistry: The glass ionomer cement. *Br Dent J* 132:133–135, 1972.

34. Mount GJ: Adhesion of glass ionomer cement in the clinical environment. *Oper Dent* 16:141–148, 1991.

35. Swift EJ: Effects of glass ionomers on recurrent caries. *Oper Dent* 14:40–43, 1989.

36. Mickenautsch S, Yengopal V, Leal SC, et al: Absence of carious lesions at margins of glass-ionomer and amalgam restorations: A meta-analysis. *Ped Dent* 10(1):41–46, 2009.

37. Wilder AD, Boghosian AA, Bayne SC, et al: Effect of powder/liquid ratio on the clinical and laboratory performance of resin-modified glass ionomers. *J Dent* 26:369–377, 1998.

38. Combe EC, Burke FJT, Douglas WH: Thermal properties. In Combe EC, Burke FJT, Douglas WH, editors: *Dental biomaterials*, Boston, 1999, Kluwer Academic Publishers.

39. Collins CJ, Bryant RW, Hodge KL: A clinical evaluation of posterior composite resin restorations: 8-year findings. *J Dent* 26:311–317, 1998.

40. Mair LH: Ten-year clinical assessment of three posterior resin composites and two amalgams. *Quintessence Int* 29:483–490, 1998.

41. Jörgensen KD, Matono R, Shimokobe H: Deformation of cavities and resin fillings in loaded teeth. *J Dent Res* 84:46–50, 1976.

42. Lee WC, Eakle WS: Possible role of tensile stress in the etiology of cervical erosive lesions of teeth. *J Prosthet Dent* 52:374–380, 1984.

43. Ehrnford L, Derand T: Cervical gap formation in Class II composite resin restorations. *Swed Dent J* 8:15–19, 1984.

44. Torstenson B, Brännström M: Composite resin contraction gaps measured with a fluorescent resin technique. *Dent Mater* 4:238–242, 1988.

45. Andersson-Wenckert IE, van Dijken JW, Hörstedt P: Modified Class II open sandwich restorations: Evaluation of interfacial adaptation and influence of different restorative techniques. *Eur J Oral Sci* 110:270–275, 2002.

46. Besnault C, Attal JP: Simulated oral environment and microleakage of Class II resin-based composite and sandwich restorations. *Am J Dent* 16:186–190, 2003.

47. Donly KJ: Enamel and dentin demineralization inhibition of fluoride-releasing materials. *J Dent* 7:1221–1224, 1994.

48. Loguercio AD, Alessandra R, Mazzocco KC, et al: Microleakage in Class II composite resin restorations: Total bonding and open sandwich technique. *J Adhes Dent* 4:137–144, 2002.

49. Murray PE, Hafez AA, Smith AJ, et al: Bacterial microleakage and pulp inflammation associated with various restorative materials. *Dent Mater* 18:470–478, 2002.

50. Nagamine M, Itota T, Torii Y, et al: Effect of resin-modified glass ionomer cements on secondary caries. *Am J Dent* 10:173–178, 1997.

51. Souto M, Donly JK: Caries inhibition of glass ionomers. *Am J Dent* 7: 122–124, 1994.

52. Feilezer AJ, De Gee AJ, Davidson CL: Setting stress in composite resin in relation to configuration of the restoration. *J Dent Res* 66:1636–1639, 1987.

53. Heymann HO: The artistry of conservative esthetic dentistry. *J Am Dent Assoc (special issue)* December:14E–23E, 1987.

54. Sturdevant CM: *The art and science of operative dentistry*, ed 1, New York, 1968, McGraw-Hill.

55. Ikemi T, Nemoto K: Effects of lining materials on the composite resin's shrinkage stresses. *Dent Mater* 13:1–8, 1994.

56. Tolidis K, Nobecourt A, Randall RC: Effect of a resin-modified glass ionomer liner on volumetric polymerization shrinkage of various composites. *Dent Mater* 14:417–423, 1998.

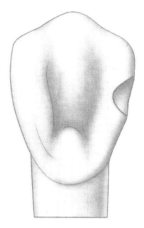

Fig. 9-4 A small, scoop-shaped Class III tooth preparation.

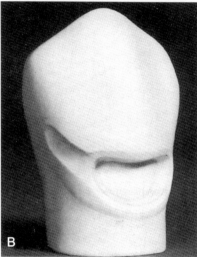

Fig. 9-5 **A,** Decalcified area extending mesially from cavitated Class V lesion. **B,** Completed Class V preparation with conservative mesial extension.

caries removal, completion of the preparation, and insertion of the restorative material (see Fig. 9-3, *D*). No effort is made to prepare the walls that are perpendicular to the enamel surface; for small preparations, the walls may diverge externally from the axial depth in a scooped shape, resulting in a beveled marginal design and conservation of internal tooth structure (Fig. 9-4). For larger preparations, the initial tooth preparation still is as conservative as possible, but the preparation walls may not be as divergent from the axial wall. Subsequent beveling or flaring of accessible enamel areas may be required. Despite the size of the lesion, the objective of the initial tooth preparation is the same: to prepare the tooth as conservatively as possible by extending the outline form just enough to include the peripheral extent of the lesion. Sometimes, the incorporation of an enamel bevel also may be used to extend the final outline form to include the caries lesion (Fig. 9-5). If possible, the outline form should not (1) include the entire proximal contact area, (2) extend onto the facial surface, or (3) be extended subgingivally. Extensions should be minimal, including only the tooth structure that is compromised by the extent of the caries lesion or defect. Some undermined enamel can be left in nonstress areas, but very friable enamel at the margins should be removed.

The extension axially also is dictated by the extent of the fault or caries lesion and usually is not uniform in depth. As noted earlier, most initial composite restorations (primary caries) use a scooped or concave preparation design (Fig. 9-6, *A* and *B*). Because a caries lesion that requires a restoration usually extends into dentin, many Class III preparations are done to an initial axial wall depth of 0.2 mm into dentin (Fig. 9-7). No attempt is made, however, to prepare distinct or uniform axial preparation walls; rather, the objective is to include only the infected carious area as conservatively as possible by "scooping out" the defective tooth structure. Additional caries excavation (deeper than the initial stage of 0.2 mm pulpal to the dentinoenamel junction [DEJ]) or marginal refinement may be necessary later.

The axial wall must provide access for the removal of infected dentin and the application of the adhesive and composite. If the preparation outline extends gingivally onto the root surface, the gingival floor should form a cavosurface margin of 90 degrees, and the depth of the gingivoaxial line angle should be not more than 0.75 mm at this initial stage of tooth preparation. The external walls are prepared perpendicular to the root surface. In this area of the tooth, apical of the cementoenamel junction (CEJ), the external walls are composed entirely of dentin and cementum. Another consideration could be the use of a resin-modified glass ionomer (RMGI) liner on the root surface portion before composite placement to help maintain the seal.[12-15]

When completed, the initial tooth preparation extends the outline form to include the entire fault unless it is anticipated that the incorporation of an additional enamel bevel would complete that objective. Small preparations typically have a beveled marginal configuration from the initial tooth preparation.

Little may need to be done in the final tooth preparation stage for these preparations. Final tooth preparation steps for a Class III direct composite restoration are, when indicated, (1) removal of infected dentin; (2) pulp protection; (3) bevel placement on accessible enamel margins; and (4) final procedures of cleaning and inspecting. All remaining infected

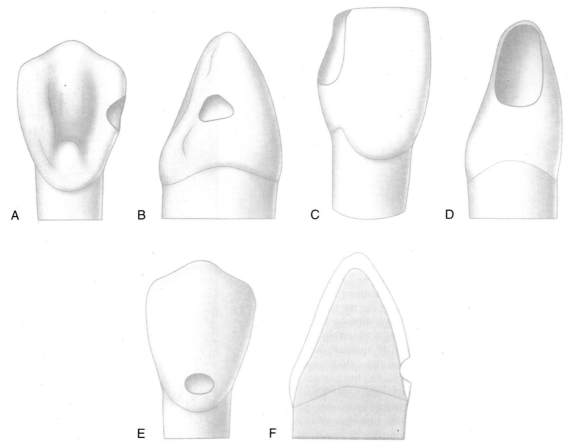

Fig. 9-6 Preparation designs for Class III (*A* and *B*), Class IV (*C* and *D*), and Class V (*E* and *F*) initial composite restorations (primary caries).

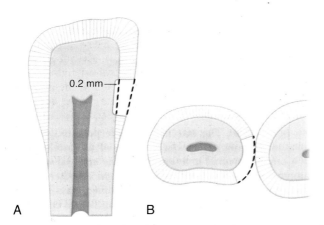

Fig. 9-7 Ideal initial axial wall preparation depth. **A,** Incisogingival section showing axial wall 0.2 mm into dentin. **B,** Faciolingual section showing facial extension and axial wall following the contour of the tooth.

dentin is removed using round burs, small spoon excavators, or both. Particular care must be exercised not to weaken the walls or incisal angles that are subject to masticatory forces.

Larger preparations may require additional beveling of the accessible enamel walls to enhance retention by bonding (Figs. 9-8, *A* and *B*, and 9-9). These enamel margins are beveled with a flame-shaped or round diamond instrument. The bevel is prepared by creating a 45-degree angle to the external surface and to a width of 0.5 to 2.0 mm, depending on the size of the preparation, location of the margin, and esthetic requirements of the restoration (Fig. 9-10; see Fig. 9-9). If the gingival floor has been extended gingivally to a position where the remaining enamel thickness is minimal or nonexistent, the bevel is omitted from this area to preserve the remaining enamel margin or maintain 90-degree cavosurface margin in dentin. Likewise, a bevel on the lingual enamel margin of a maxillary incisor may be precluded because of the presence of occlusal contact.

Remaining old restorative material on the axial wall should be removed if any of the following conditions are present: (1) the old material is amalgam, and its color would negatively affect the color of the new restoration; (2) clinical or radiographic evidence of caries under the old material is present; (3) the tooth pulp was symptomatic preoperatively; (4) the periphery of the remaining restorative material is not intact (i.e., some breach has occurred in the junction of the material with the adjacent tooth structure, which may indicate caries under the material); or (5) the use of the underlying dentin is necessary to effect a stronger bond for retention purposes. If none of these conditions is present, the operator may elect to leave the remaining restorative material, rather than risk unnecessary excavation nearer to the pulp and subsequent irritation or exposure of the pulp. A RMGI base is applied only

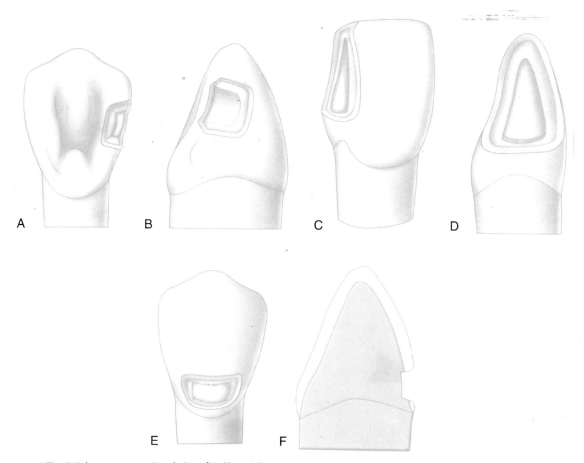

Fig. 9-8 Larger preparation designs for Class III (*A* and *B*), Class IV (*C* and *D*), and Class V (*E* and *F*) restorations.

if the remaining dentin thickness is judged to be less than 1.5 mm and in the deepest portions of the preparation.[16] Calcium hydroxide liners are used only in cases of pulp exposures or near-exposures as a direct pulp-capping material.[16] If used, the calcium hydroxide liner should always be covered with a RMGI base, sealing the area and preventing the etchant (applied later) from dissolving the liner.[16,17]

When replacing an existing failed Class III restoration, the tooth preparation for the replacement restoration normally will have the same general form of the previous tooth preparation. As discussed previously, usually retention is obtained by bonding to enamel and dentin, and no groove retention is necessary. When replacing a large restoration or restoring a large Class III lesion, however, the operator may decide that retention form should be enhanced by placing groove (at gingival) cove (at incisal) retention features in addition to bonding.

For Class III direct composite preparations with *facial access*, with a few exceptions, the same stages and steps of tooth preparation are followed as for lingual access. The procedure is simplified because direct vision is used (Fig. 9-11).

It is expeditious to prepare and restore approximating caries lesions or faulty restorations on adjacent teeth at the same appointment. Usually, one of the preparations is larger (more extended outline form) than the other. When the larger outline form is developed first, the second preparation usually can be more conservative because of the improved access

provided by the larger preparation. The reverse order would be followed when the restorative material is inserted.

A large Class III lesion on the distal surface of a maxillary right central incisor is shown in Fig. 9-12, *A*. The rubber dam is placed after the anesthetic has been administered and the shade has been selected. A wedge is inserted in the gingival embrasure to depress the rubber dam and underlying soft tissue, improving gingival access (see Fig. 9-12, *B*). Using a carbide bur or diamond instrument rotating at high speed and with air-water spray, the outline form is prepared with appropriate extension and the initial, limited pulpal depth previously described in the lingual approach preparation (see Fig. 9-12, *C*). Caries removal with a spoon excavator and an explorer is shown (see Fig. 9-11, *D* and *E*). Some undermined enamel can be left if it is not in a high-stress area.

When a proximal caries lesion or defective restoration extends onto the facial *and* the lingual surfaces, access may be accomplished from either a facial approach or a lingual approach. An example of an extensive Class III initial tooth preparation that allows such choice is illustrated in Fig. 9-13.

Restorative Technique
Matrix Application

A matrix is a device that is applied to a prepared tooth before the insertion of the restorative material. Its purposes include (1) confining the restorative material excess and (2) assisting

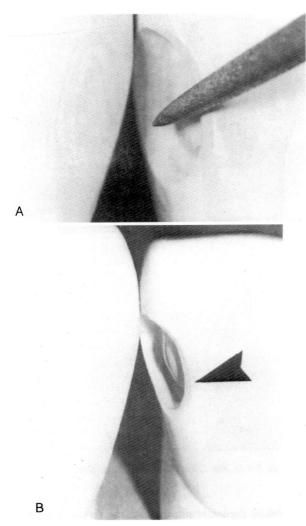

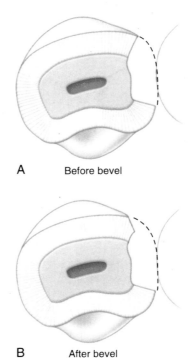

Fig. 9-10 Cross-section of facial approach Class III before (*A*) and after (*B*) 45-degree cavosurface bevel on the facial margin.

Fig. 9-9 Large Class III tooth preparation. **A,** Beveling. The cavosurface bevel is prepared with a flame-shaped or round diamond, resulting in an angle approximately 45 degrees to the external tooth surface. **B,** Completed cavosurface bevel (*arrowhead*).

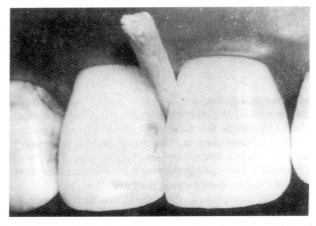

Fig. 9-11 Completed Class III tooth preparation (facial approach), with the bevel marked.

in the development of the appropriate axial tooth contours. The matrix usually is applied and stabilized with a wedge before application of the adhesive because it helps contain the adhesive components to the prepared tooth. Care must be taken, however, to avoid pooling of adhesive adjacent to the matrix.

A properly contoured and wedged matrix is a prerequisite for a restoration involving the entire proximal contact area, unless the adjacent tooth is missing in which case the restoration can be completed using a free-hand final approach. When correctly used, not only would a matrix aid in placing and contouring the composite restorative material, but it may also reduce the amount of excess material, thus minimizing the finishing time.

A properly contoured thin Mylar strip matrix is used for most Class III and IV preparations. Because the proximal surface of a tooth is usually convex incisogingivally and the strip may be flat, it is necessary to shape the strip to conform to the desired tooth contour. One way to contour a Mylar strip is by drawing it along a hard, rounded, object (Fig. 9-14). The

amount of convexity placed in the strip depends on the size and contour of the anticipated restoration. Several pulls of the strip with heavy pressure across the rounded end of the operating pliers may be required to obtain enough convexity. The contoured strip is positioned between teeth so that the convex area conforms to the desired tooth contour (Fig. 9-15, *A*). The matrix strip is extended at least 1 mm beyond the prepared gingival and incisal margins. Sometimes, the strip does not slide through or is distorted by a tight contact or preparation margin. In such instances, a wedge is lightly positioned in the gingival embrasure before the strip is inserted. Care must be taken not to injure the interproximal tissues and induce bleeding. When the strip is past the binding area, it may be necessary to loosen the wedge to place the strip past the gingival

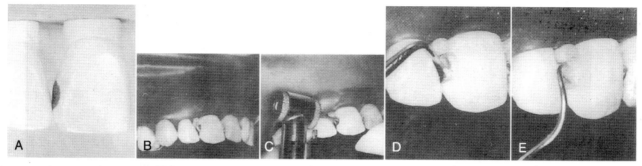

Fig. 9-12 Class III initial preparation (facial approach). **A,** Large proximal caries with facial involvement. **B,** Isolated area of operation. **C,** Entry and extension with No. 2 bur or diamond. **D,** Caries removal with spoon excavator. **E,** Explorer point removes caries at the dentinoenamel junction (DEJ).

margin (between the wedge and margin). Then the wedge is re-inserted tightly (see Fig. 9-15, *B*).

A wedge is needed at the gingival margin to (1) hold the Mylar strip in position, (2) provide slight separation of the teeth, and (3) prevent a gingival overhang of the composite material. A wedge must be used to separate teeth sufficiently to compensate for the thickness of the matrix if the completed restoration is to contact the adjacent tooth properly.

Several types of commercial wedges are available in assorted sizes. A triangular-shaped wedge (in cross-section) is indicated for preparations with margins that are deep in the gingival sulcus. An end of a round wooden toothpick usually is an excellent wedge for preparations with margins coronal to the gingival sulcus. The wedge is kept as short as possible to avoid conflict with access during insertion of the restorative material.

The wedge is placed using No. 110 pliers from the facial approach for lingual access preparations, and vice versa for facial access, just apical to the gingival margin. When isolation is accomplished with the rubber dam, wedge placement may be aided by a small amount of water-soluble lubricant on the tip of the wedge. The rubber dam is first stretched gingivally (on the side from which the wedge is inserted), then released gradually during wedge insertion (Fig. 9-16). Subsequently, a trial opening and closing of the matrix strip is helpful. It must open enough for access to insert the adhesive and composite and close sufficiently to ensure a proper contour. It may be necessary to shorten the wedge or insert it from the opposite embrasure to optimize access.

Placement of the Adhesive

Adhesive placement steps are accomplished with strict adherence to the manufacturer's directions for the particular adhesive being used.

The usual technique for adhesive placement when using an etch-and-rinse adhesive is as follows: First, the proximal surface of the adjacent unprepared tooth should be protected from inadvertent etching by placing a Mylar strip, if not yet applied, or a Teflon tape. Then, phosphoric acid gel etchant is applied to all of the prepared tooth structure, approximately 0.5 mm beyond the prepared margins onto the adjacent unprepared tooth. The etchant typically is left undisturbed for 15 seconds. The area is rinsed thoroughly to remove the etchant. If dentin is exposed, rather than air-dry the rinsed

area, it may be better to use a damp cotton pellet, a foam pellet, or a disposable brush to remove the excess water. If the area is dried, it can be re-moistened with water, a re-wetting agent, or a desensitizing agent such as glutaraldehyde-containing desensitizers. Glutaraldehyde-containing desensitizers have been shown to have no adverse effects on bond strength and have been shown to reduce postoperative sensitivity by reducing dentin permeability.[18-21] Ultimately, the dentin surface should appear moist, as evidenced by a glistening appearance. Over-drying or pooling of excess water should be avoided.

If the bonding system combines the primer and the adhesive, as in a one-bottle etch-and-rinse adhesive, the solution is applied next on all of the tooth structure that has been etched. Every effort should be made to prevent the adhesive from pooling in remote areas of the preparation or against the Mylar strip, if used (Fig. 9-17, *A*). When applied, the adhesive is air-dried to evaporate any solvent (acetone, alcohol, or water), then light-activated, as directed. Because these materials are resin-based, they generally exhibit an oxygen-inhibited layer on the surface after polymerization. The composite material bonds directly to the polymerized adhesive, unless the oxygen-inhibited layer is contaminated. The application of the adhesive and the composite should occur in a timely manner.

Insertion and Light-Activation of the Composite

The composite bonds chemically with the adhesive, forming a strong attachment between the tooth and the restorative material. Although self-cured composites are available, they are very rarely used today for Class III direct composite restorations. The following paragraphs provide the restorative technique for light-activated composites.

The mesial surface of a maxillary left lateral incisor is used to illustrate facial insertion of a light-activated composite (see Fig. 9-17, *A* through *C*). The matrix strip is contoured, placed interproximally, and wedged at the gingival margin. The lingual aspect of the strip is secured with the index finger, while the thumb reflects the facial portion out of the way (see Fig. 9-17). Light-activated materials do not have to be mixed and are not dispensed until ready for use.

The composite is inserted by a hand instrument or syringe. Light-activated composites are usually available in two forms: (1) a threaded syringe for manual dispensing and hand instrument insertion or (2) a self-contained compule that is placed

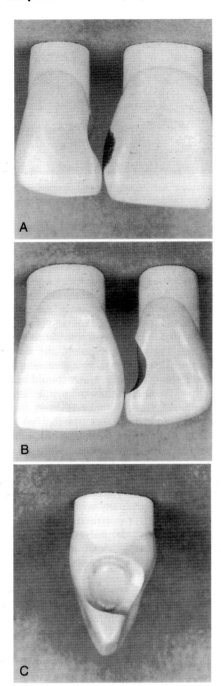

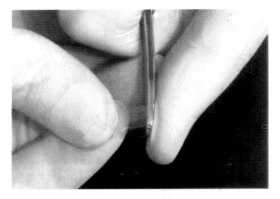

Fig. 9-14 Contouring Mylar strip matrix. *(Courtesy Aldridge D. Wilder, DDS.)*

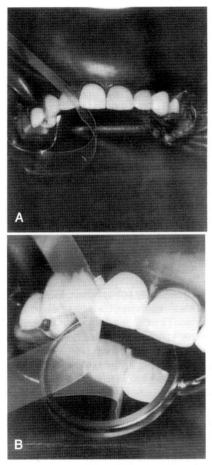

Fig. 9-13 Large Class III tooth preparation extending onto root surface. **A,** Facial view. **B,** Lingual view. **C,** Mesial view showing gingival and incisal retention, which is only used when deemed necessary to increase retention. The tooth preparation is now ready for beveling of the enamel walls.

Fig. 9-15 Inserting and wedging Mylar strip matrix. **A,** Strip with concave area next to the preparation is positioned between teeth. **B,** Strip in position and wedge inserted. The length of the Mylar strip can be reduced, as needed.

into an injection syringe for dispensing or insertion. If a threaded syringe is used, a hand instrument is used to cut off an amount of composite that would restore the preparation onto a paper pad or plastic container. The composite also can be dispensed from the compule, if so desired. The composite should be protected from ambient light to prevent premature polymerization. Likewise, the threaded syringe (or compule

tip) should be recapped immediately to prevent setting of the composite at the end of the syringe. The composite is picked up with the blade end of the hand instrument and wiped into the tooth preparation. If the composite is to be injected directly into the preparation, the selected compule is placed into the injection syringe, and the composite is injected directly into the preparation. The operator uses the plugger

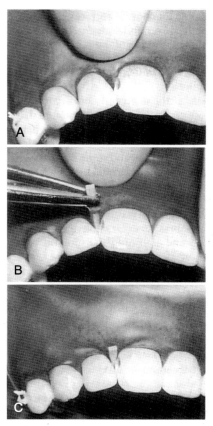

Fig. 9-16 Using a triangular wood wedge to expose gingival margin of large proximal preparation. **A,** The dam is stretched facially and gingivally with the fingertip. **B,** Insertion of wedge (the dam is released during wedge insertion). **C,** Wedge in place.

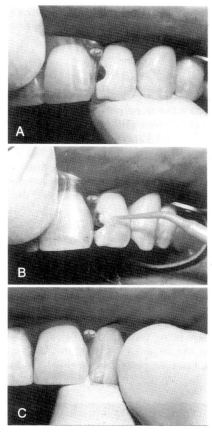

Fig. 9-17 Insertion of light-activated composite. **A,** Bonding adhesive is applied and light-activated. **B,** The lingual aspect of the strip is secured with the index finger, while the facial portion is reflected away for access. **C,** After insertion of the composite, the matrix strip is closed, and the material is activated through the strip.

end of the hand instrument to press the material into the preparation. If the composite has a tendency to stick to the instrument, a sparing amount of bonding resin or a gauze dampened in alcohol can be used to lubricate the instrument. Most modern composites will not stick to a clean instrument. A second increment of composite is applied, if needed, to fill the preparation completely and provide a slight excess so that positive pressure can be applied with the matrix strip when closed. Any gross excess is removed quickly with the blade of the insertion instrument or an explorer tine before closing the matrix.

The operator closes the lingual end of the strip over the composite and holds it with the index finger. Next, the operator pulls the matrix toward the facial direction to cover the facial margin with the composite. This step will provide the best composite–tooth adaptation at that margin. Before light-activating the composite, the operator closes the facial end of the strip over the tooth with the thumb and index finger of the other hand, tightening the gingival aspect of the strip ahead of the incisal portion. The matrix is held in such a way that light can reach the composite. The matrix can be held in this manner until light activation is complete.

When the material has been inserted, it is light-activated through the strip as directed (see Fig. 9-17, *C*). The strip should not be touched with the tip of the light initially because it could distort the contour of the restoration. The operator

removes the index finger and light-activates the lingual surface. Longer light exposures usually are required for the polymerization of dark and opaque shades. If the restoration is under-contoured, more composite can be added to the previously placed composite and light-activated. No etching or adhesive is required between layers if the surface has not been contaminated, and the oxygen-inhibited layer remains.

With large restorations, it is better to add and light-activate the composite in several increments to reduce the effects of polymerization shrinkage and to ensure complete light activation in remote regions. Adjacent proximal tooth preparations should be restored one at a time. Techniques have been suggested for inserting two approximating restorations simultaneously, but these procedures may result in matrix movement, poor adaptation, open contact, overhangs, and faulty contours (Fig. 9-18). If two adjacent preparations are present, the preparation with the least access (usually the one prepared second) is restored first. If too much convexity is present on the first proximal restoration, the excess must be removed before the second restoration is inserted. If too little contour is present, more material is added to correct the contour. The proximal surface of the first restoration should be contoured completely before the second restoration is started. Because the second tooth preparation has been contaminated, it must be cleaned before bonding materials and composite are applied and the composite are inserted. During these procedures, a Mylar strip or Teflon tape should be in place to protect the first restoration and the tooth.

Contouring and Polishing of the Composite

Good technique and experience in inserting composites significantly reduce the amount of finishing required. Usually, a slight excess of material will need to be removed to provide the final contour and smooth finish. Coarse diamond instruments can be used to remove gross excess, but they generally are not recommended for finishing composites because of the high risk of inadvertently damaging the contiguous tooth structure. Compared with finishing burs and disks, they also leave a rough surface on the restoration and the tooth. Special fine diamond finishing instruments, 12-bladed carbide finishing burs, and abrasive finishing disks can be used to obtain excellent results if the manufacturers' instructions are followed. Care must be exercised with all rotary instruments to prevent damage to the tooth structure, especially at the gingival marginal areas.

Similar to tooth preparation rotary instruments, contouring and polishing instruments should be used according to the specific surface being contoured and polished. For example, flexible disks and finishing strips are suitable for convex and flat surfaces; finishing points and oval-shaped finishing burs are more suitable for concave surfaces; and finishing cups can be used in both convex and concave surfaces. A flame-shaped carbide finishing bur or diamond is recommended for removing excess composite on facial surfaces (Fig. 9-19, A). Medium speed with light intermittent brush strokes and air coolant are used for contouring.

Abrasive disks (the degree of abrasiveness depends on the amount of excess to be removed) mounted on a mandrel specific to the disk type, in a contra-angle handpiece at low speed, can be used instead of or after the finishing bur or diamond in facial surfaces and some interproximal and incisal embrasures (Fig. 9-20, A). Several brands of abrasive disks are available, and most are effective when used correctly. These disks are flexible and are produced in different diameters, thicknesses, and abrasive textures. Thin disks with small diameters fit into embrasure areas easily and are especially useful in contouring and polishing the gingival areas. Regardless of the type of disk chosen, disks are used sequentially from coarse to very fine grit, generating a smooth surface. The external enamel surface should act as a guide for proper contour. A constant shifting motion aids in contouring and preventing the development of a flat surface. Final polishing is achieved with rubber or silicone polishing instruments, diamond-impregnated polishers, polishing disks, and polishing pastes (see Fig. 9-19, B and D).

Excess lingual composite is removed using a round or oval-shaped 12-bladed carbide finishing bur or finishing diamond. A smoother surface is produced using a finer round or oval carbide finishing bur (with 18–24 or 30–40 blades) or fine diamond at medium speed with air coolant and light intermittent pressure (see Fig. 9-20, B). The appropriate size and shape depend on the amount of excess and shape of the lingual surface. Polishing is achieved with rubber polishing instruments and diamond-impregnated polishers.

Proximal surface contours and margins should be assessed visually and tactilely with an explorer and dental floss. The floss is positioned at the gingival margin and "shoe-shined" as it is pulled occlusally. If the floss catches or frays, additional finishing is required. A No. 12 surgical blade mounted in a Bard-Parker handle (see Fig. 9-20, C) is well suited for

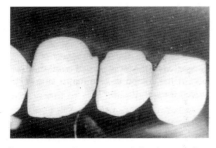

Fig. 9-18 Adjacent restorations, restored simultaneously and displaying poor contours and gingival overhangs.

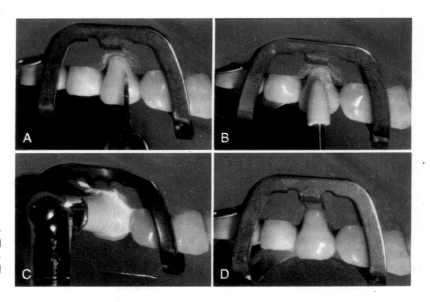

Fig. 9-19 Finishing and polishing. **A,** Flame-shaped finishing bur removing excess and contouring. **B** and **C,** Rubber polishing point (*B*) and aluminum oxide polishing paste (*C*) used for final polishing. **D,** Completed restoration.

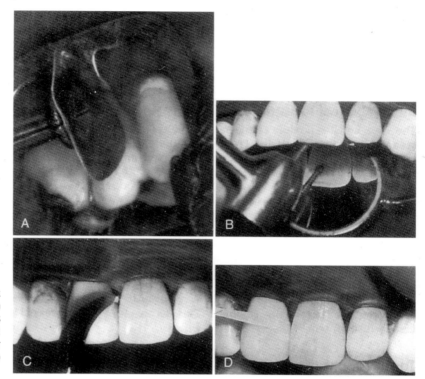

Fig. 9-20 Finishing composites. **A,** Abrasive disk mounted on mandrel can be used for finishing when access permits. **B,** The round carbide finishing bur is well suited for finishing lingual surfaces. **C,** The No. 12 surgical blade in Bard-Parker handle can be used for removing interproximal excess. **D,** The abrasive strip should be curved over the area to be finished.

removing excess material from the gingival proximal area. A No. 12 surgical blade in a Bard-Parker handle is thin and has a curved shape of the blade, making this instrument ideal for removing gingival overhangs. The instrument should be moved from the tooth to the restoration or along the margins, using light shaving strokes, keeping a portion of the cutting edge on the external enamel surface as a guide to prevent over-reduction. If a large amount of composite is removed with one stroke or in the wrong direction, it may fracture inside the tooth preparation and warrant a repair because the irregular void created may collect plaque and debris and cause discoloration or recurrent caries. The excess is gently shaved away to avoid removing a large chunk of material unintentionally. Rotary instruments especially designed for this task are also available and can be used for removing excess and opening embrasure areas. Caution must be taken with all instruments not to remove too much contour or to produce a "ledged" contact (a ledge bordering the contact area). All carbide instruments are made of carbon steel and may leave gray marks on the restoration. This discoloration is superficial and is removed easily during the final finishing by abrasive strips or disks (see Fig. 9-20, D).

Further contouring and finishing of proximal surfaces can be completed with abrasive finishing strips. Some strips have two different types of abrasives (e.g., medium and fine) on opposing ends of the strip, with a small area in-between where no abrasive is present to allow easy and safe insertion of the strip through the contact area. Thin diamond-coated metal strips also are commercially available in various grits. Different widths of strips are available. A narrow width is usually more appropriate for contouring because it allows more versatility for finishing specific areas. Wide strips tend to flatten the proximal contour, remove too much material at the contact

areas, and extend too far gingivally. This results in a poor contour and a weak or absent contact, which must be corrected.

The strip should not be drawn back-and-forth across the restoration in a "sawing" manner. It should be curved over the restoration and tooth surface in a fashion similar to that used with a shoe-shine cloth, concentrating on areas that need attention (see Fig. 9-20, D). To open the lingual embrasure or round the marginal ridge, the lingual part of the strip is held against the composite with the index finger of one hand, while the other end of the strip is pulled facially with the other hand.

Contouring and finishing the proximal surface, including the gingival margin, also develops the general embrasure form around the proximal contact. Further embrasure form development is accomplished with additional use of flame-shaped carbide finishing burs, fine diamonds, or the No. 12 surgical blade.

Finally, occlusion should be carefully checked after the rubber dam is removed, if one was used. The operator evaluates the occlusion in maximum intercuspation and eccentric movements by having the patient close on a piece of articulating paper and slide mandibular teeth over the restored area. If excess composite is present, the operator removes only a small amount at a time and rechecks with articulating paper. Usually, occlusion is adjusted until it does not differ from the original occlusion.

Instead of working sequentially by surface as described above (facial, lingual, proximal, and occlusal), the operator may elect to work by instrument sequence, that is, contour all surfaces of the restoration by using contouring instruments first and then proceed to polish all surfaces by using the polishing instruments described. This approach minimizes the amount of time necessary to change instruments between surfaces.

Clinical Technique for Class IV Direct Composite Restorations

Initial Clinical Procedures

The same initial procedure considerations presented earlier are appropriate for Class IV direct composite restorations. The preoperative assessment of the occlusion is even more important for Class IV restorations because it might influence the tooth preparation extension (placing margins in noncontact areas) and retention and resistance form features (heavy occlusion requires increased retention and resistance form).

Also, proper shade selection can be more difficult for large Class IV restorations. Use of separate translucent and opaque shades of composite is often necessary. Specific information for esthetic considerations is presented in Chapter 12.

For large Class IV lesions or fractures, a preoperative impression may be taken to be used as a template for developing the restoration contours. This technique is described later.

Tooth Preparation

Similar to the Class III preparation, the tooth preparation for a Class IV direct composite restoration involves (1) creating access to the defective structure (caries, fracture, non-carious defect), (2) removal of faulty structures (caries, defective dentin and enamel, defective restoration and base material), and (3) creating the convenience form for the restoration. The tooth preparation for large incisoproximal areas requires more attention to the retention form than that for a small Class IV defect. If a large amount of tooth structure is missing and the restoration is in a high stress area, groove retention form may be indicated even when the preparation periphery is entirely in enamel. Also, enamel bevels can be increased in width to provide greater surface area for etching, resulting in a stronger bond between the composite and the tooth and potentially better esthetic result.

The treatment of teeth with minor coronal fractures requires minimal preparation. If the fracture is confined to enamel, adequate retention usually can be attained by simply beveling the sharp cavosurface margins in the fractured area with a flame-shaped diamond instrument followed by bonding (Fig. 9-21). Regardless of its size, the extensions of the Class IV direct composite preparation is ultimately dictated by the extension of the caries lesion, fracture, or failed restoration being replaced. The outline form is prepared to include weakened, friable enamel.

A maxillary right central incisor with a large defective Class III restoration and a fractured mesio-incisal corner, which necessitates a Class IV restoration, is illustrated in Figure 9-22, A. Using a round carbide bur or diamond instrument of appropriate size at high speed with air-water coolant, the outline form is prepared. All weakened enamel is removed, and the initial axial wall depth is established. As with the Class III tooth preparation, the final tooth preparation steps for a Class IV tooth preparation are, when indicated, (1) removal of infected dentin, (2) pulp protection, (3) bevel placement on accessible enamel margins, and (4) final procedures of cleaning and inspecting. The operator bevels the cavosurface margin of all accessible enamel margins of the preparation. The bevel is prepared at a 45-degree angle to the external tooth surface with a flame-shaped or round diamond instrument (see Fig. 9-22, B). The width of the bevel should be 0.5 to 2 mm, depending on the amount of tooth structure missing and the retention perceived necessary. The use of a scalloped, nonlinear bevel sometimes helps in masking the restoration margin.

Although retention for most Class IV direct composite restorations is provided primarily by bonding of the composite to enamel and dentin, when large incisoproximal areas are being restored, additional mechanical retention may be obtained by groove-shaped or other forms of undercuts, dovetail extensions, or a combination of these. If retention undercuts are deemed necessary, a gingival retention groove is prepared using a No. $\frac{1}{4}$ round bur. It is prepared 0.2 mm inside the DEJ at a depth of 0.25 mm (half the diameter of the No. $\frac{1}{4}$ round bur) and at an angle bisecting the junction of the axial wall and gingival wall. This groove should extend the length of the gingival floor and slightly up the facioaxial and linguoaxial line angles (see Fig. 9-22, C). No retentive undercut is usually needed at the incisal area, where mostly enamel exists. An optional dovetail extension onto the lingual surface of the tooth might enhance the restoration's strength and retention, but it is less conservative and not used often. Incisal and gingival retention and dovetail extension are illustrated in Fig. 9-23. Fig. 9-22, D, illustrates the completed large Class IV tooth preparation.

Restorative Technique
Matrix Application

Most Class IV composite restorations require a matrix to confine the restorative material excess and to assist in the development of the appropriate axial tooth contours, except for very small incisal edge enamel fractures, which can be restored using a free-hand technique. The Mylar strip matrix, described previously, also can be used for most Class IV preparations, although the strip's flexibility makes control of the matrix difficult. This difficulty may result in an over-contoured or under-contoured restoration, open contact, or both. Also, composite material extrudes incisally, but this excess can be easily removed when contouring and finishing.

Creasing (folding) the matrix at the position of the lingual line angle helps reduce the potential under-contouring (rounding) of that area of the restoration. The matrix is positioned and wedged as described for the Class III composite technique. Gingival overhangs and open contacts are common with any matrix techniques that do not employ gingival wedging. A commercially available preformed plastic or celluloid crown form is usually too thick and is not recommended as a matrix. Alternatively, a custom lingual matrix may be used for large Class IV preparations.[22] Figure 9-24, A, illustrates a large defective distofacial Class IV that needs to be replaced. The shade should be selected before isolating the area and removing the restorative material (see Fig. 9-24, B). Before the existing restoration is removed, the lingual matrix is prepared by using either a polyvinyl siloxane impression putty or a fast-set silicone matrix material. The operator records the lingual contours and, if possible, incisal contours of the existing restoration by using a small amount of the

17. Goracci G, Mori G: Scanning electron microscopic evaluation of resin-dentin and calcium hydroxide-dentin interface with resin composite restorations. *Quintessence Int* 27(2):129–135, 1996.

18. Reinhardt JW, Stephens NH, Fortin D: Effect of Gluma desensitization on dentin bond strength. *Am J Dent* 8(4):170–172, 1995.

19. Ritter AV, Bertoli C, Swift EJ, Jr: Dentin bond strengths as a function of solvent and glutaraldehyde content. *Am J Dent* 14(4):221–226, 2001.

20. Ritter AV, Swift EJ, Jr, Yamauchi M: Effects of phosphoric acid and glutaraldehyde-HEMA on dentin collagen. *Eur J Oral Sci* 109(5):348–353, 2001.

21. Schüpbach P, Lutz F, Finger WJ: Closing of dentinal tubules by GLUMA desensitizer. *Eur J Oral Sci* 105:414–421, 1997.

22. Dietschi D: Free-hand bonding in the esthetic treatment of anterior teeth: Creating the illusion. *J Esthet Dent* 9(4):156–164, 1997.

23. Ritter AV, Heymann HO, Swift EJ, Jr, et al: Clinical evaluation of an all-in-one adhesive in non-carious cervical lesions with different degrees of dentin sclerosis. *Oper Dent* 33(4):370–378, 2008.

24. Tay FR, Pashley DH: Resin bonding to cervical sclerotic dentin: A review. *J Dent* 32(3):173–196, 2004.

25. Yoshiyama M, Sano H, Ebisu S, et al: Regional strengths of bonding agents to cervical sclerotic root dentin. *J Dent Res* 75(6):1404–1413, 1996.

26. Mount GJ: Adhesion of glass-ionomer cement in the clinical environment. *Oper Dent* 16(4):141–148, 1991.

27. Swift EJ, Jr: Effects of glass ionomers on recurrent caries. *Oper Dent* 14(1):40–43, 1989.

28. Markovic D, Petrovic BB, Peric TO: Fluoride content and recharge ability of five glassionomer dental materials. *BMC Oral Health* 8:21, 2008.

Class I, II, and VI Direct Composite Restorations and Other Tooth-Colored Restorations

André V. Ritter, Ricardo Walter, Theodore M. Roberson

Class I, II, and VI Direct Composite Restorations

Posterior composite restorations were introduced in the late 1960s and early 1970s.[1-7] Because of the improved physical properties of composites and bonding systems, studies typically report successful results for their use in posterior teeth.[8-15] The American Dental Association (ADA) indicates the appropriateness of composites for use as pit-and-fissure sealants, preventive resin restorations, and Class I and II restorations for initial and moderate-sized lesions, using modified conservative tooth preparations.[16] The ADA further states that "when used correctly in the primary and permanent dentition, the expected lifetime of resin-based composites can be comparable to that of amalgam in Class I, Class II, and Class V restorations."[17] The longevity of posterior composites, however, is directly related to factors such as the size of the restoration, the patient's caries risk, and operator technique.[15,18-23]

This chapter presents information about typical Class I, II, and VI direct composite restorations (Fig. 10-1), also known as *posterior composite restorations*. The chapter also presents information and techniques for pit-and-fissure sealants, preventive resin or conservative composite restorations, extensive Class II restorations, and foundations.

Pertinent Material Qualities and Properties

As presented in Chapter 8, composite is a material that has sufficient strength for Class I and II restorations. It is insulative and, in most cases, does not require pulpal protection with bases. Because composite is bonded to enamel and dentin, tooth preparations for composite can be very conservative. A composite restoration not only is retained well in the tooth, but also can strengthen the remaining unprepared tooth structure.[24,25] Class I and II composite restorations also have all the other benefits of bonding presented in Chapters 4 and 8.

Indications

Class I, II, and VI direct composite restorations are indicated for the restoration of primary caries lesions in the occlusal (Class I and VI) and proximal (Class II) surfaces of posterior teeth. When used in posterior teeth, direct composite will perform best in small- and moderate-sized restorations, preferably with enamel margins. Because composites are tooth-colored, these restorations are particularly indicated when esthetics is considered to be of primary importance. They also are indicated occasionally as large restorations that may serve as foundations for crowns. Additionally, in selected cases, large composite restorations may be used where an interim restoration is indicated or where economics or other factors preclude a more definitive restoration such as a crown.

Contraindications

The main contraindication for use of composite for Class I, II, and VI restorations is an operating area that cannot be adequately isolated. Class I and II composites also may be contraindicated for large restorations when heavy occlusal stresses are present.[26] In restorations in which the proximal box extends onto the root surface, posterior composites should only be used if absolutely required because of the difficulty in predictably bonding to the gingival wall absent an enamel margin. Extended (deep) gingival margins also can be more difficult to light-activate owing to their location. Whenever a defect extends onto the root surface, negative effects for the restoration may occur, no matter what restorative material is being used. Any extension onto the root surface requires the best and most meticulous efforts of the operator to ensure a successful,

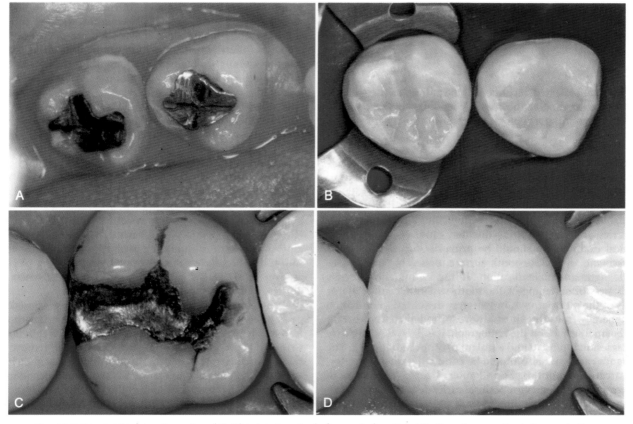

Fig. 10-1 Composite restorations. **A** and **B,** Class I composite, before and after. **C** and **D,** Class II composite, before and after.

long-lasting restoration. This chapter presents information of alternative restorative techniques for such cases.

Advantages

The advantages of composite as a Class I and II direct restorative material relative to other restorative materials are:

1. Esthetics
2. Conservative tooth structure removal
3. Easier, less complex tooth preparation
4. Insulation
5. Decreased microleakage
6. Increased short-term strength of remaining tooth structure[24,27]

Disadvantages

The disadvantages of Class I and II direct composite restorations are as follows:

1. Polymerization shrinkage effects
2. Lower fracture toughness than most indirect restorations
3. More technique-sensitive than amalgam restorations and some indirect restorations
4. Possible greater localized occlusal wear[28-30]
5. Unknown biocompatibility of some components (bisphenol A [BPA])

This chapter presents techniques for restoring the occlusal surface (including the occlusal thirds of facial and lingual surfaces) and proximal surface of posterior teeth with composite and other directly placed tooth-colored materials. The least invasive treatments are presented first, followed by progressively more involved methods of treatment. Consequently, the rationale and technique for pit-and-fissure sealants, preventive resin or conservative composite restorations, and Class VI composite restorations are presented first. Next, Class I and II composite restorations are presented, followed by composite foundations.

Pit-and-Fissure Sealants

Pits and fissures typically result from an incomplete coalescence of enamel and are particularly prone to caries. These areas can be sealed with a low-viscosity fluid resin after acid-etching. Long-term clinical studies indicate that pit-and-fissure sealants provide a safe and effective method of preventing caries.[31-33] In children, sealants are most effective when they are applied to the pits and fissures of permanent posterior teeth immediately on eruption of the clinical crowns, provided proper isolation can be achieved. Adults also can benefit from the use of sealants if the individual experiences an increase in caries susceptibility because of a change in diet, lack of adequate saliva, or a particular medical condition. Most currently used sealant materials are light-activated urethane dimethacrylate or BIS-GMA (bisphenol A–glycidyl methacrylate) resins. Opaquers and tints frequently are added to sealants to produce color contrast to aid in visual assessment.

Indications

Sealants are indicated, regardless of the patient's age, for either preventive or therapeutic uses, depending on the patient's caries risk, tooth morphology, or presence of incipient enamel caries.

In assessing the occlusal surfaces of posterior teeth as potential candidates for a sealant procedure, the primary decision is whether or not a cavitated lesion exists. This decision is based primarily on radiographic and clinical examinations, although other technologies for occlusal caries detection are available. Explorers must be used judiciously in the detection of caries, as a sharp explorer tine may cause a cavitation. The clinical examination should be primarily focused on visual assessments of a clean tooth surface, preferably under adequate light and magnification. If the examination reveals chalkiness or softening of the tooth structure at the base or walls of the pit or groove, brown-gray discoloration radiating peripherally from the pit or groove, or radiolucency beneath the enamel surface on the radiograph, it is likely that an active caries lesion is present and a sealant may not be indicated. The patient's caries risk also should be considered when considering treatment options. See Chapter 3 for a discussion of emerging technologies for occlusal caries detection and monitoring, including laser fluorescence and alternative current (AC) impedance spectroscopy.

When no cavitated caries lesion is diagnosed, the treatment decision is either to pursue no treatment or to place a pit-and-fissure sealant, particularly if the surface is at high risk for future caries. If a small caries lesion is detected, and the adjacent grooves and pits, although sound at the present time, are at risk for caries in the future, a preventive resin restoration or conservative composite restoration (which combines a small Class I composite with a sealant) may be the treatment recommendation. Before any of these treatments are initiated, the operator must be certain that no interproximal (Class II) caries or fault exists.

Although studies show that sealants can be applied over small, cavitated lesions, with no subsequent progression of caries, sealants should be used primarily for the prevention of caries rather than for the treatment of existing caries lesions.[34,35] A bitewing radiograph should be obtained and evaluated before sealant placement to ensure that no dentinal or proximal caries is evident. Only caries-free pits and fissures or incipient lesions in enamel not extending to the dentino-enamel junction (DEJ) currently are recommended for treatment with pit-and-fissure sealants.[36]

Clinical Technique

Because materials and techniques vary, it is important to follow the manufacturer's instructions for the sealant material being used. A standard method for applying sealants to posterior teeth is presented here. Each quadrant is treated separately and may involve one or more teeth. The following discussion deals with a fissure present on a mandibular first permanent molar (Fig. 10-2, A). The tooth is isolated by using a rubber dam (or another effective isolation method such as cotton rolls or Isolite). Isolation of the area is crucial to the success of the sealant. Sealant placement in younger patients is more common, and since molar teeth are often not fully erupted in these patients, isolation can be difficult. If proper isolation cannot be obtained, the bond of the sealant material to the tooth surface can be compromised, resulting in either loss of the sealant or caries under the sealant. The area is cleaned with a slurry of pumice on a bristle brush (see Fig. 10-2, B). Bristles reach into faulty areas better than a rubber prophy cup can, which tends to burnish debris and pumice into the pits and fissures. The tooth is rinsed thoroughly, while the explorer tip is used carefully to remove residual pumice or additional debris. The tooth surface is dried, and etched with 35% to 40% phosphoric acid for 15 to 30 seconds. Liquid acid etchants were used in the past, but gel etchants are more popular now because they are easier to apply and to control. However, only gels that are sufficiently fluid to penetrate the grooves and fissures should be used. Airborne particle abrasion techniques have been advocated for preparing pits and grooves before sealant placement, but their effectiveness has not been fully investigated yet.[37]

One technique that is used by many clinicians, especially in cases where occlusal caries could be present in deep grooves, is to lightly prepare the suspicious grooves with a thin flame-shaped diamond to lightly roughen the enamel, remove the fluoride-rich enamel that is more impervious to acid-etching, and open the grooves and fissures for better resin penetration. If caries is noted to extend toward the DEJ, the preparation is then approached as a preventive resin restoration (see the next section in this Chapter).

Properly acid-etched enamel surface has a lightly frosted appearance (see Fig. 10-2, C). Fluoride-rich, acid-resistant enamel may need to be etched for a longer time. Any brown stains that originally may have been in the pits and fissures still may be present and should be allowed to remain. The sealant material is then applied with an applicator or small hand instrument. The sealant is gently teased into place, to avoid entrapping air, and it should overfill slightly all pits and fissures, but it should not extend onto unetched surfaces. If too much sealant is applied, excess can be removed with a microbrush prior to light-activation. After light-activation and removal of the rubber dam, if used, the occlusion is evaluated by using articulating paper. If necessary, a round carbide finishing bur or white stone is used to remove any excess sealant. The surface usually does not require further polishing.

Preventive Resin and Conservative Composite Restorations

When restoring minimally carious pits and fissures on an unrestored tooth, an ultraconservative preparation design is recommended. This design allows for restoration of the lesion or defect with minimal removal of the tooth structure and often may be combined with the use of flowable composite or sealant to seal radiating non-carious fissures or pits that are at high risk for subsequent caries activity (Fig. 10-3). Originally referred to as a preventive resin restoration, this type of ultra-conservative restoration is now termed *conservative composite restoration* at the University of North Carolina.[38,39] An accurate diagnosis is essential before restoring the occlusal surface of a posterior tooth. The crucial factor in this clinical assessment

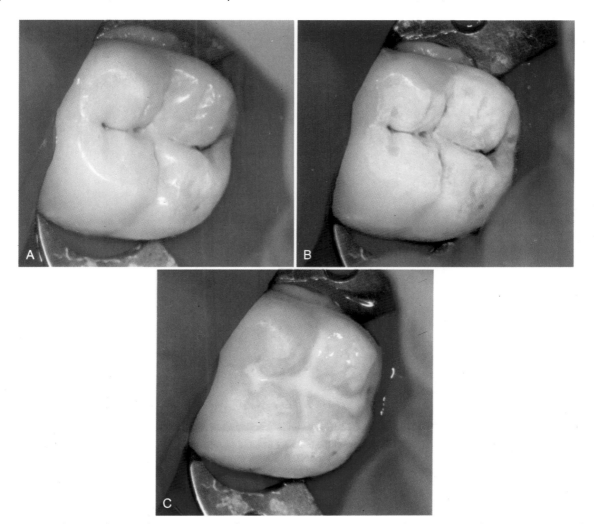

Fig.10-2 Steps in application of pit-and-fissure sealant. **A,** After isolation and thorough cleaning of the occlusal surface to be sealed. **B,** After acid-etching, rinsing, and drying. **C,** With sealant applied.

is whether or not the suspicious pit or fissure has active caries that requires restorative intervention. Usually, a conservative composite restoration is the treatment of choice for the primary occlusal caries lesion as the tooth preparation can be minimally invasive.

Sometimes, if a definitive diagnosis of caries cannot be made, an exploratory preparation of the suspicious area is performed with a small bur or diamond (Fig. 10-4). This approach is particularly indicated in patients at high risk for caries. The objective of this procedure is to explore suspicious pits or grooves with a very small bur or diamond to determine the extent of the suspected fault. As the tooth preparation is deepened, an assessment is made in the suspicious areas to determine whether or not to continue the preparation toward the DEJ (see Fig. 10-4, C). If the suspicious fault is removed or found to be sound at a shallow preparation depth (minimal dentin caries), the conservative exploratory preparation and adjacent pits and fissures are etched with 35% to 40% phosphoric acid for 15 to 30 seconds, rinsed thoroughly, and lightly dried. The etched surfaces then are treated with an adhesive, which is placed and light-activated, according to manufacturer's instructions. The conservatively prepared area can then be

restored with a flowable composite, which is placed and light-activated, according to manufacturer's instructions. The adjacent etched pits and fissures, if judged to be at risk, can then be sealed using a pit-and-fissure sealant or the same flowable composite following the technique described previously. If the suspicious area is found to be carious, the preparation depth is extended until all of the caries is removed, and the prepared area is then restored with composite as described later in this chapter (Class I direct composite restoration), and unprepared pits and fissures are sealed. In the example presented in Fig. 10-4, the preparation was restored with composite.

An example of a conservative composite restoration is illustrated in Figure 10-5, A. All initial examinations are inconclusive relative to a definitive diagnosis of active caries in this site. Figure 10-5, B through D, shows the initial, exploratory tooth preparation of the fissure. The initial depth is kept just into dentin where caries is present. Where caries is not present, the preparation stops on enamel. The occlusal extension is complete when a caries-free DEJ is reached. If dentin at the pulpal floor is judged to be infected as evidenced by a soft feel or "stick" of the explorer, a larger round bur, No. 330 bur or diamond, or No. 245 bur or diamond is used to extend the

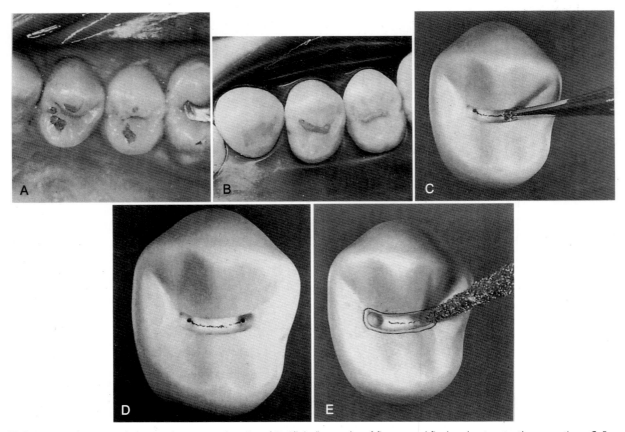

Fig. 10-5 Conservative composite restoration preparation. **A** and **B,** Clinical examples of fissures and final exploratory tooth preparations. **C,** Preparation is made with a No. 1 or No. 2 bur or similar diamond. **D,** Initial extensions. Pit remnants remain. **E,** Carious pits excavated and preparation roughened (*margins highlighted*).

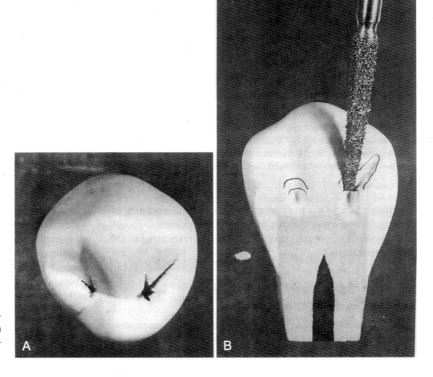

Fig. 10-6 Conservative composite restoration preparation. **A,** Two small, faulty pits are often present on a mandibular first premolar. **B,** Preparations are accomplished with coarse diamond.

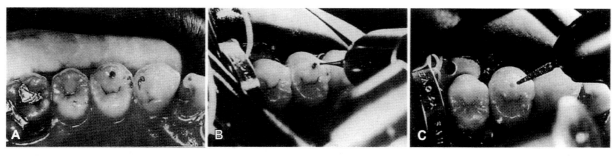

Fig. 10-7 Class VI tooth preparation for composite restoration. **A,** Class VI preparation on the facial cusp tip of the maxillary premolar. **B,** Entry with small round bur or diamond. **C,** Preparation roughened with diamond, if necessary.

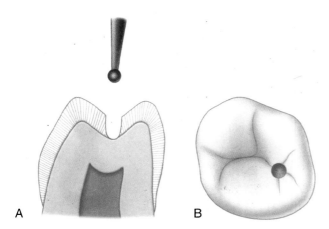

Fig. 10-8 Faciolingual cross-section of small Class I tooth preparation using round diamond.

angle may be more flared (obtuse) than if an elongated pearl instrument is used (Fig. 10-8).

Various cutting instruments may be used for Class I and II tooth preparations; the size and shape of the instrument generally are dictated by the size of the lesion or other defect or by the type of defective restoration being replaced. Both carbide and diamond instruments can be used effectively. It should be noted that diamond instruments create a thicker smear layer, however, which might make bonding more difficult for self-etch bonding systems.[40-43]

Moderate to Large Class I Direct Composite Restorations

Moderate to large Class I direct composite restorations, especially when used for larger caries lesions or to replace existing defective amalgam restorations, will typically feature flat walls that are perpendicular to occlusal forces, as well as strong tooth and restoration marginal configurations. All of these features help resist potential fracture in less conservative tooth preparations. However, the preparation should never be excessively extended beyond removal of faulty structures to justify resistance and retention forms, as this will weaken the tooth structure and can ultimately lead to failure of the tooth-restoration unit. If the occlusal portion of the restoration is expected to be extensive, elongated pearl cutting instruments with round features are preferred because they result in strong, 90-degree cavosurface margins. However, this box-like form

preparation may increase the negative effects of the configuration factor (C-factor). (See the section on inserting and light-activating the composite for other considerations regarding the C-factor for Class I direct composite restorations.) The objective of the tooth preparation is to remove all of the caries or fault as conservatively as possible. Because the composite is bonded to the tooth structure, other less involved, or at-risk, areas can be sealed as part of the conservative preparation techniques. Sealants may be combined with the Class I composite restoration, as described previously.

In large composite restorations, the tooth is entered in the area most affected by caries, with the elongated pearl diamond or bur positioned parallel to the long axis of the crown. When it is anticipated that the entire mesiodistal length of a central groove will be prepared, it is easier to enter the distal portion first and then transverse mesially. This technique permits better vision to the operator during the preparation. The pulpal floor is prepared to an initial depth that is approximately 0.2 mm internal to the DEJ (Fig. 10-9). The instrument is moved mesially, following the central groove, and any fall and rise of the DEJ (see Fig. 10-9, *B*). Mesial, distal, facial, and lingual extensions are dictated by the caries, old restorative material, or defect, always using the DEJ as a reference for both extensions and pulpal depth. The cuspal and marginal ridge areas should be preserved as much as possible. Although the final bonded composite restoration would help restore some of the strength of weakened, unprepared tooth structure, the outline form should be as conservative as possible. Extensions toward cusp tips should be as minimal as possible. Extensions into marginal ridges should result in at least 1.5 mm of remaining tooth structure (measured from the internal extension to the proximal height of contour) for premolars and approximately 2 mm for molars (Fig. 10-10). These limited extensions help preserve the dentinal support of the marginal ridge enamel and cusp tips.

As the instrument is moved along the central groove, the resulting pulpal floor is usually moderately flat (as a result of the shape of the tip of the instrument) and follows the rise and fall of the DEJ. If extension is required toward the cusp tips, the same depth that is approximately 0.2 mm inside the DEJ is maintained, usually resulting in the pulpal floor rising occlusally (Fig. 10-11). The same uniform depth concept also is appropriate when extending a facial or lingual groove radiating from the occlusal surface. When a groove extension is through the cusp ridge, the instrument prepares the facial (or lingual) portion of the faulty groove at an axial depth of 0.2 mm inside the DEJ and gingivally to include all caries and other defects (Fig. 10-12).

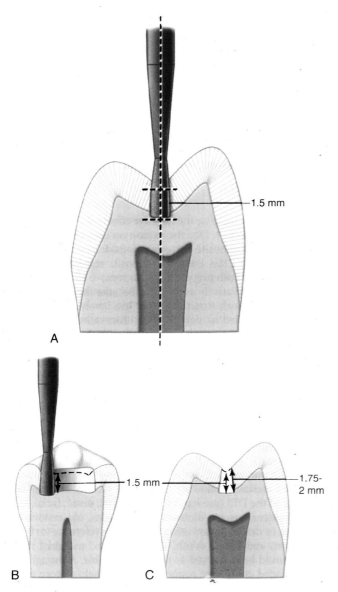

Fig. 10-9 **A,** Entry cut. Diamond or bur held parallel to the long axis of the crown. Initial pulpal depth is 1.5 mm from the central groove. When the central groove is removed, facial and lingual wall measurements usually are greater than 1.5 mm. (The steeper the wall, the greater is the height.) **B,** 1.5-mm depth from the central groove. **C,** Approximately 1.75- to 2-mm facial or lingual wall heights.

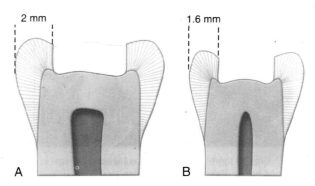

Fig. 10-10 Mesiodistal extension. Preserve dentin support of marginal ridge enamel. **A,** Molar. **B,** Premolar.

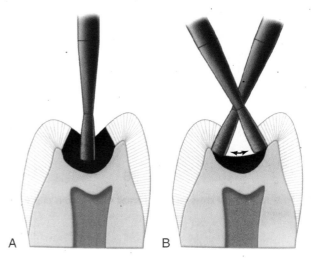

Fig. 10-11 **A,** After initial entry cut at correct initial depth (1.5 mm), the caries remains facially and lingually. **B,** Orientation of diamond or bur must be tilted as the instrument is extended facially or lingually to maintain a 1.5-mm depth.

After extending the outline form to sound tooth structure, if any caries or old restorative material remains on the pulpal floor, it should be removed with the appropriately-sized round bur or hand instrument. The occlusal margin is left as prepared. No attempt is made to place additional beveling on the occlusal margin because it may result in thin composite in areas of heavy occlusal contact. Because of the occlusal surface enamel rod direction, the ends of the enamel rods already are exposed by the preparation, which further reduces the need for occlusal bevels.

Although large, extensive posterior composite restorations may have some potential disadvantages when used routinely, "real world" dentistry sometimes necessitates esthetic treatment alternatives that may provide a needed service to the patient. Often, patients simply cannot afford a more expensive esthetic restoration, or they may have dental or medical conditions that preclude their placement. In such instances, large posterior composite restorations sometimes can be used as a reasonable alternative when more permanent options are not possible or realistic.

Restorative Technique
Placement of the Adhesive

Techniques for the placement of the adhesive are the same as described in Chapter 9. See Chapter 4 for a more extensive discussion on adhesives. When using an etch-and-rinse adhesive, over-drying the etched dentin can compromise dentin bonding.[44-46] Aqueous solutions containing glutaraldehyde and 2-hydroxyethyl methacrylate (HEMA) can be used as a re-wetting agent when using etch-and-rinse systems.[47-50] The bonding agent is applied to the entire preparation with a microbrush, in accordance with the manufacturer's instructions. After application, the adhesive is polymerized with a light-activation unit, as recommended by the manufacturer.

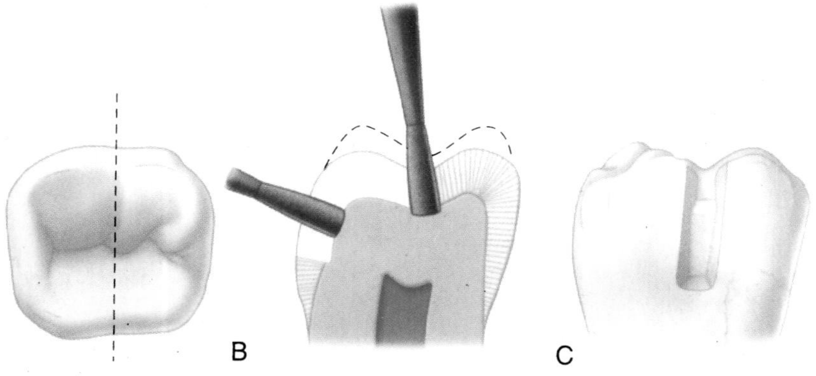

Fig. 10-12 Groove extension. **A,** Cross-section through the faciolingual groove area. **B,** Extension through cusp ridge at 1.5-mm initial pulpal depth; the facial wall depth is 0.2 mm inside the dentinoenamel junction (DEJ). **C,** Facial view.

When the final tooth preparation is judged to be near the pulp in vital teeth, the operator may elect to use a base material prior to placing the adhesive and the composite. If the remaining dentin thickness (RDT) is between 0.5 and 1.5 mm, a resin-modified glass ionomer (RMGI) base is used; if the RDT is less than 0.5 mm, a calcium hydroxide liner should be applied to the deepest aspect of the preparation, then protected with an RMGI base prior to adhesive placement.[51]

Insertion and Light-Activation of the Composite

A matrix is usually not necessary for Class I direct composite restorations, even when facial and lingual surface grooves are included. The composite should not be dispensed until it is ready to use because it may begin to polymerize from the ambient light in the operatory. Because of variations in materials, each manufacturer's specific instructions should be followed.

Composite insertion hand instruments or a compule may be used to insert the composite material. The dispenser, for example, a syringe or compule, must be kept covered when not in use to prevent premature hardening of the material. Small increments of composite material are added and successively light-activated (Fig. 10-13). It is important to place (and light-activate) the composite incrementally to maximize the polymerization depth of cure and possibly to reduce the negative effects of polymerization shrinkage.

The term "configuration factor" or "C-factor" has been used to describe the ratio of bonded to unbonded surfaces in a tooth preparation and restoration. A typical Class I tooth preparation will have a high C-factor of 5 (five bonded surfaces—pulpal, facial, lingual, mesial, and distal—vs. one unbonded surface—occlusal). The higher the C-factor of a tooth preparation, the higher the potential for composite polymerization shrinkage stress, as the composite shrinkage deformation is restricted by the bonded surfaces. Incremental insertion and light-activation of the composite may reduce the negative C-factor effects for Class I composite restorations.[52-55]

The use of an RMGI liner or a flowable composite liner also may reduce the effects of polymerization shrinkage stress because of their favorable elastic modulus (more elastic material will more effectively absorb polymerization stresses).[56,57] When composite is placed over an RMGI material, this technique is often referred to as a "sandwich" technique. The potential advantages of this technique are (1) the RMGI material bonds to the dentin without opening the dentinal tubules, reducing the potential for post-operative sensitivity;[58] (2) the RMGI material, because of its bond to dentin and potential for fluoride release (potential anti-cariogenicity), provides a better seal when used in cases where the preparation extends gingivally onto root structure;[59] and (3) the favorable elastic modulus of the RMGI reduces the effects of polymerization shrinkage stresses. These suggested advantages are considered controversial, as no published research based on longitudinal clinical trials evaluating the technique is available.

Flowable composites also are advocated as liners under posterior composite restorations. The purported primary advantage is that they may reduce some of the negative effects of polymerization shrinkage because of their very favorable elastic modulus.[60,61] Again, results are equivocal with regard to the available research.

When it is necessary to extend a composite restoration onto the root surface, the use of an RMGI liner beneath the portion of the restoration on the root surface may decrease microleakage, gap formation, and recurrent caries.[59,62-66] In those circumstances, the use of an RMGI material is a valid option. Likewise, the use of an RMGI, flowable composite, filled dentin adhesive, coupled with the incremental insertion and curing of the composite may offset the negative effects of a high C-factor for Class I composite restorations.[56,57]

Regardless of the effect of incremental placement on shrinkage stress, posterior composites should be placed incrementally to facilitate proper light-activation and development of correct anatomy. Especially in Class I direct composite restorations, the anatomic references of the occlusal unprepared tooth structure should guide the placement and shaping of the composite increments (see Figs. 10-1, *A* and *B*, 10-13, *G*, and 10-14, *I*). If needed, very deep portions of the tooth preparation are restored first, with increments of no more than 2 mm in thickness (see Fig. 10-13, *B*). The "enamel layer" of the restoration, that is, the occlusal 1.5-3 mm, should be placed using an anatomic layering technique.[20] The operator places and shapes the composite before it is light-activated so that the composite restores the occlusal anatomy of the tooth. Typically, the operator places and light-activates one increment per cusp at a time and continues to place subsequent increments until the preparation is filled and the occlusal anatomy is fully developed (see Fig. 10-13, *C* through *F*). The uncured composite can be shaped against the unprepared cusp inclines, which will result in a very natural anatomic

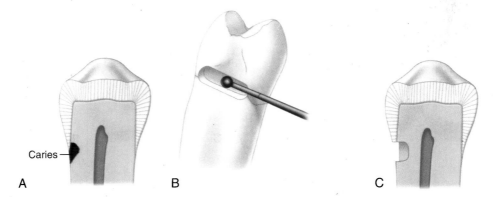

Fig.10-17 Facial or lingual slot preparation. **A,** Cervical caries on the proximal surface. **B,** The round diamond or bur enters the tooth from the accessible embrasure, oriented to the occlusogingival middle of the lesion. **C,** Slot preparation.

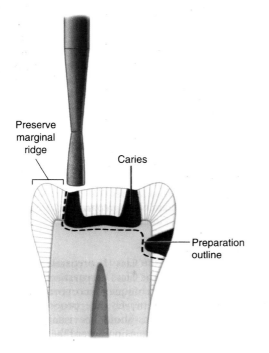

Fig. 10-18 When only one proximal surfaces is affected, the opposite marginal ridge should be maintained.

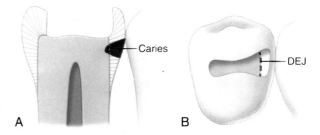

Fig.10-19 Occlusal extension into faulty proximal surface. **A** and **B,** Extension exposes the dentinoenamel junction (DEJ) but does not hit the adjacent tooth. Facial and lingual extensions as preoperatively visualized (see Fig. 10-9 for initial pulpal floor depth).

after the preparation outline, including the proximal box extensions, has been established.

Because the facial and lingual proximal extensions of the faulty proximal surface were visualized preoperatively, the occlusal extension toward that proximal surface begins to widen facially and lingually to begin to outline those extensions as conservatively as possible. Care is taken to preserve cuspal areas as much as possible during these extensions. At the same time, the instrument extends through the marginal ridge to within 0.5 mm of the outer contour of the marginal ridge. This extension exposes the proximal DEJ and protects the adjacent tooth (Fig. 10-19). At this time, the occlusal portion of the preparation is complete except for possible additional pulpal floor caries excavation. The occlusal walls

generally converge occlusally because of the inverted shape of the instrument.

PROXIMAL BOX

Typically, caries develops on a proximal surface immediately gingival to the proximal contact. The extent of the caries lesion and amount of old restorative material are two factors that dictate the facial, lingual, and gingival extensions of the proximal box of the preparation. Although it is not required to extend the proximal box beyond contact with the adjacent tooth (i.e., provide clearance with the adjacent tooth), it may simplify the preparation, matrix placement, and contouring procedures. If all of the defect can be removed without extending the proximal preparation beyond the contact, however, the restoration of the proximal contact with the composite is simplified (Fig. 10-20, *A*).

Before the instrument is extended through the marginal ridge, the proximal ditch cut is initiated. The operator holds the instrument over the DEJ with the tip of the instrument positioned to create a gingivally directed cut that is 0.2 mm inside the DEJ (see Fig. 10-20, *B* through *D*). For a No. 245 instrument with a tip diameter of 0.8 mm, this would require one-fourth of the instrument's tip positioned over the dentin side of the DEJ (the other three fourths of the tip over the enamel side). The instrument is extended facially, lingually, and gingivally to include all of the caries or old material, or both. The faciolingual cutting motion follows the DEJ and is

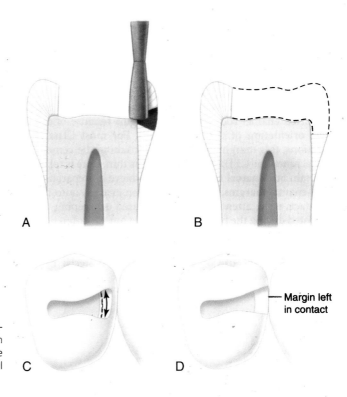

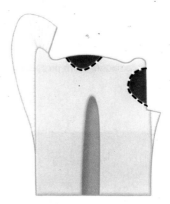

Fig. 10-20 **A,** The proximal wall may be left in contact with the adjacent tooth. **B,** Proximal ditch cut. The instrument is positioned such that gingivally directed cut creates the axial wall 0.2 mm inside the dentinoenamel junction (DEJ). **C,** Faciolingual direction of axial wall preparation follows the DEJ. **D,** Axial wall 0.2 mm inside the DEJ.

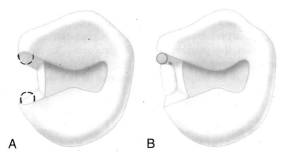

Fig. 10-21 Using a smaller instrument to prepare the cavosurface margin areas of facial and lingual proximal walls. **A,** Facial and lingual proximal margins undermined. **B,** Using a smaller instrument.

Fig. 10-22 Proximal extension. The enamel margin on the gingival floor is critical for bonding, so it should be preserved, if not compromised. Any remaining infected dentin on the axial wall (or the pulpal floor) is excavated as part of the final tooth preparation (as indicated by dotted lines).

usually in a slightly convex arc outward (see Fig. 10-21, *C*). During this entire cutting, the instrument is held parallel to the long axis of the tooth crown. The facial and lingual margins are extended as necessary and should result in at least a 90-degree margin, more obtuse being acceptable as well. If the preparation is conservative, a smaller, thinner instrument is used to complete the faciolingual wall formation, avoiding contact with the adjacent tooth (Fig. 10-21). Alternatively, a sharp hand instrument such as a chisel, hatchet, or a gingival margin trimmer can be used to finish the enamel wall. At this point, the remaining proximal enamel that was initially maintained to prevent damage to the adjacent tooth has been removed. The gingival floor is prepared flat (because of the tip of the instrument) with an approximately 90-degree cavosurface margin. Gingival extension should be as minimal as possible, in an attempt to maintain an enamel margin. The axial wall should be 0.2 mm inside the DEJ and have a slight

outward convexity. For large caries lesions, additional axial wall caries excavation may be necessary later, during final tooth preparation (Fig. 10-22).

If no carious dentin or other defect remains, the preparation is considered complete at this time (Fig. 10-23). Because the composite is retained in the preparation by micromechanical retention, no secondary preparation retention features are necessary. No bevels are placed on the occlusal cavosurface margins because these walls already have exposed enamel rod ends because of the enamel rod direction in this area. A bevel placed on an occlusal margin may result in thin composite on the occlusal surface in areas of potentially heavy contact. This feature also could result in fracture or wear of the composite in these areas. Beveled composite margins also may be more difficult to finish.

Bevels are rarely used on any of the proximal box walls because of the difficulty in restoring these areas, particularly when using inherently viscous packable composites. Bevels also are not recommended along the gingival margins of the proximal box; however, it is still necessary to remove any unsupported enamel rods along the margins because of the gingival orientation of the enamel rods. For most Class II preparations, this margin already is approaching the cementoenamel junction (CEJ), and the enamel is thin. Care is taken to maintain any enamel in this area to achieve a preparation with all-enamel margins. If the preparation extends onto the root surface, more attention must be focused on keeping the area isolated during the bonding technique, but no differences in tooth preparation are required. As noted earlier, when the gingival floor is on the root surface (no enamel at the cavo-surface margin), the use of a glass ionomer material may

decrease microleakage and recurrent caries.[59,62,63,65-67] Usually, the only remaining final tooth preparation procedure that might be necessary is additional excavation of carious dentin on either the pulpal floor or the axial wall. If necessary, a round bur or appropriate spoon excavator is used to remove any remaining caries.

Figure 10-24, *A*, illustrates an esthetic problem seen on the mesiofacial aspect of a maxillary first premolar as a result of extensive recurrent caries and existing faulty restoration. The preoperative occlusion assessment indicates that the facial cusp of the opposing mandibular premolar (which usually occludes on the mesial marginal ridge of the maxillary premolar) does not contact that area on this tooth (see Fig. 10-24, *B*). The existing occlusal amalgam on the maxillary second premolar also is determined to have extensive recurrent caries and is replaced with a composite during the same appointment.

After the operator cleans the teeth, administers local anesthetic, selects the shade of composite, and isolates the area, a wedge is placed in the gingival embrasure (see Fig. 10-24, *C*). Early wedging helps in the separation of teeth, to compensate later for the thickness of the matrix band, fulfilling one of several requirements for a good proximal contact for the composite restoration. The placement of a bitine ring preoperatively can achieve the same goal. The lack of pressure against the matrix during placement of composite compared with pressure of amalgam during its condensation dictates the need not only for increased separation by early wedging but also the need for operator alertness to verify matrix contact with the adjacent tooth before composite placement. The wedge also depresses and protects the rubber dam and gingival tissue when the proximal area is prepared. An additional, further tightening (insertion) of the wedge during tooth preparation may be helpful. The presence of the wedge during

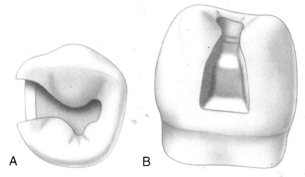

Fig. 10-23 Final Class II composite tooth preparation. **A,** Occlusal view. **B,** Proximal view.

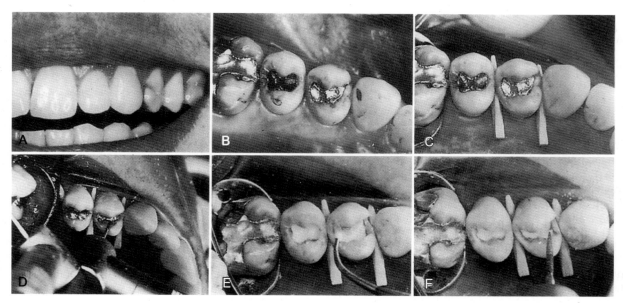

Fig. 10-24 Mesio-occlusal (MO) Class II tooth preparation for posterior composite restoration in the maxillary first premolar. **A,** Esthetic problem is caused by caries and existing amalgam restoration. **B,** In this patient, the mesial marginal ridge is not a centric holding area. **C,** Early wedging after rubber dam placement. **D,** An elongated pear bur or diamond is used for initial tooth preparations on both premolars. **E,** After extensive caries is excavated, a calcium hydroxide liner and a resin-modified glass ionomer (RMGI) base are inserted. **F,** Preparations are completed, if necessary, by roughening the prepared tooth structure with diamond instrument.

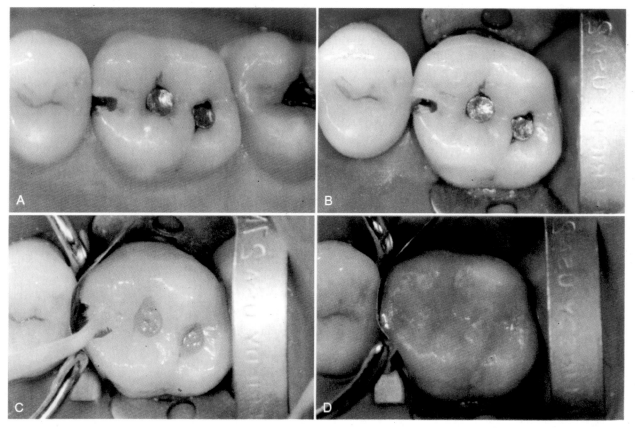

Fig. 10-25 Mesio-occlusal (MO) Class II direct composite restoration, which does not require a liner. **A,** Mesial primary caries and occlusal secondary caries exists preoperatively. **B,** Rubber dam isolation. **C,** Matrix application and placement of the adhesive. **D,** Insertion and light-activation of the composite. The completed restoration is shown in Fig. 10-28, *D*.

tooth preparation may serve as a guide to avoid overextension of the gingival floor.

A No. 245 bur or diamond is used to remove the existing amalgam restorations and to prepare the mesial surface of the first premolar in a conservative manner (see Fig. 10-24, *D*). A smaller instrument may be more appropriate if the lesion is smaller. A notable difference in the initial Class II preparation design for a composite restoration compared with that for an amalgam is the axial wall depth. When preparing the proximal box for a composite restoration, the axial wall initial depth usually is limited to 0.2 mm into dentin; this means that the tip of the No. 245 bur or diamond would be cutting approximately one-fourth in dentin and three-fourths in enamel to be most conservative. (The diameter of the No. 245 bur's tip end is 0.8 mm.) This decreased pulpal depth of the axial wall occurs because retention locks usually are unnecessary; the decreased depth provides greater conservation of the tooth structure. The occlusal walls may converge occlusally (because of the inverted shape of the No. 245 bur or diamond), and the proximal walls may be parallel or convergent occlusally. Preparing convergent proximal walls provides additional retention form, when needed.

The initial preparation is completed as previously described. With a round bur or spoon excavator, the operator removes any remaining infected dentin and any stains that show through the mesiofacial enamel. In this example, a calcium hydroxide liner and an RMGI base were applied over the

deeply excavated area (see Fig. 10-24, *E*). Because of the removal of the amalgam and extensive caries, many areas of the enamel are left unsupported by dentin but are not friable. This undermined, but not friable, enamel is not removed. At this time, the tooth preparation is complete (see Fig. 10-24, *F*).

If a composite restoration is properly bonded to the preparation walls, such as in preparations with all-enamel margins, little or no potential for microleakage and pulpal complications exists. A calcium hydroxide liner is indicated, however, to treat a near-exposure of the pulp (within 0.5 mm of the pulp), a possible micro-exposure, or an actual exposure. If used, the calcium hydroxide liner is covered with an RMGI base to protect it from dissolution during the bonding procedures.[51,68] Otherwise, neither a liner nor a base is indicated in Class II tooth preparations for composite (Fig. 10-25). It is desirable not to cover any portion of the dentinal walls with a liner, unless necessary, because the liner would decrease dentin bonding potential.

Restorative Technique
Matrix Application

One of the most important steps in restoring Class II preparations with direct composites is the selection and proper placement of the matrix. In contrast to amalgam, which can be condensed to improve the proximal contact, Class II composites are almost totally dependent on the contour and position of the matrix for establishing appropriate proximal contacts. Early wedging and re-tightening of the wedge during tooth preparation aid in achieving sufficient separation of teeth to compensate for the thickness of the matrix band. Before placing the composite material, the matrix band must be in absolute contact with (touching) the adjacent contact area.

Generally, the matrix is applied before adhesive placement. An ultra-thin metal matrix band generally is preferred for the restoration of a Class II composite because it is thinner than a typical metal band and can be contoured better than a clear polyester matrix. No significant problems are experienced in placing and light-activating composite material when using a metal matrix as long as small incremental additions (2 mm each or less) are used.

Although a Tofflemire-type matrix can be used for restoring a two-surface tooth preparation, pre-contoured sectional metallic matrices are preferable (Fig. 10-26), because only one thickness of metal matrix material is encountered instead of two, making contact generation easier. These sectional matrices are relatively easy to use, very thin, and come in different sizes that can be used according to the clinical situation. There are several systems available, and selection is based on operator preference. These systems may use a bitine ring to (1) aid in stabilizing the matrix band and (2) provide additional tooth separation while the composite is inserted. The primary benefit of these systems is a simpler method for establishing an appropriate composite proximal contour and contact. Use of these systems for restoring wide faciolingual proximal preparations requires careful application; otherwise, the bitine ring prongs may cause deformation of the matrix band, resulting in a poor restoration contour.

When both proximal surfaces are involved, a Tofflemire retainer with an ultra-thin (0.001 inch), burnishable matrix band is used. The band is contoured, positioned, wedged, and shaped, as needed, for proper proximal contacts and embrasures. Before placement, the metal matrix band for posterior composites should be burnished on a paper pad to impart proper proximal contour to the band (the same as a matrix for amalgam). Alternatively, an ultra-thin precontoured metal matrix band may be used in the Tofflemire retainer.

If the Tofflemire matrix band is open excessively along the lingual margins of the preparation (usually because of the contour of the tooth), a "tinner's joint" can be used to close the matrix band. This joint is made by grasping the lingual portion of the matrix band with No. 110 pliers and cinching the band tightly together above the height of contour of the

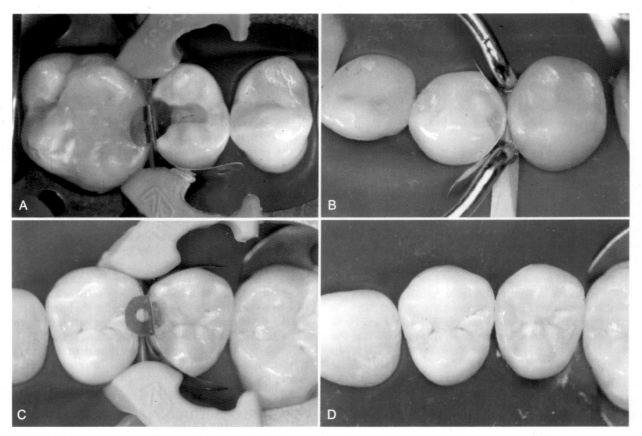

Fig. 10-26 Sectional matrix systems for posterior composites. **A,** Sectional matrix system in place with plastic wedge and bitine ring to restore the maxillary premolar with direct composite. **B,** Sectional matrix system in place with wooden wedge and bitine ring to restore the mandibular premolar with direct composite. **C,** Sectional matrix system in place with plastic wedge and bitine ring to restore the maxillary premolar with direct composite. **D,** Case presented in C after placement and light-activation of the composite, and matrix removal, before any contouring. Note minimal excess composite as a result of good matrix adaptation to facial and lingual embrasures.

completed, the occlusion is adjusted as necessary, and the restoration is polished. Because these very large restorations may stretch the limits of composite restorations, the patient should be on a frequent recall regimen.

Figure 10-31 illustrates an extensive Class II modified tooth preparation. A maxillary first premolar is badly discolored from a large, faulty, corroded amalgam restoration and caries

(see Fig. 10-31, *A* and *B*). Esthetic and economic factors resulted in the decision to replace the amalgam with a composite restoration, rather than an indirect restoration. The preparation is shown with all of the old amalgam and infected dentin removed, leaving the facial and lingual enamel walls severely weakened (see Fig. 10-31, *C*). After placement of a calcium hydroxide liner and an RMGI base over the deeply

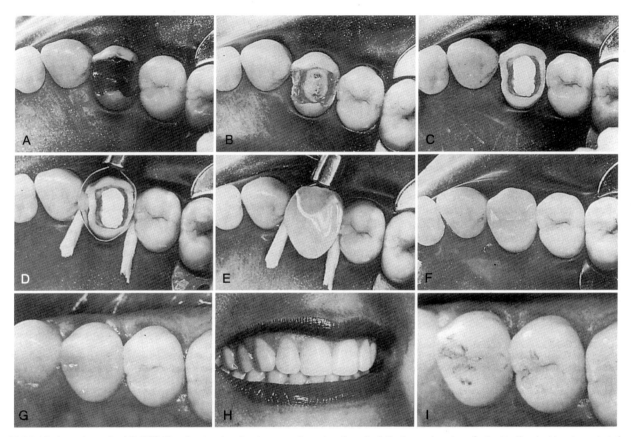

Fig. 10-31 Mesio-occluso-distal (MOD) Class II extensive direct composite restoration. **A,** Esthetics and cost are factors in the decision to replace faulty restoration with posterior composite. **B,** Amalgam and infected dentin removed. **C,** Calcium hydroxide liner and a resin-modified glass ionomer (RMGI) base inserted. **D,** Matrix in place. **E,** Composite has been placed incrementally. **F,** After inserting and polishing composite restoration. **G–I,** Occlusal (G) and facial (H) views after 5 years of service. **I,** Occlusion marked with articulating paper at 5-year follow-up appointment.

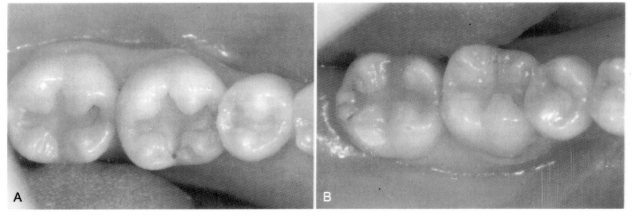

Fig. 10-32 Class I composite restorations at 30 years of service.

excavated area (see Fig. 10-31, *D*), a diamond was used to reduce the severely undermined enamel of the lingual cusp approximately 1.5 mm (functional cusp) and to place a reverse bevel with a chamfered margin on the lingual surface. The same instrument was used to reduce the facial cusp 0.75 mm (nonfunctional cusp) and to place a slight counterbevel. Figure 10-31, *E* and *F*, shows the matrix placement and composite insertion. The completed restoration is shown in Figure 10-31, *G*, and, after 5 years of service, in Figure 10-31, *H* through *I*. This extensive tooth preparation has been observed to be successful but not from controlled clinical research studies.

Summary

This chapter has presented the rationale and technique for composite use in the treatment of the occlusal and proximal surfaces of posterior teeth. The use of composite as the restorative material for many Class I and II restorations is emphasized not only by this chapter but by this entire textbook as well. This emphasis is not based on concerns about the use of amalgam as a restorative material. As subsequent chapters will show, amalgam restorations are still strongly recommended in this book. Regardless, many Class I and II lesions are best restored with composite, which presents adequate longevity when properly placed (Fig. 10-32). Typical problems, solutions, and repair techniques for composite restorations are presented in Chapter 8.

References

1. McCune RJ: Clinical comparison of anterior and posterior restorative materials. *Int Assoc Dent Res* (abstract no. 482), 1969.
2. McCune RJ: Clinical comparison of posterior restorative materials. *Int Assoc Dent Res* (abstract no. 546), 1967.
3. Ambrose ER, Leith DR, Pinchuk M, et al: Manipulation and insertion of a composite resin for anterior and posterior cavity preparations. *J Can Dent Assoc (Tor)* 37(5):188–195, 1971.
4. Denehy GE: Posterior splinting with the composite resins. *Dent Dig* 77(12):694–699, 1971.
5. Durnan JR: Esthetic dental amalgam-composite resin restorations for posterior teeth. *J Prosthet Dent* 25(3):175–176, 1971.
6. Phillips RW, Avery DR, Mehra R, et al: Observations on a composite resin for Class II restorations: Three-year report. *J Prosthet Dent* 30(6):891–897, 1973.
7. Leinfelder KF, Sluder TB, Sockwell CL, et al: Clinical evaluation of composite resins as anterior and posterior restorative materials. *J Prosthet Dent* 33(4):407–416, 1975.
8. Barnes DM, Blank LW, Thompson VP, et al: A 5- and 8-year clinical evaluation of a posterior composite resin. *Quintessence Int* 22(2):143–151, 1991.
9. Heymann HO, Wilder AD, Jr, May KN, Jr, et al: Two-year clinical study of composite resins in posterior teeth. *Dent Mater* 2(1):37–41, 1986.
10. Studervant JR, Lundeen TF, Sluder TB, et al: Five-year study of two light-cured posterior composite resins. *Dent Mater* 4:105–110, 1988.
11. Wilson NH, Norman RD: Five-year findings of a multiclinical trial for a posterior composite. *J Dent* 19(3):153–159, 1991.
12. Wilder AD, Jr, May KN, Jr, Bayne SC, et al: Seventeen-year clinical study of ultraviolet-cured posterior composite Class I and II restorations. *J Esthet Dent* 11(3):135–142, 1999.
13. Mazer RB, Isenberg BP, Wright WW, et al: Clinical evaluation of a posterior composite resin containing a new type of filler particle. *J Esthet Dent* 1:66–70, 1988.
14. Mazer RB, Leinfelder KF: Evaluating a microfill posterior composite resin. A five-year study. *J Am Dent Assoc* 123(4):32–38, 1992.
15. Opdam NJ, Bronkhorst EM, Loomans BA, et al: 12-year survival of composite vs. amalgam restorations. *J Dent Res* 89(10):1063–1067, 2010.
16. American Dental Association Council on Scientific Affairs, ADA Council on Dental Benefits and Programs: Statement on posterior resin-based composites. *J Am Dent Assoc* 126:1627–1628, 1998.
17. American Dental Association: Intervention: Pit and fissure sealants. *J Am Dent Assoc* 126:17S–18S, 1995.
18. Opdam NJ, Bronkhorst EM, Cenci MS, et al: Age of failed restorations: A deceptive longevity parameter. *J Dent*, 39(3):225–230, 2010.
19. Raj V, Macedo GV, Ritter AV: Longevity of posterior composite restorations. *J Esthet Restor Dent* 19(1):3–5, 2007.
20. Ritter AV: Posterior composites revisited. *J Esthet Restor Dent* 20(1):57–67, 2008.
21. Kohler B, Rasmusson CG, Odman P: A five-year clinical evaluation of Class II composite resin restorations. *J Dent* 28(2):111–116, 2000.
22. Soncini JA, Maserejian NN, Trachtenberg F, et al: The longevity of amalgam versus compomer/composite restorations in posterior primary and permanent teeth: Findings from the New England Children's Amalgam Trial. *J Am Dent Assoc* 138(6):763–772, 2007.
23. van Dijken JW: Durability of resin composite restorations in high C-factor cavities: A 12-year follow-up. *J Dent* 38(6):469–474, 2010.
24. Ausiello P, De Gee AJ, Rengo S, et al: Fracture resistance of endodontically-treated premolars adhesively restored. *Am J Dent* 10(5):237–241, 1997.
25. Santos MJ, Bezerra RB: Fracture resistance of maxillary premolars restored with direct and indirect adhesive techniques. *J Can Dent Assoc* 71(8):585, 2005.
26. Ferracane JL: Is the wear of dental composites still a clinical concern? Is there still a need for in vitro wear simulating devices? *Dent Mater* 22(8):689–692, 2006.
27. Liberman R, Ben-Amar A, Gontar G, et al: The effect of posterior composite restorations on the resistance of cavity walls to vertically applied occlusal loads. *J Oral Rehabil* 17(1):99–105, 1990.
28. Collins CJ, Bryant RW, Hodge KL: A clinical evaluation of posterior composite resin restorations: 8-year findings. *J Dent* 26(4):311–317, 1998.
29. Mair LH: Ten-year clinical assessment of three posterior resin composites and two amalgams. *Quintessence Int* 29(8):483–490, 1998.
30. Kramer N, Reinelt C, Richter G, et al: Nanohybrid vs. fine hybrid composite in Class II cavities: Clinical results and margin analysis after four years. *Dent Mater* 25(6):750–759, 2009.
31. Simonsen RJ: Retention and effectiveness of a single application of white sealant after 10 years. *J Am Dent Assoc* 115(1):31–36, 1987.
32. Swift EJ, Jr: The effect of sealants on dental caries: A review. *J Am Dent Assoc* 116(6):700–704, 1988.
33. Ahovuo-Saloranta A, Hiiri A, Nordblad A, et al: Pit and fissure sealants for preventing dental decay in the permanent teeth of children and adolescents. *Cochrane Database Syst Rev* (3):CD001830, 2004.
34. Handelman SL, Leverett DH, Espeland MA, et al: Clinical radiographic evaluation of sealed carious and sound tooth surfaces. *J Am Dent Assoc* 113(5):751–754, 1986.
35. Mertz-Fairhurst, EJ, Smith CD, Williams JE, et al: Cariostatic and ultraconservative sealed restorations: Six-year results. *Quintessence Int* 23(12):827–838, 1992.
36. Beauchamp J, Caufield PW, Crall JJ, et al: Evidence-based clinical recommendations for the use of pit-and-fissure sealants: A report of the American Dental Association Council on Scientific Affairs. *J Am Dent Assoc* 139(3):257–268, 2008.
37. Bendinskaite R, Peciuliene V, Brukiene V: A five years clinical evaluation of sealed occlusal surfaces of molars. *Stomatologija* 12(3):87–92, 2010.
38. Simonsen RJ: Preventive resin restorations (I). *Quintessence Int Dent Dig* 9(1):69–76, 1978.
39. Simonsen RJ: Preventive resin restorations: Three-year results. *J Am Dent Assoc* 100(4):535–539, 1980.
40. Chan KM, Tay FR, King NM, et al: Bonding of mild self-etching primers/adhesives to dentin with thick smear layers. *Am J Dent* 16(5):340–346, 2003.
41. Ogata M, Harada N, Yamaguchi S, et al: Effect of self-etching primer vs phosphoric acid etchant on bonding to bur-prepared dentin. *Oper Dent* 27(5):447–454, 2002.
42. Oliveira SS, Pugach MK, Hilton JF, et al: The influence of the dentin smear layer on adhesion: A self-etching primer vs. a total-etch system. *Dent Mater* 19(8):758–767, 2003.
43. Tani C, Finger WJ: Effect of smear layer thickness on bond strength mediated by three all-in-one self-etching priming adhesives. *J Adhes Dent* 16:340–346, 2003.
44. Gwinnett AJ: Moist versus dry dentin: Its effect on shear bond strength. *Am J Dent* 5(3):127–129, 1992.
45. Gwinnett AJ, Kanca JA, 3rd: Micromorphology of the bonded dentin interface and its relationship to bond strength. *Am J Dent* 5(2):73–77, 1992.

46. Heymann HO, Bayne SC: Current concepts in dentin bonding: Focusing on dentinal adhesion factors. *J Am Dent Assoc* 124(5):26–36, 1993.

47. Hansen EK, Asmussen E: Improved efficacy of dentin-bonding agents. *Eur J Oral Sci* 105(5 Pt 1):434–439, 1997.

48. Reinhardt JW, Stephens NH, Fortin D: Effect of Gluma desensitization on dentin bond strength. *Am J Dent* 8(4):170–172, 1995.

49. Schüpbach P, Lutz F, Finger WJ: Closing of dentinal tubules by GLUMA desensitizer. *Eur J Oral Sci* 105:414–421, 1997.

50. Ritter AV, Bertoli C, Swift EJ, Jr: Dentin bond strengths as a function of solvent and glutaraldehyde content. *Am J Dent* 14(4):221–226, 2001.

51. Ritter AV, Swift EJ: Current restorative concepts of pulp protection. *Endod Topics* 5:41–48, 2003.

52. Tantbirojn D, Pfeifer CS, Braga RR, et al: Do low-shrink composites reduce polymerization shrinkage effects? *J Dent Res* 90(5):596–601, 2011.

53. Versluis A, Douglas WH, Cross M, et al: Does an incremental filling technique reduce polymerization shrinkage stresses? *J Dent Res* 75(3):871–878, 1996.

54. Versluis A, Tantbirojn D: Theoretical considerations of contraction stress. *Compend Contin Educ Dent Suppl* (25):S24–S32; quiz S73, 1999.

55. Versluis A, Tantbirojn D, Pintado MR, et al: Residual shrinkage stress distributions in molars after composite restoration. *Dent Mater* 20(6):554–564, 2004.

56. Ikemi T, Nemoto K: Effects of lining materials on the composite resins shrinkage stresses. *Dent Mater J* 13(1):1–8, 1994.

57. Tolidis K, Nobecourt A, Randall RC: Effect of a resin-modified glass ionomer liner on volumetric polymerization shrinkage of various composites. *Dent Mater* 14(6):417–423, 1998.

58. Browning WD: The benefits of glass ionomer self-adhesive materials in restorative dentistry. *Compend Contin Educ Dent* 27(5):308–314; quiz 315–316, 2006.

59. Loguercio AD, Alessandra R, Mazzocco KC, et al: Microleakage in class II composite resin restorations: Total bonding and open sandwich technique. *J Adhes Dent* 4(2):137–144, 2002.

60. Chuang SF, Jin YT, Liu JK, et al: Influence of flowable composite lining thickness on Class II composite restorations. *Oper Dent* 29(3):301–308, 2004.

61. Olmez A, Oztas N, Bodur H: The effect of flowable resin composite on microleakage and internal voids in class II composite restorations. *Oper Dent* 29(6):713–719, 2004.

62. Andersson-Wenckert IE, van Dijken JW, Horstedt P: Modified Class II open sandwich restorations: Evaluation of interfacial adaptation and influence of different restorative techniques. *Eur J Oral Sci* 110(3):270–275, 2002.

63. Besnault C, Attal JP: Simulated oral environment and microleakage of class II resin-based composite and sandwich restorations. *Am J Dent* 16:186–190, 2003.

64. Donly KJ: Enamel and dentin demineralization inhibition of fluoride-releasing materials. *Am J Dent* 7(5):275–278, 1994.

65. Nagamine M, Itota T, Torii Y, et al: Effect of resin-modified glass ionomer cements on secondary caries. *Am J Dent* 10(4):173–178, 1997.

66. Souto M, Donly KJ: Caries inhibition of glass ionomers. *Am J Dent* 7(2):122–124, 1994.

67. Murray PE, Hafez AA, Smith AJ, et al: Bacterial microleakage and pulp inflammation associated with various restorative materials. *Dent Mater* 18(6):470–478, 2002.

68. Goracci G, Mori G: Scanning electron microscopic evaluation of resin-dentin and calcium hydroxide-dentin interface with resin composite restorations. *Quintessence Int* 27(2):129–135, 1996.

69. Elsayad I: Cuspal movement and gap formation in premolars restored with preheated resin composite. *Oper Dent* 34(6):725–731, 2009.

70. Fróes-Salgado NR, Silva LM, Kawano Y, et al: Composite pre-heating: Effects on marginal adaptation, degree of conversion and mechanical properties. *Dent Mater* 26(9):908–914, 2010.

71. Wagner WC, Aksu MN, Neme AM, et al: Effect of pre-heating resin composite on restoration microleakage. *Oper Dent* 33(1):72–78, 2008.

72. da Costa J, McPharlin R, Hilton T, et al: Effect of heat on the flow of commercial composites. *Am J Dent* 22(2):92–96, 2009.

73. Daronch M, Rueggeberg FA, Hall G, et al: Effect of composite temperature on in vitro intrapulpal temperature rise. *Dent Mater* 23(10):1283–1288, 2007.

74. Rueggeberg FA, Daronch M, Browning WD, et al: In vivo temperature measurement: Tooth preparation and restoration with preheated resin composite. *J Esthet Restor Dent* 22(5):314–322, 2010.

75. Sanares AM, Itthagarun A, King NM, et al: Adverse surface interactions between one-bottle light-cured adhesives and chemical-cured composites. *Dent Mater* 17(6):542–556, 2001.

76. Swift EJ, Jr, May KN, Jr, Wilder AD, Jr: Effect of polymerization mode on bond strengths of resin adhesive/cement systems. *J Prosthodont* 7(4):256–260, 1998.

Chapter 11

Dental Caries: Etiology, Clinical Characteristics, Risk

Edward J. Swift, Jr., John R. Sturdevant, Lee W. Boushell

Class I and II Indirect Tooth-Colored Restorations

Chapters 8, 9, and 10 describe *direct* tooth-colored composite restorations. Teeth also can be restored using *indirect* techniques, in which restorations are fabricated outside of the patient's mouth. Indirect restorations are made on a replica of the prepared tooth in a dental laboratory or by using computer-aided design/computer-assisted manufacturing (CAD/CAM) either chairside or in the dental laboratory (Fig. 11-1). This chapter reviews the indications, contraindications, advantages, disadvantages, and clinical techniques for Class I and II indirect tooth-colored restorations.

Indications

The indications for Class I and II indirect tooth-colored restorations are based on a combination of esthetic demands and restoration size and include the following:

- *Esthetics:* Indirect tooth-colored restorations are indicated for Class I and II restorations (inlays and onlays) located in areas of esthetic importance for the patient.
- *Large defects or previous restorations:* Indirect tooth-colored restorations should be considered for restoration of large Class I and II defects or replacement of large compromised existing restorations, especially those that are wide faciolingually or require cusp coverage. Large intracoronal preparations are best restored with adhesive restorations that strengthen the remaining tooth structure.[1-3] The contours of large restorations are more easily developed using indirect techniques. Wear resistance of direct composite resins has improved greatly over the years and is not a concern with small- to moderate-sized restorations.[4] However, in larger restorations, indirect restorative materials should be considered.[5]

Contraindications

Contraindications for indirect tooth-colored restorations include the following:

- *Heavy occlusal forces:* Ceramic restorations can fracture when they lack sufficient thickness or are subject to excessive occlusal stress, as in patients who have bruxing or clenching habits.[6] Heavy wear facets or a lack of occlusal enamel are good indicators of bruxing and clenching habits (Fig. 11-2).
- *Inability to maintain a dry field:* Despite limited research suggesting that some contemporary dental adhesives might counteract certain types of contamination, adhesive techniques require near-perfect moisture control to ensure successful long-term clinical results.[7-9]
- *Deep subgingival preparations:* Although this is not an absolute contraindication, preparations with deep subgingival margins generally should be avoided. These margins are difficult to record with an elastomeric or even a digital impression and are difficult to evaluate and finish. Additionally, dentin bond strengths at gingival floors are not particularly good, so bonding to enamel margins is greatly preferred, especially along gingival margins of proximal boxes.[10,11]

Advantages

Except for the higher cost and increased time, the advantages of indirect tooth-colored restorations are similar to the advantages of direct composite restorations. Indirect tooth-colored restorations have the following additional advantages:

- *Improved physical properties:* A wide variety of high-strength tooth-colored restorative materials, including laboratory-processed and computer-milled ceramics, can be used with indirect techniques. These have better physical properties than direct composite materials because they are fabricated under relatively ideal laboratory conditions. For CAD/CAM restorations, although some are fabricated chairside, the materials themselves are manufactured under nearly ideal industrial conditions.[12]

- *Variety of materials and techniques:* Indirect tooth-colored restorations can be fabricated with ceramics using traditional laboratory processes or using chairside or laboratory CAD/CAM methods.
- *Wear resistance:* Ceramic restorations are more wear resistant than direct composite restorations, an especially important factor when restoring large occlusal areas of posterior teeth.
- *Reduced polymerization shrinkage:* Polymerization shrinkage and its resulting stresses are a major shortcoming of direct composite restorations. With indirect techniques, the bulk of the preparation is filled with the indirect tooth-colored restoration, and stresses are reduced because little resin cement is used during cementation. Although shrinkage of resin materials in thin bonded layers can produce relatively high stress, clinical studies indicate ceramic

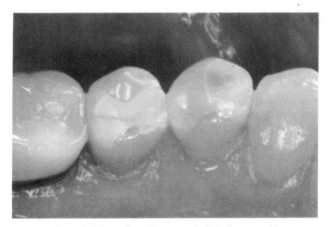

Fig. 11-1 Ceramic inlays after 23 years of clinical service. These were fabricated with an early computer-aided design/computer-assisted manufacturing (CAD/CAM) device.

inlays and onlays have better marginal adaptation, anatomic form, color match, and overall survival rates than do direct composite restorations.[5,13,14]

- *Support of remaining tooth structure:* Teeth weakened by caries, trauma, or preparation can be strengthened by adhesively bonding indirect tooth-colored restorations.[1-3] The reduced polymerization shrinkage stress associated with the indirect technique also is desirable when restoring such weakened teeth.
- *More precise control of contours and contacts:* Indirect techniques usually provide better contours (especially proximal contours) and occlusal contacts than do direct restorations because of the improved access and visibility outside the mouth.
- *Biocompatibility and good tissue response:* Ceramics are considered chemically inert materials with excellent biocompatibility and soft tissue response.[15] The pulpal biocompatibility of the indirect techniques is related more to the resin cements than to the ceramic materials used.
- *Increased auxiliary support:* Most indirect techniques allow the fabrication of the restoration to be delegated totally or partially to the dental laboratory. Such delegation allows for more efficient use of the dentist's time.

Disadvantages

The following are disadvantages of indirect tooth-colored restorations:

- *Increased cost and time:* Most indirect techniques, except for chairside CAD/CAM methods, require two patient appointments plus fabrication of a provisional restoration. These factors, along with laboratory fees, contribute to the higher cost of indirect restorations in comparison with direct restorations. Although indirect tooth-colored inlays and onlays are more expensive than amalgam or direct composite restorations, they are usually less costly than more invasive esthetic alternatives such as all-ceramic or porcelain-fused-to-metal (PFM) crowns.
- *Technique sensitivity:* Restorations made using indirect techniques require a high level of operator skill. A devotion

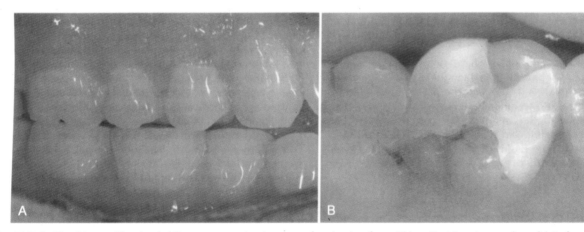

Fig. 11-2 A, Clenching and bruxing habits can cause extensive wear of occlusal surfaces. This patient is not a good candidate for ceramic inlays. **B,** Example of a fractured onlay in a patient with heavy occlusion.

to excellence is necessary during preparation, impression, try-in, bonding, and finishing the restoration.

- *Difficult try-in and delivery:* Indirect composite restorations can be polished intraorally using the same instruments and materials used to polish direct composites, although access to some marginal areas can be difficult. Ceramics are more difficult to polish because of potential resin-filled marginal gaps and the hardness of the ceramic surfaces.
- *Brittleness of ceramics:* A ceramic restoration can fracture if the preparation does not provide adequate thickness to resist occlusal forces or if the restoration is not appropriately supported by the resin cement and the preparation. With weaker ceramic materials, fractures can occur even during try-in and bonding procedures.[16]
- *Wear of opposing dentition and restorations:* Some ceramic materials can cause excessive wear of opposing enamel or restorations.[17] Improvements in materials have reduced this problem, but ceramics, particularly if rough and unpolished, can wear opposing teeth and restorations.
- *Short clinical track record:* Compared with traditional methods such as cast gold or even amalgam restorations, bonded indirect tooth-colored restorations have a relatively short record of clinical service. They have become popular only in recent years, and relatively few controlled clinical trials are available, although these are increasing in number.[5,18-35]
- *Low potential for repair:* When a partial fracture occurs in a ceramic inlay or onlay, repair is usually not a definitive treatment. The actual procedure (mechanical roughening, etching with hydrofluoric [HF] acid, and application of a silane coupling agent before restoring with adhesive and composite) is relatively simple. However, because many ceramic inlays and onlays are indicated in areas where occlusal wear, esthetics, and fracture resistance are important, composite repairs frequently are not appropriate or successful.

Types of Ceramic Inlays and Onlays

Although some laboratory-processed composite systems have been available, and at least one machinable composite (Paradigm MZ100, 3M ESPE, St. Paul, MN) is available for CAD/CAM, most tooth-colored indirect posterior restorations are fabricated from ceramic materials.[12] Therefore, this chapter will address ceramic inlays and onlays only, with the understanding that the techniques for composite inlays and onlays are generally similar.

Ceramic inlays and onlays have become popular not only because of patient demand for esthetic, durable restorative materials but also because of improvements in materials, fabrication techniques, adhesives, and resin-based cements. Among the ceramic materials used are feldspathic porcelain, leucite-reinforced pressed ceramics, lithium disilicate, and various types of machinable (milled) ceramics designed for use with either chairside or laboratory CAD/CAM systems.[36]

Feldspathic Porcelain

Dental porcelains are partially crystalline minerals (feldspar, silica, alumina) dispersed in a glass matrix.[36] Porcelain restorations are made from finely ground ceramic powders that are mixed with distilled water or a special liquid, shaped into the desired form, and then fired and fused together to form a translucent material that looks like tooth structure. Currently, some ceramic inlays and onlays are fabricated in the dental laboratory by firing dental porcelains on refractory dies, but more are fabricated by pressing or milling methods, which are described later. The fabrication steps for fired ceramic inlays and onlays are summarized as follows:

- After tooth preparation, an impression is made, and a die-stone master working cast is poured (Fig. 11-3, *A*).
- The die is duplicated and poured with a refractory investment capable of withstanding porcelain firing temperatures. The duplication method must result in the master die and the refractory die being accurately interchangeable (see Fig. 11-3, *B*).
- Porcelain is added into the preparation area of the refractory die and fired in an oven. Multiple increments and firings are necessary to compensate for sintering shrinkage (see Fig. 11-3, *C*).
- The ceramic restoration is recovered from the refractory die, cleaned of all investment, and seated on the master die and working cast for final adjustments and finishing (see Fig. 11-3, *D*).

Although feldspathic porcelain inlays and onlays are less popular than in the past, some dental laboratories continue to use this method because of its low startup cost. The ceramic powders and investments are relatively inexpensive, and the technique is compatible with most existing ceramic laboratory equipment such as firing furnaces. The major disadvantage is its technique sensitivity, both for the technician and the dentist. Inlays and onlays fabricated with this technique must be handled gently during try-in and bonding to avoid fracture. Feldspathic porcelains are weak, so even after bonding, the incidence of fracture can be relatively high.[36]

Pressed Glass-Ceramics

Over 40 years ago, it was discovered that certain glasses could be modified with nucleating agents and, on heat treatment, be changed into ceramics with organized crystalline forms. Such "glass-ceramics" were stronger, had a higher melting point than noncrystalline glass, and had variable coefficients of thermal expansion.[37] At first, these glass-ceramics were developed primarily for cookware and other heat-resistant products. However, in 1984, the glass-ceramic material Dicor (DENTSPLY International, York, PA) was patented and became a popular ceramic for dental restorations. A major disadvantage of Dicor was its translucency, which necessitated external application of all shading.

Dicor restorations were made using a lost-wax, centrifugal casting process. Newer leucite-reinforced glass-ceramic systems (e.g., IPS Empress, Ivoclar Vivadent, Amherst, NY) also use the lost-wax method, but the material is heated to a high temperature and pneumatically pressed, rather than centrifuged, into a mold. Although some studies indicate that hot pressed ceramics are not substantially stronger than fired feldspathic porcelains, they do provide better clinical service.[28,29,38,39] The fabrication steps for one type of

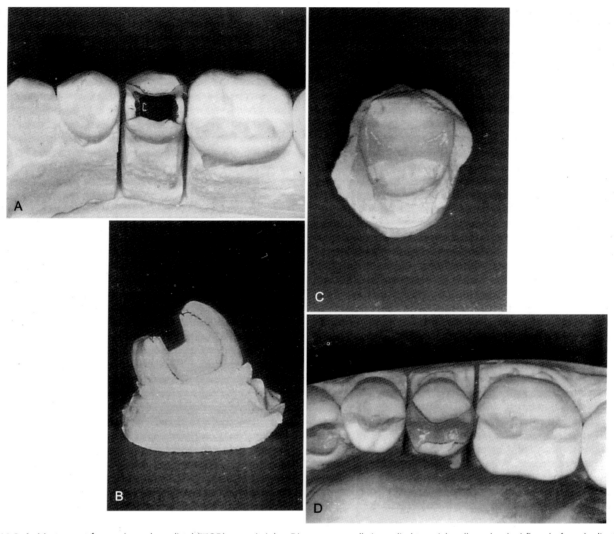

Fig. 11-3 A, Master cast for mesio-occluso-distal (MOD) ceramic inlay. Die spacer usually is applied to axial walls and pulpal floor before duplication. **B,** Master die is impressed, and then a duplicate die is poured with refractory investment. **C,** Dental porcelains are added and fired in increments until the inlay is the correct shape. **D,** The inlay is cleaned of all investment and then seated on master die for final adjustments and finishing. The ceramic inlay is now ready for delivery. (**D,** Courtesy of Dr. G. Sheen)

leucite-reinforced pressed ceramic restoration (IPS Empress) are summarized as follows:

1. After tooth preparation, an impression is made, and a working cast is poured in die-stone. A wax pattern of the restoration is made using conventional techniques (Fig. 11-4, A).
2. After spruing (see Fig. 11-4, B), investing, and wax pattern burnout, a shaded ceramic ingot and aluminum oxide plunger are placed into a special furnace (see Fig. 11-4, C). The shade and opacity of the selected ingot (see Fig 11-4, D) are based on the information provided by the clinician, specifically the desired shade of the final restoration and the shade of the prepared tooth.
3. At approximately 2012°F (1100°C), the ceramic ingot becomes plastic and is slowly pressed into the mold by an automated mechanism.

4. After being separated from the mold, the restoration is seated on the master die and working cast for final adjustments and finishing.
5. To reproduce the tooth shade accurately, a heavily pigmented surface stain is typically applied. The ceramic ingots are relatively translucent and available in a variety of shades, so staining for hot pressed ceramic inlay and onlay restorations is typically minimal.

The advantages of leucite-reinforced pressed ceramics are their (1) similarity to traditional "wax-up" processes, (2) excellent marginal fit, (3) moderately high strength, and (4) surface hardness similar to that of enamel.[40,41] Although pressed ceramic inlays and onlays are stronger than porcelain inlays made on refractory dies, they are still somewhat fragile during try-in and must be bonded rather than conventionally cemented. IPS Empress inlays and onlays have performed well in clinical trials ranging up to 12 years in duration.[22,24,28,29,42]

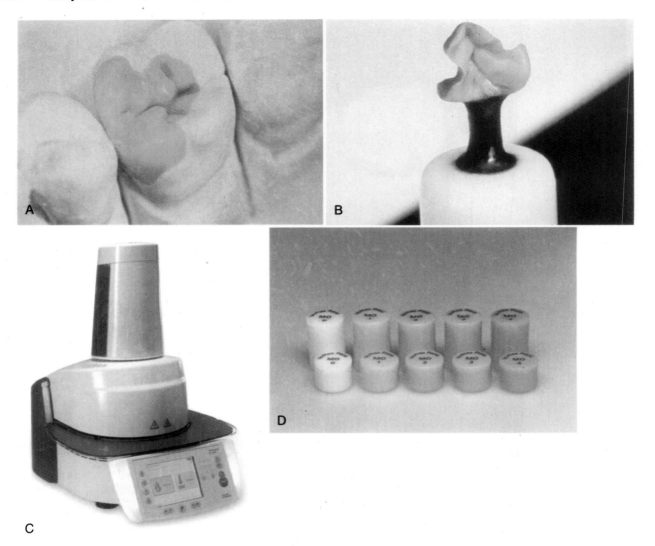

Fig. 11-4 Fabrication of a pressed ceramic onlay. **A,** Wax pattern. **B,** Wax pattern on sprue base, ready to be invested. **C,** Device for pressing heated ceramic (Programat EP 5000). **D,** Selection of ceramic ingots used for forming the restoration. *(Courtesy of Ivoclar Vivadent Inc., Amherst, NY.)*

Lithium Disilicate

A newer type of ceramic, lithium disilicate (e.max, Ivoclar Vivadent Inc., Amherst, NY), is available in both pressed (IPS e.max Press) and machinable (IPS e.max CAD) forms, and either can be used to fabricate inlays and onlays.[43] The two forms of e.max are slightly different in composition, but lithium disilicate is a moderately high-strength glass ceramic that also can be used for full crowns or ultra-thin veneers. In vitro testing of this ceramic material has shown very positive results, and it has become a highly popular alternative for inlays and onlays. However, because the material is relatively new, long-term clinical studies to demonstrate superior performance are lacking.

CAD/CAM

Improvements in technology have spawned increasingly sophisticated computerized devices that can fabricate restorations from high-quality ceramics in a matter of minutes. Some CAD/CAM systems are expensive laboratory-based units requiring the submission of an elastomeric or digital impression of the prepared tooth. The CEREC system was the first commercially available CAD/CAM system developed for the rapid chairside design and fabrication of ceramic restorations. The most popular dental CAD/CAM systems in use today are the CEREC 3D (Sirona Dental Systems, LLC, USA, Charlotte, NC) and E4D (D4D Technologies, LLC, Richardson, TX) (Fig. 11-5).

Generation of a chairside CAD/CAM restoration begins after the dentist prepares the tooth and uses a scanning device to collect information about the shape of the preparation and its relationship with the surrounding structures (Fig. 11-6). This step is termed *optical impression*. The system projects an image of the preparation and surrounding structures on a monitor, allowing the dentist or the auxiliary personnel to use the CAD portion of the system to design the restoration. The operator must input or confirm some of the restoration design such as the position of the gingival margins (Fig. 11-7).

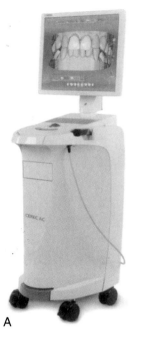
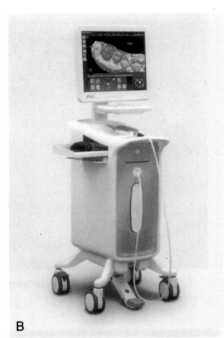

Fig. 11-5 CEREC AC (*A*) and E4D (*B*) computer-aided design/ computer-assisted manufacturing (CAD/CAM) devices. These chairside units are compact and mobile. (*A, Courtesy Sirona Dental Systems LLC, Charlotte, NC. B, Courtesy D4D Technologies, LLC, Richardson, TX.*)

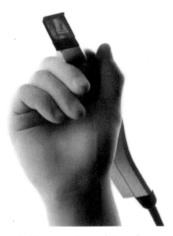

Fig. 11-6 A small handheld scanner is used to make an optical impression of the tooth preparation. (*Courtesy of Sirona Dental Systems LLC, Charlotte, NC.*)

include the feldspathic glass ceramics Vitablocs Mark II (Vident, Brea, CA) and CEREC Blocs (Sirona, manufactured by Vita Zahnfabrik, Bad Säckingen, Germany). The ceramic blocks are available in various shades and opacities, and some are even layered to mimic the relative opacity or translucency in different areas of a tooth.[12]

Two leucite-reinforced glass ceramics are available—IPS Empress CAD (Ivoclar Vivadent) and Paradigm C (3M ESPE). As mentioned above, lithium disilicate also is available in machinable form as IPS e.max CAD blocks. Although newer materials are stronger than the original ceramics, less is known about their long-term clinical performance.[12]

The major disadvantages of chairside CAD/CAM systems are the high initial cost and the need for special training. CAD/CAM technology is changing rapidly, however, with each new generation of devices having more capability, accuracy, and ease of use.[45] In addition, clinical studies have reported good results on the longevity of CAD/CAM ceramic restorations.[30,46-50]

Clinical Procedures

Many of the clinical procedures described are common to laboratory-fabricated and chairside CAD/CAM restorations. Some specific procedural details for CAD/CAM restorations are described in the section below on CAD/CAM techniques.

Tooth Preparation

Preparations for specific types of indirect tooth-colored inlays and onlays may vary because of differences in fabrication steps for each commercial system and variations in the physical properties of the restorative materials. Before beginning any procedure, the clinician must decide which type of restoration

After the restoration has been designed, the computer directs a milling device (CAM portion of the system) that mills the restoration out of a block of high-quality ceramic or composite in minutes (Fig. 11-8). The restoration is removed from the milling device and is ready for try-in, any needed adjustment, bonding, and polishing.

A major advantage of CAD/CAM systems, both laboratory and chairside, is the quality of the restorative material.[12,44] Manufacturers make blocks of "machinable ceramics" or "machinable composites" specifically for computer-assisted milling devices. Because these materials are fabricated under ideal industrial conditions, their physical properties have been optimized. Several different types of ceramics are available for chairside CAD/CAM restoration fabrication. These

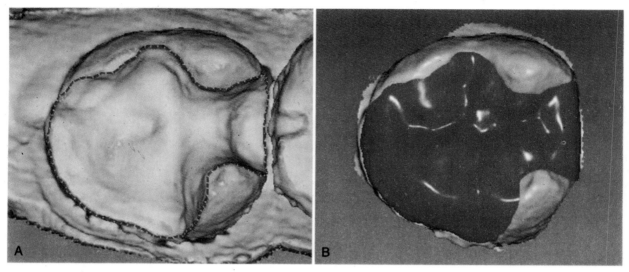

Fig. 11-7 Screen captures of two phases of an onlay restoration design. *(Courtesy of D4D Technologies, LLC, Richardson, TX.)*

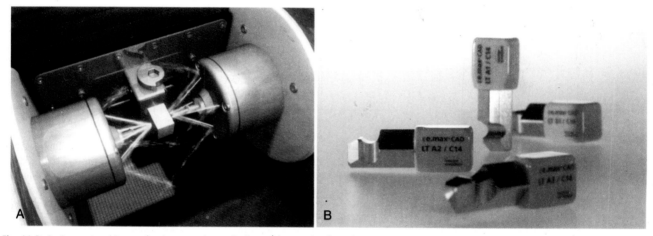

Fig. 11-8 A, Computer-driven software controls small, diamond-coated milling devices that mill the restoration out of a block of high-quality ceramic (as shown in *B*). *(Courtesy of D4D Technologies, LLC, Richardson, TX.)*

is indicated, according to the factors discussed in the previous sections in this chapter. If the clinician is not familiar with the technique, it is helpful to consult the manufacturer's literature and, if necessary, the dental laboratory to ensure the best results.

As a first clinical step, the patient is anesthetized and the area is isolated, preferably using a rubber dam. The compromised restoration (if present) is completely removed, and all caries is excavated. During preparation, stains on the external walls, such as those often left by corrosion products of old amalgam restorations, should be removed. Such stains could appear as black or gray lines at the margin after cementation. (This comment does not apply to stained but noncarious dentin on pulpal and axial walls.)

Preparations for indirect tooth-colored inlays and onlays are designed to provide adequate thickness for the restorative material and a passive insertion pattern with rounded internal angles and well-defined margins. All margins should have a 90-degree butt-joint cavosurface angle to ensure marginal

strength of the restoration. All line and point angles, internal and external, should be rounded to avoid stress concentrations in the restoration and tooth, reducing the potential for fractures (Figs. 11-9, 11-10, and 11-11).

The carbide bur or diamond used for tooth preparation should be a tapered instrument that creates occlusally divergent facial and lingual walls (Fig. 11-12), which allows for passive insertion and removal of the restoration. The junction of the sides and tip of the cutting instrument should have a rounded design to avoid creating sharp, stress-inducing internal angles in the preparation. Although the optimal gingival–occlusal divergence of the preparation is unknown, it should be greater than the 2 to 5 degrees per wall recommended for cast gold inlays and onlays. Divergence can and should be increased because the tooth-colored restoration is adhesively bonded and because only light pressure is applied during try-in and bonding. However, resistance and retention form are required to help preserve the adhesive interface, so excessive divergence must be avoided.

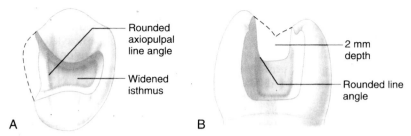

Fig. 11-9 **A,** Mesio-occlusal (MO) onlay preparation for tooth-colored inlay in maxillary first premolar (occlusal view). Isthmus should be at least 2 mm wide to prevent inlay fracture. The axiopulpal line angle should be rounded to avoid seating errors and to lower stress concentrations. **B,** Mesio-occluso-distal (MOD) onlay preparation for tooth-colored inlay in the maxillary first premolar (proximal view). The pulpal floor should be prepared to a depth of 2 mm, and the axiopulpal line angles should be rounded. The proximal margins should be extended to allow at least 0.5 mm clearance of contact with the neighboring tooth. Gingival margins in enamel are greatly preferred.

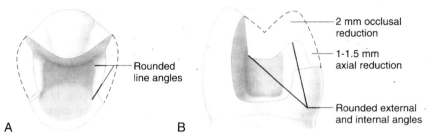

Fig. 11-10 Occlusal (*A*) and proximal (*B*) views of mesio-occluso-disto-lingual (MODL) onlay preparation on maxillary first premolar. The lingual cusp has been reduced and the lingual margin extended beyond any possible contact with opposing tooth by preparing a "collar." Functional cusps require 2 mm of occlusal reduction. All internal and external line angles are rounded.

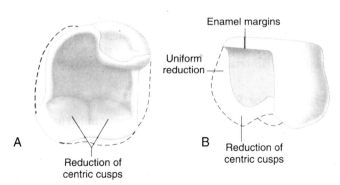

Fig. 11-11 Mesio-occluso-disto-facio-lingual (MODFL) onlay preparation on the maxillary right first molar. Distofacial (DF), mesiolingual (ML), and distolingual (DL) cusps are reduced. **A,** Occlusal view. **B,** Facial view.

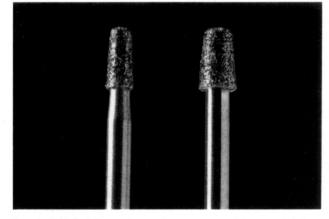

Fig. 11-12 Typical diamond rotary instruments used for ceramic inlay or onlay tooth preparations.

Throughout preparation, the cutting instruments used to develop vertical walls are oriented to a single path of draw, usually the long axis of the tooth crown. The occlusal portion of the preparation should be 2 mm deep. Based on input from laboratory technicians, many failures of ceramic inlays and onlays can be attributed to insufficient thickness resulting from insufficient occlusal reduction. Most ceramic systems require that any isthmus be at least 2 mm wide to decrease the possibility of fracture of the restoration. The facial and lingual walls should be extended to sound tooth structure and should go around the cusps in smooth curves. Ideally, there should be no undercuts that would prevent the insertion or removal of the restoration. Small undercuts, if present, can be blocked out using a resin-modified glass ionomer (RMGI) liner. The pulpal floor should be smooth and relatively flat. After removal of extensive caries or previous restorative material from any internal wall, the floor is restored to more nearly ideal form with a material that has a reasonably high compressive strength such as an RMGI liner or base.

The facial, lingual, and gingival margins of the proximal boxes should be extended to clear the adjacent tooth by at least 0.5 mm. These clearances provide adequate access to the margins for the impression and for finishing and polishing instruments. For all walls, a 90-degree cavosurface margin is ideal because ceramic materials are fragile in thin sections. The gingival margin should be extended as minimally as possible because margins in enamel are greatly preferred for bonding and because deep gingival margins are difficult to impress and to isolate properly during bonding. When a portion of the facial or lingual surface is affected by caries or other defect, it might be necessary to extend the preparation (with a gingival shoulder) around the transitional line angle to include the defect. The axial wall of the shouldered extension should be prepared to allow for adequate restoration thickness (i.e., 1–1.5 mm).

When extending through or along the cuspal inclines to reach sound tooth structure, a cusp usually should be capped if the extension is two-thirds or greater than the distance from any primary groove to the cusp tip (see Figs. 11-10 and 11-11). If the cusps must be capped, they should be reduced by 2 mm and should have a 90-degree cavosurface angle. When capping cusps, especially centric holding cusps, it might be necessary to prepare a shoulder to move the facial or lingual cavosurface margin away from any possible contact with the opposing tooth, either in maximum intercuspal position or during functional movements. Contacts directly on margins can lead to premature deterioration of marginal integrity. The axial wall of the resulting shoulder should be sufficiently deep to allow for adequate thickness of the restorative material and should have the same path of draw as the main portion of the preparation.

Impression

Tooth-colored inlay or onlay systems require an elastomeric or optical impression of the prepared tooth and the adjacent teeth and interocclusal records, which allow the restoration to be fabricated on a working cast in the laboratory. Of course, with chairside CAD/CAM systems, no working cast is necessary.

Provisional Restoration

A provisional or temporary restoration is necessary when using indirect systems that require two appointments. The provisional restoration protects the pulp–dentin complex in vital teeth, maintains the position of the prepared tooth in the arch, and protects the soft tissues adjacent to the prepared areas. The provisional can be made using conventional techniques and bis-acryl composite materials. Care should be taken to avoid bonding of the temporary material to the preparation at this phase of the procedure. A lubricant of some sort (e.g., glycerin) can be applied to the preparation, if desired, especially if a resin-based material was used to block out undercuts or level the floor of the preparation. Temporary restorations for PFM and cast gold restorations typically are cemented with eugenol-based temporary cements. Eugenol is believed to interfere with resin polymerization, however, and potentially could reduce the adhesion of the permanent composite cement to tooth structure.[51,52] Although some studies report this does not occur if the tooth is thoroughly cleaned using pumice, excavator, or air abrasion before cementation of the permanent restoration, use of a non-eugenol temporary cement is recommended.[53,54] For

exceptionally nonretentive preparations, or when the temporary phase is expected to last longer than 2 to 3 weeks, zinc phosphate or polycarboxylate cement can be used to increase retention of the provisional restoration. Resin-based temporary cements are also available (e.g., TempBond Clear, Kerr Corporation, Orange, CA).

CAD/CAM Techniques

Clinical procedures for CAD/CAM systems differ somewhat from the procedures previously described. Tooth preparations for CAD/CAM inlays must reflect the capabilities of the CAD software and hardware and the CAM milling devices that fabricate the restorations. One example of how preparations are modified when using the CEREC system pertains to undercuts. Laboratory-fabricated indirect systems require the preparation to have a path of draw that allows insertion and removal of the restoration without interferences from undercuts. In contrast, the CEREC system automatically "blocks out" any undercuts during the optical impression (Fig. 11-13). Of course, large undercuts should be avoided.

Using a chairside CAD/CAM system, an experienced dentist can prepare the tooth, fabricate an inlay, and deliver it in approximately 1 hour (Fig. 11-14). This system eliminates the need for a conventional impression, provisional restoration, and multiple patient appointments.

Try-in and Bonding

Try-in and bonding of tooth-colored inlays or onlays are more demanding than those for cast gold restorations because of (1) the relatively fragile nature of some ceramic materials, (2) the requirement of near-perfect moisture control, and (3) the use of resin cements. Occlusal evaluation and adjustment generally are delayed until after the restoration is bonded, to avoid fracture of the ceramic material.[16]

Preliminary Steps

The use of a rubber dam is strongly recommended to prevent moisture contamination of the conditioned tooth or restoration surfaces during cementation and to improve access and visibility during delivery of the restoration. After removing the provisional restoration, all of the temporary cement is cleaned from the preparation walls.

Restoration Try-in and Proximal Contact Adjustment

The inlay or onlay is placed into the preparation using light pressure to evaluate its fit. If the restoration does not seat completely, the most likely cause is an over-contoured proximal surface (Fig. 11-15). Using the mouth mirror, where needed, the embrasures should be viewed from the facial, lingual, and occlusal aspects to determine where the proximal contour needs adjustment to allow final seating of the restoration, while producing the correct position and form of the contact. Passing thin dental floss through the contact reveals tightness and position of the proximal contact, signifying to the experienced operator the degree and location of excess contact. Articulating paper also can be used successfully to identify overly tight proximal contacts. Abrasive disks or

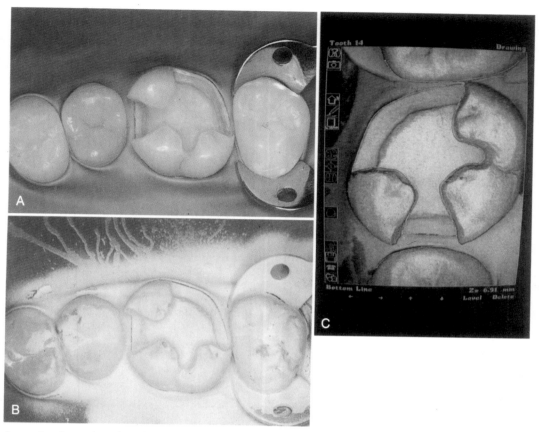

Fig. 11-13 **A,** Preparation for mesio-occluso-disto-facial (MODF) ceramic onlay on maxillary first molar. **B,** Preparation coated with special powder for capture with optical impression by CEREC device. **C,** Optical impression.

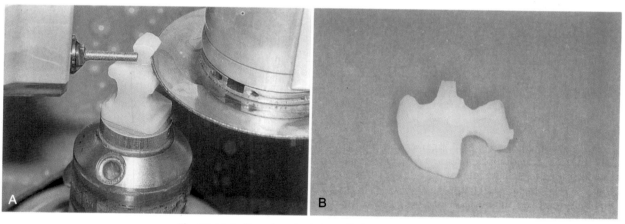

Fig. 11-14 **A,** Ceramic onlay being milled. **B,** Milled onlay.

points are used to adjust the proximal contour and contact relationship. While adjusting the intensity and location of the proximal contacts, increasingly finer grits of abrasive instruments are used to polish the proximal surfaces because they will be inaccessible for polishing after cementation.

If the proximal contours are not over-contoured and the restoration still does not fit completely, the preparation should be checked again for residual temporary materials or debris. If the preparation is clean, internal or marginal interferences also might prevent the restoration from seating completely. When these interferences have been identified through careful visual inspection of the margins or using "fit-checker" materials, they can be adjusted on the restoration, in the preparation, or both. These interferences are rare because contemporary impression materials and ceramic fabrication systems are accurate. In the event of a significant discrepancy between the preparation and the restoration, a new impression must be taken.

Repair of Ceramic Inlays and Onlays

Minor defects in ceramic restorations can be repaired, but before initiating any repair procedure, the operator should determine whether replacement, rather than repair, is the appropriate treatment. If repair is appropriate, the dentist should attempt to identify the cause of the problem and correct it, if possible. For example, a small fracture resulting from occlusal trauma might indicate that some adjustment of the opposing occlusion is required.

The repair procedure is initiated by mechanical roughening of the involved surface. Although a coarse diamond may be used, a better result is obtained with the use of airborne particle abrasion using aluminum oxide particles and a special intraoral device.[65] This initial mechanical roughening is followed by brief (typically 2 minutes) application of 5% to 10% HF acid gel. HF acid etches the surface, creating further micro-defects to facilitate mechanical bonding. The next step in the repair procedure is application of a silane coupling agent. Silanes mediate chemical bonding between ceramics and resins and may improve the predictability of resin–resin repairs.[59] The manufacturer's guidelines should be followed when using silanes because they can differ substantially from one product to another. After the silane has been applied, a resin adhesive is applied and light-cured. A composite of the appropriate shade is placed, cured, contoured, and polished.

Summary

Advances in ceramic, polymer, and adhesive technologies have resulted in the development of a variety of tooth-colored indirect Class I and II restorations. These restorations offer an excellent alternative to direct composite restorations, especially for large restorations, and are more conservative than full-coverage restorations. Because the clinical procedures are relatively technique-sensitive, however, proper case selection, operator skill, and attention to detail are crucial to success.

Acknowledgement

The authors thank Mr. David Avery, CDT of Drake Precision Dental Laboratory (Charlotte, NC) for his input during the revision of this chapter.

References

1. Ausiello P, De Gee AJ, Rengo S, et al: Fracture resistance of endodontically-treated premolars adhesively restored. *Am J Dent* 10:237–241, 1997.
2. Burke FJT, Wilson NH, Watts DC: The effect of cuspal coverage on the fracture resistance of teeth restored with indirect composite resin restorations. *Quintessence Int* 24:875–880, 1993.
3. Camacho GB, Gonçalves M, Nonaka T, et al: Fracture strength of restored premolars. *Am J Dent* 20:121–124, 2007.
4. Ferracane JL: Is there still a need for in vitro wear simulating devices? *Dent Mater* 22:689–692, 2006.
5. Lange RT, Pfeiffer P: Clinical evaluation of ceramic inlays compared to composite restorations. *Oper Dent* 34:263–272, 2009.
6. van Dijken JW, Hasselrot L: A prospective 15-year evaluation of extensive dentin-enamel-bonded pressed ceramic coverages. *Dent Mater* 26:929–939, 2010.
7. El-Kalla IH, Garcia-Godoy F: Saliva contamination and bond strength of single-bottle adhesives to enamel and dentin. *Am J Dent* 10:83–87, 1997.

8. Sheikh H: Effect of saliva contamination and cleansing on the bond strengths of self-etch adhesives to dentin. *J Esthet Restor Dent* 22:402–411, 2010.
9. Meyer A, Jr., Cardoso LC, Araujo E, et al: Ceramic inlays and onlays: Clinical procedures for predictable results. *J Esthet Restor Dent* 15:338–351, 2003.
10. Purk JH: In vitro microtensile bond strength of four adhesives tested at the gingival and pulpal walls of Class II restorations. *J Am Dent Assoc* 137:1414–1418, 2006.
11. Ferrari M, Mason PN, Fabianelli A, et al: Influence of tissue characteristics at margins on leakage of Class II indirect porcelain restorations. *Am J Dent* 12:134–142, 1999.
12. Fasbinder DJ: Materials for chairside CAD/CAM restorations. *Compend Cont Educ Dent* 31:702–709, 2010.
13. Feilzer AJ, De Gee AJ, Davidson CL: Increased wall-to-wall curing contraction in thin bonded layers. *J Dent Res* 68:48–50, 1989.
14. Manhart J, Chen H, Hamm G, et al: Buonocore Memorial Lecture. Review of the clinical survival of direct and indirect restorations in posterior teeth of the permanent dentition. *Oper Dent* 29:481–508, 2004.
15. St. John KR: Biocompatibility of dental materials. *Dent Clin N Am* 51:747–760, 2007.
16. Magne P, Paranhos MP, Schlichting LH: Influence of material selection on the risk of inlay fracture during pre-cementation functional occlusal tapping. *Dent Mater* 27:109–113, 2011.
17. al-Hiyasat AS, Saunders WP, Smith GM: Three-body wear associated with three ceramics and enamel. *J Prosthet Dent* 82:476–481, 1999.
18. Arnelund CF, Johansson A, Ericson M, et al: Five-year evaluation of two resin-retained ceramic systems: A retrospective study in a general practice setting. *Int J Prosthodont* 17:300–306, 2004.
19. El-Mowafy O, Brochu JF: Longevity and clinical performance of IPS-Empress ceramic restorations—a literature review. *J Can Dent Assoc* 8:233–237, 2002.
20. Fabianelli A, Goracci C, Bertelli E, et al: A clinical trial of Empress II porcelain inlays luted to vital teeth with a dual-curing adhesive system and a self-curing resin cement. *J Adhes Dent* 8:427–431, 2006.
21. Fasbinder DJ, Dennison JB, Heys DR, et al: The clinical performance of CAD/CAM-generated composite inlays. *J Am Dent Assoc* 136:1714–1723, 2005.
22. Frankenberger R, Taschner M, Garcia-Godoy F, et al: Leucite-reinforced glass ceramic inlays and onlays after 12 years. *J Adhes Dent* 10:393–398, 2008.
23. Fuzzi M, Rappelli G: Ceramic inlays: Clinical assessment and survival rate. *J Adhes Dent* 1:71–79, 1999.
24. Galiatsatos AS, Bergou D: Six-year clinical evaluation of ceramic inlays and onlays. *Quintessence Int* 39:407–412, 2008.
25. Guess PC, Strub JR, Steinhart N, et al: All-ceramic partial coverage restorations—midterm results of a 5-year prospective clinical splitmouth study. *J Dent* 37:627–637, 2009.
26. Hayashi M, et al: Eight-year clinical evaluation of fired ceramic inlays. *Oper Dent* 25:473–481, 2000.
27. Haywood VB, Heymann HO, Kusy RP, et al: Polishing porcelain veneers: An SEM and specular reflectance analysis. *Dent Mater* 4:116–121, 1988.
28. Krämer N, Taschner M, Lohbauer U, et al: Totally bonded ceramic inlays and onlays after eight years. *J Adhes Dent* 10:307–314, 2008.
29. Krämer N, Frankenberger R: Clinical performance of bonded leucite-reinforced glass ceramic inlays and onlays after eight years. *Dent Mater* 21:262–271, 2005.
30. Krejci I, Lutz F, Reimer M, et al: Wear of ceramic inlays, their enamel antagonists, and luting cements. *J Prosthet Dent* 69:425–430, 1993.
31. Naeselius K, Arnelund CF, Molin MK: Clinical evaluation of all-ceramic onlays: A 4-year retrospective study. *Int J Prosthodont* 21:40–44, 2008.
32. Roulet J-F: Longevity of glass ceramic inlays and amalgam—results up to 6 years. *Clin Oral Invest* 1:40–46, 1997.
33. Schulz P, Johansson A, Arvidson K: A retrospective study of Mirage ceramic inlays over up to 9 years. *Int J Prosthodont* 16:510–514, 2003.
34. Thordrup M, Isidor F, Hörsted-Bindslev P: A prospective clinical study of indirect and direct composite and ceramic inlays: Ten-year results. *Quintessence Int* 37:139–144, 2006.
35. van Dijken JW, Höglund-Aberg C, Olofsson AL: Fired ceramic inlays: A 6-year follow-up. *J Dent* 26:219–225, 1998.
36. Giordano R, McLaren EA: Ceramics overview: Classification by microstructure and processing methods. *Compend Cont Educ Dent* 31:682–697, 2010.
37. MacCulloch WT: Advances in dental ceramics. *Br Dent J* 124:361–365, 1968.
38. Cattell MJ, Clarke RL, Lynch EJ: The transverse strength, reliability and microstructural features of four dental ceramics—Part I. *J Dent* 25:399–407, 1997.
39. Cattell MJ, Clarke RL, Lynch EJ: The biaxial flexure strength and reliability of four dental ceramics—Part II. *J Dent* 25:409–414, 1997.

40. Guazzato M: Strength, fracture toughness and microstructure of a selection of all-ceramic materials. Part I. Pressable and alumina glass-infiltrated ceramics. *Dent Mater* 20:441–448, 2004.

41. Seghi RR, Denry IL, Rosenstiel SF: Relative fracture toughness and hardness of new dental ceramics. *J Prosthet Dent* 74:145–150, 1995.

42. Fradeani M, Aquilano A, Bassein L: Longitudinal study of pressed glass-ceramic inlays for four and a half years. *J Prosthet Dent* 78:346–353, 1997.

43. Ritter RG: Multifunctional uses of a novel ceramic—lithium disilicate. *J Esthet Restor Dent* 22:332–341, 2010.

44. Charlton DG, Roberts HW, Tiba A: Measurement of select physical and mechanical properties of 3 machinable ceramic materials. *Quintessence Int* 39:573–579, 2008.

45. Liu P-R, Essig ME: A panorama of dental CAD/CAM restorative systems. *Compend Cont Educ Dent* 29:482–493, 2008.

46. Berg NG, Derand T: A 5-year evaluation of ceramic inlays (CEREC). *Swed Dent J* 21:121–127, 1997.

47. Otto T, De Nisco S: Computer-aided direct ceramic restorations: A 10-year prospective clinical study of Cerec CAD/CAM inlays and onlays. *Int J Prosthodont* 15:122–128, 2002.

48. Pallesen U, van Dijken JW: An 8-year evaluation of sintered ceramic and glass ceramic inlays processed by the Cerec CAD/CAM system. *Eur J Oral Sci* 108: 239–246, 2000.

49. Reich SM, Wichmann M, Rinne H, et al: Clinical performance of large, all-ceramic CAD/CAM-generated restorations after three years: A pilot study. *J Am Dent Assoc* 135:605–612, 2004.

50. Sjögren G, Molin M, van Dijken JW: A 10-year prospective evaluation of CAD/CAM-manufactured (Cerec) ceramic inlays cemented with a chemically cured or dual-cured resin composite. *Int J Prosthodont* 17:241–246, 2004.

51. Rosenstiel SF, Gegauff AG: Effect of provisional cementing agents on provisional resins. *J Prosthet Dent* 59:29–33, 1988.

52. Erkut S, Küçükesmen HC, Eminkahyagil N, et al: Influence of previous provisional cementation on the bond strength between two definitive resin-based luting and dentin bonding agents and human dentin. *Oper Dent* 32:84–93, 2007.

53. Abo-Hamar SE, Federlin M, Hiller KA, et al: Effect of temporary cements on the bond strength of ceramic luted to dentin. *Dent Mater* 21:794–803, 2005.

54. Schwartz R, Davis R, Hilton TJ: Effect of temporary cements on the bond strength of a resin cement. *Am J Dent* 5:147–150, 1992.

55. Frankenberger R, Lohbauer U, Schaible RB, et al: Luting of ceramic inlays in vitro: Marginal quality of self-etch and etch-and-rinse adhesives versus self-etch cements. *Dent Mater* 24:185–191, 2008.

56. Sturdevant JR, Bayne SC, Heymann HO: Margin gap size of ceramic inlays using second-generation CAD/CAM equipment. *J Esthet Dent* 11:206–214, 1999.

57. Naves LZ: Surface/interface morphology and bond strength to glass ceramic etched for different periods. *Oper Dent* 35:420–427, 2010.

58. Fabianelli A, Pollington S, Papacchini F, et al: The effect of different surface treatments on bond strength between leucite reinforced feldspathic ceramic and composite resin. *J Dent* 38:39–43, 2010.

59. Filho AM, Vieira LC, Araújo E, et al: Effect of different ceramic surface treatments on resin microtensile bond strength. *J Prosthodont* 13:28–35, 2004.

60. Behr M, Hansmann M, Rosentritt M, et al: Marginal adaptation of three self-adhesive resin cements vs. a well-tried adhesive luting agent. *Clin Oral Invest* 13:459–464, 2009.

61. Taschner M, Frankenberger R, García-Godoy F, et al: IPS Empress inlays luted with a self-adhesive resin cement after 1 year. *Am J Dent* 22:55–59, 2009.

62. Abo-Hamar SE, Hiller KA, Jung H, et al: Bond strength of a new universal self-adhesive resin luting cement to dentin and enamel. *Clin Oral Invest* 9:161–167, 2005.

63. Cadenaro M, Navarra CO, Antoniolli F, et al: The effect of curing mode on extent of polymerization and microhardness of dual-cured, self-adhesive resin cements. *Am J Dent* 23:14–18, 2010.

64. Borges GA, Agarwal P, Miranzi BA, et al: Influence of different ceramics on resin cement Knoop Hardness Number. *Oper Dent* 33:622–628, 2008.

65. Panah FG, Rezai SM, Ahmadian L: The influence of ceramic surface treatments on the micro-shear bond strength of composite resin to IPS Empress 2. *J Prosthodont* 17:409–414, 2008.

Chapter 12

Additional Conservative Esthetic Procedures

Harald O. Heymann

Significant improvements in tooth-colored restorative materials and adhesive techniques have resulted in numerous conservative esthetic treatment possibilities. Although restorative dentistry is a blend of art and science, conservative esthetic dentistry truly emphasizes the artistic component. As Goldstein stated, "Esthetic dentistry is the art of dentistry in its purest form."[1] As with many forms of art, conservative esthetic dentistry provides a means of artistic expression that feeds on creativity and imagination. Dentists find performing conservative esthetic procedures enjoyable, and patients appreciate the immediate esthetic improvements rendered, often without the need for local anesthesia.

One of the greatest assets a person can have is a smile that shows beautiful, natural teeth (Fig. 12-1). Children and teenagers are especially sensitive about unattractive teeth. When teeth are discolored, malformed, crooked, or missing, often the person makes a conscious effort to avoid smiling and tries to "cover up" his or her teeth. Correction of these types of dental problems can produce dramatic changes in appearance, which often result in improved confidence, personality, and social life. The restoration of a smile is one of the most appreciated and gratifying services a dentist can render. The positive psychological effects of improving a patient's smile often contribute to an improved self-image and enhanced self-esteem. These improvements make conservative esthetic dentistry particularly gratifying for the dentist and represent a new dimension of dental treatment for patients.

This chapter presents conservative esthetic procedures in the context of their clinical applications. The principles and clinical steps involved in adhesive bonding for the treatment alternatives discussed in this chapter are similar to those described in Chapters 8 to 10. Only specific conservative esthetic clinical procedures or variations from previously described techniques are presented in this chapter.

Artistic Elements

Regardless of the result desired, certain basic artistic elements must be considered to ensure an optimal esthetic result. In conservative esthetic dentistry, these elements include the following:

- Shape or form
- Symmetry and proportionality
- Position and alignment
- Surface texture
- Color
- Translucency

Some or all of these elements are common to virtually every conservative esthetic dental procedure; a basic knowledge and understanding of these artistic elements is required to attain esthetic results consistently.

Shape or Form

The shape of teeth largely determines their esthetic appearance. To achieve optimal dental esthetics, it is imperative that natural anatomic forms be achieved. A basic knowledge of normal tooth anatomy is fundamental to the success of any conservative esthetic dental procedure.

When viewing the clinical crown of an incisor from a facial (or lingual) position, the crown outline is trapezoidal. Subtle variations in shape and contour produce very different appearances, however. Rounded incisal angles, open incisal and facial embrasures, and softened facial line angles typically characterize a youthful smile. A smile characteristic of an older individual having experienced attrition secondary to aging, typically exhibits incisal embrasures that are more closed and incisal angles that are more prominent (i.e., less rounded). Frequently, minor modification of existing tooth contours, sometimes referred to as *cosmetic contouring*, can effect a significant esthetic change (see section on alterations of shape of natural teeth). Reshaping enamel by rounding incisal angles, opening incisal embrasures, and reducing prominent facial line angles can produce a more youthful appearance (Fig. 12-2).

Significant generalized esthetic changes are possible when treating all anterior teeth (and occasionally the first

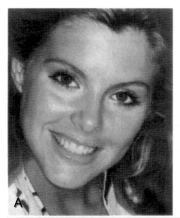

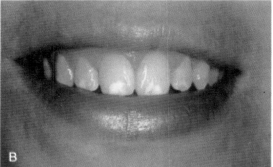

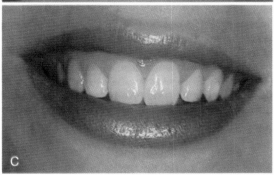

Fig. 12-1 Examples of conservative esthetic procedures. **A,** A beautiful radiant smile is one of the greatest assets a person can have. **B,** The appearance of this aspiring young model was marred by hypocalcified areas of maxillary anterior teeth. **C,** A simple treatment consisted of removing part of the discolored enamel, acid etching the preparations, and restoring with direct-composite partial veneers. *(Courtesy of Dr. C. L. Sockwell.)*

premolars) visible in the patient's smile. This fact is particularly true when placing full-coverage facial restorations such as veneers (see the section on Veneers). With this treatment method, the dentist can produce significant changes in tooth shapes and forms to yield a variety of different appearances.

Although less extensive, restoring an individual tooth rather than all anterior teeth simultaneously may require greater artistic ability. Generalized restoration of all anterior teeth with full facial veneers affords the dentist significant control of the contours generated. When treating an isolated tooth, however, the success of the result is determined largely by how well the restored tooth esthetically matches the surrounding natural teeth. The contralateral tooth to the one being restored should be examined closely for subtle characterizing features such as developmental depressions, embrasure form, prominences, or other distinguishing characteristics of form. A high degree of realism must be reproduced artfully to achieve optimal esthetics when restoring isolated teeth or areas.

Illusions of shape also play a significant role in dental esthetics. The border outline of an anterior tooth (i.e., facial view) is primarily two-dimensional (i.e., length and width). The third dimension of depth is crucial, however, in creating illusions, especially those of apparent width and length.

Prominent areas of contour on a tooth typically are highlighted with direct illumination, making them more noticeable, whereas areas of depression or diminishing contour are shadowed and less conspicuous. By controlling the areas of light reflection and shadowing, full facial coverage restorations (in particular) can be esthetically contoured to achieve various desired illusions of form.

The apparent size of a tooth can be changed by altering the position of facial prominences or heights of contour without changing the actual dimension of the tooth. Compared with normal tooth contours (Fig. 12-3, *A*), a tooth can be made to appear narrower by positioning the mesiofacial and distofacial line angles closer together (see Fig. 12-3, *B*). Developmental depressions also can be positioned closer together to enhance the illusion of narrowness. Similarly, greater apparent width can be achieved by positioning the line angles and developmental depressions further apart (see Fig. 12-3, *C*).

Although more difficult, the apparent length of teeth also can be changed by illusion. Compared with normal tooth contours (Fig. 12-4, *A*), a tooth can be made to appear shorter by emphasizing the horizontal elements such as gingival perikymata and by positioning the gingival height of contour further incisally (see Fig. 12-4, *B*). Slight modification of the

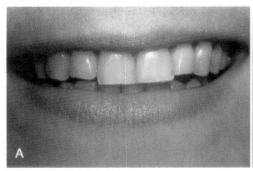

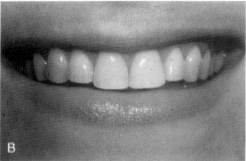

Fig. 12-2 Cosmetic contouring. **A,** Anterior teeth before treatment. **B,** By reshaping teeth, a more youthful appearance is produced.

incisal area, achieved by moving the incisal height of contour further gingivally, also enhances the illusion of a shorter tooth. The opposite tenets are true for increasing the apparent length of a tooth. The heights of contour are moved farther apart incisogingivally, and vertical elements such as developmental depressions are emphasized (see Fig. 12-4, *C*).

Used in combination, these illusionary techniques are particularly valuable for controlling the apparent dimension of teeth in procedures that result in an actual increased width of teeth, such as in diastema (i.e., space) closure (see the section on Correction of Diastemas). By contouring the composite additions in such a way that the original positions of the line angles are maintained, the increased widths of the restored teeth are less noticeable (Fig. 12-5). If full facial coverage

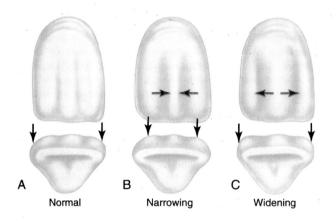

Fig. 12-3 Creating illusions of width. **A,** Normal width. **B,** A tooth can be made to appear narrower by positioning mesial and distal line angles closer together and by more closely approximating developmental depressions. **C,** Greater apparent width is achieved by positioning line angles and developmental depressions farther apart.

restorations are placed in conjunction with a diastema closure, vertical elements can be enhanced and horizontal features de-emphasized to control further the apparent dimension of teeth.

Symmetry and Proportionality

The overall esthetic appearance of a human smile is governed largely by the symmetry and proportionality of the teeth that constitute the smile. Asymmetric teeth or teeth that are out of proportion to the surrounding teeth disrupt the sense of balance and harmony essential for optimal esthetics. Assuming that the patient's teeth are aligned normally (i.e., rotations or faciolingual positional defects are not present), dental symmetry can be maintained if the sizes of contralateral teeth are equivalent. A dental caliper should be used in conjunction with any conservative esthetic dental procedure that would alter the mesiodistal dimension of teeth. This recommendation is particularly true for procedures such as diastema closure or other procedures involving augmentation of proximal surfaces with composite. By first measuring and recording the widths of the interdental space and the teeth to be augmented, the appropriate amount of contour to be generated with composite resin addition can be determined (Fig. 12-6). In this manner, symmetric and equal tooth contours can be generated (see the section on Correction of Diastemas). When dealing with restorations involving the midline, particular attention also must be paid to the incisal and gingival embrasure forms; the mesial contours of both central incisors must be mirror images of one another to ensure an optimally symmetric and esthetic result.

In addition to being symmetric, anterior teeth must be in proper proportion to one another to achieve maximum esthetics. The quality of proportionality is relative and varies greatly, depending on other factors (e.g., tooth position, tooth

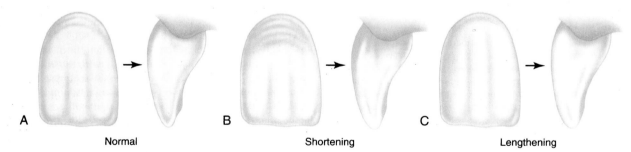

Fig. 12-4 Creating illusions of length. **A,** Normal length. **B,** A tooth can be made to appear shorter by emphasizing horizontal elements and by positioning the gingival height of contour farther incisally. **C,** The illusion of length is achieved by moving the gingival height of contour gingivally and by emphasizing vertical elements, such as developmental depressions.

Fig. 12-5 Controlling apparent tooth size when adding proximal dimension. **A,** Teeth before treatment. **B,** By maintaining original positions of the facial line angles (see areas of light reflection), increased widths of teeth after composite augmentations are less noticeable.

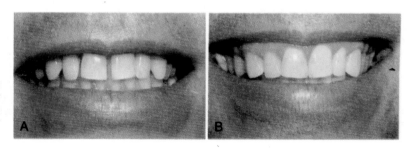

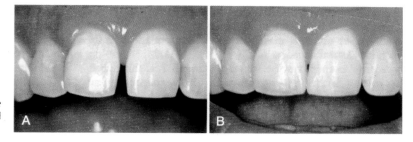

Fig. 12-6 Diastema closure. **A,** Teeth before composite additions. **B,** Symmetrical and equal contours are achieved in the final restorations.

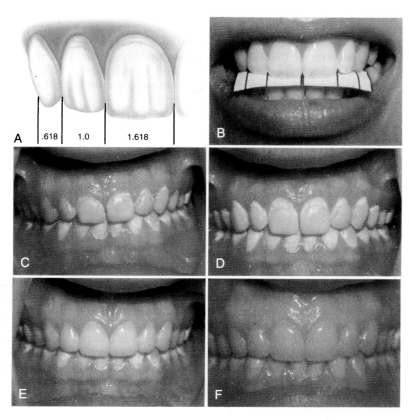

Fig. 12-7 Tooth proportions. **A,** The rule of the golden proportion. The exact ratios of proportionality. **B,** The anterior teeth of this patient are in golden proportion to one another. **C,** Width-to-length ratios. Pre-operative view reveals width-to-length ratio of 1:1. **D,** Following a periodontal surgical crown lengthening procedure, a more esthetic width-to-length ratio of 0.80 exists. **E,** Final result with etched porcelain veneers. A width-to-length ratio of 0.80 is maintained. **F,** A 7-year post-operative view reveals a stable and esthetic long-term result.

alignment, arch form, configuration of the smile). One long-accepted theorem of the relative proportionality of maxillary anterior teeth typically visible in a smile involves the concept of *the golden proportion*.[2] Originally formulated as one of Euclid's elements, this theorem has been relied on through the ages as a geometric basis for proportionality in the beauty of art and nature.[3] On the basis of this formula, a smile, when viewed from the front, is considered to be esthetically pleasing if each tooth in that smile (starting from the midline) is approximately 60% of the size of the tooth immediately mesial to it. The exact proportion of the distal tooth to the mesial tooth is 0.618 (Fig. 12-7, *A*). These recurring esthetic dental proportions are based on the apparent sizes of teeth when viewed straight on and not the actual sizes of individual teeth. An example of an esthetically pleasing smile that meets the golden proportion can be seen in Figure 12-7, *B*.

Although the golden proportion is not the absolute determinant of dental esthetics, it does provide a practical and proven guide for establishing proportionality when restoring anterior teeth, especially if these teeth are considered long. However,

according to a study by Preston, only 17% of the population naturally exhibits smiles that meet the golden proportion as the recurring esthetic dental proportion.[4] According to a survey of dentists by Ward, a recurring esthetic dental proportion of 70% (as opposed to 61.8 % as with the golden proportion) is preferred when teeth are of normal dimension.[5]

Little scientific information is available regarding the proper proportions of individual anterior teeth. A study by Sterrett et al. revealed that the average width-to-length ratio for a maxillary central incisor in men was 0.85 and in women was 0.86.[6] The actual width-to-length ratios found in this same study for maxillary lateral incisors in men and women were 0.76 and 0.79, respectively. Another study by Magne et al. reported average width-to-length ratios of 0.87 for worn maxillary central incisors and 0.78 for unworn maxillary central incisors.[7] An accepted theorem for achieving esthetically pleasing central incisors maintains that the ideal width-to-length ratio should be 0.75 to 0.80.[8] This ratio represents the ideal proportions needed to optimize the esthetic result and can help guide the treatment planning process. Considering the range of recommended width-to-length ratios, 0.80 seems to be a good benchmark for achieving optimally esthetic results when restoring maxillary central incisors and 0.75 for maxillary lateral incisors.

A good example can be seen in Figure 12-7, *C* through *F*. Because of altered passive eruption, this teenaged patient exhibited a preoperative width-to-length ratio of 1:1 for her maxillary central incisors (see Fig. 12-7, *C*). She revealed excessive gingival tissues relative to the display of her anterior teeth. To achieve a more esthetic appearance, it was determined that a width-to-length ratio of 0.80 would be desirable. After a periodontal surgical crown-lengthening procedure, a more esthetic width-to-length ratio of 0.80 was attained (see Fig. 12-7, *D*). After placement of eight etched porcelain veneers for the treatment of fluorosis discoloration, the same 0.80 width-to-length ratio can be seen (see Fig. 12-7, *E*). A 7-year postoperative photograph reveals the long-term esthetic result (see Fig. 12-7, *F*).

Because central incisors are the dominant focal point in dental composition, the dentist must avoid narrow, elongated, or short-and-wide contours. Adequate treatment planning and a fundamental knowledge of the importance of the ideal width-to-length ratios can optimize the final esthetic outcome. The importance of interdisciplinary treatment involving orthodontics, periodontics, or both cannot be underestimated.

Position and Alignment

The overall harmony and balance of a smile depend largely on proper position of teeth and their alignment in the arch. Malposed or rotated teeth disrupt the arch form and may interfere with the apparent relative proportions of teeth. Orthodontic treatment of such defects always should be considered, especially if other positional or malocclusion problems exist in the mouth. If orthodontic treatment is either impractical or unaffordable, however, minor positional defects often can be treated with composite augmentation or full facial veneers indirectly made from composite or porcelain. Only problems that can be treated conservatively without significant alteration of the occlusion or gingival contours of teeth should be treated in this manner.

Minor rotations can be corrected by reducing the enamel in the area of prominence and augmenting the deficient area with composite resin (Fig. 12-8, *A* and *B*). Care must be taken to restrict all recontouring of prominent areas to enamel. If the rotation is to be treated with an indirectly fabricated composite or porcelain veneer, an intra-enamel preparation is recommended, with greater reduction provided in the area of prominence. This preparation allows subsequent restoration to appropriate physiologic contours.

Malposed teeth are treated in a similar manner. Teeth in mild linguoversion can be treated by augmentation with full facial veneers placed directly with composite or made indirectly from processed composite or porcelain (see Fig. 12-8, *C* and *D*). Care must be exercised in maintaining physiologic gingival contours that do not impinge on tissue or result in an emergence profile of the restoration that is detrimental to gingival health. A functional incisal edge should be maintained by appropriate contouring of the restoration (an excessively thick incisal edge should be avoided). If the occlusion allows, limited reduction of enamel on the lingual aspect can be accomplished to reduce the faciolingual dimension of the incisal portion of the tooth. Lingual areas participating in protrusive functional contact should not be altered, however. Individual teeth that are significantly displaced facially (i.e., facioversion) are best treated orthodontically.

Surface Texture

The character and individuality of teeth are determined largely by their surface texture and existing characteristics. Realistic restorations closely mimic the subtle areas of stippling, concavity, and convexity that are typically present on natural teeth. Teeth in young individuals characteristically exhibit significant surface characterization, whereas teeth in older individuals tend to possess a smoother surface texture caused by abrasional wear. Even in older patients, however, restorations that are devoid of surface characterizations are rarely indicated.

The surfaces of natural teeth typically break up light and reflect it in many directions. Consequently, anatomic features (e.g., developmental depressions, prominences, facets, perikymata) should be examined closely and reproduced to the extent that they are present on the surrounding surfaces. The restored areas of teeth should reflect light as in the unrestored adjacent surfaces. In addition, as alluded to earlier, by controlling areas of light reflection and shadowing, various desired illusions also can be created.

Color

Color is the most complex and least understood artistic element. It is an area in which numerous interdependent

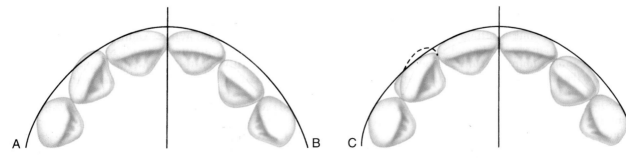

Fig. 12-8 Position and alignment. **A,** A minor rotation is first treated by reducing enamel in the area of prominence. **B,** The deficient area is restored to proper contour with composite. **C,** Maxillary lateral incisor is in slight linguoversion. **D,** Restorative augmentation of facial surface corrects malposition.

factors exist, all of which contribute to the final esthetic outcome of the restoration. Although complex, a basic knowledge of color is imperative to producing consistently esthetic restorations.

Three fundamental elements of color are *hue, value,* and *chroma.* Hue is the intrinsic quality or shade of the color. Value refers to the relative lightness or darkness of a hue. It is determined by the amount of white or black in a hue. Chroma is the intensity of any particular hue. Some current shade guides are based first on value because of the importance of this element of color.

Dentists also must understand the coloration of natural teeth to select the appropriate shades of restorative materials accurately and consistently. Teeth typically are composed of a multitude of colors. A gradation of color usually occurs from the gingival region to the incisal region, with the gingival region being typically darker because of thinner enamel. Use of several different shades of restorative material may be required to restore a tooth esthetically. Exposed root surfaces are particularly darker (i.e., dentin colored) because of the absence of overlying enamel. In most individuals, canines are slightly darker than are incisors.

Young individuals with thick enamel characteristically exhibit lighter teeth. Individuals with darker complexions usually appear to have lighter teeth because of the contrast that exists between teeth and the surrounding facial structures. Women can enhance the apparent lightness of their teeth simply by using a darker shade of makeup or lipstick. By increasing the contrast between teeth and the surrounding facial tissue, the illusion of lighter teeth can be created.

Color changes associated with aging also occur, primarily owing to wear. As the facial enamel is worn away, the underlying dentin becomes more apparent, resulting in a darker tooth. Incisal edges are often darker because of the thinning of enamel or the exposure of dentin because of normal attrition. Cervical areas also tend to darken because of abrasion.

An understanding of normal tooth coloration enhances the dentist's ability to create a restoration that appears natural. Several clinical factors also must be considered, however, to enhance the color-matching quality of the restoration. Many shade guides for composite materials are inaccurate. Not only are they often composed of a material dissimilar to that of the composite, but they also do not take into consideration color changes that occur from batch to batch or changes caused by aging of the composite. Accurate shade selection is best attained by applying and curing a small amount of the composite restorative material in the area of the tooth that may need restoration. Shade selection should be determined before isolating teeth so that color variations that can occur as a result of drying and dehydration of teeth are avoided.

Problems in color perception also complicate selection of the appropriate shade of restorative material. Various light sources produce different perceptions of color. This phenomenon is referred to as *metamerism.*[9] The color of the surrounding environment influences what is seen in the patient's mouth. Color perception also is influenced by the physiologic limitations of the dentist's eye. On extended viewing of a particular tooth site, eyes experience color fatigue, resulting in a loss of sensitivity to yellow-orange shades.[7] By looking away at a blue object or background (i.e., the complementary color), the dentist's eyes quickly recover and are able to distinguish subtle variations in yellow-orange hues again. Because of the many indirect factors that influence color perception, it is recommended that the dentist, the assistant, and especially the patient all be involved in shade selection.

Translucency

Translucency is another factor that affects the esthetic quality of the restoration. The degree of translucency is related to how deeply light penetrates into the tooth or restoration before it is reflected outward. Normally, light penetrates through enamel into dentin before being reflected outward (Fig. 12-9, *A*); this affords the realistic esthetic vitality characteristic of normal, unrestored teeth. Shallow penetration of light often results in loss of esthetic vitality. This phenomenon is a common problem encountered when treating severely intrinsically stained teeth such as teeth affected by tetracycline with direct or indirect veneers. Although opaque resin media can mask the underlying stain, esthetic vitality is usually lost because of reduced light penetration (see Fig. 12-9, *B*). Indirect veneers of processed composite or porcelain fabricated to include inherent opacity also may have this problem.

Illusions of translucency also can be created to enhance the realism of a restoration. Color modifiers (also referred to as *tints*) can be used to achieve apparent translucency and tone down bright stains or to characterize a restoration. Figure 12-10 shows a case in which the maxillary right central incisor with intrinsic yellow staining caused by trauma to the tooth warranted restoration. When bleaching treatments were unsuccessful because of calcific metamorphosis, a direct composite veneer was used in this patient. After an intra-enamel

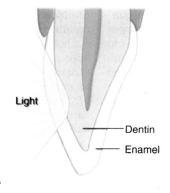

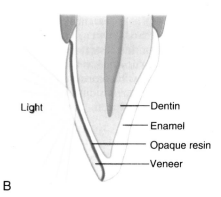

Fig. 12-9 Translucency and light penetration. **A,** Light normally penetrates deeply through enamel and into dentin before being reflected outward. This affords realistic esthetic vitality. **B,** Light penetration is limited by opaquing resin media under veneers. Esthetic vitality is compromised.

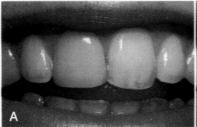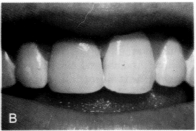

Fig. 12-10 Use of internally placed color modifiers. **A,** The maxillary right central incisor exhibits bright intrinsic yellow staining as a result of calcific metamorphosis. **B,** Color modifiers under direct-composite veneer reduce brightness and intensity of stain and simulate vertical areas of translucency.

preparation and acid-etching, a violet color modifier (the complementary color of yellow) was applied to the prepared facial surface to reduce the brightness and intensity of the underlying yellow tooth. Additionally, a mixture of gray and violet color modifiers was used to simulate vertical areas of translucency. The final restoration is shown in Figure 12-10, *B*. Color modifiers also can be incorporated in the restoration to simulate maverick colors, to check lines, or to surface spots for further characterization. Color modifiers always should be placed within a composite restoration, not on its surface.

Clinical Considerations

Although an understanding of basic artistic elements is imperative to successfully placing esthetic restorations, certain clinical considerations must be addressed concomitantly to ensure the overall quality of the restoration. In addition to being esthetic, restorations must be functional. Dawson stated, "Esthetics and function go hand in hand. The better the esthetics, the better the function is likely to be and vice versa."[10]

The occlusion always must be assessed before any conservative esthetic procedure. Anterior guidance, in particular, must be maintained and occlusal harmony ensured when treating areas involved in occlusion. Another requirement of all conservative esthetic restorations is that they possess physiologic contours that promote good gingival health. Particular care must be taken in all treatments to finish the gingival areas of the restoration adequately and to remove any gingival excess of material. Emergence angles of the restorations must be physiologic and not impinge on gingival tissue.

Conservative Alterations of Tooth Contours and Contacts

Many unsightly tooth contours and diastemas can be corrected or the appearance greatly improved by several conservative methods. Often, these procedures can be incorporated into routine restorative treatment. The objective is to improve esthetics and yet preserve as much healthy tooth structure as possible, consistent with the acceptable occlusion and health of surrounding tissue. These procedures include reshaping natural teeth, correcting embrasures, and closing diastemas.

Alterations of Shape of Natural Teeth

Some esthetic problems can be corrected conservatively without the need for tooth preparation and restoration.

Consideration always should be given to reshaping and polishing natural teeth to improve their appearance and function (Fig. 12-11). In addition, the rounding of sharp angles can be considered a prophylactic measure to reduce stress and to prevent chipping and fractures of the incisal edges.

Etiology

Attrition of the incisal edges often results in closed incisal embrasures and angular incisal edges (see Fig. 12-11, *A*). Anterior teeth, especially maxillary central incisors, often are fractured in accidents. Other esthetic problems, including attrition and abnormal wear from poor dental habits (e.g., biting fingernails, holding objects with teeth), often can be corrected or the appearance improved by reshaping natural teeth.

Treatment

Consultation and examination are necessary before any changes are made to the shapes of teeth. Photographs, study models, line drawings, and esthetic imaging devices enable the patient to envision the potential improvement before any changes are made.

As noted earlier, cosmetic contouring to achieve youthful characteristics often includes rounding incisal angles, reducing facial line angles, and opening incisal embrasures. The opposite characteristics typically are considered more mature features. Cosmetic reshaping to smooth rough incisal edges and improve symmetry is equally beneficial to women and men.

The patient must understand what is involved and must want to have the alteration made. If reshaping is desired, it is helpful to mark, by using a pencil or alcohol-marking pen, an outline of the areas of the teeth to be reshaped (see Fig. 12-11, *B*). By marking the anticipated areas for enamel reshaping, the patient is provided some indication of what the post-operative result may look like (see Fig. 12-11, *C*). If available, esthetic computer imaging also can be used to illustrate the possible result before treatment.

Because all reshaping is restricted to enamel, anesthesia is not required. A cotton roll is recommended for isolation. Diamond instruments and abrasive disks and points are used for contouring, finishing, and polishing (see Fig. 12-11, *D* and *E*). Through careful reshaping of appropriate enamel surfaces, a more esthetic smile (characterized by youthful features) is attained. Rounded incisal edges also are less likely to chip or fracture (see Fig. 12-11, *F*).

A second example involves the irregular, fractured incisal surfaces of maxillary central incisors (Fig. 12-12, *A*). An esthetic result can be accomplished by slightly shortening the

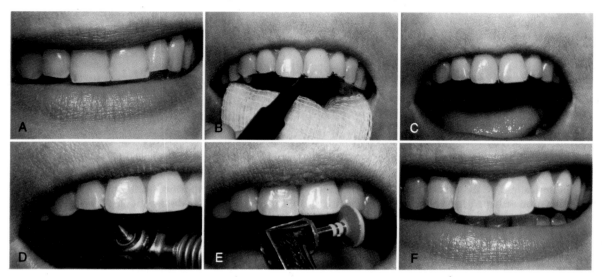

Fig. 12-11 Reshaping natural teeth. **A,** Maxillary anterior teeth with worn incisal edges. **B,** Areas to be reshaped are outlined. **C,** Outlined areas give the patient an idea of what the final result will look like. **D,** A diamond instrument is used to reshape the incisal edges. **E,** A rubber abrasive disk is used to polish the incisal edges. **F,** Reshaping results in a more youthful smile.

Fig. 12-12 Irregular incisal edges. **A,** Central incisors have rough, fractured incisal edges. **B,** Esthetic result is obtained by recontouring incisal edges.

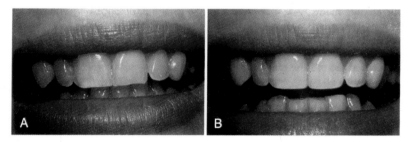

Fig. 12-13 Loss of incisal embrasures from attrition. Before (*A*) and after (*B*) recontouring teeth to produce a more youthful appearance and improve resistance to fracture.

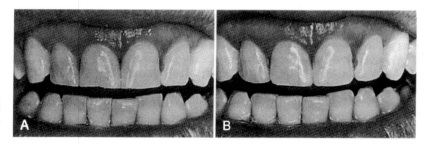

incisal edges and reshaping both teeth to a symmetrical form. Photographs, line drawings, esthetic imaging, or marking the outline on the patient's teeth enables the patient to envision the potential improvement before any changes are made. Protrusive function always should be evaluated to prevent inadvertent elimination of this occlusal contact. Conservative treatment consists of using diamond instruments and abrasive disks and points for contouring and polishing the central incisors. The finished result is illustrated in Figure 12-12, *B*.

As some patients grow older or have the habit of bruxism, the incisal surfaces often wear away, leaving sharp edges that chip easily. This is also accompanied by loss of the incisal

embrasures (Fig. 12-13, *A*). To lessen the chance of more fractures and to create a more youthful smile, the incisal embrasures are opened, and the incisal angles of teeth are rounded (see Fig. 12-13, *B*).

Alterations of Embrasures
Etiology

Anterior teeth can have embrasures that are too open as a result of the shape or position of teeth in the arch. When the permanent lateral incisors are congenitally missing, canines and posterior teeth may drift mesially, or the space may be

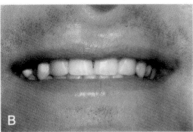

Fig. 12-14 Closing incisal embrasures. **A,** Maxillary canines moved to close spaces left by missing lateral incisors. The mesial incisal embrasures are too open. **B,** Canines reshaped to appear like lateral incisors.

closed orthodontically. The facial surface and cusp angle of some canines can be reshaped to appear like lateral incisors. In many instances, the mesio-incisal embrasures remain too open (Fig. 12-14, *A*).

Treatment

Composite can be added to establish an esthetic contour and correct the open embrasures. Evaluation of the occlusion before restoration determines if the addition would be compatible with functional movements. The patient should understand the procedures involved and should want to have the change made. Line drawings, esthetic imaging, or photographs of similar examples are often helpful in explaining the procedure and allaying patient concerns. Another patient aid involves adding ivory-colored wax or composite to teeth (unetched) to fill the embrasure temporarily to simulate the final result.

Preliminary procedures include cleaning the involved teeth, selecting the shade, and isolating the area. Local anesthesia usually is not required because the preparation does not extend subgingivally and involves only enamel. A coarse, flame-shaped diamond instrument is used to remove overly convex enamel surfaces (if present) and to roughen the enamel surface area to be augmented with composite material. It may be necessary to place a wedge and use an abrasive strip to prepare the proximal surface. The final contour of the restoration should be envisioned before the preparation is made so that all areas to be bonded are adequately roughened.

A polyester strip is inserted to protect the adjacent tooth during acid etching. After etching, rinsing, and drying, the contoured strip is positioned. A light-cured composite material is inserted, and the strip is closed during polymerization. The incisal embrasures of both canines are corrected, and both restorations are finished by routine procedures (see Fig. 12-14, *B*). The occlusion should be evaluated to assess centric contacts and functional movements, and any adjustments or corrections should be made, if indicated.

Correction of Diastemas
Etiology

The presence of diastemas between anterior teeth is an esthetic problem for some patients (Fig. 12-15). Before treatment, a diagnosis of the cause is made, including an evaluation of the occlusion. Probably the most frequent site of a diastema is between maxillary central incisors. A prominent labial frenum with non-elastic fibers extending proximally often prevents the normal approximation of erupting central incisors.[11] Other causative factors include congenitally missing teeth,

undersized or malformed teeth, interarch tooth size discrepancies (i.e., Bolton discrepancy), supernumerary teeth, and heredity. Diastemas also may result from other problems such as tongue thrusting, periodontal disease, or posterior bite collapse. Diastemas should not be closed without first recognizing and treating the underlying cause, as merely treating the cause may correct the diastema.

Treatment

Traditionally, diastemas have been treated by surgical, periodontal, orthodontic, and prosthetic procedures. These types of corrections can be impractical or unaffordable and often do not result in permanent closure of the diastema. In carefully selected cases, a more practical alternative is use of the acid-etch technique and composite augmentation of proximal surfaces (see Figs. 12-5 and Fig. 12-6). All treatment options (including no treatment) should be considered before resorting immediately to composite augmentation. Line drawings, photographs, computer imaging, models with spaces filled, and direct temporary additions of ivory-colored wax or composite material on natural teeth (unetched) are important preliminary procedures.

The correction of a diastema between maxillary central incisors is described and illustrated in Figure 12-15. After the teeth are cleaned and the shade selected, a Boley gauge or other suitable caliper is used to measure the width of the diastema and the individual teeth (see Fig. 12-15, *B* and *C*). Occasionally, one central incisor is wider, requiring a greater addition to the narrower tooth. Assuming the incisors are of equal width, symmetrical additions can be ensured by using half of the total measurement of the diastema to gauge the width of the first tooth restored. Cotton rolls, instead of a rubber dam, are recommended for isolation because of the importance of relating the contour of the restoration directly to the proximal tissue. Usually, the restoration must begin slightly below the gingival crest to appear natural and to be confluent with the tooth contours.

With cotton rolls in place, a gingival retraction cord of an appropriate size is tucked in the gingival crevice of each tooth from midfacial mesially to midlingual (see Fig. 12-15, *D*). The cord retracts the soft tissue and prevents seepage from the crevice. In some instances, the retraction cord may need to be inserted for one tooth at a time to prevent strangulation of interproximal tissue during preparation and restorative procedures. To enhance retention of the composite, a coarse, flame-shaped diamond instrument is used to roughen the proximal surfaces, extending from the facial line angle to the lingual line angle (see Fig. 12-15, *E*). More extension may be needed to correct the facial or lingual contours, depending on

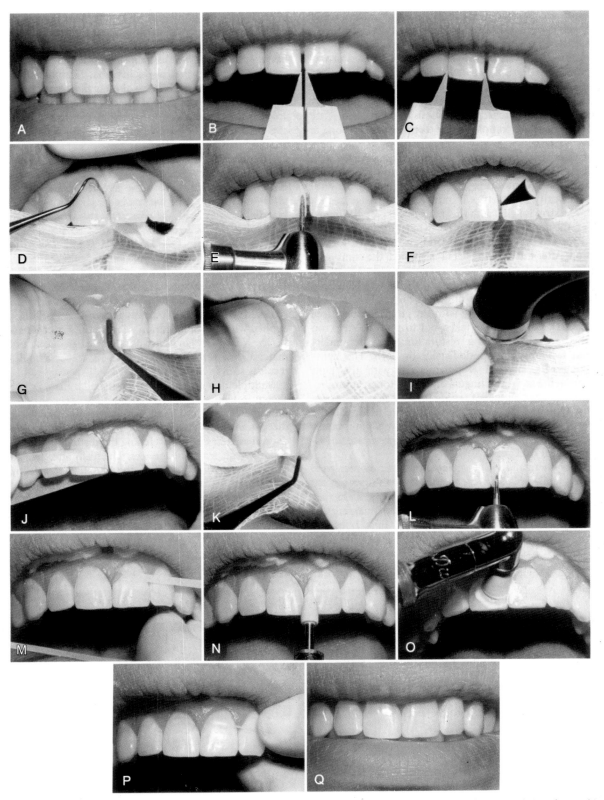

Fig. 12-15 Diastema closure. **A,** Esthetic problem created by space between central incisors. **B** and **C,** Interdental space and size of central incisors measured with caliper. **D,** Teeth isolated with cotton rolls and retraction cord tucked into the gingival crevice. **E,** A diamond instrument is used to roughen enamel surfaces. **F,** Etched enamel surface indicated by arrow. **G,** Composite inserted with composite instrument. **H,** Matrix strip closed with thumb and forefinger. **I,** Composite addition is cured. **J,** Finishing strip used to finalize contour of first addition. **K,** A tight contact is attained by displacing the second tooth being restored in a distal direction with thumb and forefinger, while holding matrix in contact with adjacent restoration. **L,** Flame-shaped finishing bur used to contour restoration. **M,** Finishing strip used to smooth the subgingival areas. **N,** The restoration is polished with a rubber abrasive point. **O,** Final luster attained with polishing paste applied with Prophy cup. **P,** Unwaxed floss used to detect any excess composite. **Q,** Diastema closed with symmetrical and equal additions of composite.

the anatomy and position of the individual tooth. The enamel is acid-etched approximately 0.5 mm past the prepared, roughened surface. The acid should be applied gingivally only to the extent of the anticipated restoration. After rinsing and drying, the etched enamel should display a lightly frosted appearance (see Fig. 12-15, *F*). A 2 × 2 inch (5 × 5 cm) gauze is draped across the mouth and tongue to prevent inadvertent contamination of the etched preparations by the patient. After both preparations are completed, the teeth are restored one at a time.

A polyester strip is contoured and placed proximally, with the gingival aspect of the strip extending below the gingival crest. Additional contouring may be required to produce enough convexity in the strip. In most cases, a wedge cannot be used. The strip is held (with the index finger) on the lingual aspect of the tooth to be restored, while the facial end is reflected for access. A light-cured composite is used for the restoration. After the bonding agent is applied, the composite material is inserted with a hand instrument (see Fig. 12-15, *G*). Careful attention is given to pressing the material lingually to ensure confluence with the lingual surface. The matrix is gently closed facially, beginning with the gingival aspect (see Fig. 12-15, *H*). Care must be taken not to pull the strip too tightly because the resulting restoration may be under-contoured faciolingually, mesiodistally, or both. The light-cured composite material is polymerized with the light directed from the facial and lingual directions for an appropriate amount of time. Note that curing times may vary according to the type of light source, the composite used, and the thickness of the material (see Fig. 12-15, *I*). Initially, it is better to over-contour the first restoration slightly to facilitate finishing it to an ideal contour.

When polymerization is complete, the strip is removed. Contouring and finishing are achieved with appropriate carbide finishing burs, fine diamonds, or abrasive disks (see Fig. 12-15, *L*). Finishing strips are invaluable for finalizing the proximal contours (see Fig. 12-15, *J* and *M*). Final polishing is deferred until the contralateral restoration is completed. It

is imperative for good gingival health that the cervical aspect of the composite addition be immaculately smooth and continuous with the tooth structure. Overhangs must not be present. Removal of the gingival retraction cord facilitates inspection and smoothing of this area. Flossing with a length of unwaxed floss verifies that the gingival margin is correct and smooth if no fraying of the floss occurs (see Fig. 12-15, *P*). It is important that the correct mesiodistal dimension of the first tooth be established before the second tooth is restored.

After etching, rinsing, and drying, the second restoration is completed. A tight proximal contact can be attained by displacing the second tooth being restored in a distal direction (with the thumb and the index finger) while holding the matrix in contact with the adjacent restoration (see Fig. 12-15, *K*). Contouring is accomplished with a 12-fluted carbide bur and finishing strips (see Fig. 12-15, *L* and *M*). Articulating paper should be used to evaluate the patient's occlusion to ensure that the restorations are not offensive in centric or functional movements; adjustments can be made with a carbide finishing bur or abrasive disks. Final polishing is achieved with rubber polishing points or polishing paste applied with a Prophy cup in a low-speed handpiece (see Fig. 12-15, *N* and *O*). Unwaxed floss is used to detect any excess material or overhang (see Fig. 12-15, *P*). The final esthetic result is seen in Figure 12-15, *Q*.

Multiple diastemas among the maxillary anterior teeth are shown in Figure 12-16, *A*. Closing the spaces by orthodontic movement was considered in this patient; however, because the patient's teeth were under-contoured mesiodistally, the diastemas were closed by etching the teeth and bonding composite to the proximal surfaces. The teeth after treatment are shown in Figure 12-16, *B*. In the presence of defective Class III restorations or proximal caries, it is recommended that the teeth be restored with the same composite used for closing the diastema. Often, these restorations can be performed at the same time the diastema is closed with composite additions (Fig. 12-17).

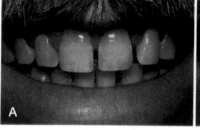
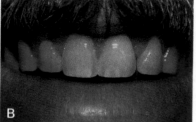

Fig. 12-16 Multiple diastemas occurring among maxillary anterior teeth. **A,** Before correction. **B,** Appearance after diastemas are closed with composite augmentation.

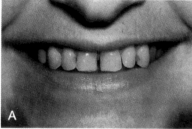
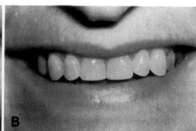

Fig. 12-17 **A,** Diastema closure and cosmetic contouring. **B,** Significant esthetic improvement is achieved by replacing defective Class III restorations and closing diastemas with conservative-composite additions and cosmetically reshaping teeth.

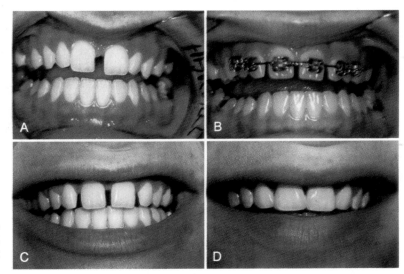

Fig. 12-18 Space distribution. **A,** Midline diastema too large for simple closure with composite additions. **B** and **C,** Space distributed among four incisors with orthodontic treatment. **D,** Final result after composite additions.

Occasionally, diastemas are simply too large to close esthetically with composite augmentation alone (Fig. 12-18, *A*). Closing a large space of this magnitude with composite would merely create an alternative esthetic problem, that is, excessively large central incisors, which would further exacerbate the existing discrepancy in proportionality among anterior teeth. In such cases, large spaces are best redistributed orthodontically among anterior teeth so that symmetric and equal composite additions can be made to the central and lateral incisors (see Fig. 12-18, *B* and *C*). This approach that involves space distribution results in improved proportionality among anterior teeth (see the earlier section on Artistic Elements). The final result, immediately after completion, is shown in Figure 12-18, *D*.

Conservative Treatments for Discolored Teeth

One of the most frequent reasons patients seek dental care is discolored anterior teeth. Patients with teeth of normal color request whitening procedures. Treatment options include removal of surface stains, bleaching, microabrasion or macroabrasion, veneering, and placement of porcelain crowns. Many dentists recommend porcelain crowns as the best solution for badly discolored teeth. If crowns are done properly with the highly esthetic ceramic materials currently available, they have great potential for being esthetic and long lasting. Increasing numbers of patients do not want their teeth "cut down" for crowns and choose an alternative, conservative approach such as veneers (see the subsequent section on Veneers) that preserves as much of the natural tooth as possible. This treatment is performed with the understanding that the corrective measures may be less permanent.

Discolorations are classified as extrinsic or intrinsic. Extrinsic stains are located on the outer surfaces of teeth, whereas intrinsic stains are internal. The etiology and treatment of extrinsic and intrinsic stains are discussed in the following sections.

Extrinsic Discolorations
Etiology

Stains on the external surfaces of teeth (referred to as *extrinsic discolorations*) are common and may be the result of numerous factors. In young patients, stains of almost any color can be found and are usually more prominent in the cervical areas of teeth (Fig. 12-19, *A*). These stains may be related to remnants of Nasmyth's membrane, poor oral hygiene, existing restorations, gingival bleeding, plaque accumulation, eating habits, or the presence of chromogenic microorganisms.[12] In older patients, stains on the surfaces of teeth are more likely to be brown, black, or gray and occur on areas adjacent to gingival tissue. Poor oral hygiene is a contributing factor, but coffee, tea, and other types of chromogenic foods or medications can produce stains (even on plaque-free surfaces). Tobacco stains also are observed frequently. Existing restorations may be discolored for the same reasons.

An example of one of the most interesting and unusual types of external staining is illustrated in Figure 12-19, *B*. In Southeast Asia, some women traditionally dye their teeth with betel nut juice to match their hair and eyes as a sign of beauty.[13] Slices of lemon are held in contact with the teeth before applying the betel nut juice to make the staining process more effective. This example was probably one of the first applications of the acid-etch technique. A weak acid, such as that found in citrus fruits, is known to cause rapid decalcification of enamel.

Treatment

Most surface stains can be removed by routine prophylactic procedures (Fig. 12-20). Some superficial discolorations on tooth-colored restorations and decalcified areas on teeth, however, cannot be corrected by such cleaning. Conservative correction may be accomplished by mild microabrasion or by surfacing the thin, outer, discolored layer with a flame-shaped, carbide finishing bur or diamond instrument (i.e., macroabrasion), followed by polishing with abrasive disks or points to obtain an acceptable result. (See subsequent sections on

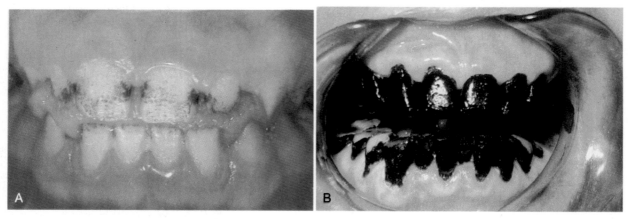

Fig. 12-19 Extrinsic stains. **A,** Surface stains on facial surfaces in a young patient. **B,** Exotic decoration of anterior teeth by etching with citrus fruit juice and applying black pigment (betel nut stain). (**A,** Courtesy of Dr. Tim Wright. **B,** From Daniel SJ, Harfst SA, Wilder RS: Mosby's dental hygiene: Concepts, cases, and competencies, ed 2, St. Louis, Mosby, 2008, Courtesy of Dr. George Taybos, Jackson, MS.)

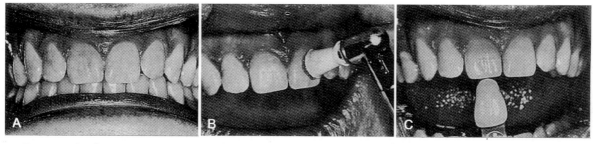

Fig. 12-20 Treatment of surface stains. **A,** Tobacco stains. **B,** Pumicing teeth with rubber cup. **C,** Shade guide used to confirm normal color of natural teeth.

Fig. 12-21 Intrinsic stains. **A,** Staining by tetracycline drugs. **B,** Staining of the maxillary left central incisor from tooth trauma and degeneration of the pulp.

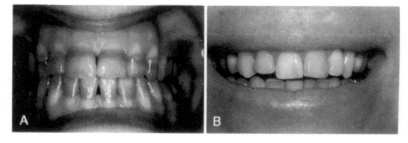

Microabrasion and Macroabrasion for details of clinical technique.)

Intrinsic Discolorations
Etiology

Intrinsic discolorations are caused by deeper (not superficial) internal stains or enamel defects; these stains are more complex to treat than are external types. Teeth with vital or non-vital pulps as well as root canal–treated teeth can be affected. Vital teeth may be discolored at the time the crowns are forming, and the abnormal condition usually involves several teeth. Causative factors include hereditary disorders, medications (particularly tetracycline preparations), excess fluoride, high fevers associated with early childhood illnesses, and other types of trauma.[12] The staining may be located in enamel or

dentin. Discolorations restricted to dentin still may show through enamel. Discoloration also may be localized or generalized, involving the entire tooth.

Various preparations of the antibiotic drug tetracycline can cause the most distracting, generalized type of intrinsic discoloration (Fig. 12-21, *A*).[14] The severity of the staining depends on the dose, the duration of exposure to the drug, and the type of tetracycline analogue used. Different types of tetracyclines induce different types of discoloration, varying from yellow-orange to dark blue-gray. Dark blue-gray, tetracycline-stained teeth are considerably more difficult to treat than are teeth with mild yellow-orange discolorations. Staining from tetracycline-type drugs most frequently occurs at an early age and is caused by ingestion of the drug concomitant with the development of permanent teeth. Studies indicate that permanent teeth in adults also can experience a graying discoloration, however, as a result of long-term exposure to minocycline, a tetracycline analogue.[14]

The presence of excessive fluoride in drinking water and other sources at the time of teeth formation can result in another type of intrinsic stain called *fluorosis*. The staining usually is generalized. Localized areas of discoloration may occur on individual teeth because of enamel or dentin defects induced during tooth development. High fevers and other forms of trauma can damage the tooth during its development, resulting in unesthetic hypoplastic defects. Additionally, localized areas of dysmineralization, or the failure of the enamel to calcify properly, can result in hypocalcified white spots. After eruption, poor oral hygiene also can result in decalcified white spots. Poor oral hygiene during orthodontic treatment frequently results in these types of decalcified defects. White or discolored spots with intact enamel surface (i.e., surface not soft) are often evidence of intraoral remineralization, however, and such spots are not indications for invasive treatment (unless for esthetic concerns). Additionally, caries, metallic restorations, corroded pins, and leakage or secondary caries around existing restorations can result in various types of intrinsic discoloration.

As noted earlier, aging effects also can result in yellowed teeth. As patients grow older, the tooth enamel becomes thinner because of wear and allows underlying dentin to become more apparent. Also, often, continuing deposition of secondary dentin occurs in older individuals, resulting in greater dentin thickness. This deposition results in a yellowing effect, depending on the intrinsic color of dentin. Additionally, the permeability of teeth usually allows the infusion (over time) of significant organic pigments (from chromogenic foods, drinks, and tobacco products) that produce a yellowing effect.

Nonvital teeth also can become discolored intrinsically. These stains usually occur in individual teeth after eruption has taken place. The pulp may become infected or degenerate as a result of trauma, deep caries, or irritation from restorative procedures. If these teeth are properly treated by root canal therapy, they usually retain their normal color. If treatment is delayed, discoloration of the crown is more likely to occur. The degenerative products from the pulp tissue stain dentin, and this is readily apparent because of the translucency of enamel (see Fig. 12-21, *B*). Trauma resulting in calcific metamorphosis (i.e., calcification of the pulp chamber, root canal, or both) also can produce significant yellowing of the tooth. This condition is extremely difficult to treat (see Fig. 12-10).

Treatment

Some people definitely have esthetic problems because of intrinsic stains, but some others worry needlessly about the overall color of their teeth. In the latter instance, the dentist must decide if the color of teeth can be improved enough to justify treatment, even though the patient insists on having something done. Individuals with light complexions may believe that their teeth are too dark, when actually they are normal in color (Fig. 12-22, *A*). Positioning a shade tab from a shade guide of tooth colors next to such teeth often shows these patients that the color of their teeth is well within the normal range of shades. As stated earlier, tanned skin, darker makeup, or darker lipstick usually make teeth appear much

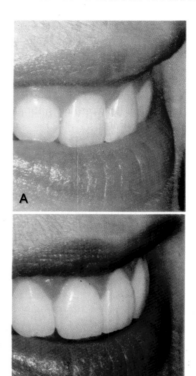

Fig. 12-22 Illusion of a lighter appearance of teeth by use of darker makeup. **A,** Before. **B,** After. (From Freedman G: Contemporary esthetic dentistry, St. Louis, Mosby, 2012.)

whiter by increasing the contrast between teeth and the surrounding facial features (see Fig. 12-22, *B*).

The patient should be told that many discolorations can be corrected or the appearance of teeth greatly improved through conservative methods such as bleaching, microabrasion or macroabrasion, and veneering. Mild discolorations are best left untreated, are bleached, or are treated conservatively with microabrasion or macroabrasion because no restorative material is as good as the healthy, natural tooth structure. The patient should be informed that the gingival tissue adjacent to restorative material will never be as healthy as that next to normal tooth structure.

Color photographs of previously treated teeth with intrinsic staining (i.e., before and after treatment) are excellent adjuncts to help the patient make an informed decision. Esthetic imaging with modern computer simulation of the postoperative result also can be an effective educational tool. Patients appreciate knowing what the cause of the problem is, how it can be corrected, how much time is involved, and what the cost will be. They also should be informed of the life expectancy of the various treatment alternatives suggested. Vital bleaching usually results in tooth lightening for only 1 to 3 years, whereas an etched porcelain veneer should last 10 to 15 years or longer. With continuous improvements in materials and techniques, a much longer lifespan may be possible with any of these procedures. The clinical longevity of esthetic restorations also is enhanced in patients with good oral hygiene, proper diet, a favorable bite relationship, and little or no contact with agents that cause discoloration or deterioration.

Correction of intrinsic discolorations caused by failing restorations entails replacement of the faulty portion or the entire restoration. Correction of discolorations caused by carious lesions requires appropriate restorative treatment. Esthetic inserts for metal restorations are described later in this chapter. For the other types of intrinsic discolorations previously discussed, detailed treatment options are presented in the following three sections.

Bleaching Treatments

The lightening of the color of a tooth through the application of a chemical agent to oxidize the organic pigmentation in the tooth is referred to as *bleaching*. In keeping with the overall conservative philosophy of tooth restoration, consideration should be given first to bleaching anterior teeth when intrinsic discolorations are encountered. Bleaching techniques may be classified as to whether they involve vital or non-vital teeth and whether the procedure is performed in the office or outside the office. Bleaching of non-vital teeth was first reported in 1848; in-office bleaching of vital teeth was first reported in 1868.[15] By the early 1900s, in-office vital bleaching had evolved to include the use of heat and light for activation of the process. Although a 3% ether and peroxide mouthwash used for bleaching in 1893 has been reported in the literature, the "dentist-prescribed, home-applied" technique (also referred to as *nightguard vital bleaching* or *at-home bleaching*) for bleaching vital teeth outside the office began around 1968, although it was not commonly known until the late 1980s.[16]

Most bleaching techniques use some form or derivative of hydrogen peroxide in different concentrations and application techniques. The mechanism of action of bleaching teeth with hydrogen peroxide is considered to be oxidation of organic pigments, although the chemistry is not well understood. Bleaching generally has an approximate lifespan of 1 to 3 years, although the change may be permanent in some situations.

With all bleaching techniques, a transitory decrease occurs in the potential bond strength of composite when it is applied to bleached enamel and dentin. This reduction in bond strength results from residual oxygen or peroxide residue in the tooth that inhibits the setting of the bonding resin, precluding adequate resin tag formation in the etched enamel. No loss of bond strength is noted if the composite restorative treatment is delayed at least 1 week after cessation of any bleaching.[17]

Nonvital Bleaching Procedures

The primary indication for nonvital bleaching is to lighten teeth that have undergone root canal therapy. Discoloration may be a result of bleeding into dentin from trauma before root canal therapy, degradation of pulp tissue left in the chamber after such therapy, or staining from restorative materials and cements placed in the tooth as a part of the root canal treatment. Most posterior teeth that have received root canal therapy require full-coverage restorations that encompass the tooth to prevent subsequent fracture. Anterior teeth needing restorative treatment and that are largely intact may be restored with composite rather than with partial-coverage or

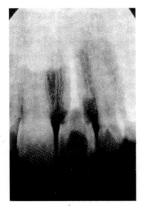

Fig. 12-23 Radiograph revealing the presence of extensive cervical resorption.

full-coverage restorations without significantly compromising the strength of the tooth.[18] This knowledge has resulted in a resurgence in the use of non-vital bleaching techniques. Non-vital bleaching techniques include an in-office technique and an out-of-office procedure referred to as *walking bleach*. (See the following sections for details of these two techniques.)

Although nonvital bleaching is effective, a slight potential (i.e., 1%) exists for a deleterious side effect termed *external cervical resorption* (Fig. 12-23).[19] This sequela requires prompt and aggressive treatment. In animal models, cervical resorption has been observed most when using a thermocatalytic technique with high heat.[20] The walking bleach technique or an in-office technique that does not require the use of heat is preferred for nonvital bleaching. To reduce the possibility of resorption, immediately after bleaching, a paste of calcium hydroxide powder and sterile water is placed in the pulp chamber as described in the following sections.[21] Also, sodium perborate alone, rather than in conjunction with hydrogen peroxide, should be used as the primary bleaching agent. Although sodium perborate may bleach more slowly, it is safer and less offensive to the tooth.[22] Periodic radiographs should be obtained after bleaching to screen for cervical resorption, which generally has its onset in 1 to 7 years.[23]

In-Office Nonvital Bleaching Technique

The in-office bleaching for nonvital teeth historically has involved a thermocatalytic technique consisting of the placement of 35% hydrogen peroxide liquid into the debrided pulp chamber and acceleration of the oxidation process by placement of a heating instrument into the pulp chamber. The thermocatalytic technique is not recommended, however, because of the potential for cervical resorption.[19] A more current technique uses 30% to 35% hydrogen peroxide pastes or gels that require no heat. This technique is frequently the preferred in-office technique for bleaching non-vital teeth. In both techniques, it is imperative that a sealing cement (resin-modified glass ionomer [RMGI] cement is recommended) be placed over the exposed root canal filling before application of the bleaching agent to prevent leakage and penetration of the bleaching material in an apical direction. It is also recommended that the bleaching agent be applied in the coronal portion of the tooth incisal to the level of the periodontal ligament (not down into the root canal space) to prevent unwanted

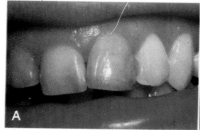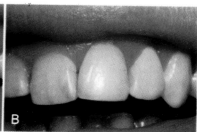

Fig. **12-24** Indication for bleaching root canal–filled tooth. **A,** Before. **B,** After intracoronal, nonvital bleaching.

leakage of the bleaching agent through the lateral canals or canaliculi to the periodontal ligament.

Walking Bleach Technique

Before beginning the walking bleach technique, the dentist needs to evaluate the potential for occlusal contact on the area of the root canal access opening. The dentist places a rubber dam to isolate the discolored tooth and removes all materials in the coronal portion of the tooth (i.e., access opening). The dentist removes gutta-percha (to approximately 1–2 mm apical of the clinical crown) and enlarges the endodontic access opening sufficiently to ensure complete debridement of the pulp chamber. Next, the dentist places an RMGI liner to seal the gutta-percha of the root canal, filling from the coronal portion of the pulp chamber. After this seal has hardened, the dentist trims any excess material from the seal so that the discolored dentin is exposed peripherally.

Sodium perborate is used with this technique because it is deemed extremely safe.[24] Using a cement spatula, with heavy pressure on a glass slab, one drop of saline or sterile anesthetic solution is blended with enough sodium perborate to form a creamy paste. A spoon excavator or similar instrument is used to fill the pulp chamber (with the bleaching mixture) to within 2 mm of the cavosurface margin, avoiding contact with the enamel cavosurface margins of the access opening. The dentist uses a cotton pellet to blot the mixture and places a temporary sealing material (e.g., Intermediate Restorative Material [DENTSPLY Caulk, Milford, DE], or Cavit [3M ESPE, St. Paul, MN]) to seal the access opening. The area should remain isolated for approximately 5 minutes after closure to evaluate the adequacy of the seal of the temporary restoration. If bubbles appear around the margins of the temporary material indicating leakage, the temporary restoration must be replaced. If no bubbles appear, the dentist removes the rubber dam and checks the occlusion to assess the presence or absence of contact on the temporary restoration.

The sodium perborate should be changed weekly. On successful bleaching of the tooth, the chamber is rinsed and filled to within 2 mm of the cavosurface margin with a paste consisting of calcium hydroxide powder in sterile saline. (The enamel walls and margins are kept clean and free of the calcium hydroxide paste.) As noted earlier, a paste of calcium hydroxide powder and sterile water is placed immediately after bleaching in the pulp chamber to reduce the possibility of resorption.[21] The dentist reseals the access opening with a temporary restorative material, as previously described, and allows the calcium hydroxide material to remain in the pulp chamber for 2 weeks. Subsequently, the dentist removes the temporary restorative material, rinses away the calcium

hydroxide, and dries the pulp chamber. Next, the dentist etches enamel and dentin and restores the tooth with a light-cured composite (Fig. 12-24).

Occasionally, a tooth that has been bleached by using the walking bleach technique and sealed with a composite restoration may subsequently become discolored. In this instance, the alternative treatment option should be an attempt to bleach the tooth externally with one of the external bleaching techniques (see next section).

Vital Bleaching Procedures

Generally, the indications for the different vital bleaching techniques are similar, with patient preference, cost, compliance, and difficulty in the removal of certain discolorations dictating the choice of treatment or combination of treatments. Indications for vital bleaching include teeth intrinsically discolored because of aging, trauma, or certain medications. External vital bleaching techniques are alternative treatment options for a failed, nonvital, walking bleach procedure. Vital bleaching also is often indicated before and after restorative treatments to harmonize the shades of the restorative materials with those of natural teeth.

Teeth exhibiting yellow or orange intrinsic discoloration seem to respond best to vital bleaching, whereas teeth exhibiting bluish gray discolorations often are considerably more difficult to treat in this manner. Other indications for external bleaching include teeth that have been darkened by trauma but are still vital or teeth that have a poor endodontic prognosis because of the absence of a radiographically visible canal (i.e., calcific metamorphosis). Brown fluorosis stains also are often responsive to treatment, but white fluorosis stains may not be resolved effectively (although they can be made less obvious if the surrounding tooth structure can be significantly whitened).

Vital bleaching techniques include an in-office technique referred to as *power bleaching* and an out-of-office alternative that is a "dentist-prescribed, home-applied" technique (i.e., nightguard vital bleaching, or simply "at-home bleaching").[25,26] These techniques may be used separately or in combination with one another. (Details are provided in subsequent sections.) Some over-the-counter bleaching materials, particularly products involving a trayless strip delivery system, also are effective for whitening teeth, but these are not discussed in this chapter.[27]

Overall, vital bleaching has been proven to be safe and effective when performed by, or under the supervision of, a dentist. With short-term treatment, no appreciable effect has been observed on existing restorative materials, either in loss of material integrity or in color change, with one exception:

Polymethyl methacrylate restorations exhibit a yellow-orange discoloration on exposure to carbamide peroxide. For this reason, temporary crowns should be made from bisacryl materials, rather than polymethyl methacrylate crown and bridge resin, if exposure to carbamide peroxide is anticipated.

Because hydrogen peroxide has such a low molecular weight, it easily passes through enamel and dentin. This characteristic is thought to account for the mild tooth sensitivity occasionally experienced during treatment. This effect is transient, however, and no long-term harm to the pulp has been reported.

Often, the dentist has to decide whether to use an in-office bleaching technique or prescribe a home-applied technique. The advantages of the in-office vital bleaching technique are that (although it uses very caustic chemicals) it is totally under the dentist's control, soft tissue is generally protected from the process, and the technique has the potential for bleaching teeth more rapidly. Disadvantages primarily relate to the cost, the unpredictable outcome, and the unknown duration of the treatment. The features that warrant concern and caution include the potential for soft tissue damage to both patient and provider, discomfort caused by the rubber dam or other isolation devices, and the potential for post-treatment sensitivity. The advantages of the dentist-prescribed, home-applied technique are the use of a lower concentration of peroxide (generally 10%–15% carbamide peroxide), ease of application, minimal side effects, and lower cost because of the reduced chair time required for treatment. The disadvantages are reliance on patient compliance, longer treatment time, and the (unknown) potential for soft tissue changes with excessively extended use.

In-Office Vital Bleaching Technique

In-office vital bleaching requires an excellent rubber dam technique and careful patient management. Vaseline or cocoa butter may be placed on the patient's lips and gingival tissue before application of the rubber dam to help protect these soft tissues from any inadvertent exposure to the bleaching agent. Anterior teeth (and sometimes the first premolars) are isolated with a heavy rubber dam to provide maximum retraction of tissue and an optimal seal around teeth. A good seal of the dam is ensured by ligation of the dam with waxed dental tape or the use of a sealing putty or varnish. Light-cured, resin-based "paint-on" rubber dam isolation media are available for use with in-office bleaching materials but cannot provide the same degree of protection and isolation as a conventionally applied rubber dam. Etching of teeth with 37% phosphoric acid, once considered a required part of this technique, is unnecessary.[28]

Numerous commercially available bleaching agents are available for in-office bleaching procedures. Most consist of paste or gel compositions that most commonly contain 30% to 35% hydrogen peroxide. Other additives, such as metallic ion–producing materials or alkalinizing agents that can speed up the oxidation reaction, also are commonly found in these commercially available whitening products. The dentist places the hydrogen peroxide–containing paste or gel on teeth. The patient is instructed to report any sensations of burning of the lips or gingiva that would indicate a leaking dam and the need to terminate treatment.

Most of the credible research indicates that the addition of light during the bleaching procedure does not improve the whitening result beyond what the bleach alone can achieve.[29] Use of a light to generate heat may accelerate the oxidation reaction of the hydrogen peroxide and expedite treatment through a thermocatalytic effect. PAC lights and high-output quartz halogen lights have been commonly used for this purpose. Use of lights to heat the bleaching agent, however, causes a greater level of tooth dehydration. This effect not only can increase tooth sensitivity but also results in an immediate apparent whitening of the tooth owing to dehydration that makes the actual whitening result more difficult to assess. Use of carbon dioxide laser to heat the bleaching mixture and accelerate the bleaching treatment has not been recommended, according to a report of the American Dental Association (ADA) because of the potential for hard or soft tissue damage.[30] On completion of the treatment, the dentist rinses the patient's teeth, removes the rubber dam or isolation medium, and cautions the patient about postoperative sensitivity. A nonsteroidal analgesic and anti-inflammatory drug may be administered if sensitivity is anticipated.

Contrary to the claims of some manufacturers, optimal whitening typically requires more than one bleaching treatment.[31] Bleaching treatments generally are rendered weekly for two to six treatments, with each treatment lasting 30 to 45 minutes. Patients may experience transient tooth sensitivity between appointments, but no long-term adverse effects of bleaching teeth with otherwise healthy pulps have been reported in the literature. Because the enamel is not acid-etched, it is not necessary to polish the teeth after they have been bleached, and it is not essential to provide any fluoride treatment.

Dentist-Prescribed, Home-Applied Technique

The dentist-prescribed, home-applied technique (i.e., nightguard vital bleaching) is much less labor intensive and requires substantially less in-office time. An impression of the arch to be treated is made and poured in cast stone. It should be ensured that the impression is free of bubbles on or around teeth by wiping the impression material onto teeth and the adjacent gingival areas before inserting the impression. After appropriate infection control procedures, the dentist rinses the impression vigorously and pours with cast stone. Incomplete rinsing of the impression may cause a softened surface on the stone, which may result in a nightguard (bleaching tray) that is slightly too small and that may irritate tissue. The dentist trims the cast around the periphery to eliminate the vestibule and thin out the base of the cast palatally (until a hole is produced). Generally, the cast must be lifted from the table of the cast-trimming machine to remove the vestibule successfully without damaging teeth. The dentist allows the cast to dry and blocks out any significant undercuts by using a block-out material (e.g., putty, clay, light-activated spacer material).

The nightguard is formed on the cast with the use of a heated vacuum-forming machine. After the machine has warmed up for 10 minutes, a sheet of 0.020- to 0.040-inch (0.75- to 1.5-mm) soft vinyl nightguard material is inserted and allowed to be softened by heat until the material sags approximately by 1 inch. The top portion of the machine is closed slowly and gently, and the vacuum is allowed to form the heat-softened material around the cast. After sufficient time has been allowed for adaptation of the material, the dentist turns off the machine and allows the material to cool.

Next, the dentist uses scissors or a No. 11 surgical blade in a Bard-Parker handle to trim in a smooth, straight cut about 3 to 5 mm from the most apical portion of the gingival crest of teeth (facially and lingually). This excess material is removed first. The horseshoe-shaped nightguard is removed from the cast. The dentist trims the facial edges of the nightguard in a scalloped design, following the outline of the free gingival crest and using sharp, curved scissors. Scalloping of the lingual surface is optional because the bleaching material is applied primarily to the facial aspects of teeth. Alternatively (on the lingual aspect), the nightguard may be trimmed apically to within 2 mm of the free gingival crest in a smooth, horseshoe-shaped configuration. This scalloped design is preferred because it allows the tray to cover only teeth and prevents entrapment of the bleaching material between gingival tissue and the nightguard. The nightguard is completed and is ready for delivery to the patient (Fig. 12-25).

The dentist inserts the nightguard into the patient's mouth and evaluates it for adaptation, rough edges, or blanching of tissue. A properly fitting nightguard is shown in Figure 12-26. Further shortening (i.e., trimming) may be indicated in problem areas. The dentist evaluates the occlusion on the nightguard with the patient in maximum intercuspation. If the patient is unable to obtain a comfortable occlusion because of premature posterior tooth contacts, the nightguard is trimmed to exclude coverage of the terminal posterior teeth, as needed (to allow optimal tooth contact in maximum intercuspation). In addition, if no lingual scalloping is done, the edges of the guard on the palate should terminate in grooves or valleys, where possible, rather than on the heights of soft tissue contours (e.g., in the area of the incisive papilla).

A 10% to 15% carbamide peroxide bleaching material generally is recommended for this bleaching technique.

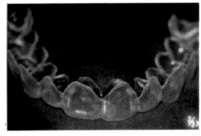

Fig. 12-25 Vacuum-formed, clear plastic nightguard used for vital bleaching (i.e., scalloped version).

Commercial bleaching products are available as clear gels and white pastes. Carbamide peroxide degrades into 3% hydrogen peroxide (active ingredient) and 7% urea. Bleaching materials containing carbopol are recommended because carbopol thickens the bleaching solution and extends the oxidation process. On the basis of numerous research studies, carbamide peroxide bleaching materials seem to be safe and effective when administered by or under the supervision of a dentist.[22]

The patient is instructed in the application of the bleaching gel or paste into the nightguard. A thin bead of material is extruded into the nightguard along the facial aspects corresponding to the area of each tooth to be bleached. Usually, only the anterior six to eight teeth are bleached. The clinician should review proper insertion of the nightguard with the patient. After inserting the nightguard, excess material is wiped from the soft tissue along the edge with a soft-bristled toothbrush. No excess material should be allowed to remain on soft tissue because of the potential for gingival irritation. The patient should be informed not to drink liquids or rinse during treatment and to remove the nightguard for meals and oral hygiene.

Although no single treatment regimen is best for all patients, most patients prefer an overnight treatment approach because of the convenience. If the nightguard is worn at night, a single application of bleaching material at bedtime is indicated. In the morning, the patient should remove the nightguard, clean it under running water with a toothbrush, and store it in the container provided. Total treatment time using an overnight approach is usually 1 to 2 weeks. If patients cannot tolerate overnight bleaching, the bleaching time and frequency can be adjusted to accommodate the patient's comfort level. In addition, in these cases, tolerance to the nightguard and bleaching material generally are improved if the patient gradually increases the wearing time each day.

If either of the two primary adverse effects occurs (i.e., sensitive teeth or irritated gingiva), the patient should reduce or discontinue treatment immediately and contact the dentist so that the cause of the problem can be determined and the treatment approach modified. The dentist may prescribe desensitizing agents to help alleviate sensitivity associated with bleaching.

It is recommended that only one arch be bleached at a time, beginning with the maxillary arch. Bleaching the maxillary arch first allows the untreated mandibular arch to serve as a constant standard for comparison. Restricting the bleaching to one arch at a time reduces the potential for occlusal problems that could occur if the thicknesses of two mouthguards were interposed simultaneously. Figure 12-27 illustrates a typical case before and after treatment with nightguard vital bleaching.

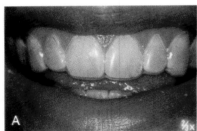
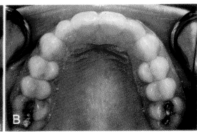

Fig. 12-26 Nightguard for vital bleaching. **A** and **B,** Clear plastic nightguard properly seated and positioned in the mouth (scalloped on facial, unscalloped on lingual).

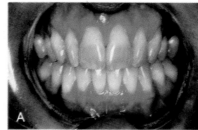
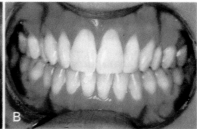

Fig. 12-27 Nightguard vital bleaching. **A,** Before bleaching treatment. **B,** After treatment.

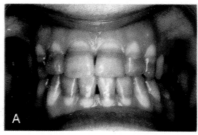
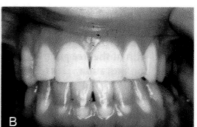

Fig. 12-28 Bleaching tetracycline-stained teeth. **A,** Before nonvital bleaching. **B,** After treatment. *(Courtesy of Dr. Wayne Mohorn.)*

Tetracycline-stained teeth typically are much more resistant to bleaching. Teeth stained with tetracycline require prolonged treatment durations of several months before any results are observed. Often, tetracycline-stained teeth are unresponsive to the procedure, especially if the stains are blue-gray in color. Tetracycline-stained teeth may approach, but never seem to achieve, the appearance of normal teeth. A single tetracycline-stained tooth with previous endodontic therapy or a different pulp size may respond differently from other teeth in the arch to the bleaching technique.

Because bleaching tetracycline-stained teeth is difficult, some clinicians advocate intentional endodontic therapy along with the use of an intracoronal nonvital bleaching technique to overcome this problem (Fig. 12-28). Although the esthetic result appears much better than that obtained from external bleaching, this approach involves all the inherent risks otherwise associated with root canal treatment. External bleaching techniques offer a safer alternative, although they may not be as rapid or effective. Veneers or full crowns are alternative esthetic treatment methods for difficult tetracycline-stained teeth but involve irreversible restorative techniques (see the section on Indirect Veneer Techniques). No one bleaching technique is effective in all cases, and all successes are not equal. Often, with vital bleaching, a combination of the in-office technique and the dentist-prescribed, home-applied technique has better results than either technique used alone.

Microabrasion and Macroabrasion

Microabrasion and *macroabrasion* represent conservative alternatives for the reduction or elimination of superficial discolorations. As the terms imply, the stained areas or defects are abraded away. These techniques result in the physical removal of the tooth structure and are indicated only for stains or enamel defects that do not extend beyond a few tenths of a millimeter in depth. If the defect or discoloration remains even after treatment with microabrasion or macroabrasion, a restorative alternative is indicated.

Microabrasion

In 1984, McCloskey reported the use of 18% hydrochloric acid swabbed on teeth for the removal of superficial fluorosis stains.[32] Subsequently, in 1986, Croll and Cavanaugh modified the technique to include the use of pumice with hydrochloric acid to form a paste applied with a tongue blade.[33] This technique is called *microabrasion* and involves the surface dissolution of the enamel by acid along with the abrasiveness of the pumice to remove superficial stains or defects. Since that time, Croll further modified the technique, reducing the concentration of the acid to approximately 11% and increasing the abrasiveness of the paste using silicon carbide particles (in a water-soluble gel paste) instead of pumice.[34] This product, marketed as Prema compound (Premier Dental Products Co., Plymouth Meeting, PA) or Opalustre (Ultradent Products, Inc., South Jordan, UT), represents an improved and safer means for the removal of superficial stains or defects. This technique involves the physical removal of tooth structure and does not remove stains or defects through any bleaching phenomenon.

Before treatment, the clinician should evaluate the nature and extent of the enamel defect or stain and differentiate between nonhereditary developmental dysmineralization (i.e., abnormal mineralization) defects (e.g., white or light brown fluoretic enamel and the idiopathic white or light brown spot) versus incipient carious lesions. Incipient carious lesions usually are located near the gingival margin. These lesions have a smooth surface and appear opaque or chalky white when dried but are less visible when hydrated.

Incipient caries is reversible if treated immediately. Changing the oral environment through oral hygiene practices and dietary adjustments allows remineralization to occur. If the caries lesion has progressed to have a slightly roughened surface, however, microabrasion coupled with a

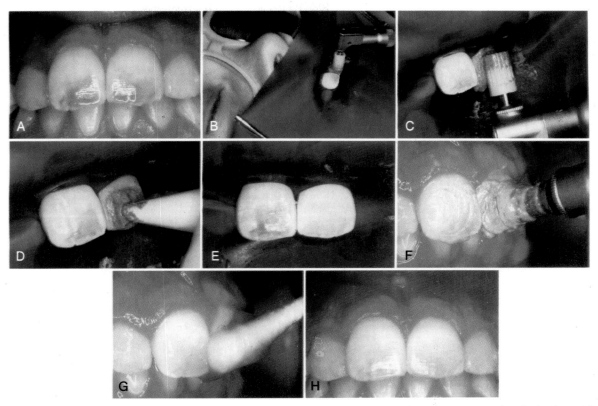

Fig. 12-29 Microabrasion. **A,** Young patient with unesthetic fluorosis stains on central incisors. **B** and **C,** Prema compound applied with special rubber cup with fluted edges. Protective glasses and rubber dam are needed for the safety of the patient. **D,** Hand applicator for applying Prema compound. **E,** Stain removed from the left central incisor after microabrasion. **F,** Treated enamel surfaces polished with prophylactic paste. **G,** Topical fluoride applied to treated enamel surfaces. **H,** Final esthetic result. *(Courtesy of Dr. Ted Croll.)*

remineralization program is an initial option. If this approach is unsuccessful, it can be followed by a restoration. Cavitation of the enamel surface is an indication for restorative intervention. As the location of smooth-surface enamel caries nears the cementoenamel junction (CEJ), then enamel is too thin to permit microabrasion or macroabrasion as a treatment option.

A developmental discolored spot (opaque white or light brown) is the result of an unknown, local traumatic event during amelogenesis and is termed *idiopathic*. Its surface is intact, smooth, and hard. It usually is located in the incisal (occlusal) half of enamel, which contributes to the unsightly appearance. The patient (or the patient's parents in the case of a child) must be informed that an accurate prognosis for microabrasion cannot be given but that microabrasion will be applied first. If microabrasion is unsuccessful because of the depth of the defect exceeding 0.2 to 0.3 mm, the tooth will be restored with a tooth-colored restoration. Surface discolorations resulting from fluorosis also can be removed by microabrasion if the discoloration is within the 0.2- to 0.3-mm removal depth limit.

Figure 12-29, *A*, shows a young patient with fluorosis stains on teeth No. 8 and No. 9. A rubber dam is placed to isolate the teeth to be treated and to protect the gingival tissues from the acid in the Prema paste or compound (Premier Dental Products). Protective glasses should be worn by the patient to shield the eyes from any spatter. The Prema paste is applied to the defective area of the tooth with a special rubber cup that has fluted edges (see Fig. 12-29, *B* and *C*). The abrasive

compound can be applied with either the side or the end of the rubber cup. A 10× gear reduction, low-speed handpiece (similar to that used for placing pins) is recommended for the application of the Prema compound to reduce the possibility of removing too much tooth structure and to prevent spatter. Moderately firm pressure is used in applying the compound.

For small, localized, idiopathic white or light brown areas, a hand application device also is available for use with the Prema compound (see Fig. 12-29, *D*). Periodically, the paste is rinsed away to assess the extent of defect removal. The facial surface also is viewed with a mirror from the incisal aspect to determine how much tooth structure has been removed. Care must be taken not to remove too much tooth structure. The procedure is continued until the defect is removed or until it is deemed imprudent to continue further (see Fig. 12-29, *E*). The treated areas are polished with a fluoride-containing Prophy paste to restore surface luster (see Fig. 12-29, *F*). Immediately after treatment, a topical fluoride is applied to teeth to enhance remineralization (see Fig. 12-29, *G*). Results are shown in Figure 12-29, *H*.

Macroabrasion

An alternative technique for the removal of localized, superficial white spots (not subject to conservative, remineralization therapy) and other surface stains or defects is called *macroabrasion*. Macroabrasion simply uses a 12-fluted composite finishing bur or a fine grit finishing diamond in a

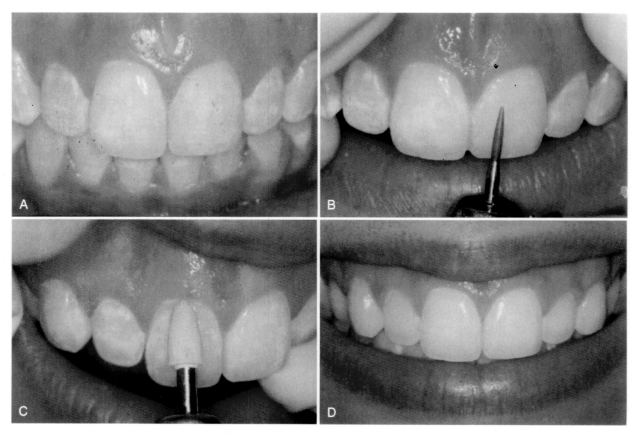

Fig. 12-30 Macroabrasion. **A,** Outer surfaces of maxillary anterior teeth are unesthetic because of superficial enamel defects. **B** and **C,** Removal of discoloration by abrasive surfacing and polishing procedures. **D,** Completed treatment revealing conservative esthetic outcome.

high-speed handpiece to remove the defect (Fig. 12-30, *A* and *B*). Care must be taken to use light, intermittent pressure and to monitor the removal of tooth structure carefully to avoid irreversible damage to the tooth. Air-water spray is recommended, not only as a coolant but also to maintain the tooth in a hydrated state to facilitate the assessment of defect removal. Teeth that have white spot defects are particularly susceptible to dehydration resulting in other apparent white spots that are not normally seen when the tooth is hydrated. Dehydration exaggerates the appearance of white spots and makes defect removal difficult to assess. After removal of the defect or on termination of any further removal of tooth structure, a 30-fluted, finishing bur is used to remove any facets or striations created by the previous instruments. Final polishing is accomplished with an abrasive rubber point (see Fig. 12-30, *C*). The results are shown in Figure 12-30, *D*.

Comparable results can be achieved with microabrasion and macroabrasion. Both treatments have advantages as well as disadvantages. Microabrasion has the advantage of ensuring better control of the removal of tooth structure. High-speed instrumentation used in macroabrasion is technique sensitive and can have catastrophic results if the clinician fails to use extreme caution. Macroabrasion is considerably faster and does not require the use of a rubber dam or special instrumentation. Defect removal also is easier with macroabrasion compared with microabrasion if an air-water spray is used during treatment to maintain hydration of teeth. Nonetheless, microabrasion is recommended over macroabrasion for the

treatment of superficial defects in children because of better operator control and superior patient acceptance. To accelerate the process, a combination of macroabrasion and microabrasion also may be considered. Gross removal of the defect is accomplished with macroabrasion, followed by final treatment with microabrasion.

Veneers

A veneer is a layer of tooth-colored material that is applied to a tooth to restore localized or generalized defects and intrinsic discolorations (see Figs. 12-7, 12-33, 12-34, 12-35, and 12-41). Typically, veneers are made of directly applied composite, processed composite, porcelain, or pressed ceramic materials. Common indications for veneers include teeth with facial surfaces that are malformed, discolored, abraded, or eroded or have faulty restorations (Fig. 12-31).

Two types of esthetic veneers exist: (1) partial veneers and (2) full veneers (Fig. 12-32). Partial veneers are indicated for the restoration of localized defects or areas of intrinsic discoloration (Fig. 12-33; see also Fig. 12-1). Full veneers are indicated for the restoration of generalized defects or areas of intrinsic staining involving most of the facial surface of the tooth (see Figs. 12-7, 12-35, 12-36, 12-37, and 12-41). Several important factors, including patient age, occlusion, tissue health, position and alignment of teeth, and oral hygiene, must be evaluated before pursuing full veneers as a treatment

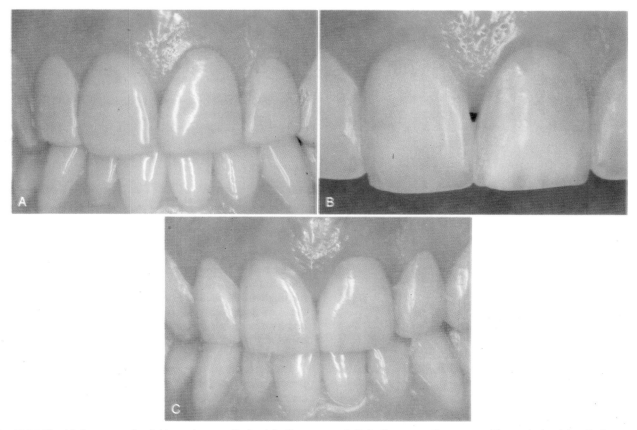

Fig. 12-35 Direct full veneers using light-cured composite for defective veneers. **A,** Defective composite veneers with marginal staining. **B,** Conservative intra-enamel preparation. **C,** New direct composite veneers on maxillary anterior teeth *(Courtesy Dr. Robert Margeas).*

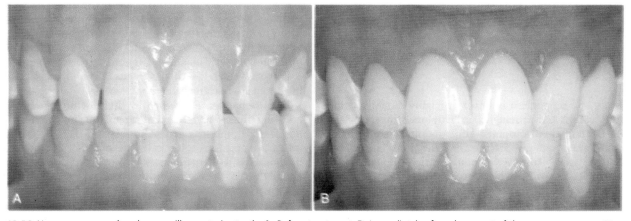

Fig. 12-36 No-prep veneers placed on maxillary anterior teeth. **A,** Before treatment. **B,** Immediately after placement of the no-prep veneers. *(Courtesy of Dr. Patricia Pereira.)*

However, no-prep veneers can be problematic. First, no-prep veneers are inherently made thinner and, consequently, are more prone to fracture, especially during the try-in phase. Second, for indirect no-prep veneers, interproximal areas are difficult to access for proper finishing. And third, as noted earlier, if case selection is not done properly and the teeth are already of normal contour, the resulting veneers inevitably will be over-contoured. Veneers that are over-contoured are not generally esthetic and often can result in impingement of gingival tissue, as noted earlier (see Fig.

12-31, *D*). For these reasons, it is advisable, in most cases, to use a conservative, intra-enamel preparation for the use of indirect veneers, as noted below.

Etched Porcelain Veneers

The preferred type of indirect veneer is the etched porcelain (i.e., feldspathic) veneer. Porcelain veneers etched with hydrofluoric acid are capable of achieving high bond strengths to the etched enamel via a resin-bonding medium.[39-41] This

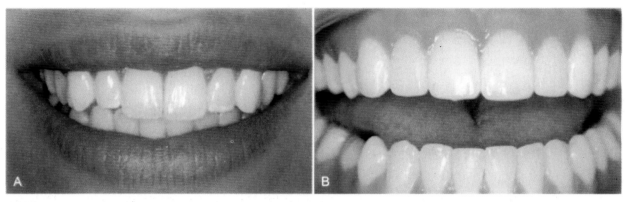

Fig. 12-37 No-prep veneers placed to restore undersized maxillary lateral incisors. **A,** Before treatment. **B,** After placement of the no-prep veneers. *(Courtesy of Dr. Gary Radz.)*

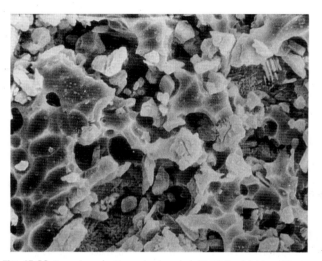

Fig. 12-38 Scanning electron micrograph (×31,000) of feldspathic porcelain etched with hydrofluoric acid. *(Courtesy of Dr. Steven Bayne.)*

porcelain etching pattern is shown in Figure 12-38. In addition to the high bond strengths, etched porcelain veneers are highly esthetic, stain resistant, and periodontally compatible. The incidence of cohesive fracture for etched porcelain veneers is also very low.[36] However, as noted earlier, the key to the long-term success with etched porcelain veneers is the use of a *conservative intra-enamel preparation.* Preparations into dentin should be avoided because virtually all problems associated with etched porcelain veneers (debonding, accelerated marginal staining, tooth sensitivity, etc.) occur when excessive amounts of dentin are exposed in the veneer preparation.

TOOTH PREPARATION

Because the most important consideration in determining the success of etched porcelain veneers is tooth preparation, a systematic approach will be presented first, using a dentiform series, prior to reviewing the associated clinical procedures (Fig. 12-39). A veneer design using a butt-joint incisal edge will be illustrated first. The tooth used to illustrate the preparation sequence has intentionally been colored blue to allow better visualization of the involved steps. However, it is not recommended that this tooth marking be done clinically.

The veneer preparation is made with a tapered, rounded-end diamond instrument. It is critical that the tip diameter of the diamond be measured because the diamond will serve as the measuring tool in gauging proper reduction depth. A diamond with a tip diameter of 1.0 to 1.2 mm is recommended. The tip diameter of the diamond used in this series is 1.2 mm.

The first step in the veneer preparation is establishing the peripheral outline form. Position the diamond to half its depth (approximately 0.6 mm in this example) just facial to the proximal contact on either proximal surface, and then extend the bur, while maintaining its occluso-gingival orientation, around the gingival area and then back up the opposite proximal area, again keeping the diamond positioned just facial to the proximal contact area (see Fig. 12-39, *A* and *B*). In this example, a supragingival marginal position was maintained. Recall that clinically, the position of the gingival margin is determined by lip position (and the resulting display of teeth) and the gingival extent of the facial discoloration or defect being treated, as noted previously. If possible, a supragingival margin position is always considered desirable because it minimizes the potential for an adverse gingival response.

Facial reduction is achieved by first identifying and then reducing three separate facial zones: the incisal third, the middle third, and the gingival third (see Fig. 12-39, *C*), in that order. To prepare the incisal zone of facial reduction, the diamond first is aligned parallel with the facial surface of the incisal third of the tooth. The diamond is then moved mesio-distally from line angle to line angle until the desired depth of approximately 0.6 mm is attained. Again, the tip of the diamond is used to gauge this reduction. Reduction depth can be verified by viewing the tip of the diamond in proximity to the unprepared tooth structure gingival to this reduced area when viewed from the proximal, facial, and incisal aspects (see Fig. 12-39, *D* and *E*). Care also must be taken to round the mesial and distal facial line angles during this reduction sequence to ensure uniform facial reduction.

The middle third is reduced in a similar manner. By carefully watching the striations being created by the diamond mesiodistally during the reduction of the middle third, it is easy to see when the level of the previous incisal third reduction is reached (see Fig. 12-39, *F*). When a similar reduction level has been reached, the striations in the middle one third will then extend into the area previously reduced in the incisal

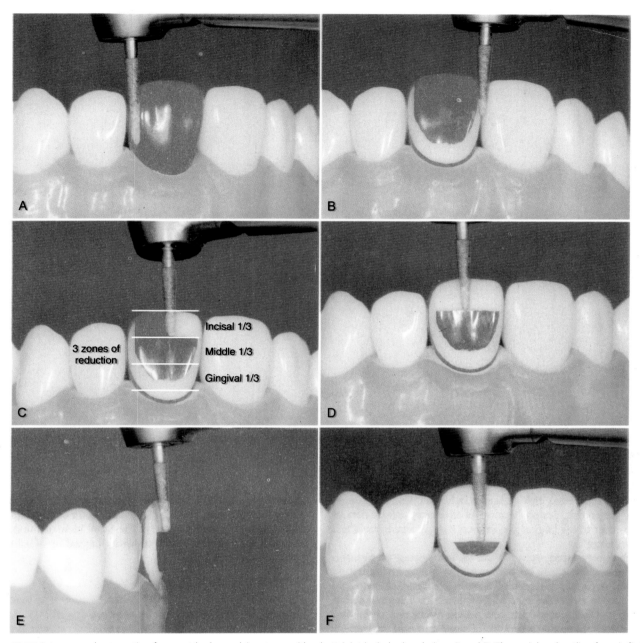

Fig. 12-39 Intra-enamel preparation for an etched porcelain veneer with a butt-joint incisal edge design. **A** and **B,** The peripheral outline form is first established using a rounded-end diamond instrument. **C–H,** Facial reduction is achieved by first identifying and then reducing three separate facial zones: the incisal third, the middle third, and the gingival third (see Fig. 12-39, C), in that order.

third. Stop immediately. *Do not go deeper.* Again, a reduction depth of approximately 0.6 mm is desirable. Moreover, the reduction depth again can be verified by viewing the tip of the diamond in proximity to the unprepared tooth structure gingival to this reduced area when viewed from the proximal, facial, and incisal aspects. Care also must be taken to round the mesial and distal facial line angles during this reduction sequence to ensure uniform facial reduction.

Reduction of the gingival one third is straightforward and simply involves removal of the remaining "island" of unprepared tooth structure to a level consistent with the surrounding previously prepared tooth structure (see Fig. 12-39, G and H).

Incisal reduction is made by orienting the diamond perpendicular to the incisal edge and then reducing the incisal edge to attain a *minimum* reduction of 1 mm or, more desirably, 1.5 mm (see Fig. 12-39, I). Clinically, this reduction in depth will be gauged using an incisal reduction index. In this dentiform example, a minimum 1-mm incisal reduction depth was generated. Finally, round the facio-incisal line angle with the side of the diamond to reduce internal stresses in the porcelain veneer. The final intra-enamel preparation for an etched porcelain veneer using a butt-joint incisal edge design is seen in Figure 12-39, J.

Frequently, an incisal lapping preparation is preferred. If the patient has worn or defective areas on the lingual aspect

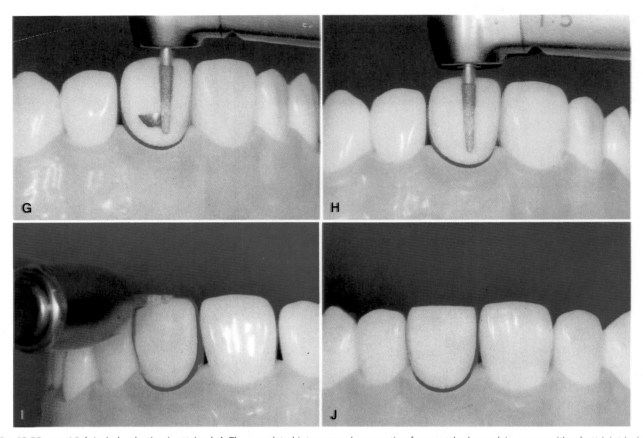

Fig. 12-39, cont'd **I,** Incisal reduction is attained. **J,** The completed intra-enamel preparation for an etched porcelain veneer with a butt-joint incisal edge.

of the incisal edge, this design is indicated. Some operators also prefer this design because of enhanced adaptation of the veneer to the lingual preparation margin attributable to a "lap sliding" fit.

The preparation steps for the incisal lapping preparation are identical to those for the butt-joint design, including the steps for incisal reduction. However, additional steps are required to attain the incisal lapping feature. The first step in achieving this preparation design is to notch the mesial and distal incisal angles. The tip of the same diamond instrument used for the earlier steps of the veneer preparation is used to establish these notches. Using the diamond, extend the notches completely through the incisal angles faciolingually to a depth incisogingivally consistent with the desired amount of lapping of the lingual surface (Fig. 12-40, *A*). For example, if a 0.5-mm lap of the lingual surface is desired, as in this example, the notches are prepared to a depth of 0.5 mm each accordingly (see Fig. 12-40, *B*).

Once the incisal notches have been generated incisogingivally to a depth consistent with the desired amount of lingual lapping, the preparation of the lingual lap is made. Position the diamond into the tooth to a depth of approximately 0.6 mm (less if remaining faciolingual thickness of the incisal edge enamel is compromised) and extend the preparation across the lingual surface from notch to notch (see Fig. 12-40, *C*). The resulting sharp incisal angles must then be rounded to finish the incisal lapping portion of the preparation. Care must be taken to include any desired lingual defect. The

gingival extent of the incisal lap is determined by the extent of any lingual defect. The final lapping portion of the preparation is seen in Figure 12-40, *D*. The facial view of the completed incisal lapping preparation with a lingual lap of 0.5 mm is seen in Figure 12-40, *E*.

CLINICAL PROCEDURES

The case of a patient with generalized fluorosis is used to illustrate the clinical procedures involved (Fig. 12-41, *A*). A consult appointment is always recommended prior to initiating the veneer procedures. At this appointment, the actual procedures are discussed in detail, appropriate consents are obtained, and any needed records are generated, including shade selection, intraoral photographs, and impressions for diagnostic models and occlusal records. Laboratory communications are greatly enhanced through the inclusion of digital photographs. An excellent series of baseline photographs, including some with shade tabs positioned in the photographic field to document the preoperative shapes and shades of the involved teeth, should be made.

Although intra-enamel preparations will be used, it is always recommended that patients be anesthetized during the appointment for tooth preparation to ensure maximum comfort for the patient and the dentist. Once the anesthetic is administered, preoperative records such as an incisal reduction index and those needed to facilitate temporization are made. An incisal reduction index is always recommended to accurately gauge the amount of incisal reduction during the

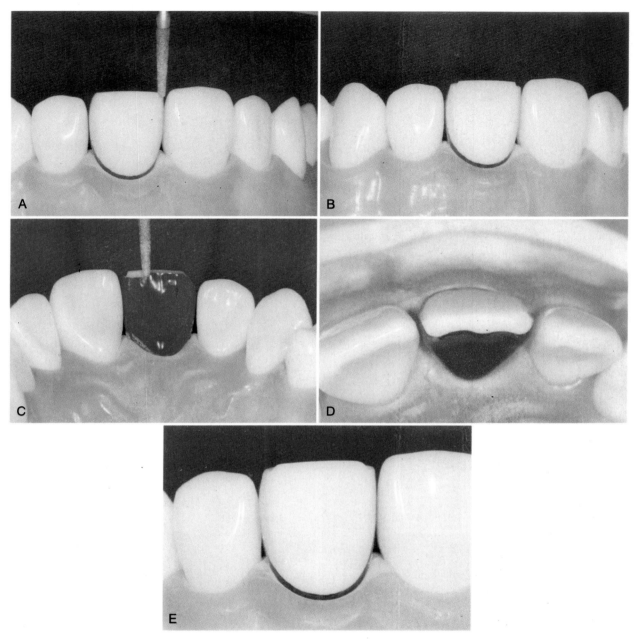

Fig. 12-40 Intra-enamel preparation steps for an etched porcelain veneer with an incisal-lapping design. **A** and **B,** Incisal notches. **C,** Preparing the lingual lapping portion of the prep. **D** and **E,** The completed intra-enamel preparation viewed from the lingual and facial aspects for an etched porcelain veneer with an incisal-lapping design.

preparation of teeth for etched porcelain veneers (Fig. 12-42; see also Fig. 12-41, *B* through *H*). An incisal reduction index is made by recording the lingual and incisal contours of the anterior teeth to be prepared or the contours generated in a diagnostic wax-up. Typically, a fast setting silicone or polyvinyl siloxane elastomeric material is used to generate this record. If a diagnostic model has been made in which the incisal edge positions of the final veneers will be different from the current teeth, the incisal reduction index should be made using the diagnostic model (see Fig. 12-42, *A* and *B*). As in this case, if no change in the incisal edge positions of the involved teeth is desired, the reduction index can be made directly in the patient's mouth by recording the existing contours of the

involved teeth. Once the facial excess has been trimmed away with a No. 12 surgical blade in a Bard-Parker handle, the incisal reduction index should be tried in the mouth to verify the accuracy of the index (see Fig. 12-41, *B*).

The patient in this case has a high smile line and generalized defects that involve the entire facial surfaces of anterior teeth. Therefore, a small diameter gingival retraction cord is placed in anticipation of veneer margins that will be placed at the level of the free gingival margins (see Fig. 12-41, *C*).

Incisal lapping preparations for porcelain veneers are made on the maxillary central and lateral incisors consistent with the systematic step-by-step preparation procedures described earlier. The intra-enamel preparations are made with a tapered,

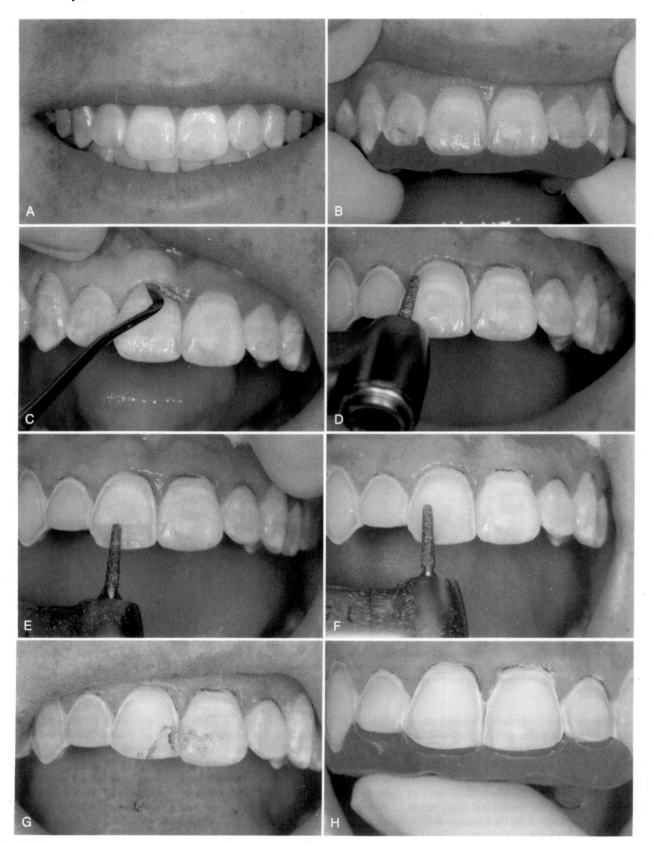

Fig. 12-41 Etched porcelain veneers using an intra-enamel preparation. **A,** A patient with severe dental fluorosis. **B,** An incisal reduction index is made intraorally, since no significant change in incisal edge position is desired. **C,** Retraction cord is placed. **D,** The outline form is first established. **E–G,** Facial reduction is attained by using three zones of facial reduction. **H,** Incisal reduction is verified using the incisal reduction index.

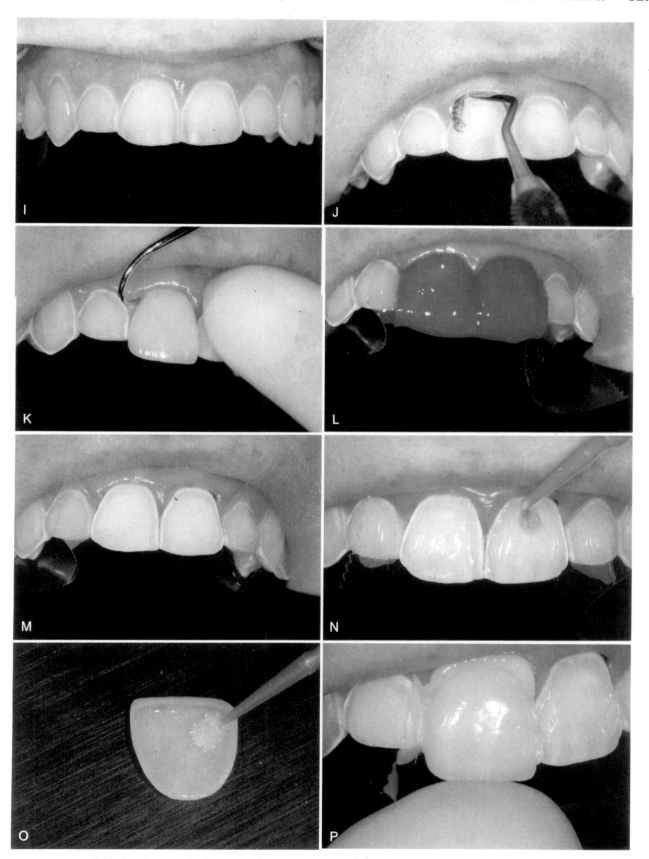

Fig. 12-41, cont'd **I,** Finished preparations for intra-enamel preparations. Note the window preparations on canines and premolars. **J,** Retraction cord is placed for isolation. **K,** The fit of the veneer is assessed. **L** and **M,** Etching of the prepared maxillary central incisors. **N** and **O,** Adhesive is applied to the etched enamel and the tooth side of the porcelain veneer. **P,** The veneer is loaded with resin cement and seated on the tooth.

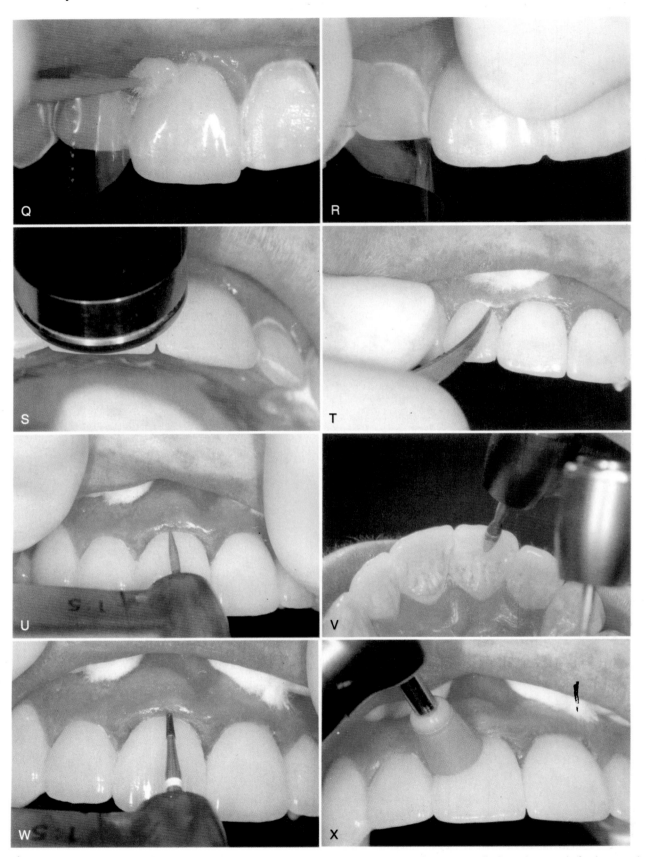

Fig. 12-41, cont'd **Q,** Excess cement is removed with a microbrush. **R,** Excess cement is removed interproximally through removal of polyester strip. **S,** Resin cement cured with intense curing light. **T,** No. 12 surgical blade in a Bard-Parker handle is used for removing excess cured resin cement. **U** and **V,** Diamond instruments used to "dress" marginal areas. **W** and **X,** 30-fluted carbide burs and diamond impregnated polishing instruments used to finish and polish veneer margins.

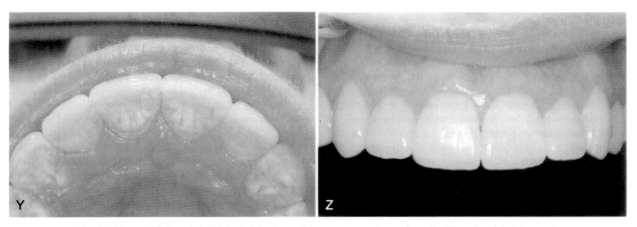

Fig. 12-41, cont'd **Y** and **Z,** Finished etched porcelain veneers as viewed from the lingual and facial aspects.

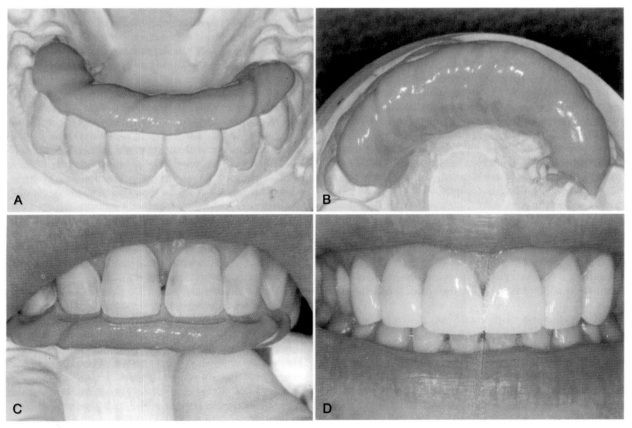

Fig. 12-42 Incisal reduction index made from a diagnostic model. **A** and **B,** A fast-set elastomeric material is used to record the lingual and incisal contours of the diagnostic model. **C,** Incisal reduction index is used to verify proper incisal preparation of teeth. **D,** Finished etched porcelain veneers.

rounded-end diamond instrument to a depth of approximately 0.5 to 0.75 mm midfacially, diminishing to a depth of 0.3 to 0.5 mm along the gingival margins, depending on enamel thickness. The outline form is first established as noted earlier (see Fig. 12-41, *D*). Facial reduction is attained by using three zones of facial reduction as previously described (see Fig. 12-41, *E* through *G*). Veneer interproximal margins should extend into the facial and gingival embrasures, without engaging an undercut, and yet should be located just facial to the proximal contacts.

Since this patient is young with beautifully shaped canines and also exhibits a canine-guided occlusion, a window type of preparation design was employed when preparing the maxillary canines. By restricting the window prep veneers to the facial surface entirely, functional contact will be maintained solely on tooth structure, thereby preventing accelerated wear of opposing teeth. Adequate incisal reduction is verified using the incisal reduction index as noted earlier (see Fig. 12-41, *H*). The finished preparations are shown in Figure 12-41, *I*.

After the preparations are completed, an elastomeric impression is made and appropriate occlusal records generated. Digital photos of the prepared teeth (with and without appropriate shade tabs in the photographic field) also are recommended. In most cases, temporaries are fabricated for the prepared teeth, as described in the subsequent section on temporization (see Veneer Temporization). If a diagnostic wax-up was generated, veneer temporaries are necessary to assess the tooth contours generated in the wax-up intraorally. If no diagnostic wax-up was needed, occasionally, temporary restorations are not required, if the patient consents, because the preparations are shallow and involve only enamel. In these cases, the patient should be instructed to avoid biting hard foods, objects, keep the areas clean with a soft bristled brush, and expect the possibility of some mild sensitivity to hot and cold. It should be noted that the vast majority of veneer cases will warrant temporization.

After they have been fabricated in the laboratory, the porcelain veneers are returned to the dentist for cementation at the second appointment. The completed veneers must be inspected for cracks, overextended margins, and adequate internal etching (as evidenced by a frosted appearance). Marginal areas, in particular, should be inspected for proper etching so that an adequate seal occurs in these areas. Overextended marginal areas interproximally may preclude full seating of adjacent veneers. These areas can be trimmed carefully with a micron-finishing diamond instrument or flexible abrasive disk. Unless severe or inaccessible, most minor overextensions should be trimmed only after bonding the veneer to the tooth because of the risk of fracturing the porcelain.

After the prepared teeth are cleaned with a pumice slurry, rinsed, and dried, isolation is accomplished with a lip retractor (optional) and cotton rolls. A 2 × 2 inch cotton gauze is placed across the back of the patient's mouth to protect against aspiration or swallowing of an inadvertently dropped veneer. If the veneer margins closely approximate the gingiva, a small diameter retraction cord should be placed in the gingival crevice during try-in and cementation to prevent inadvertent contamination of the bonds from crevicular fluids (see Fig. 12-41, J).

The fit of each veneer is evaluated on the respective individual tooth and adjusted if necessary. A No. 2 explorer should be used to assess marginal fit (see Fig. 12-41, K). All of the veneers should be tried in place not only individually but also in adjacent pairs to ensure the fit of adjacent seated veneers. Veneers should be tried in place only on clean, dry teeth to eliminate any potential for contamination. If accidental contamination occurs, the veneer should be cleaned thoroughly with alcohol or acid etchant, rinsed, and dried before bonding.

Prior to cementation, a silane agent can optionally be applied to the internal surfaces of the veneers. The silane acts as a coupling agent, forming a chemical bond between the porcelain and the resin that increases bond strength of the resin to the porcelain.[42] It also improves the wettability of the porcelain. The primary source of retention with porcelain veneers still remains the etched porcelain surface itself. Only a modest increase in bond strength results from silanation of the porcelain; however, it is recommended because it also may reduce marginal leakage and discoloration.

A light-cured resin cement is recommended for bonding the veneer to the tooth because light-cured resins are more color stable and provide additional working time over the self-cured or dual-cured versions. Shade selection of the bonding medium is determined after the fit of the individual veneers has been evaluated and confirmed. Water can be used as an optical medium for try-in to assess the appearance of the veneers. With this technique, water is placed in a single central incisor veneer (or both central incisor veneers), placed on clean, dry teeth, and the appearance assessed. If the veneers are deemed acceptable in appearance, an untinted shade of the bonding resin is indicated. For the vast majority of etched porcelain veneers, an untinted shade of the bonding resin is recommended. Because etched porcelain veneers can be fabricated with inherent color gradients, characterizations and even additional opaques when further masking of stains is needed, it is unusual that alternative shades or opaque resin bonding media are needed. Nonetheless, alternative shades or opaque versions of resin bonding cements are sometimes preferred by some dentists.

If alternative shades of resin cements are needed, shade selection is made by first placing a uniform layer of a selected shade of resin cement, approximately 0.5 mm in thickness, on the tooth side of a single veneer. Typically, a central incisor veneer is used to facilitate shade determination of the cement. The operatory light is turned away during shade assessment to prevent premature and inadvertent curing of the resin cement. The veneer is seated on a clean, dry, unetched tooth; the excess resin cement is removed with a brush; and the overall shade of the veneer is evaluated. After try-in, the veneer is removed quickly and stored in a container that is impervious to light to prevent curing of the cement. If the shade of the cement is determined to be appropriate, more of the same shade is added to the veneer just before bonding. If a different shade is deemed necessary, the existing shade is wiped from the inner aspect of the veneer with a disposable microbrush, and a new shade of resin cement is placed in the veneer. In the meantime, the assistant can remove residual cement of the previous shade from the tooth with a cotton pellet or brush. The veneer loaded with the new shade of cement is reseated and evaluated, as previously described.

Water-soluble try-in pastes that correspond to the same shades of resin cements also are available with many veneer bonding kits. These try-in pastes allow shade assessment without the risk of inadvertent premature curing of the cement because the try-in pastes are not capable of setting. However, after the try-in process with these try-in pastes, the veneers must be thoroughly cleaned, according to the manufacturer's instructions, to ensure that optimal bonding occurs. A light-cured resin cement of the same shade is used for final cementation.

The inherent shade of the veneer, characterization, and internal opaquing must be accomplished primarily during the fabrication of the veneer itself in the laboratory. Some additional masking can be accomplished chairside using an opaque resin-bonding medium at the time of bonding. However, excess use of opaque bonding resins also can reduce the "esthetic vitality" of the veneer, resulting in a poor esthetic outcome. Also, the overall shade of the veneer can be modified only slightly by the shade of cement selected. Significant changes in shading or masking ability cannot be accomplished chairside.

Prior to cementation of the veneers, the retraction cords are evaluated to ensure that they are tucked adequately into the gingival crevice. The tooth used for try-in to assess the shade of the resin bonding medium should be cleaned again with a slurry of pumice to remove any residual resin or try-in paste that may preclude proper acid etching of the enamel.

A technique recommended for applying the veneers one at a time is presented here. Polyester strips are placed interproximally to prevent inadvertent bonding to the adjacent tooth, followed by etching, rinsing, and drying procedures. It is recommended that the two central incisors be etched and their veneers bonded first because of their critical importance esthetically. Etch the teeth to be bonded with a 35% to 37% phosphoric acid gel (see Fig. 12-41, *L*). Following etching, rinsing, and drying, the preparations should exhibit a frosted appearance as evidence of an appropriately etched enamel surface (see Fig. 12-41, *M*). An adhesive is applied to the etched enamel and the tooth side of the silane-primed porcelain veneer (see Fig. 12-41, *N* and *O*). Next, a thin layer (0.5 mm) of the selected shade of light-cured resin cement is placed on the tooth side of the veneer, taking care not to entrap air. The first veneer is placed on the tooth and vibrated (carefully and lightly) into position with a blunt instrument or light finger pressure (see Fig. 12-41, *P*). The margins of the veneer are examined with a No. 2 explorer to verify accurate seating. Next, the excess resin cement is removed with a disposable microbrush, always directing the microbrush in a gingival direction to prevent displacement of the veneer (see Fig. 12-41, *Q*). The second veneer is placed and cleaned of excess cement in like manner. If a veneer cement with thick viscosity is used, the polyester strips can be carefully removed to facilitate removal of interproximal resin prior to curing (see Fig. 12-41, *R*). However, the resin cement should be cured only after visual inspection reveals no excess resin remains in these critical interproximal areas.

Veneer margins are evaluated again before the veneer is exposed to the curing light. To ensure complete polymerization, the veneer should be cured for a minimum of 20 to 40 seconds each from the facial and lingual directions with a high-intensity blue LED (light-emitting diode) light (see Fig. 12-41, *S*). A light stream of air can be directed on the tooth during the curing sequence to prevent overheating from the curing light. After positioning and bonding of the first two veneers on the central incisors, the remaining veneers can be positioned carefully and bonded in like manner. Following proper positioning and bonding of all the veneers, any residual resin cement can be removed. A No. 12 surgical blade in a Bard-Parker handle is ideal for removing excess cured resin cement remaining around the margins (see Fig. 12-41, *T*). Care must be exercised to ensure that the surgical blade is used only with a secure finger rest and using short shaving strokes, always directed parallel to the veneer margins. Removal of the

retraction cord at this time facilitates access and visibility to the subgingival areas. If the marginal fit of the porcelain veneers is deemed acceptable and a favorable emergence profile exists, only removal of the excess cement is required.

If the porcelain margins are overextended beyond the cavosurface angles, an overhang is present, or the marginal areas are too bulbous, recontouring of these areas is required (especially along the gingival margins) to ensure proper physiologic contours and gingival health. A flame-shaped fine diamond instrument is used to carefully recontour and "dress" these areas (see Fig. 12-41, *U*). Marginal areas should be confluent with the surrounding unprepared tooth surfaces when assessed with a No. 2 explorer. The lingual areas are always finished with an oval-shaped fine diamond instrument (see Fig. 12-41, *V*). Because the use of a diamond instrument breaks the glazed surface, a series of appropriate instruments is used to restore a smooth surface texture. First, a rounded end or bullet-shaped (or oval for lingual surfaces), 30-fluted carbide finishing bur (Midwest No. 9803 or Brasseler No. 7801) is used to plane the porcelain surface and to remove the striations created by the diamond instruments (see Fig. 12-41, *W*). Studies show that the best results occur if the diamond instruments are used with air and water coolant, whereas the 30-fluted bur should be used dry.[43] Second, the porcelain is smoothed and polished with a series of abrasive rubber, porcelain polishing cups, and points (Dialite Porcelain Polishing Kit; Brasseler USA, Savannah, GA) (see Fig. 12-41, *X*). Final surface luster is imparted by using a porcelain-polishing paste, applied with either a rubber Prophy cup or a felt wheel. This step is optional if a suitable polish has been attained with the polishing points and cups. The completed veneers are shown from incisal and facial views in Figure 12-41, *Y* and *Z*.

Etched porcelain veneers also can be used effectively to restore malformed anterior teeth conservatively. Malformed lateral incisors are shown in Figure 12-43, *A*. Incisal, lapping preparations that are extended well onto the lingual surface are used (see Fig. 12-43, *B*). The resulting restorations are virtually comparable with "three-quarter crowns" in porcelain. The final esthetic results are shown in Figure 12-43, *C*.

Darkly discolored teeth are more difficult to treat with porcelain veneers. Several modifications in the veneering technique can be used to enhance the final esthetic result. First, opaque porcelain can be incorporated during the fabrication of the veneers to achieve more inherent masking. If the veneers are not inherently opaque, little chance exists for adequate masking of a darkly stained tooth. Typically, 5% to 15% opaque porcelain is required to achieve optimal masking. Exceeding 15% opaque porcelain dramatically reduces light penetration and results in a significant loss of esthetic vitality;

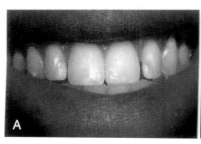
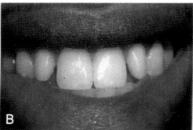
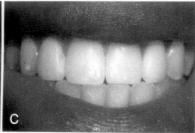

Fig. 12-43 Treatment of malformed teeth with porcelain veneers. **A,** Malformed lateral incisors. **B,** An incisal-lapping preparation similar to a three quarters crown in enamel is used. **C,** Final esthetic results.

the esthetic vitality or the realistic appearance of teeth depends on light penetration (see the section on Artistic Elements, Translucency). Second, a slightly deeper tooth preparation can be used to allow greater veneer thickness. The preparation should always be restricted to enamel, however, to ensure optimal bonding of the veneer to the tooth. Even with improved dentin-bonding agents, the bonds to dentin are less predictable or durable than the bonds to enamel because of the high variability and dynamic nature of dentin. Bonds to etched enamel are highly predictable and very durable.

Third, the laboratory can be instructed to use several coats of a die-spacing medium on the laboratory model to allow a slightly greater thickness of the resin-bonding medium. The die-spacing medium must not be extended closer than 1 mm to the margins to ensure adequate positioning of the veneer to the preparation during try-in and bonding and to provide for a slight internal space. A typical case of darkly discolored teeth showing prepared teeth and postoperative result is shown in Figure 12-44.

Patients who have darkly stained teeth always should be informed that although porcelain (or composite) veneers can result in improved esthetics, they may not entirely eliminate or mask extremely dark stains. Because of the limited thickness of the veneers and the absolute necessity of incorporating intrinsic opacity, the realistic translucency or esthetic vitality of veneered teeth may never be comparable with that of natural, unaffected teeth (see Fig. 12-9). Full porcelain coverage with all-ceramic crowns may be indicated in some

patients with severe discoloration because of the crown's greater capacity to restore esthetic vitality. Nonetheless, porcelain veneers are a viable option, in most cases, for patients who desire esthetic improvement without significant tooth reduction.

Pressed Ceramic Veneers

Another esthetic alternative for veneering teeth is the use of pressed ceramics (e.g., IPS Empress or e.max [Ivoclar Vivadent]). In contrast to etched porcelain veneers that are fabricated by stacking and firing feldspathic porcelain, pressed ceramic veneers are literally cast using a lost wax technique. Excellent esthetics is possible using pressed ceramic materials for most cases involving mild to moderate discoloration. Because of the more translucent nature of pressed ceramic veneers, however, dark discolorations are best treated with etched porcelain veneers. The clinical technique for placing pressed ceramic veneers (e.g., IPS Empress) is not markedly different from that for feldspathic porcelain veneers, other than the need for a slightly greater tooth reduction depth.

The procedures for tooth preparation, try-in, and bonding of pressed veneers are the same as for etched porcelain veneers except that the marginal fit is superior. For that reason, often little marginal finishing is necessary. Only the excess bonding medium needs to be removed. A typical case involving pressed ceramic veneers, with before and after treatment views, is shown in Figure 12-45.

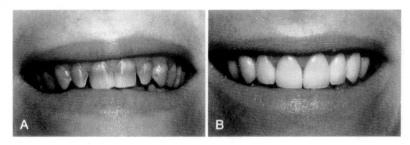

Fig. 12-44 Darkly stained teeth treated with porcelain veneers. **A,** Tetracycline-stained teeth seen after preparation for porcelain veneers. **B,** After view of completed veneers.

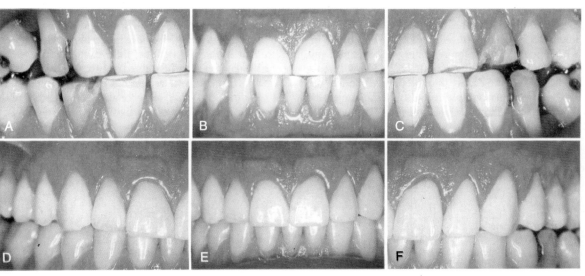

Fig. 12-45 Pressed ceramic veneers (IPS Empress). **A–C,** Before treatment, facial views. **D–F,** Esthetic result after completed veneers. *(Courtesy of Dr. ...tieri.)*

Veneers Temporization

Because intra-enamel preparations for etched porcelain veneers are by design very conservative, the resulting temporaries are inherently thin. Furthermore, they cannot be bonded in a similar manner to conventional temporaries for crowns, for example, because of the lack of inherent retention form. Moreover, since they are very thin, they cannot be made in the mouth and removed for trimming and subsequent cementing because of the high probability of fracture. Therefore, veneers temporaries must be made and placed simultaneously intraorally.

Figure 12-46 illustrates a typical case involving the fabrication of temporaries for etched porcelain veneers for maxillary anterior teeth. A clear polyvinyl siloxane material is used to make the preoperative impression from which the temporaries will be made. If no diagnostic model is needed and the existing contours of the teeth are to be replicated, the impression for the temporaries is made directly in the mouth. However, as in this case, if a diagnostic wax-up was generated (see Fig. 12-46, A and B), the clear polyvinyl siloxane impression is made from this diagnostic model. Making the temporary from the diagnostic wax-up enables the clinician to see the contours of the wax-up manifested intraorally in the resulting temporaries. As seen in Figure 12-46, C, the impression itself is removed from the outer tray (no tray adhesive is used) and set aside for future use.

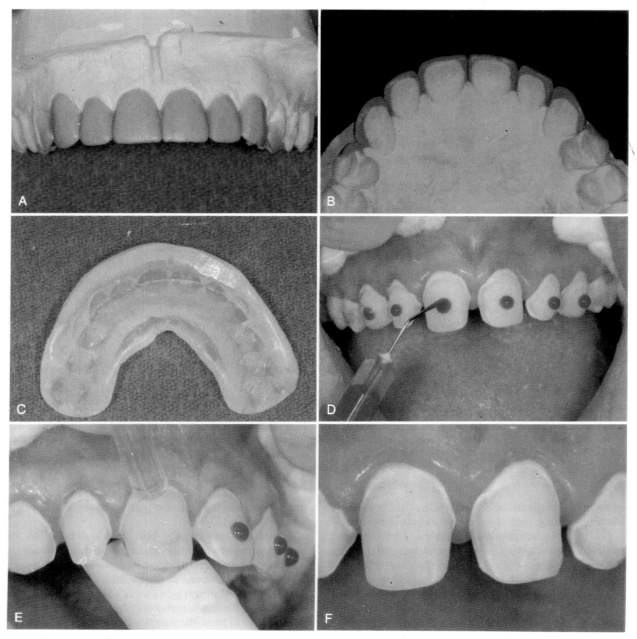

Fig. 12-46 Temporization for etched porcelain veneers. **A** and **B,** Diagnostic models in anticipation of etched porcelain veneers. **C,** Clear polyvinyl siloxane (PVS) impression made from diagnostic model. **D–F,** Spot-etched areas for retention of temporary veneers.

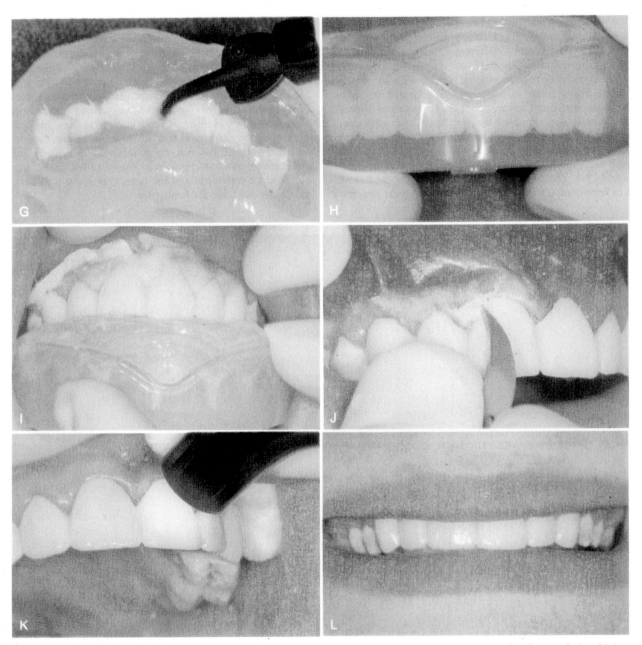

Fig. 12-46, cont'd G and **H,** Clear PVS impression is quickly loaded with bis-acryl temporary material, and positioned in the mouth. **I** and **J,** Impression is removed, and No. 12 blade in a Bard-Parker surgical handle is used to remove excess material. **K,** Glazing agent placed and cured. **L** and **M,** Final facial and lingual views of veneer temporaries.

Following the preparation and impression of the teeth for porcelain veneers, the teeth to be temporized are "spot-etched" with 35% to 37% phosphoric acid. Only a 2-mm circle of enamel should be etched on the facial surface of each tooth to be veneered (see Fig. 12-46, *D* and *E*). Because of the low viscosity of the bis-acryl temporary material, no bonding agent is required for bonding. The bis-acryl material will infiltrate the etched areas for micromechanical bonding. These "spot-etched" areas will be the only areas to which the veneer temporaries will be bonded. If the entire tooth were etched, the veneer temporaries could not be readily removed. After etching," only small etched circles evidenced by a frosted

appearance should be present on the surface of each prepared tooth (see Fig. 12-46, *F*).

The etched teeth must be kept clean and dry at this point. The clear polyvinyl siloxane impression is quickly loaded with a self-curing bis-acryl temporary material and thereafter is immediately positioned in the mouth (see Fig. 12-46, *G* and *H*). Once seated, finger pressure is applied to the peripheral areas of the flexible impression (since no outer hard tray is present) to express the excess material and "thin out" the resulting resin "flash."

When the bis-acryl temporary material has set, the clear impression is removed (see Fig. 12-46, *I*). The gross excess

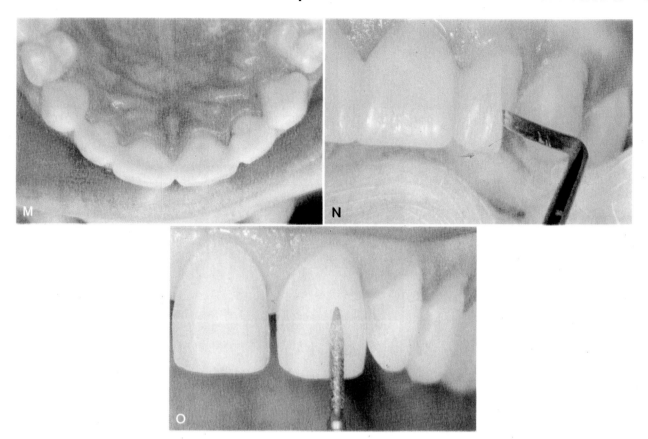

Fig. 12-46, cont'd **N** and **O,** At delivery appointment, temporary veneers are removed with Black's spoon, and the spot-etched and bonded areas are relieved with a diamond.

"flash" material facially and lingually is removed with cotton pliers. Thereafter, a No. 12 blade held in a Bard-Parker surgical handle is used to *carefully* trim the excess temporary material around the margins of each tooth (see Fig. 12-46, *J*). The same No. 12 blade is used to carefully trim excess material in the gingival embrasure areas as well.

A sharp large discoid applied parallel to the lingual margins is used to remove resin "flash" in the lingual concave areas. The temporary veneers are all joined together interproximally, increasing their collective strength and enhancing retention. A light-cured resin glazing agent is applied and cured to generate a smooth surface texture (see Fig. 12-46, *K*). Final views of the finished temporaries are seen in Figure 12-46, *L* and *M*.

Appropriate adjustments can then be made intraorally in the temporaries to optimize occlusion and esthetics. A digital photograph of the final temporaries should be shared with the laboratory as a template for the final veneers. Patients must be instructed that they should not bite anything of any substance because of the weak nature of these veneers. These provisional veneers literally are more to accommodate esthetics and not function during the interim time until delivery of the final veneers.

As demonstrated in a different case, once the patient returns for the final try-in and cementation of the veneers, the temporaries are carefully removed by prying them from each tooth using a Black's spoon (see Fig. 12-46, *N*). The temporaries can readily be removed, since the only area where they

actually are bonded to the tooth is the very small "spot-etched" 2-mm circle on the facial surface of each prepared tooth. Once the veneer temporaries are removed, the areas that had been "spot-etched" and bonded need to be lightly resurfaced with a flame-shaped diamond to ensure no residual resin bonding agent is present that could preclude proper seating and bonding of the final veneers (see Fig. 12-46, *O*).

Veneers for Metal Restorations

Esthetic inserts (i.e., partial or full veneers) of a tooth-colored material can be placed on the facial surface of a tooth previously restored with a metal restoration. For new castings, plans are made at the time of tooth preparation and during laboratory development of the wax pattern to incorporate a vene into the cast restoration. After such a casting has be cemented, the veneer can be inserted, as described in the n section, except that the portion of mechanical retention of veneer into the casting has been provided in the wax pa stage.

Veneers for Existing Metal Restorations

Occasionally, the facial portion of an existing metal tion (amalgam or gold) is judged to be distracting (F *A*). A careful examination, including a radiograph, *i* to determine that the existing restoration is sound

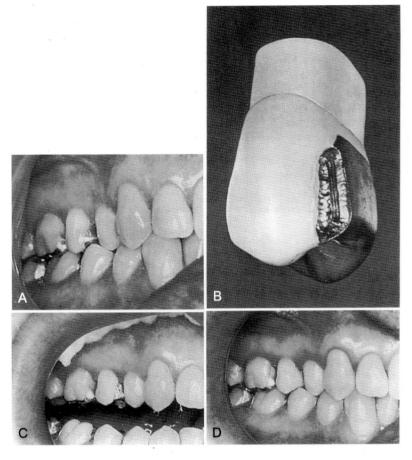

Fig. 12-47 Veneer for existing cast restoration. **A,** Mesio-facial portion of onlay is distracting to patient. **B,** Model of tooth and preparation. Note 90-degree cavosurface angle and retention prepared in gold and the cavosurface bevel in enamel. **C,** Clinical preparation ready for composite resin. **D,** Completed restoration.

esthetic correction is made. The size of the unesthetic area determines the extent of the preparation. Anesthesia is not usually required because the preparation is in metal and enamel. Preliminary procedures consist of cleaning the area with pumice, selecting the shade, and isolating the site with a cotton roll. When the unesthetic metal extends subgingivally, the level of the gingival tissue is marked on the restoration with a sharp explorer, and a retraction cord is placed in the gingival crevice. Rubber dam isolation may be required in some instances.

A No. 2 carbide bur rotating at high speed with an air-water spray is used to remove the metal, starting at a point midway between the gingival and occlusal margins. The preparation is made perpendicular to the surface (a minimum of approximately 1 mm in depth), leaving a butt joint at the cavosurface margins. The 1-mm depth and butt joint should be maintained as the preparation is extended occlusally. All of the metal along the facial enamel is removed, and the preparation is extended into the facial and occlusal embrasures just enough for the veneer to hide the metal. The contact areas on the proximal or occlusal surfaces must not be included in the preparation. To complete the outline form, the preparation is extended gingivally approximately 1 mm past the mark indicating the clinical level of the gingival tissue.

The final preparation should have the same features as those described for veneers in new cast restorations. Mechanical retention is placed in the gingival area with a No. 1/4 carbide bur (using air coolant to enhance vision) 0.25 mm

deep along the gingivoaxial and linguoaxial angles. Retention and esthetics are enhanced by beveling the enamel cavosurface margin (approximately 0.5 mm wide) with a coarse, flame-shaped diamond instrument oriented at 45 degrees to the external tooth surface (see Fig. 12-47, *B*). After it is etched, rinsed, and dried, the preparation is complete (see Fig. 12-47, *C*). Adhesive resin liners containing 4-methyloxy ethyl trimellitic anhydride (4-META), capable of bonding composite to metal, also may be used but are quite technique sensitive.[44] Manufacturers' instructions should be followed strictly to ensure optimal results with these materials. The composite material is inserted and finished in the usual manner (see Fig. 12-47, *D*).

Repairs of Veneers

Failures of esthetic veneers occur because of breakage, discoloration, or wear. Consideration should be given to conservative repairs of veneers if the examination reveals that the remaining tooth and restoration are sound. It is not always necessary to remove all of the old restoration. The material most commonly used for making repairs is light-cured composite.

Veneers on Tooth Structure

Small chipped areas on veneers often can be corrected recontouring and polishing. When a sizable area is broken

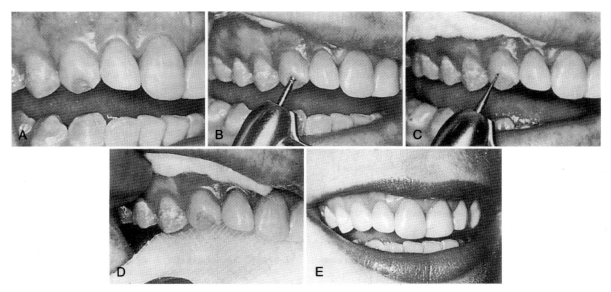

Fig. 12-48 Repairing a direct composite veneer. **A,** Fractured veneer on the maxillary canine. **B,** Preparation with rounded-end diamond instrument. **C,** Undercuts placed in existing veneer with a No. 1/4 bur. **D,** Completed preparation is shown isolated and etched. **E,** Veneer restored to original color and contour.

usually can be repaired if the remaining portion is sound (Fig. 12-48, *A*). For direct composite veneers, repairs ideally should be made with the same material that was used originally. After cleaning the area and selecting the shade, the operator should roughen the damaged surface of the veneer or tooth or both with a coarse, tapered, rounded-end diamond instrument to form a chamfered cavosurface margin (see Fig. 12-48, *B*). Roughening with micro-etching (i.e., sandblasting) also is effective. For more positive retention, mechanical locks may be placed in the remaining composite material with a small, round bur (see Fig. 12-48, *C*). Acid etchant is applied to clean the prepared area and to etch any exposed enamel, which is then rinsed and dried (see Fig. 12-48, *D*). Next, an adhesive is applied to the preparation (i.e., existing composite and enamel) and polymerized. Composite is added, cured, and finished in the usual manner (see Fig. 12-48, *E*).

To repair porcelain veneers, a hydrofluoric acid gel, suitable for intraoral use (but only with a rubber dam in place), must be used to etch the fractured porcelain. Hydrofluoric acid gels are available in approximately 10% buffered concentrations that can be used for intraoral porcelain repairs if proper isolation with a rubber dam is used. Although caution still must be taken when using hydrofluoric acid gels intraorally, the lower acid concentration allows for relatively safe intraoral use. Full-strength hydrofluoric acid should *never* be used intraorally for etching porcelain. Isolation of the porcelain veneer to be repaired should always be accomplished with a rubber dam to protect gingival tissue from the irritating effects of the hydrofluoric acid. The manufacturer's instructions must be followed regarding application time for the hydrofluoric acid gel to ensure optimal porcelain etching. A lightly frosted appearance, similar to that of etched enamel, should be seen if the porcelain has been properly etched. A silane coupling agent may be applied to the etched porcelain surface before the adhesive is applied. Composite material is added, cured, and finished in the usual manner. Large fractures are best treated by replacing the entire porcelain veneer.

Acknowledgments

Portions of the section on artistic elements were reprinted with permission from Heymann HO: The artistry of conservative esthetic dentistry, *J Am Dent Assoc* 115(12E; special issue):14, 1987.

References

1. Goldstein RE: *Esthetics in dentistry*, Philadelphia, 1976, JB Lippincott.
2. Levin EI: Dental esthetics and the golden proportion. *J Prosthet Dent* 40:244, 1978.
3. Borissavlievitch M: *The golden number*, London, 1964, Alec Tiranti.
4. Preston JD: The golden proportion revisited. *J Esthet Dent* 5:247–251, 1993.
5. Ward DH: A study of dentists' preferred maxillary anterior tooth width proportions: comparing recurring esthetic dental proportions to other mathematical and naturally occurring proportions. *J Esthet Rest Dent* 19(6):324–339, 2007.
6. Sterrett JD, Oliver T, Robinson F, et al: Width/length ratios of normal clinical crowns of maxillary anterior teeth. *J Clin Periodontol* 26:153–157, 1999.
7. Magne P, Gallucci GO, Belser UC: Anatomic crown width/length ratios of unworn and worn maxillary teeth in white subjects. *J Prosthet Dent* 89:453–461, 2003.
8. Chiche GJ, Pinault A: *Esthetics of anterior fixed prosthodontics*, Chicago, 1994, Quintessence.
9. Sproull RC: Understanding color. In Goldstein RE, editor: *Esthetics in dentistry*, Philadelphia, 1976, JB Lippincott.
10. Dawson PE: *Evaluation, diagnosis, and treatment of occlusal problems*, ed 2, St. Louis, 1989, Mosby.
11. Graber TM, Vanarsdall RL: *Orthodontics: Current principles and techniques*, ed 3, St. Louis, 2000, Mosby.
12. Hattab FN, Qudeimat MA, al-Rimawi HS: Dental discolorations: An overview. *J Esthet Dent* 11:291, 1999.
13. Flynn M: Black teeth: A primitive method of caries prevention in southeast Asia. *J Am Dent Assoc* 95:96, 1977.
14. Carver CC, Heymann HO: Dental and oral discolorations associated with minocycline and other tetracycline analogs. *J Esthet Dent* 11:43, 1999.
15. Haywood VB: History, safety, and effectiveness of current bleaching techniques and applications of the nightguard vital bleaching technique. *Quintessence Int* 23:471, 1992.
16. Haywood VB: Nightguard vital bleaching: A history and products update: Part 1. *Esthetic Dent Update* 2:63, 1991.

17. Titley KC, Torneck CD, Ruse ND: The effect of carbamide-peroxide gel on the shear bond strength of a microfill resin to bovine enamel. *J Dent Res* 71:20, 1992.

18. Sorensen JA, Martinoff JT: Intracoronal reinforcement and coronal coverage: A study of endodontically treated teeth. *J Prosthet Dent* 51:780, 1984.

19. Harrington GW, Natkin E: External resorption associated with bleaching of pulpless teeth. *J Endod* 5:344, 1979.

20. Madison S, Walton R: Cervical root resorption following bleaching of endodontically treated teeth. *J Endod* 16:570, 1990.

21. Lado EA: Bleaching of endodontically treated teeth: An update on cervical resorption. *Gen Dent* 36:500, 1988.

22. Haywood VB, Heymann HO: Nightguard vital bleaching: How safe is it? *Quintessence Int* 22:515, 1991.

23. Lado EA, Stanley HR, Weisman MI: Cervical resorption in bleached teeth. *Oral Surg* 55:78, 1983.

24. Holmstrup G, Palm AM, Lambjerg-Hansen H: Bleaching of discolored root-filled teeth. *Endod Dent Traumatol* 4:197, 1988.

25. Feinman RA, Goldstein RL, Garber DA: *Bleaching teeth*, Chicago, 1987, Quintessence.

26. Haywood VB, Heymann HO: Nightguard vital bleaching. *Quintessence Int* 20:173, 1989.

27. Sagel PA, Odioso LL, McMillan DA, et al: Vital tooth whitening with a novel hydrogen peroxide strip system: Design, kinetics, and clinical response, *Compend Cont Educ Dent* 29(Suppl):S10–S15, 2000.

28. Hall DA: Should etching be performed as a part of a vital bleaching technique? *Quintessence Int* 22:679, 1991.

29. Papathanasiou A, Kastali S, Perry RD, et al: Clinical evaluation of a 35% hydrogen peroxide in-office whitening system. *Compend Cont Educ Dent* 23:335–346, 2002.

30. American Dental Association Council on Scientific Affairs: Report on laser bleaching. *J Am Dent Assoc* 129:1484, 1998.

31. Shethri SA, Matis BA, Cochran MA, et al: A clinical evaluation of two in-office bleaching products. *Oper Dent* 28:488–495, 2003.

32. McCloskey RJ: A technique for removal of fluorosis stains. *J Am Dent Assoc* 109:63, 1984.

33. Croll TP, Cavanaugh RR: Enamel color modification by controlled hydrochloric acid-pumice abrasion: Part 1. Technique and examples. *Quintessence Int* 17:81, 1986.

34. Croll TP: Enamel microabrasion for removal of superficial dysmineralization and decalcification defects. *J Am Dent Assoc* 120:411, 1990.

35. Dumfahrt H, Schaffer H: Porcelain laminate veneers: A retrospective evaluation after 1-10 years of service. *Int J Prosthodont* 13:9–18, 2000.

36. Friedman MJ: A 15-year review of porcelain veneer failure: A clinician's observation, *Compend Cont Educ Dent* 19:625–636, 1998.

37. Hashimoto M, Ohno H, Kaga M, et al: Resin-tooth interfaces after long-term function. *Am J Dent* 14:211–215, 2001.

38. Meiers JC, Young D: Two-year composite/dentin durability. *Am J Dent* 14:141–144, 2001.

39. Calamia JR: Etched porcelain facial veneers: A new treatment modality based on scientific and clinical evidence. *N Y J Dent* 53:255, 1983.

40. Friedman MJ: The enamel ceramic alternative: porcelain veneers vs. metal ceramic crowns. *CDA J* 20:27, 1992.

41. Stangel I, Nathanson D, Hsu CS: Shear strength of the composite bond to etched porcelain. *J Dent Res* 66:1460, 1987.

42. Bayne SC, Taylor DF, Zardiackas LD: *Biomaterials science*, Chapel Hill, NC, 1991, Brightstar.

43. Haywood VB, Heymann HO, Kusy RP, et al: Polishing porcelain veneers: An SEM and specular reflectance analysis. *Dent Mater* 4:116, 1988.

44. Cooley RL, Burger KM, Chain MC: Evaluation of a 4-META adhesive cement. *J Esthet Dent* 3:7, 1991.

Chapter 13

Introduction to Amalgam Restorations

Lee W. Boushell, Terrence E. Donovan, Theodore M. Roberson

Amalgam

Dental amalgam is a metallic restorative material composed of a mixture of silver–tin–copper alloy and mercury. The unset mixture is pressed (condensed) into a specifically prepared undercut tooth form and contoured to restore the tooth's form and function. When the material hardens, the tooth is functional again, restored with a silver-colored restoration (Fig. 13-1). Dental amalgam is described in detail in Online Chapter 18. In this book, dental amalgam is referred to as *amalgam*. Amalgam has been the primary direct restorative material for more than 150 years in the United States. It has been the subject of intense research and has been found to be safe and beneficial as a direct restorative material.[1-3] Many people have benefited from amalgam restorations, which restore a tooth in the most cost-effective manner. The U.S. Public Health Service stated, "In fact, hundreds of millions of teeth have been retained that otherwise would have been sacrificed because restorative alternatives would have been too expensive for many people."[4]

In addition to being cost-effective, amalgam is the most user-friendly direct restorative material. This is a result of a mechanism that ensures self-sealing of the amalgam to the prepared cavity walls. This quality occurs as a result of percolation of oral fluids between the amalgam and the tooth, which results in corrosion and the buildup of corrosion products in the microscopic interface. The corrosion products self-seal the restoration and reduce microleakage. This process is self-limiting and takes about 2 months.

History

Amalgam was introduced to the United States in the 1830s. Initially, amalgam restorations were made by dentists filing silver coins and mixing the filings with mercury, creating a putty-like mass that was placed into the defective tooth. As knowledge increased and research intensified, major advancements in the formulation and use of amalgam occurred. Concerns about mercury toxicity in the use of amalgam were, however, expressed in many countries; concerns reached major proportions in the early 1990s. The American Dental Association (ADA) and the U.S. Public Health Service have issued many statements expressing their support for the use and safety of amalgam as a restorative material.[1,4]

Current Status

Today, the popularity of amalgam as a direct restorative material has decreased.[5,6] This decline is attributed, in part, to the reduction in caries rates and to esthetic concerns. However, the primary cause of the reduction in the use of amalgam is the recognition of the benefits and improved esthetics of composite as a restorative material. Thus, concerns about the use of amalgam restorations relate primarily to poor esthetics and the greater potential for the weakening of the tooth structure: Dental amalgams inherently require greater removal of tooth structure to accommodate its strength requirements.

Because of environmental concerns about mercury contamination, the use of amalgam as a restorative material already has decreased in many countries. Legislation restricting and, in some cases, phasing out the use of amalgam has been implemented in Japan, Denmark, Canada, Sweden, and Germany.

Even with the concern about the disposal of mercury, this textbook advocates the continued use of amalgam as a direct restorative material, especially in light of the finding that bonded composite resin restorations have an increased risk of development of secondary caries.[7,8] Research repeatedly has shown the safety of amalgam and the success of restorations made from amalgam. Although the scope of the clinical uses of amalgam presented in this book are narrower than in the past, amalgam still is recognized as an excellent material for restoring many defects in teeth.

Types of Amalgam Restorative Materials
Low-Copper Amalgam

Low-copper amalgams were prominent before the early 1960s. When the setting reaction occurred, the material was subject to corrosion because a tin–mercury phase (gamma-two) formed. This corrosion led to the rapid breakdown of amalgam restorations. Subsequent research for improving amalgam led

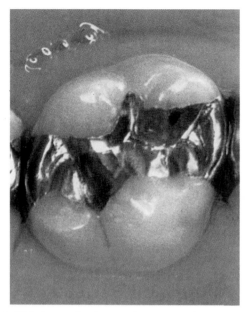

Fig. 13-1 Clinical example of an amalgam restoration. *(From Hatrick CD, Eakle WS, Bird WF: Dental materials: Clinical applications for dental assistants and dental hygienists,* ed 2, St. Louis, Saunders, 2011.)

to the development of high-copper amalgam materials. Low-copper amalgams are used very seldom in the United States.

High-Copper Amalgam

High-copper amalgams are the materials predominantly used today in the United States. In this book, unless otherwise specified, the term *amalgam* refers to high-copper dental amalgam. The increase in copper content to 12% or greater designates an amalgam as a high-copper type. The advantage of the added copper is that it preferentially reacts with the tin and reduces the formation of the more corrosive phase (gamma-two) within the amalgam mass. This change in composition reduces possible deleterious corrosion effects on the restoration. However, enough corrosion occurs at the amalgam–tooth interface to result in the successful sealing of the restoration.[9,10] These materials can provide satisfactory performance for more than 12 years.[11,12] High-copper materials can be either spherical or admixed in the composition.

Spherical Amalgam

A spherical amalgam contains small, round alloy particles that are mixed with mercury to form the mass that is placed into the tooth preparation. Because of the shape of the particles, the material is condensed into the tooth preparation with little condensation pressure. This advantage is combined with its high early strength to provide a material that is well suited for very large amalgam restorations such as complex amalgams or foundations.[13]

Admixed Amalgam

An admixed amalgam contains irregularly shaped and sized alloy particles, sometimes combined with spherical shapes, which are mixed to form the mass that is placed into the tooth preparation. The irregular shape of many of the particles makes a mass that requires more condensation pressure (which many dentists prefer) and permits this heavier condensation pressure to assist in displacing matrix bands to generate proximal contacts more easily.

New Amalgam Alloys

Because of the concern about mercury toxicity, many new compositions of amalgam are being promoted as mercury-free or low-mercury amalgam restorative materials. Alloys with gallium or indium or alloys using cold-welding techniques are presented as alternatives to mercury-containing amalgams. None of these new alloys shows sufficient promise to become a universal replacement for current amalgam materials.[14-16]

Important Properties

The linear coefficient of the thermal expansion of amalgam is 2.5 times greater than that of tooth structure, but it is closer than the linear coefficient of thermal expansion of composite.[17-19] Although the compressive strength of high-copper amalgam is similar to tooth structure, the tensile strength is lower, making amalgam restorations prone to fracture.[8,20,21] Usually, high-copper amalgam fracture is a bulk fracture, not a marginal fracture. All amalgams are brittle and have low edge strength. The amalgam material must have sufficient bulk (usually 1 to 2 mm, depending on the position within the tooth) and a 90-degree or greater marginal configuration.

Creep and flow relate to the deformation of a material under load over time. High-copper amalgams exhibit no clinically relevant creep or flow.[22,23] Because amalgam is metallic in structure, it also is a good thermal conductor. An amalgam restoration should not be placed close to the pulpal tissues of the tooth without the use of a liner or base (or both) between the pulp and the amalgam.

Amalgam Restorations

Amalgam functions as a direct restorative material because of its easy insertion into a tooth preparation and, when hardened, its ability to restore the tooth to proper form and function. The tooth preparation form not only must remove the fault in the tooth and remove weakened tooth structure, but it must also be formed to allow the amalgam material to function properly. The required tooth preparation form must allow the amalgam to (1) possess a uniform specified minimum thickness for strength, (2) produce a 90-degree amalgam angle (butt-joint form) at the margin, and (3) be mechanically retained in the tooth (Fig. 13-2). Without this preparation form, the amalgam possibly could be dislodged or could fracture. After desensitizing the prepared tooth structure, mixing, inserting, carving, and finishing the amalgam are relatively fast and easy (Fig. 13-3, *A*). For these reasons, it is a user-friendly material that is less technique sensitive or operator sensitive compared with composite.

Some practitioners have continued to use bonded amalgam restorations in their practice (see Fig. 13-3, *B*). As noted

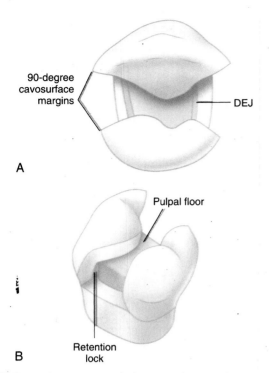

Fig. 13-2 A and **B,** Diagrams of Class II amalgam tooth preparations illustrating uniform pulpal and axial wall depths, 90-degree cavosurface margins, and convergence of walls or prepared retention form or both.

previously, this book no longer promotes the use of bonded amalgams.[24-27] The mechanism of bonding an amalgam restoration is similar to that for bonding a composite restoration in some aspects, but it is different in others. A bonded amalgam restoration, done properly, may seal the prepared tooth structure and may strengthen the remaining unprepared tooth structure. The retention gained by bonding, however, is minimal; consequently, bonded amalgam restorations still require the same tooth preparation retention form as do non-bonded amalgam restorations.[28,29] Isolation requirements for a bonded amalgam restoration are the same as for a composite restoration.

Another amalgam technique uses light-cured adhesive to seal the dentin under the amalgam material (see Fig. 13-3, *C*). This procedure, as is true of all procedures that use adhesive technology, requires proper isolation. The prepared tooth structure is etched, primed, and sealed with adhesive. The adhesive is polymerized before insertion of the amalgam. (Usually, a one-bottle sealer material that combines the primer and the adhesive is used.) This technique seals the dentinal tubules effectively.[30,31]

Uses

Because of its strength and ease of use, amalgam provides an excellent means for restoring large defects in non-esthetic areas.[32] A review of almost 3500 4-surface and 5-surface amalgams revealed successful outcomes at 5 years for 72% of the four-surface and 65% of the five-surface amalgams. This result compared favorably with the 5-year success rates for gold and porcelain crowns, which were 84% and 85%, respectively.[33]

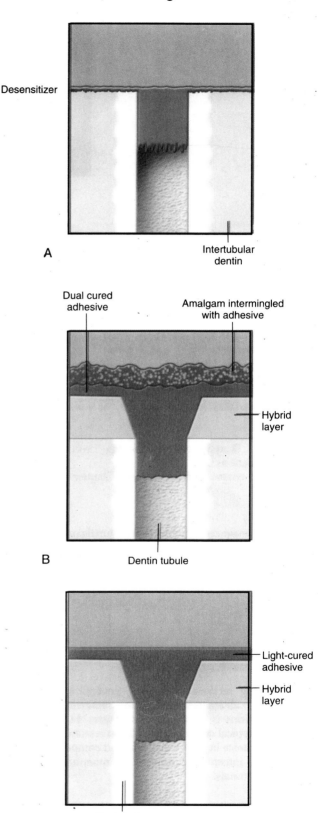

Fig. 13-3 Types of amalgam restorations. **A,** Conventional amalgam restoration with desensitizer (5% glutaraldehyde + 35% hydroxy-ethyl methacrylate [HEMA]). **B,** Bonded amalgam (amalgam intermingled with adhesive resin). **C,** Sealed amalgam (adhesive resin placed and cured before amalgam placement).

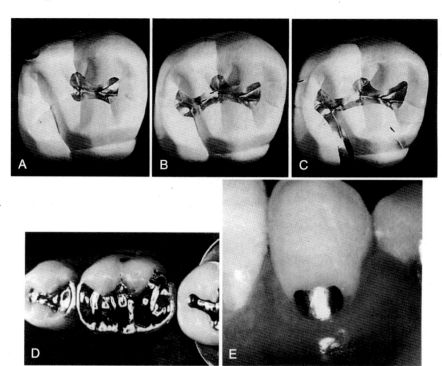

Fig. 13-4 Amalgam restorations. **A–C,** Class I. **D,** Class II. **E,** Class V. (Most practitioners would restore all of these teeth with composite, except tooth No. 30.)

Generally, amalgams can be used for the following clinical procedures:

1. Class I, II, and V restorations (Fig. 13-4)
2. Foundations (Fig. 13-5)
3. Caries-control restorations (see Chapter 2)

Handling

Because of the concern about mercury, amalgam restorations require meticulous handling to avoid unnecessary mercury exposure to the environment, the office, the personnel, or the patient. Proper mercury hygiene procedures are described in Online Chapter 1 and in the subsequent chapters on amalgam restorations.

General Considerations for Amalgam Restorations

The following sections summarize general considerations with regard to all amalgam restorations. Information for specific applications is presented in Chapters 14, 15, and 16. Because the typical decision about direct restorative materials is usually a choice between amalgam and composite, some of the following information involves a comparative analysis of these two materials.

Indications
Occlusal Factors

Amalgam has greater wear resistance than does composite.[2,34] It may be indicated in clinical situations that have heavy occlusal functioning. It also may be more appropriate when a restoration restores all of the occlusal contacts of a tooth.

Isolation Factors

Minor contamination of an amalgam during the insertion procedure may not have as adverse an effect on the final restoration as the same contamination would produce for a composite restoration.

Operator Ability and Commitment Factors

The tooth preparation for an amalgam restoration is very exacting. It requires a specific form with uniform depths and a precise marginal form. Many failures of amalgam restorations may be related to inappropriate tooth preparations. The insertion and finishing procedures for amalgam are much easier than for composite.

Clinical Indications for Direct Amalgam Restorations

Because of the factors already presented, amalgam is considered most appropriate for the following indications:

1. Moderate to large Class I and II restorations (especially restorations that involve heavy occlusion, cannot be isolated well, or extend onto the root surface) (see Fig. 13-4, A and B).
2. Class V restorations (including restorations that are not esthetically critical, cannot be well isolated, or are located entirely on the root surface) (see Fig. 13-4, C).
3. Temporary caries-control restorations (including teeth that are badly broken and require a subsequent assessment of pulpal health before a definitive restoration) (see Chapter 2).
4. Foundations (including for badly broken teeth that require increased retention and resistance forms in

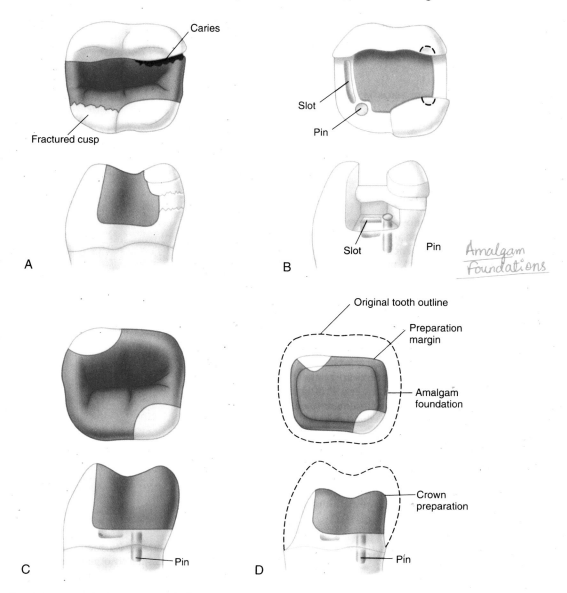

Fig. 13-5 Amalgam foundation. **A,** Defective restoration (defective amalgam, mesiolingual fractured cusp, mesiofacial caries). **B,** Tooth preparation with secondary retention and bonding, using pin and slot. **C,** Amalgam foundation placed. **D,** Tooth prepared for crown with amalgam foundation.

anticipation of the subsequent placement of a crown or metallic onlay) (see Fig. 13-5).

Contraindications

Amalgams are contraindicated in patients who are allergic to the alloy components. The use of amalgam in more prominent esthetic areas of the mouth is usually avoided. These areas include anterior teeth, premolars, and, in some patients, molars. Occasionally, a Class III amalgam restoration may be done if isolation problems exist. Likewise, in rare clinical situations, Class V amalgam restorations may be indicated in anterior areas where esthetics is not an important consideration. Amalgam should not be used when composite resin would offer better conservation of the tooth structure and equal clinical performance.

Advantages

Some of the advantages of amalgam restorations already have been stated, but the following list presents the primary reasons for the successful use of amalgam restorations for many years:

1. Ease of use
2. High compressive strength
3. Excellent wear resistance
4. Favorable long-term clinical research results
5. Lower cost than for composite restorations

Disadvantages

The primary disadvantages of amalgam restorations relate to esthetics and increased tooth structure removal during tooth preparation. The following is a list of these and other disadvantages of amalgam restorations:

1. Noninsulating
2. Non-esthetic
3. Less conservative (more removal of tooth structure during tooth preparation)
4. More difficult tooth preparation
5. Initial marginal leakage[16]

Clinical Technique

Initial Clinical Procedures

A complete examination, diagnosis, and treatment plan must be finalized before the patient is scheduled for operative appointments (except in emergencies). A brief review of the chart (including medical factors), treatment plan, and radiographs should precede each restorative procedure. At the beginning of each appointment, the dentist should also examine the operating site carefully to confirm the diagnosis of the tooth or teeth scheduled for treatment.

Local Anesthesia

Because most amalgam tooth preparations are relatively more extensive, local anesthesia usually is necessary. Profound anesthesia contributes to a comfortable and uninterrupted operation and usually results in a marked reduction in salivation.

Isolation of the Operating Site

Complete instructions for the control of moisture are given in Chapter 7. Isolation for amalgam restorations can be accomplished with a rubber dam or cotton rolls, with or without a retraction cord.

Other Pre-operative Considerations

A pre-operative assessment of the occlusion should be made. This step should occur before rubber dam placement; and the dentist should identify not only the occlusal contacts of the tooth to be restored but also the contacts on opposing and adjacent teeth. Knowing the pre-operative location of occlusal contacts is important in planning the restoration outline form and in establishing the proper occlusal contacts on the restoration. Remembering the location of the contacts on adjacent teeth provides guidance in determining when the restoration contacts have been correctly adjusted and positioned.

A wedge placed pre-operatively in the gingival embrasure is useful when restoring a posterior proximal surface. This step causes separation of the operated tooth from the adjacent tooth and may help protect the rubber dam and the interdental papilla.

For smaller amalgam restorations, it also is important to visualize pre-operatively the anticipated extension of the tooth preparation. Because the tooth preparation requires specific depths, extensions, and marginal forms, the connection of the various parts of the tooth preparation should result in minimal tooth structure removal (i.e., as little as is necessary), while maintaining the strength of the cuspal and marginal ridge areas of the tooth as much as possible (Fig. 13-6). The

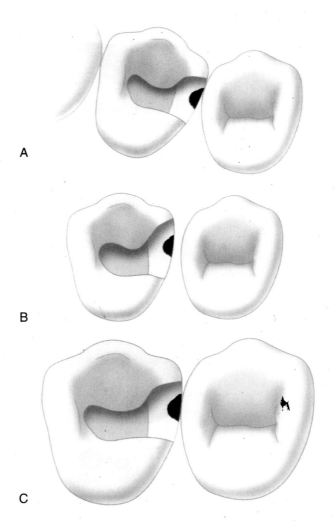

Fig. 13-6 Pre-operative visualization of tooth preparation extensions when caries is present gingival to the proximal contact and in the central groove area. **A,** Rotated tooth (lingual extension owing to faulty central groove). **B,** Open proximal contact (preparation extended wider faciolingually to develop a proximal contact with appropriate physiologic proximal contours). **C,** Normal relationship.

projected facial and lingual extensions of a proximal box should be visualized before preparing the occlusal portion of the tooth, reducing the chance of over-preparing the cuspal area while maintaining a butt-joint form of the facial or lingual proximal margins.

Tooth Preparation for Amalgam Restorations

Detailed descriptions of specific amalgam tooth preparations are presented in Chapters 5, 14, 15, and 16. As discussed in Chapter 5, the stages and steps of tooth preparation are important for amalgam tooth preparations. For an amalgam restoration to be successful, numerous steps must be accomplished correctly. After an accurate diagnosis is made, the dentist must create a tooth preparation that not only removes the defect (e.g., caries, old restorative material, malformed structure) but also leaves the remaining tooth structure in as strong a state as possible. Making the tooth preparation form appropriate for the use of amalgam as the restorative material is equally important. Because of amalgam's physical properties, it must (1) be placed into a tooth preparation that provides for a 90-degree or greater restoration angle at the cavosurface margin (because of the amalgam's limited edge strength), (2) have a minimum thickness of 1.5 to 2 mm for adequate compressive strength (because most amalgams fail by bulk fracture), and (3) be placed into a prepared undercut form in the tooth to be mechanically retained (because of the amalgam's lack of bonding to the tooth). After appropriate tooth preparation, the success of the final restoration depends on proper insertion, carving, and finishing of the amalgam material.

Requirements

The preparation features that relate specifically to the use of amalgam as the restorative material include the following:

1. Amalgam margin 90 degrees or greater (butt-joint form)
2. Adequate depth (thickness of amalgam)
3. Adequate mechanical retention form (undercut form)

Principles

The basic principles of tooth preparation must be followed for amalgam tooth preparations to ensure clinical success. The procedure is presented in two stages, academically, to facilitate student understanding of proper extension, form, and caries removal. The initial stage (1) places the tooth preparation extension into sound tooth structure at the marginal areas (not pulpally or axially); (2) extends the depth (pulpally or axially or both) to a prescribed, uniform dimension; (3) provides an initial form that retains the amalgam in the tooth; and (4) establishes the tooth preparation margins in a form that results in a 90-degree amalgam margin when the amalgam is inserted. The second and final stage of tooth preparation removes any remaining defect (caries or old restorative material) and incorporates any additional preparation features (grooves, slots, pins, steps, or amalgam pins) to achieve the appropriate retention and resistance forms. The following sections briefly describe certain aspects of tooth preparation that pertain to all amalgam restorations. The initial tooth preparation steps, although discussed separately, are performed at the same time. Extension, depth, tooth preparation wall shape, and marginal configuration are accomplished simultaneously.

INITIAL TOOTH PREPARATION DEPTH

All initial depths of a tooth preparation for amalgam relate to the dentinoenamel junction (DEJ) except in the following two instances: (1) when the occlusal enamel has been significantly worn thinner and (2) when the preparation extends onto the root surface. The initial depth pulpally is 0.2 mm inside (internal to) the DEJ or 1.5 mm as measured from the depth of the central groove (Fig. 13-7), whichever results in the greatest thickness of amalgam. The initial depth of the axial wall is 0.2 mm inside the DEJ when retention grooves are not used and 0.5 mm inside the DEJ when retention grooves are used (Fig. 13-8). The deeper extension allows placement of the

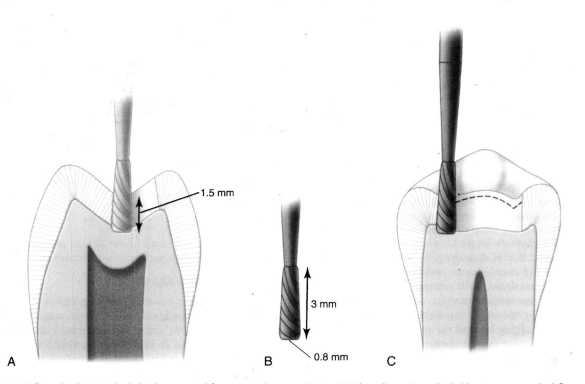

A

B   3 mm

0.8 mm   C

Fig. 13-7 Pulpal floor depth. **A,** Pulpal depth measured from central groove. **B,** No. 245 bur dimensions. **C,** Guides to proper pulpal floor depth: (1) one-half the length of the No. 245 bur, (2) 1.5 mm, or (3) 0.2 mm inside (internal to) the dentinoenamel junction (DEJ).

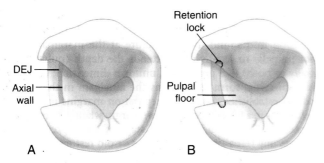

Fig. 13-8 Axial wall depth. **A,** If no retention grooves needed, axial depth 0.2 mm inside (internal to) the dentinoenamel junction (DEJ). **B,** If retention grooves needed, axial depth 0.5 mm inside (internal to) the DEJ.

retention groove without undermining marginal enamel. Axial depths on the root surface should be 0.75 to 1 mm deep so as to provide room for placement of a retention groove or cove.

OUTLINE FORM

The initial extension of the tooth preparation should be visualized preoperatively by estimating the extent of the defect, the preparation form requirements of the amalgam, and the need for adequate access to place the amalgam into the tooth. Because of the structure of enamel, enamel margins must be left in a form of 90 degrees or greater. Otherwise, enamel is subject to fracture. For enamel strength, the marginal enamel rods should be supported by sound dentin. These requirements for enamel strength must be combined with marginal requirements for amalgam (90-degree butt joint) when establishing the periphery of the tooth preparation (see Fig. 14-46).

The preparation extension is dictated primarily by the existing amount of caries, old restorative material, or defect. Adequate extension to provide access for tooth preparation, caries removal, matrix placement, and amalgam insertion also must be considered. When making the preparation extensions, every effort should be made to preserve the strength of cusps and marginal ridges. When possible, the outline form should be extended around cusps and avoid undermining the dentinal support of the marginal ridge enamel.

When viewed from the occlusal, the facial and lingual proximal cavosurface margins of a Class II preparation should be 90 degrees (i.e., perpendicular to a tangent drawn through the point of extension facially and lingually) (Fig. 13-9). In most instances, the facial and lingual proximal walls should be extended just into the facial or lingual embrasure. This extension provides adequate access for performing the preparation (with decreased risk of damaging the adjacent tooth), easier placement of the matrix band, and easier condensation and carving of the amalgam. Such extension provides a clearance between the cavosurface margin and the adjacent tooth (Fig. 13-10). For the more experienced operator, extending the proximal margins beyond the proximal contact into the respective embrasure is not always necessary. The less the outline form is extended, the more conservative is the resulting preparation and the less the tooth structure removed.

Factors dictating the outline form are presented in greater detail in Chapter 5. They include caries, old restorative

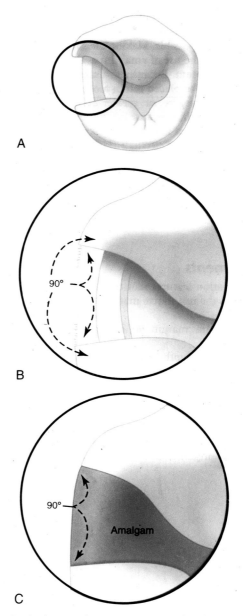

Fig. 13-9 Proximal cavosurface margins. **A,** Facial and lingual proximal cavosurface margins prepared at 90-degree angles to a tangent drawn through the point on the external tooth surface. **B,** A 90-degree proximal cavosurface margin produces a 90-degree amalgam margin. **C,** 90-degree amalgam margins.

material, inclusion of all of the defect, proximal or occlusal contact relationship, and the need for convenience form.

CAVOSURFACE MARGIN

Enamel must have a marginal configuration of 90 degrees or greater, and the amalgam must have the same. With marginal angles less than 90 degrees, enamel and amalgam will be subject to fracture, as both these materials are brittle structures. Preparation walls on vertical parts of the tooth (facial, lingual, mesial, or distal) should result in 90-degree enamel walls (representing a strong enamel margin; see Fig. 13-9) that meet the inserted amalgam at a butt joint (enamel and

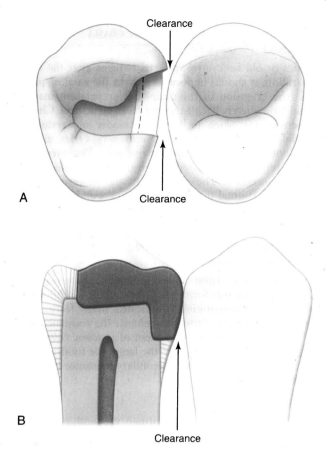

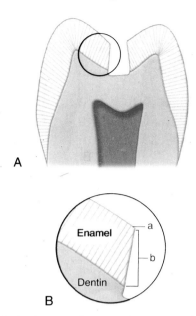

Fig. 13-11 Occlusal cavosurface margins. **A,** Tooth preparation. **B,** Occlusal margin representing the strongest enamel margin. Full-length enamel rods (*a*) and shorter enamel rods (*b*).

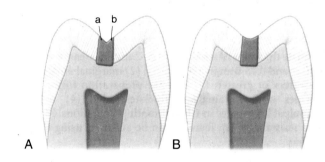

Fig. 13-10 Proximal box preparation clearance of adjacent tooth. **A,** Occlusal view. **B,** Lingual view of a cross-section through the central groove.

amalgam having 90-degree margins). Preparation walls on the occlusal surface should provide 90-degree or greater amalgam margins and usually have obtuse enamel margins (representing the strongest enamel margin; Fig. 13-11). The 90-degree occlusal amalgam margin results from the amalgam carving in the central groove area being more rounded (Fig. 13-12).

PRIMARY RETENTION FORM

Retention form preparation features lock or retain the restorative material in the tooth. For composite restorations, micromechanical bonding provides most of the retention needed. Amalgam restorations must be mechanically locked inside the tooth. Amalgam retention form (Fig. 13-13) is provided by (1) mechanical locking of the inserted amalgam into the surface irregularities of the preparation (even though the desired texture of the preparation walls is smooth) to allow proper adaptation of the amalgam to the tooth; (2) preparation of the vertical walls (especially facial and lingual walls) that converge occlusally; and (3) special retention features such as grooves, coves, slots, pins, steps, or amalgam pins that are placed during the final stage of tooth preparation. The first two of these are considered primary retention form features and are provided by the orientation and type of the preparation instrument. The third is a secondary retention form feature and is discussed in a subsequent section. A pear-shaped carbide bur

Fig. 13-12 Amalgam form at occlusal cavosurface margins. **A,** Amalgam carved too deep resulting in acute angles *a* and *b* and stress concentrations within the amalgam, increasing the potential for fracture. **B,** Amalgam carved with appropriate anatomy, resulting in an amalgam margin close to 90 degrees, although the enamel cavosurface margin is obtuse.

(No. 330 or No. 245) provides the desired wall shape and texture (see Fig. 13-7, *B*).

PRIMARY RESISTANCE FORM

Resistance form preparation features help the restoration and the tooth resist fracturing caused by occlusal forces. Resistance features that assist in preventing the tooth from fracturing include (1) maintaining as much unprepared tooth structure as possible (preserving cusps and marginal ridges); (2) having pulpal and gingival walls prepared perpendicular to the occlusal forces, when possible; (3) having rounded internal preparation angles; (4) removing unsupported or weakened tooth structure; and (5) placing pins into the tooth as part of the final stage of tooth preparation. The last of these features is considered a secondary resistance form feature and is discussed in a subsequent section. Resistance form features that assist in preventing the amalgam from fracturing include (1)

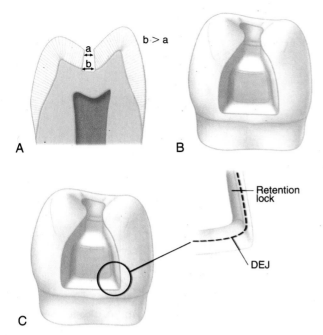

Fig. 13-13 Typical amalgam tooth preparation retention form features. **A** and **B**, Occlusal convergence of prepared walls (primary retention form). **C**, Retention grooves in proximal box (secondary retention form).

adequate thickness of amalgam (1.5–2 mm in areas of occlusal contact and 0.75 mm in axial areas); (2) marginal amalgam of 90 degrees or greater; (3) box-like preparation form, which provides uniform amalgam thickness; and (4) rounded axiopulpal line angles in Class II tooth preparations. Many of these resistance form features can be achieved using the No. 245 bur.

CONVENIENCE FORM

Convenience form preparation features are features that make the procedure easier or the area more accessible. The convenience form may include arbitrary extension of the outline form so that the marginal form can be established; caries can be accessed for removal; matrix can be placed; or amalgam can be inserted, carved, and finished. Convenience form features also may include extending the proximal margins to provide clearance from the adjacent tooth and extension of the other walls to provide greater access for caries excavation.

For simplification in teaching, all of these steps in the tooth preparation (outline, retention, resistance, and convenience forms) constitute what is referred to as *the initial stage of tooth preparation.* Although each step is an important consideration, they are accomplished simultaneously. In academic institutions, assessing the tooth preparation after the initial preparation stage provides an opportunity to evaluate a student's knowledge and ability to extend the preparation properly and establish the proper depth. If the student were to excavate extensive caries before any evaluation, the attending faculty would not know whether the prepared depths were obtained because of appropriate excavation or inappropriate overcutting of the tooth. The following factors constitute the final stage of tooth preparation.

REMOVAL OF THE REMAINING FAULT AND PULP PROTECTION

If caries or old restorative material remains after the initial preparation, it should be located only in the axial or pulpal walls (the extension of the peripheral preparation margins should have already been to sound tooth structure). Chapter 5 discusses (1) when to leave or remove old restorative material, (2) how to remove the remaining caries, and (3) what should be done to protect the pulp. Placement of a desensitizer on the prepared dentin is recommended before amalgam insertion. The objective of the desensitizer is to occlude the dentinal tubules. (Use of liners and bases under amalgam restorations is discussed in Online Chapter 18 and Chapter 5.)

SECONDARY RESISTANCE AND RETENTION FORMS

If it is determined (from clinical judgment) that insufficient retention or resistance forms are present in the tooth preparation, additional preparation is indicated. Many features that enhance the retention form also enhance the resistance form. Such features include the placement of grooves, coves, pins, slots, or amalgam pins. Usually, the larger the tooth preparation, the greater is the need for secondary resistance and retention forms.

FINAL PROCEDURES

After the previous steps are performed, the tooth preparation should be viewed from all angles. Careful assessment should be made to ensure that all caries has been removed, the depths are proper, the margins provide for correct amalgam and tooth preparation angles, and the tooth is cleaned of any residual debris.

Preparation Designs

The typical tooth preparation for amalgam is referred to as *conventional tooth preparation.* Other types include box-only and tunnel preparations for amalgam restorations. Figure 13-14 illustrates various preparation designs. Appropriate details of specific tooth preparations are presented in subsequent chapters.

Restorative Technique for Amalgam Restorations

After tooth preparation, the tooth must be readied for the insertion of amalgam. A desensitizer, which contains 5% glutaraldehyde and 35% hydroxy ethyl methacrylate (HEMA), is placed on the prepared dentin (see Fig. 13-3). This step may occur before or after the matrix application.

Matrix Placement

A matrix primarily is used when a proximal surface is to be restored. The objectives of a matrix are to (1) provide proper contact, (2) provide proper contour, (3) confine the restorative material, and (4) reduce the amount of excess material. For a matrix to be effective, it should (1) be easy to apply and remove, (2) extend below the gingival margin, (3) extend above the marginal ridge height, and (4) resist deformation

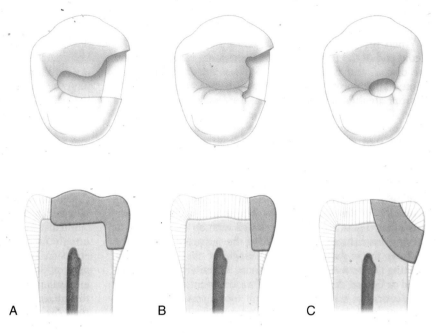

Fig. 13-14 Types of amalgam tooth preparations. **A,** Conventional. **B,** Box-only. **C,** Tunnel.

during material insertion. Chapters 14, 15, and 16 describe matrix placement for specific amalgam restorations and illustrate some of the types of matrices available.

In some clinical circumstances, a matrix may be necessary for Class I or V amalgam restorations. Examples of Class I matrices are shown in Chapter 14; examples of Class V matrices are shown in Chapter 15. Matrix application might be beneficial during tooth preparation to help protect the adjacent tooth from being damaged. The matrix, when used for this reason, would be placed on the adjacent tooth (or teeth).

Mixing (Triturating) the Amalgam Material

The manufacturer's directions should be followed when mixing the amalgam material. The speed and time of mix are factors in the setting reaction of the material. Alterations in either may cause changes in the properties of the inserted amalgam.

Inserting the Amalgam

Manipulating the amalgam during insertion is described in Online Chapter 18 as well as in Chapters 14, 15, and 16. Lateral condensation (facially and lingually directed condensation) is important in the proximal box portions of the preparation to ensure confluence of the amalgam with the margins. Spherical amalgam is more easily condensed than admixed (lathe-cut) amalgam, but some practitioners prefer the handling properties of the admixed type. Generally, smaller amalgam condensers are used first; this allows the amalgam to be properly condensed into the internal line angles and secondary retention features. Subsequently, larger condensers are used. When the amalgam is placed to slight excess with condensers, it should be precarved burnished with a large egg-shaped burnisher to finalize the condensation, remove excess mercury-rich amalgam, and initiate the carving process.

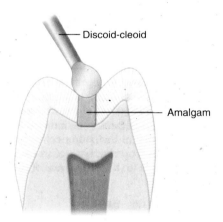

Fig. 13-15 Carving the occlusal margins.

Carving the Amalgam

The amalgam material selected for the restoration has a specific setting time. After precarve burnishing has been accomplished, the remainder of the accessible restoration must be contoured to achieve proper form and function. The insertion (condensation) and carving of the material must occur before the material has hardened so much as to be uncarvable.

OCCLUSAL AREAS

A discoid–cleoid instrument is used to carve the occlusal surface of an amalgam restoration. The rounded end (discoid) is positioned on the unprepared enamel adjacent to the amalgam margin and pulled parallel to the margin (Fig. 13-15). This removes any excess at the margin while not allowing the marginal amalgam to be over-carved (too much removed). The pointed end (cleoid) can be used to define the primary grooves, pits, and cuspal inclines. The Hollenbeck carver is also useful in carving these areas.

When the pit and groove anatomy is initiated with the cleoid end of the instrument, the instrument is switched, and the discoid end is used to smooth out the anatomic form. Some semblance of pits and grooves is necessary to provide appropriate sluiceways for the escape of food from the occlusal table. The mesial and distal pits are carved to be inferior to the marginal ridge height, helping prevent food from being wedged into the occlusal embrasure. Having definite but rounded occlusal anatomy also helps achieve a 90-degree amalgam margin on the occlusal surface (see Fig. 13-12, *B*).

For large Class II or foundation restorations, the initial carving of the occlusal surface should be rapid, concentrating primarily on the marginal ridge height and occlusal embrasure areas. These areas are developed with an explorer tip or carving instrument by mimicking the adjacent tooth. The explorer tip is pulled along the inside of the matrix band, creating the occlusal embrasure form. When viewed from the facial or lingual direction, the embrasure form created should be identical to that of the adjacent tooth, assuming that the adjacent tooth has appropriate contour. Likewise, the height of the amalgam marginal ridge should be the same as that of the adjacent tooth (see Figs. 14-94 and 14-97). If both these areas are developed properly, the potential for fracture of the marginal ridge area of the restoration is significantly reduced. Placing the initial carving emphasis on the occlusal areas for a large restoration permits the operator to remove the matrix more quickly and carve any extensive axial surfaces of the restoration, especially the interproximal areas. Some of these areas may be relatively inaccessible and must be carved while the amalgam material is still not fully set. The remaining carving or contouring necessary on the occlusal surface can be done later, and if the amalgam is too hardened to carve, the use of rotary instruments in the handpiece may be required. When the initial occlusal carving has occurred, the matrix is removed to provide access to the other areas of the restoration that require carving.

FACIAL AND LINGUAL AREAS

Most facial and lingual areas are accessible and can be carved directly. A Hollenbeck carver is useful in carving these areas. The base of the amalgam knife (scaler 34/35) also is appropriate. With regard to the cervical areas, it is important to remove any excess and develop the proper contour of the restoration. Usually, the contour is convex; care must be exercised in carving this area. The convexity is developed by using the occlusal and gingival unprepared tooth structure as guides for initiating the carving (see Fig. 15-41). The marginal areas are blended together, resulting in the desired convexity and providing the physiologic contour that promotes good gingival health.

PROXIMAL EMBRASURE AREAS

The development of the occlusal embrasure already has been described. The amalgam knife (or scaler) is an excellent instrument for removing proximal excess and developing proximal contours and embrasures (see Figs. 14-95 and 14-96). The knife is positioned below the gingival margin, and the excess is carefully shaved away. The knife is drawn occlusally to refine the proximal contour (below the contact) and the gingival embrasure form. The sharp tip of the knife also is beneficial

in developing the facial and lingual embrasure forms. Care must be exercised in not carving away any of the desired proximal contact. If the amalgam is hardening, the amalgam knife must be used to shave, rather than cut the excess away. If a cutting motion is used, the possibility of breaking or chipping the amalgam is increased.

Developing a proper proximal contour and contact is important for the physiologic health of interproximal soft tissue. Likewise, developing a smooth proximal junction between the tooth and the amalgam is important. An amalgam overhang (excess of amalgam) may result in compromised gingival health. Voids at the cavosurface margins may result in recurrent caries.

The proximal portion of the carved amalgam is evaluated by visual assessment (reflecting light into the contact area to confirm a proximal contact) and placement of dental floss into the area. If dental floss is used, it must be used judiciously, ensuring that the contact area is not inadvertently removed. A piece of floss can be inserted through the contact and into the gingival embrasure area by initially wrapping the floss around the adjacent tooth and exerting pressure on that tooth rather than the restored tooth while moving the floss through the contact area. When the floss is into the gingival embrasure area, it is wrapped around the restored tooth and moved occlusally and gingivally to determine whether excess exists and to smooth the proximal amalgam material. If excess material is detected along the gingival margin, the amalgam knife should be used again until a smooth margin is obtained.

Finishing the Amalgam Restoration

When the carving is completed, the restoration is visualized from all angles, and the thoroughness of the carving is assessed. If a rubber dam was used, it is removed, and the occlusal relationship of the restoration is assessed. Knowing the preoperative occlusal relationship of the restored tooth and adjacent teeth is helpful in developing appropriate contacts in the restoration; the tooth should be restored to appropriate occlusal contacts. Initially, the patient should be instructed to close very lightly, stopping when any contact is noted. At this point, the operator should assess the occlusion visually. If spacing is seen between adjacent teeth and their opposing teeth, the area of premature occlusal contact on the amalgam should be identified and relieved. Articulating paper is used to identify contact areas requiring adjustment, which continues until the proper occlusal relationship is accomplished. After the occlusion is adjusted, the discoid–cleoid can be used to smooth the accessible areas of the amalgam. A lightly moistened cotton pellet held in the operative pliers can be used to smooth the accessible parts of the restoration. If the carving and smoothing are done properly, no subsequent polishing of the restoration is needed, and good long-term clinical performance results.

Repairing an Amalgam Restoration

If an amalgam restoration fractures during insertion, the defective area must be re-prepared as if it were a small restoration. Appropriate depth and retention form must be generated, sometimes entirely within the existing amalgam restoration. If necessary, another matrix must be placed. A new mix of amalgam can be condensed directly into the defect, and it adheres to the amalgam already present if no intermediary material has been placed between the two amalgams. A desensitizer can be placed on any exposed dentin, but it should not be placed on the amalgam preparation walls.

Controversial Issues

Constant changes are occurring because the practice of operative dentistry is dynamic. New products and techniques have been developed, but their effectiveness cannot be assessed until appropriately designed research protocols have tested them. Numerous such developments are occurring at any time, many of which do not have the necessary documentation to prove their effectiveness, even though they receive much publicity. Varied opinions tend to generate controversy. Examples of such controversies follow.

Safety of Amalgam Restoration

A number of independent health agencies have extensively reviewed the issues of safety and efficacy of amalgam in recent years and have all concluded that available data does not justify either the discontinuance of use of amalgam or the removal of existing amalgam restorations. These agencies include the U.S. Food and Drug Administration (FDA) in 1991 and 2002 (http://fda.gov/cdrh/consumer/amalgams); the World Health Organization (WHO) along with the FDA in 1997; The National Institutes of Health (NIH) and the National Institute of Dental Research (NIDR) in 1991; and the U.S. Public Health Service (USPHS) in 1993. The National Council Against Health Fraud (NCAHF) warns consumers about dentists recommending unnecessary removal of serviceable amalgam restorations and states: "Promoting a dental practice as mercury free is unethical because it falsely implies that amalgam fillings are dangerous and that mercury-free methods are superior" (see www.ncahf.org).

The Life Sciences Research Organization (LSRO), a nonprofit scientific organization in Bethesda, MD, released results of its independent review of all articles published on this topic between 1996 and 2003. Of the 950 published articles, 300 were accepted on the basis of scientific methodology. The report concluded: "There is little evidence to support a causal relationship between silver fillings and human health problems" (see http://www.LSRO.org/).

An analysis of available data leads to the conclusion that mercury in amalgam restorations poses absolutely no problem for dental patients. This conclusion has been reached by experts in the field, by consumer interest groups, and by thorough reviews by governmental agencies. The authors of this textbook strongly agree with this conclusion.

Online Chapter 18 specifically addresses amalgam restoration safety as well and presents facts that indicate that amalgam restorations are safe. Likewise, the USPHS has reported the safety of amalgam restorations. In spite of these assessments, the mercury content in the current amalgam restorations still causes concerns, legitimate and otherwise. Proper handling of mercury in mixing the amalgam mass, removal of old amalgam restorations, and amalgam scrap disposal are paramount. Using the best management practices for amalgam waste as presented by the American Dental Association results in appropriate amalgam use.[35]

Proximal Retention Grooves

The need for proximal retention grooves for all Class II amalgam tooth preparations is debatable. This book endorses the use of proximal retention grooves for large amalgam restorations; their use for smaller restorations is not deemed necessary. However, because correct placement of proximal retention grooves is difficult, this book presents many illustrations of grooves placed in smaller restorations, primarily to promote the operator gaining sufficient experience in their use.

Summary

Amalgam is a safe and effective direct restorative material. An amalgam restoration is relatively easy to accomplish, and adherence to tooth preparation and material handling requirements results in clinical success.

References

1. American Dental Association Council on Scientific Affairs: Dental amalgam: Update on safety concerns. *J Am Dent Assoc* 129:494–503, 1998.
2. Collins CJ, Bryant RW, Hodge KL: A clinical evaluation of posterior composite resin restorations: 8-year findings. *J Dent* 26:311–317, 1998.
3. Lauterbach M, Martins IP, Castro-Caldas A, et al: Neurological outcomes in children with and without amalgam-related mercury exposure: Seven years of longitudinal observations in a randomized trial. *J Am Dent Assoc* 139:138–145, 2008.
4. Corbin SB, Kohn WG: The benefits and risks of dental amalgam: Current findings reviewed. *J Am Dent Assoc* 125:381–388, 1994.
5. Berry TG, Summitt JB, Chung AK, et al: Amalgam at the new millennium. *J Am Dent Assoc* 129:1547–1556, 1998.
6. Dunne SM, Gainsford ID, Wilson NH: Current materials and techniques for direct restorations in posterior teeth: Silver amalgam: Part 1. *Int Dent J* 47:123–136, 1997.
7. Bernando M, Luis H, Martin MD, et al: Survival and reasons for failure of amalgam versus composite restorations placed in a randomized clinical trial. *J Am Dent Assoc* 138:775–783, 2007.
8. Opdam NJM, Bronkhorst EM, Loomans BA, et al: 12-year survival of composite vs. amalgam restorations. *J Dent Res* 89:1063–1067, 2010.
9. Ben-Amar A, Cardash HS, Judes H: The sealing of the tooth/amalgam interface by corrosion products. *J Oral Rehabil* 22:101–104, 1995.
10. Liberman R, Ben-Amar A, Nordenberg D, et al: Long-term sealing properties of amalgam restorations: An in vitro study. *Dent Mater* 5:168–170, 1989.
11. Letzel H, van 't Hof MA, Marshall GW, et al: The influence of the amalgam alloy on the survival of amalgam restorations: A secondary analysis of multiple controlled clinical trials. *J Dent Res* 76:1787–1798, 1997.
12. Mahler DB: The high-copper dental amalgam alloys. *J Dent Res* 76:537–421, 1997.
13. Suchatlampong C, Goto S, Ogura H: Early compressive strength and phase-formation of dental amalgam. *Dent Mater* 14:143–151, 1995.
14. Osborne JW: Photoelastic assessment of the expansion of direct-placement gallium restorative alloys. *Quintessence Int* 30:185–191, 1999.
15. Osborne JW, Summitt JB: Direct-placement gallium restorative alloy: A 3-year clinical evaluation. *Quintessence Int* 30:49–53, 1999.
16. Venugopalan R, Broome JC, Lucas LC: The effect of water contamination on dimensional change and corrosion properties of a gallium alloy. *Dent Mater* 14:173–178, 1998.
17. Bullard RH, Leinfelder KF, Russell CM: Effect of coefficient of thermal expansion on microleakage. *J Am Dent Assoc* 116:871–874, 1988.
18. Williams PT, Hedge GL: Creep-fatigue as a possible cause of dental amalgam margin failure. *J Dent Res* 64:470–475, 1985.
19. Combe EC, Burke FJT, Douglas WH: Thermal properties. In Combe EC, Burke FJT, Douglas WH, editors: *Dental biomaterials*, Boston, 1999, Kluwer Academic Publishers.
20. Bryant RW: The strength of fifteen amalgam alloys. *Austr Dent J* 24:244–252, 1979.

21. Murray GA, Yates JL: Early compressive and diametral tensile strengths of seventeen amalgam alloy systems. *J Pedod* 5:40–50, 1980.

22. Mahler DB, Adey JD: Factors influencing the creep of dental amalgam. *J Dent Res* 70:1394–1400, 1991.

23. Vrijhoef MM, Letzel H: Creep versus marginal fracture of amalgam restorations. *J Oral Rehabil* 13:299–303, 1986.

24. Dias de Souza GM, Pereira GD, Dias CT, et al: Fracture resistance of teeth restored with the bonded amalgam technique. *Oper Dent* 26:511, 2001.

25. Mahler DB, Engle JH: Clinical evaluation of amalgam bonding in class I and II restorations. *J Am Dent Assoc* 131:43, 2000.

26. Smales RJ, Wetherell JD: Review of bonded amalgam restorations and assessment in a general practice over five years. *Oper Dent* 25:374, 2000.

27. Summitt JB, Burgess JO, Berry TG, et al: Six-year clinical evaluation of bonded and pin-retained complex amalgam restorations. *Oper Dent* 29:261, 2004.

28. Gorucu J, Tiritoglu M, Ozgünaltay G: Effects of preparation designs and adhesive systems on retention of class II amalgam restorations. *J Prosthet Dent* 78:250–254, 1997.

29. Winkler MM, Moore BK, Allen J, et al: Comparison of retentiveness of amalgam bonding agent types. *Oper Dent* 22:200–208, 1997.

30. Ben-Amar A, Liberman R, Rothkoff Z, et al: Long term sealing properties of Amalgam bond under amalgam restorations. *Am J Dent* 7:141–143, 1994.

31. Olmez A, Ulusu T: Bond strength and clinical evaluation of a new dentinal bonding agent to amalgam and resin composite. *Quintessence Int* 26:785–793, 1995.

32. Plasmans P, Creugers NH, Mulder J: Long-term survival of extensive amalgam restorations. *J Dent Res* 77:453–460, 1998.

33. Martin JA, Bader JD: Five-year treatment outcomes for teeth with large amalgams and crowns. *Oper Dent* 22:72–78, 1997.

34. Mair LH: Ten-year clinical assessment of three posterior resin composites and two amalgams. *Quintessence Int* 29:483–490, 1998.

35. American Dental Association: Amalgam waste: ADA's best management practices. *ADA News* 35:1, 2004.

Chapter 14

Class I, II, and VI Amalgam Restorations

Lee W. Boushell, Theodore M. Roberson, Aldridge D. Wilder, Jr.

Amalgam is used for the restoration of many carious or fractured posterior teeth and in the replacement of failed restorations. Understanding the physical properties of amalgam and the principles of tooth preparation is necessary to produce amalgam restorations that provide optimal service. If properly placed, an amalgam restoration provides many years of service.[1-6] Although improved techniques and materials are available, amalgam failures do occur. Much clinical time is spent replacing restorations that fail as a result of recurrent caries, marginal deterioration (i.e., ditching), fractures, or poor contours.[7,8] Attention to detail throughout the procedure can significantly decrease the incidence of failures, however, and extend the life of any restoration.[9-11] Careful evaluation of existing amalgams is important because they have the potential to provide long-term clinical service and should not be replaced unless an accurate diagnosis is made.[12]

This chapter presents the techniques and procedures for Class I, II, and VI amalgam restorations (Fig. 14-1). Class I restorations restore defects on the occlusal surface of posterior teeth, the occlusal thirds of the facial and lingual surface of molars, and the lingual surfaces of maxillary anterior teeth. Class II restorations restore defects that affect one or both of the proximal surfaces of posterior teeth. Class VI restorations restore rare defects affecting the cusp tips of posterior teeth or the incisal edges of anterior teeth.

Pertinent Material Qualities and Properties

Pertinent material qualities and properties for Class I, II, and VI amalgam restorations include the following:

- Strength
- Longevity
- Ease of use
- Clinically proven success

In addition, amalgam is the only restorative material with an interfacial seal that improves over time.[13-15]

Indications

Amalgam is indicated for the restoration of a Class I, II, and VI defect when the defect (1) is not in an area of the mouth where esthetics is highly important, (2) is moderate to large, (3) is in an area that will have heavy occlusal contacts, (4) cannot be well isolated, (5) extends onto the root surface, (6) will become a foundation for a full coverage restoration, and (7) is in a tooth that serves as an abutment for a removable partial denture.

Contraindications

Although amalgam has no specific contraindications for use in Class I, II, and VI restorations, relative contraindications for use include (1) esthetically prominent areas of posterior teeth, (2) small to moderate Class I and II defects that can be well isolated, and (3) small Class VI defects.

Advantages

Primary advantages are the ease of use and the simplicity of the procedure. As noted in the following sections, the placing and contouring of amalgam restorations are generally easier than those for composite restorations.[16]

Disadvantages

The primary disadvantages of using amalgam for Class I, II, and VI defects are (1) amalgam use requires more complex

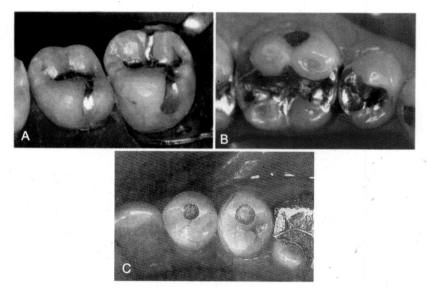

Fig. 14-1 Clinical examples of Class I, II, and VI amalgam restorations. **A,** Class I amalgam in the occlusal surface of the first molar. **B,** Class II amalgams in a premolar and molar. **C,** Class VI amalgams in premolars.

and larger tooth preparations than composite resin, and (2) amalgams may be considered to have a non-esthetic appearance by some patients.

Clinical Technique for Class I Amalgam Restorations

This section describes the use of amalgam in conservative and extensive Class I restorations.

Conservative Class I Amalgam Restorations

Conservative tooth preparation is recommended to protect the pulp, preserve the strength of the tooth, and reduce deterioration of the amalgam restoration.[17-21] Such conservative preparation saves the tooth structure, minimizing pulpal irritation and leaving the remaining tooth crown as strong as possible.[22,23] Conservative preparation also enhances marginal integrity and restoration longevity.[20,21,24] The procedural description for a small, conservative Class I amalgam restoration clearly and simply presents the basic information relating to the entire amalgam restoration technique, including tooth preparation and placement and contouring of the restoration. This basic procedural information can be expanded to describe extensive Class I restorations where amalgam use may be indicated.

Initial Clinical Procedures

After the onset of profound anesthesia, isolation with the rubber dam is recommended to gain control over the operating field and for mercury hygiene.[25,26] For a single maxillary tooth, where caries is not extensive, adequate control of the operating field may be achieved with cotton rolls and high-volume evacuation. A pre-operative assessment of the occlusal relationship of the involved and adjacent teeth also is necessary.

Tooth Preparation

This section describes the specific technique for preparing the tooth for a conservative Class I amalgam restoration. It is divided into initial and final stages.

INITIAL TOOTH PREPARATION

Initial tooth preparation is defined as establishing the outline form by extension of the external walls to sound tooth structure while maintaining a specified, limited depth (usually just inside the dentinoenamel junction [DEJ]) and providing resistance and retention forms. The outline form for the Class I occlusal amalgam tooth preparation should include only the defective occlusal pits and fissures (in a way that sharp angles in the marginal outline are avoided). The ideal outline form for a conservative amalgam restoration (Fig. 14-2, *A*) incorporates the following resistance form principles that are basic to all amalgam tooth preparations of occlusal surfaces. These principles allow margins to be positioned in areas that are sound and subject to minimal forces while conserving structure to maintain the strength and health of the tooth. The resistance principles are as follows:

- Extending around the cusps to conserve tooth structure and prevent the internal line angles from approaching the pulp horns too closely
- Keeping the facial and lingual margin extensions as minimal as possible between the central groove and the cusp tips
- Extending the outline to include fissures, placing the margins on relatively smooth, sound tooth structure
- Minimally extending into the marginal ridges (only enough to include the defect) without removing dentinal support
- Eliminating a weak wall of enamel by joining two outlines that come close together (i.e., <0.5 mm apart)
- Extending the outline form to include enamel undermined by caries

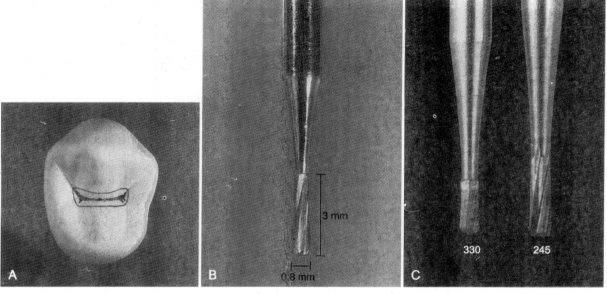

Fig. 14-2 Outline and entry. **A,** Ideal outline includes all occlusal pits and fissures. **B,** Dimensions of head of a No. 245 bur. **C,** No. 330 and No. 245 burs compared.

- Using enameloplasty on the terminal ends of shallow fissures to conserve tooth structure
- Establishing an optimal, conservative depth of the pulpal wall

A No. 245 bur with a head length of 3 mm and a tip diameter of 0.8 mm or a smaller No. 330 bur is recommended to prepare the conservative Class I tooth preparation (Fig. 14-2, *B* and *C*). The silhouette of the No. 245 bur reveals sides slightly convergent toward the shank. This produces an occlusal convergence of the facial and lingual preparation walls, providing adequate retention form for the tooth preparation. The slightly rounded corners of the end of the No. 245 bur produce slightly rounded internal line angles that render the tooth more resistant to fracture from occlusal force.[27] The No. 330 bur is a smaller version of the No. 245 bur. It is indicated for the most conservative amalgam preparations (see Fig. 14-2, *C*).

Class I occlusal tooth preparation is begun by entering the deepest or most carious pit with a punch cut using the No. 245 carbide bur at high speed with air-water spray.[28] A punch cut is performed by orienting the bur such that its long axis parallels the long axis of the tooth crown (Fig. 14-3, *A* and *B*). The bur is inserted directly into the defective pit. When the pits are equally defective, the distal pit should be entered as illustrated. Entering the distal pit first provides increased visibility for the mesial extension. The bur should be positioned such that its distal aspect is directly over the distal pit, minimizing extension into the marginal ridge (see Fig. 14-3, *C*). The bur should be rotating when it is applied to the tooth and should not stop rotating until it is removed from the tooth. Dentinal caries initially spreads at the DEJ; therefore, the goal of the initial cut is to reach the DEJ. On posterior teeth, the approximate depth of the DEJ is located at 1.5 to 2 mm from the occlusal surface. As the bur enters the pit, an initial target depth of 1.5 mm should be established. This is one-half the length of the cutting portion of the No. 245 bur. The 1.5 mm pulpal depth is measured at the central fissure (Fig. 14-3, *D*

and *E*). Depending on the cuspal incline, the depth of the prepared external walls is 1.5 to 2 mm (Fig. 14-3, *D* and *E*). The depth of the preparation is modified as needed so that the pulpal wall is established 0.1-0.2 mm into dentin. The length of the blades of an unfamiliar entry bur should be measured before it is used as a depth gauge.

Distal extension into the distal marginal ridge to include a fissure or caries occasionally requires a slight tilting of the bur distally (≤10 degrees). This creates a slight occlusal divergence to the distal wall to prevent undermining the marginal ridge of its dentin support (Fig. 14-4, *A* through *C*). Because the facial and lingual prepared walls converge, this slight divergence does not present any retention form concerns. For premolars, the distance from the margin of such an extension to the proximal surface usually should not be less than 1.6 mm, or two diameters of the end of the No. 245 bur (Fig. 14-4, *B*) measured from a tangent to the proximal surface (i.e., the proximal surface height of contour). For molars, this minimal distance is 2 mm. A minimal distal (or mesial) extension often does not require changing the orientation of the bur's axis from being parallel to the long axis of the tooth crown; the mesial and distal walls are parallel to the long axis of the tooth crown (or slightly convergent occlusally).

While maintaining the bur's orientation and depth, the preparation is extended distofacially or distolingually to include any fissures that radiate from the pit (see Fig. 14-4, *D*). When these fissures require extensions of more than a few tenths of a millimeter, however, consideration should be given to changing to a bur of smaller diameter, or to using enameloplasty. Both of these approaches conserve the tooth structure and minimize weakening of the tooth.

The bur's orientation and depth are maintained while extending along the central fissure toward the mesial pit, following the DEJ (see Fig. 14-4, *E*). When the central fissure has minimal caries, one pass through the fissure at the prescribed depth provides the desired minimal width to the isthmus. Ideally, the width of the isthmus should be just wider than the

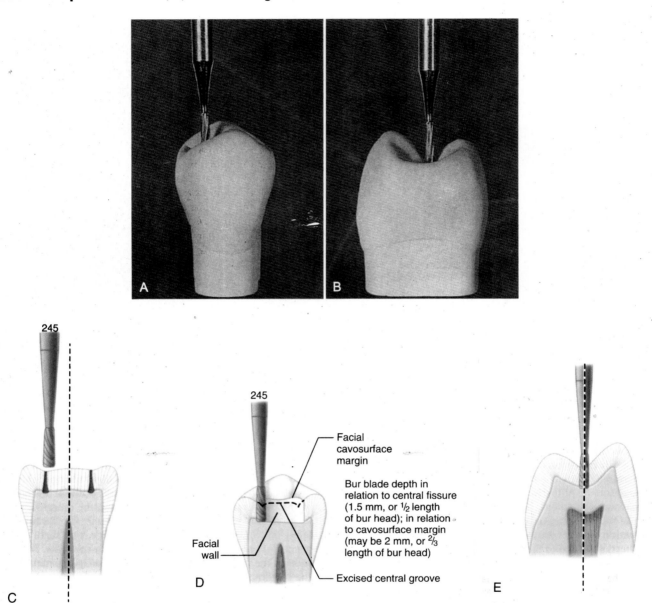

Fig. 14-3 A, No. 245 bur oriented parallel to long axis of tooth crown for entry as viewed from lingual aspect. **B,** The bur positioned for entry as viewed from the distal aspect. **C,** The bur is positioned over the most carious pit (distal) for entry. The distal aspect of the bur is positioned over the distal pit. **D,** Mesiodistal longitudinal section. Relationship of head of No. 245 bur to excised central fissure and cavosurface margin at ideal pulpal floor depth, which is just inside the dentinoenamel junction (DEJ). **E,** Faciolingual longitudinal section. Dotted line indicates the long axis of tooth crown and the direction of the bur.

diameter of the bur. It is well established that a tooth preparation with a narrow occlusal isthmus is less prone to fracture.[29,30] As previously described for the distal margin, the orientation of the bur should not change as it approaches the mesial pit if the mesial extension is minimal. If the fissure extends farther onto the marginal ridge, the long axis of the bur should be changed to establish a slight occlusal divergence to the mesial wall if the marginal ridge would be otherwise undermined of its dentinal support. Figure 14-5 illustrates the correct and incorrect preparation of the mesial and distal walls. The remainder of any occlusal enamel defects is included in the outline, and the facial and lingual walls are extended, if necessary, to remove enamel undermined by caries.[31] The

strongest and ideal enamel margin should be composed of full-length enamel rods attached to sound dentin, supported on the preparation side by shorter rods, also attached to sound dentin (Fig. 14-6).

The conservative Class I tooth preparation should have an outline form with gently flowing curves and distinct cavosurface margins. A faciolingual width of no more than 1 to 1.5 mm and a depth of 1.5 to 2 mm are considered ideal, but this goal is subject to the extension of the caries. The pulpal floor, depending on the enamel thickness, is almost always in dentin (see Fig. 14-4, C). Although conservation of the tooth structure is important, the convenience form requires that the extent of the preparation provides adequate access and visibility.

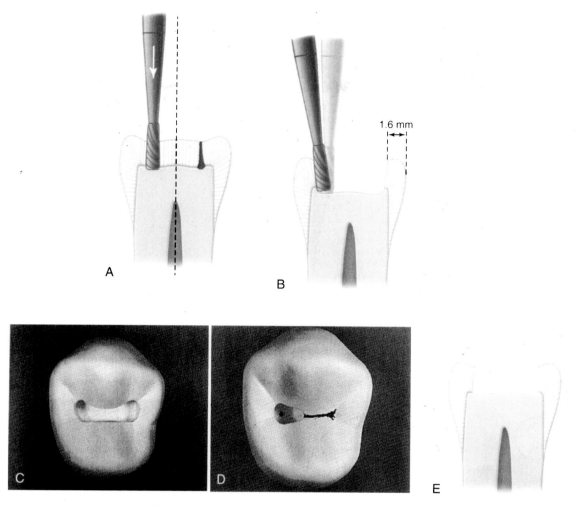

Fig. 14-4 A, Enter the pit with a punch cut to just inside the dentinoenamel junction (DEJ) (depth of 1.5 to 2 mm or one-half to two-thirds the head length of bur). The 1.5-mm depth is measured at central fissure; the measurement of same entry cut (but of prepared external wall) is 2 mm. **B,** Incline the bur distally to establish proper occlusal divergence to distal wall to prevent removal of the dentin supporting the marginal ridge enamel when the pulpal floor is in dentin, and distal extension is necessary to include a fissure or caries. For such an extension on premolars, the distance from the margin to the proximal surface (i.e., imaginary projection) must not be less than 1.6 mm (i.e., two diameters of end of bur). **C,** Occlusal view of the initial tooth preparation that has mesial and distal walls that diverge occlusally. **D,** Distofacial and distolingual fissures that radiate from the pit are included before extending along the central fissure. **E,** Mesiodistal longitudinal section. The pulpal floors are generally flat but may follow the rise and fall of the occlusal surface.

This completes the initial amalgam preparation for Class I caries. The extension should ensure that all caries is removed from the DEJ, resulting in a very narrow peripheral seat of healthy dentin on the pulpal wall surrounding the caries. For the initial tooth preparation, the pulpal wall should remain at the initial ideal depth, even if any restorative material or caries remains in the central area of the pulpal wall (Fig. 14-7). The remaining caries (and usually old restorative material) is removed during the final tooth preparation.

The primary resistance form is provided by the following:

- Sufficient area of relatively flat pulpal floor in sound tooth structure to resist forces directed in the long axis of the tooth and to provide a strong, stable seat for the restoration
- Minimal extension of external walls, which reduces weakening of the tooth
- Strong, ideal enamel margins

- Sufficient depth (i.e., 1.5 mm) that results in adequate thickness of the restoration, providing resistance to fracture and wear

The parallelism or slight occlusal convergence of two or more opposing, external walls provides the primary retention form.

Usually, the No. 245 bur is used for extensions into the mesial and distal fissures. During such extensions, the remaining depth of the fissure can be viewed in cross-section by looking at the wall being extended. When the remaining fissure is no deeper than one-quarter to one-third the thickness of enamel, enameloplasty is indicated. Enameloplasty refers to eliminating the developmental fault by removing it with the side of a flame-shaped diamond stone, leaving a smooth surface (Fig. 14-8, *A* through *C*). This procedure frequently reduces the need for further extension. The extent to which enameloplasty should be used cannot be determined

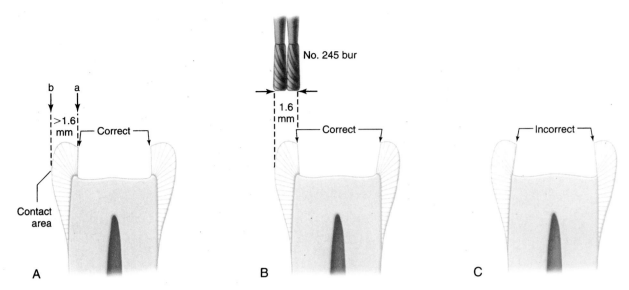

Fig. 14-5 The direction of the mesial and distal walls is influenced by the remaining thickness of the marginal ridge as measured from the mesial or distal margin (*a*) to the proximal surface (i.e., imaginary projection of proximal surface) (*b*). **A,** Mesial and distal walls should converge occlusally when the distance from *a* to *b* is greater than 1.6 mm. **B,** When the operator judges that the extension will leave only 1.6-mm thickness (two diameters of No. 245 bur) of marginal ridge (i.e., premolars) as illustrated here and in Figure 14-4, *B* and *C,* the mesial and distal walls must diverge occlusally to conserve ridge-supporting dentin. **C,** Extending the mesial or distal walls to a two-diameter limit without diverging the wall occlusally undermines the marginal ridge enamel.

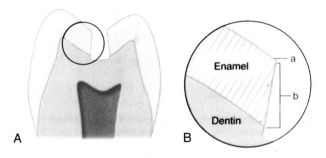

Fig. 14-6 A and **B,** The ideal and strongest enamel margin is formed by full-length enamel rods (*a*) resting on sound dentin supported on the preparation side by shorter rods, also resting on sound dentin (*b*).

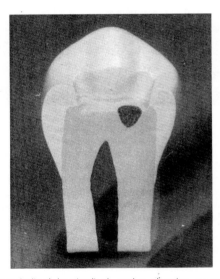

Fig. 14-7 Mesiodistal longitudinal section showing example of the pulpal floor in dentin and caries that is exposed after the initial tooth preparation. The carious lesion is surrounded by sound dentin on the pulpal floor for the resistance form.

exactly until the process of extending into the fissured area occurs, at which time the depth of the fissure into enamel can be observed. The surface left by enameloplasty should meet the tooth preparation wall, preferably with a cavosurface angle no greater than approximately 100 degrees; this would produce a distinct margin for amalgam of no less than 80 degrees (see Fig. 14-8, *D*). During carving, amalgam should be removed from areas of enameloplasty. Otherwise, thin amalgam left in these areas may fracture because of its low edge strength. If enameloplasty is unsuccessful in eliminating a mesial (or distal) fissure that extends to the crest of a marginal ridge or beyond, three alternatives exist:

1. Make no further change in the outline form
2. Extend through the marginal ridge when margins would be lingual to the contact (Fig. 14-9)
3. Include the fissure in a conservative Class II tooth preparation

The first alternative usually should be strongly considered except in patients at high risk for caries. Enameloplasty is not indicated if an area of centric contact is involved. In this case, the choices are either to consider the preparation completed (an option for patients at low risk for caries) or to extend the preparation to include the fissure as previously described.

FINAL TOOTH PREPARATION

The final tooth preparation includes (1) removal of remaining defective enamel and infected dentin on the pulpal floor; (2)

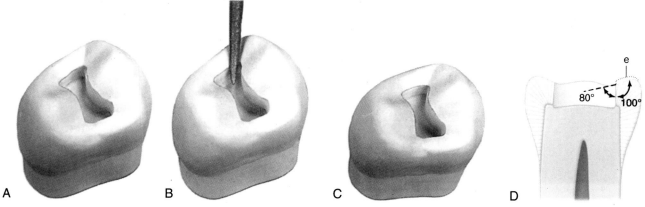

Fig. 14-8 Enameloplasty. **A,** Developmental defect at terminal end of fissure. **B,** Fine-grit diamond stone in position to remove the defect. **C,** Smooth surface after enameloplasty. **D,** The cavosurface angle should not exceed 100 degrees, and the margin–amalgam angle should not be less than 80 degrees. Enamel external surface (e) before enameloplasty.

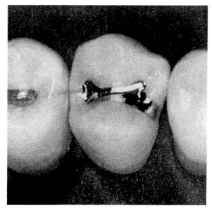

Fig. 14-9 Mesial fissure that cannot be eliminated by enameloplasty may be included in the preparation if the margins can be lingual of contact.

pulp protection, where indicated; (3) procedures for finishing the external walls; and (4) final procedures of cleaning and inspecting the prepared tooth. The use of desensitizers or bonding systems is considered the first step of the restorative technique.

If several enamel pit-and-fissure remnants remain in the floor, or if a central fissure remnant extends over most of the floor, the floor should be deepened with the No. 245 bur to eliminate the defect or to uncover the caries (Fig. 14-10). If these remnants are few and small, they can be removed with an appropriate carbide bur (Fig. 14-11). Removal of the remaining infected dentin (i.e., caries that extends pulpally from the established pulpal floor) is best accomplished using a discoid-type spoon excavator or a slowly revolving round carbide bur of appropriate size (Fig. 14-12, *A* and *B*). Using the largest instrument that fits the carious area is safest because it is least likely to penetrate the tooth in an uncontrolled manner. When removing infected dentin, the excavation should be stopped when the tooth structure feels hard or firm (i.e., the same feel as sound dentin). This situation often occurs before all lightly stained or discolored dentin is removed.[32] A sharp explorer or hand instrument is more reliable than a rotating bur for judging the adequacy of removal

of infected dentin. These instruments should be used judiciously, however, in areas of possible pulpal exposure.

The removal of carious dentin should not affect the resistance form further because the periphery would not need further extension. In addition, it should not affect the resistance form if the restoration is to rest on the pulpal wall peripheral to the excavated area or areas. The peripheral pulpal floor should be at the previously described initial pulpal floor depth just inside the DEJ (see Fig. 14-12, *C* and *D*).

If the tooth preparation is of ideal or shallow depth, no liner or base is indicated. In deeper caries excavations (where the remaining dentin thickness is judged to be 0.5 to 1 mm), a thin layer (i.e., 0.5–0.75 mm) of a light-activated, resin-modified glass ionomer (RMGI) material should be placed.[33,34] The RMGI insulates the pulp from thermal changes, bonds to dentin, releases fluoride, is strong enough to resist the forces of condensation, and reduces microleakage.[34-36] The RMGI is applied only over the deepest portion of the excavation. The entire dentin surface should not be covered (Fig. 14-13). Dentin peripheral to the liner should be available for support of the restoration.[37] The external walls already have been finished during earlier steps in this conservative tooth preparation for amalgam. An occlusal cavosurface bevel is contraindicated in the tooth preparation for an amalgam restoration.[38] It is important to provide an approximate 90- to 100-degree cavosurface angle, which should result in 80- to 90-degree amalgam at the margins.[31] This butt-joint margin of enamel and amalgam is the strongest for both. Amalgam is a brittle material with low edge strength and tends to chip under occlusal stress if its angle at the margins is less than 80 degrees.

The completed tooth preparation should be inspected and cleaned before restoration. The tooth preparation should be free of debris after the tooth has been rinsed with the air-water syringe. Disinfectants that are available may be used for cleaning the tooth preparation, but this is not considered essential.[28,39] A cotton pellet or a commercially available applicator tip moistened only with water is generally used.

OTHER CONSERVATIVE CLASS I AMALGAM PREPARATIONS

Several other conservative Class I preparations may be restored with composite because of their small size and the maximal

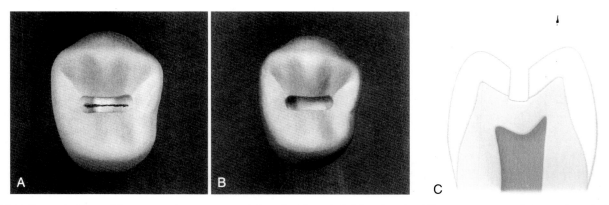

Fig. 14-10 Removal of enamel fissure extending over most of the pulpal floor. **A,** Full-length occlusal fissure remnant remaining on the pulpal floor after the initial tooth preparation. **B** and **C,** The pulpal floor is deepened to a maximum depth of 2 mm to eliminate the fissure or uncover dentinal caries.

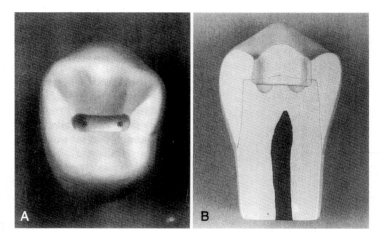

Fig. 14-11 Removal of enamel pit and fissure and infected dentin that is limited to a few small pit-and-fissure remnants. **A,** Two pit remnants remain on the pulpal floor after the initial tooth preparation. **B,** Defective enamel and infected dentin have been removed.

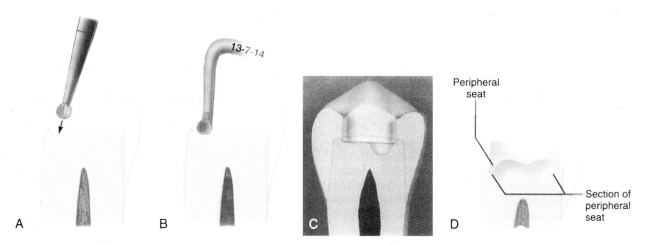

Fig. 14-12 A and **B,** Removal of dentinal caries is accomplished with round burs (*A*) or spoon excavators (*B*). **C** and **D,** The resistance form may be improved with a flat floor peripheral to the excavated area or areas.

thickness of enamel available for bonding around their periphery. However, these preparations could also be restored with amalgam. The preparations include the following:

- Facial pit of the mandibular molar
- Lingual pit of the maxillary lateral incisor
- Occlusal pits of the mandibular first premolar
- Occlusal pits and fissures of the maxillary first molar
- Occlusal pits and fissures of the mandibular second premolar

Examples of some of these types of preparations and restorations are provided in Figures 14-14 through 14-19.

Restorative Technique for Class I Amalgam Preparations

DESENSITIZER PLACEMENT

A dentin desensitizer is placed in the preparation before amalgam condensation (Fig. 14-20).[40] The dentin desensitizer is applied onto the prepared tooth surface according to manufacturer's recommendations; excess moisture is removed

without desiccating the dentin; and then the amalgam is condensed into place. The dentin desensitizer precipitates protein and forms lamellar plugs in the dentinal tubules.[41] These plugs are thought to be responsible for reducing the permeability and sensitivity of dentin. Dentin may not be totally sealed by a desensitizing agent because no hybrid layer is formed as in bonding procedures. If amalgam adhesives are used, a separate desensitizing agent is usually unnecessary. However, concerns exist about the long-term durability of amalgam adhesives and whether resin adhesives may interfere with the self-sealing capability of the amalgam.[15,42-44]

MATRIX PLACEMENT

Generally, matrices are unnecessary for a conservative Class I amalgam restoration except as specified in later sections.

INSERTION AND CARVING OF THE AMALGAM

Because of its superior clinical performance, high-copper amalgam is recommended. Pre-proportioned, disposable capsules are available in sizes ranging from 400 to 800 mg. Some pre-capsulated brands require activation of the capsules before trituration. Amalgam should be triturated (i.e., mixed) according to the manufacturer's directions. It is often necessary to

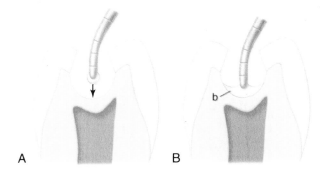

Fig. 14-13 Base application. **A,** Inserting resin-modified glass ionomer (RMGI) with periodontal probe. **B,** In moderately deep excavations, a base (*b*) thickness of 0.5 to 0.75 mm is indicated.

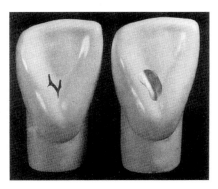

Fig. 14-15 Carious lingual pit and fissure and restoration on the maxillary lateral incisor.

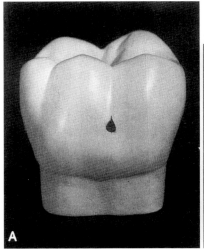
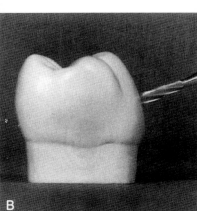
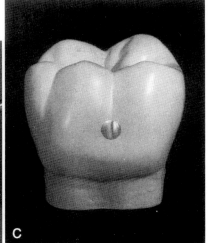

Fig. 14-14 Mandibular molar. **A,** Carious facial pit. **B,** The bur positioned perpendicular to the tooth surface for entry. **C,** Outline of restoration.

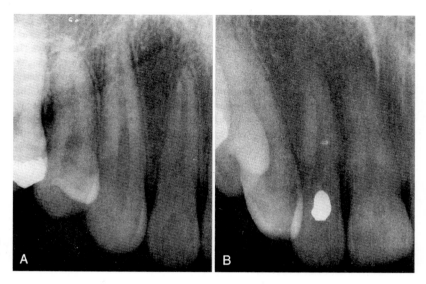

Fig. 14-16 Maxillary lateral incisor. **A,** Pre-operative radiograph of dens in dente. **B,** Radiograph of restoration after 13 years. *(Courtesy of Dr. Ludwig Scott.)*

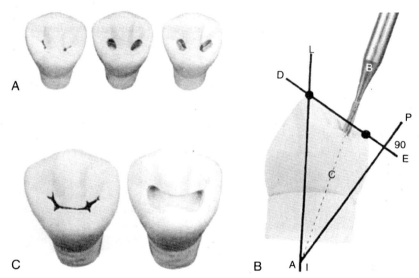

Fig. 14-17 A, Preparation design and restoration of carious occlusal pits on the mandibular first premolar. **B,** Bur tilt for entry. The cutting instrument is held such that its long axis (*broken line, CI*) is parallel with the bisector (*B*) of the angle formed by the long axis of the tooth (*LA*) and the line (*P*) that is perpendicular to the plane (*DE*) drawn through the facial and lingual cusp points. This dotted line (*CI*) is the bur position for entry. **C,** Conventional outline, including occlusal pits and central fissure.

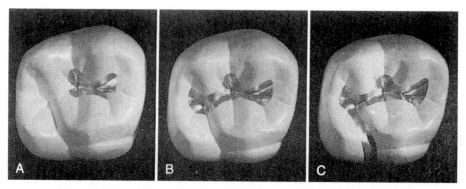

Fig. 14-18 Maxillary first molar. **A,** Outline necessary to include the mesial and central pits connected by the fissure. **B,** Preparation outline extended from outline in *A* to include distal pit and connecting deep fissure in oblique ridge. **C,** Preparation outline extended from outline in *B* to include distal oblique and lingual fissures.

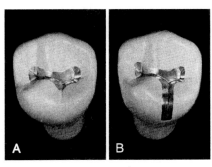

Fig. 14-19 Mandibular second premolar. **A,** Typical occlusal outline. **B,** Extension through the lingual ridge enamel is necessary when enamel-oplasty does not eliminate the lingual fissure.

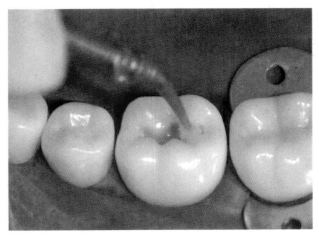

Fig. 14-20 Use of microbrush to apply the dentin desensitizer through-out tooth preparation. *(Courtesy Aldridge D. Wilder, DDS.)*

make several mixes to complete the restoration, particularly for large preparations. The triturated amalgam is emptied into an amalgam well (Fig. 14-21, *A*). Correctly mixed amalgam should not be dry and crumbly. It has a minimal, yet sufficient, "wetness" to aid in achieving a homogeneous and well-adapted restoration.[25]

The principal objectives during the insertion of amalgam are to condense the amalgam to adapt it to the preparation walls and the matrix (when used) and produce a restoration free of voids. Thorough condensation helps to reduce marginal leakage.[45,46] Optimal condensation also is necessary to minimize the mercury content in the restoration to decrease corrosion and to enhance strength and marginal integrity.[47] Condensation of amalgam that contains spherical particles requires larger condensers than are commonly used for admixed amalgam. Smaller condensers tend to penetrate a mass of spherical amalgam, resulting in less effective force to compact or adapt the amalgam within the preparation. In contrast, smaller condensers are indicated for the initial increments of admixed amalgam because it is more resistant to condensation pressure. Because the area of a circular condenser face increases by the square of the diameter, doubling the diameter requires four times more force for the same pressure on a unit area.

The outline of the tooth preparation should be reviewed before inserting amalgam to allow the formation of a mental image that will later aid in carving amalgam to the cavosurface margin. Pre-operative occlusal contact locations should be recalled (see Fig. 14-21, *B*). An amalgam carrier is used to transfer amalgam to the tooth preparation. Increments extruded from the carrier should be smaller (often only 50% or less of a full-carrier tip) for a small preparation, particularly during the initial insertion. A flat-faced, circular or elliptic condenser should be used to condense amalgam over the pulpal floor of the preparation. Amalgam should be carefully condensed into the pulpal line angles (see Fig. 14-21, *C*). Usually, a smaller condenser is used while filling the preparation and a larger one for over-packing. Each portion is thoroughly condensed prior to placement of the next increment. Each condensed increment should fill only one-third to one-half the preparation depth. Each condensing stroke should overlap the previous condensing stroke to ensure that the entire mass is well condensed. The condensation pressure required depends on the amalgam used and the diameter of the condenser nib. Condensers with larger diameter nibs require greater condensation pressure. The preparation should be over-packed 1 mm or more using heavy pressure (see Fig. 14-21, *D*); this ensures that the cavosurface margins are completely covered with well-condensed amalgam. Final condensation over cavosurface margins should be done perpendicular to the external enamel surface adjacent to the margins.

The condensation of a mix should be completed within the time specified by the manufacturer (usually 2.5 to 3.5 minutes). Otherwise, crystallization of the unused portion is too advanced to react properly with the condensed portion. The mix should be discarded if it becomes dry and another mix quickly made to continue the insertion.

To ensure that the marginal amalgam is well condensed before carving, the over-packed amalgam should be burnished immediately with a large burnisher, using heavy strokes mesiodistally and faciolingually, which is referred to as *pre-carve burnishing*. To maximize its effectiveness, the burnisher head should be large enough that in the final strokes, it contacts the cusp slopes but not the margins (see Fig. 14-21, *E*). Pre-carve burnishing produces denser amalgam at the margins of the occlusal preparations restored with high-copper amalgam alloys and initiates contouring of the restoration.[48,49]

CONTOURING AND FINISHING OF THE AMALGAM

With care, carving may begin immediately after condensation. Sharp discoid–cleoid carvers of suitable sizes are recommended. The larger end of the discoid-cleoid instrument (No. 3–No. 6) is used first, followed by the smaller instrument (No. 4 or No. 5) in regions not accessible to the larger instrument. Alternatively, the Hollenback carver can be used. All carving should be done with the edge of the blade perpendicular to the margins as the instrument is moved parallel to the margins. Part of the edge of the carving blade should rest on the unprepared tooth surface adjacent to the preparation margin (see Fig. 14-21, *F*). Using this surface as a guide helps prevent over-carving amalgam at the margins and to produce a continuity of surface contour across the margins.

Deep occlusal grooves should not be carved into the restoration because these may thin the amalgam at the margins, invite chipping, and weaken the restoration (see Fig. 14-21, *G*). Under-carving leaves thin portions of amalgam

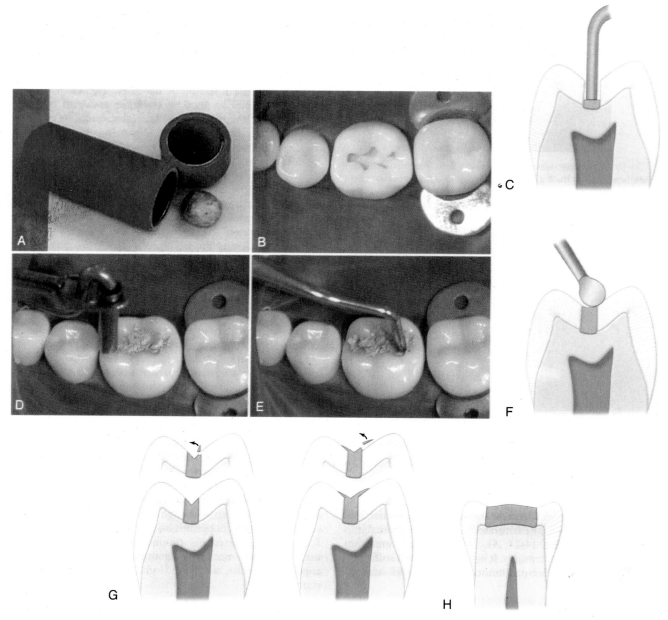

Fig. 14-21 Restoration of occlusal tooth preparation. **A,** Properly triturated amalgam is a homogeneous mass with slightly reflective surface. It flattens slightly if dropped on a tabletop. **B,** The operator should have a mental image of the outline form of the preparation before condensing amalgam to aid in locating the cavosurface margins during the carving procedure. **C,** Amalgam should be inserted incrementally and condensed with overlapping strokes. **D,** The tooth preparation should be over-packed to ensure well-condensed marginal amalgam that is not mercury-rich. **E,** Pre-carve burnishing with a large burnisher is a form of condensation. **F,** The carver should rest partially on the external tooth surface adjacent to the margins to prevent over-carving. **G,** Deep occlusal grooves invite chipping of amalgam at the margins. Thin portions of amalgam left on the external surfaces soon break away, giving the appearance that amalgam has grown out of the preparation. **H,** Carve fossae slightly deeper than the proximal marginal ridges. (**A,** From Darby ML, Walsh MM: Dental hygiene: theory and practice, ed 3, St. Louis, Saunders, 2010. **B, D, E** Courtesy of Aldridge D. Wilder, DDS.)

(subject to fracture) on the unprepared tooth surface. The thin portion of amalgam extending beyond the margin is referred to as *flash*. The mesial and distal fossae should be carved slightly deeper than the proximal marginal ridges (see Fig. 14-21, *H*).

After carving is completed, the outline of the amalgam margin should reflect the contour and location of the prepared cavosurface margin. An amalgam outline that is larger

or irregular is under-carved and requires further carving or finishing (Fig. 14-22). An amalgam restoration that is more than minimally over-carved (i.e., a submarginal defect >0.2 mm) should be replaced.[50] If the total carving time is short enough, the smoothness of the carved surface may be improved by wiping with a small, damp ball of cotton held in the operating pliers. All shavings from the carving procedure should be removed from the mouth with the aid of the oral evacuator.

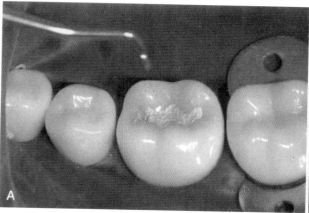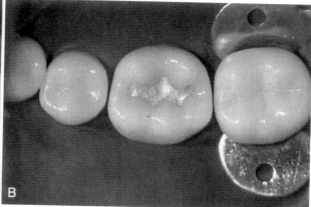

Fig. 14-22 **A,** Under-carved amalgam with flash beyond the margins. The restoration outline is irregular and larger than the preparation outline in Figure 14-21, *B.* **B,** Correctly carved amalgam restoration. *(Courtesy of Aldridge D. Wilder, DDS.)*

Some operators prefer to perform post-carve burnishing of the amalgam surface by using a small burnisher. Post-carve burnishing is done by lightly rubbing the carved surface with a burnisher of suitable size and shape to improve smoothness and produce a satin (not shiny) appearance. The surface should not be rubbed hard enough to produce grooves in the amalgam. Post-carve burnishing may improve the marginal integrity of low- and high-copper amalgams and may improve the smoothness of the restoration.[51,52] Post-carve burnishing in conjunction with pre-carve burnishing may serve as a viable substitute for conventional polishing.[53]

Next, the occlusion of the restoration must be evaluated. After completion of the carving and during the removal of the rubber dam or cotton rolls, the patient is advised not to bite because of the danger of fracturing the restoration, which is weak at this stage. Even if the carving has been carefully accomplished, the restoration occasionally is "high," indicating a premature occlusal contact. The contact potential of the restored tooth and the extent of closure are visualized, whenever possible. A piece of articulating paper is placed over the restoration, and the patient is instructed to close gently into occlusion. If the effect of anesthesia is still present, it may be difficult for the patient to tell when the teeth are in contact. After the patient has reopened the mouth and the articulating paper is removed, the following two features of the occlusal relationship suggest that the restoration is high:

1. Cusp tips of adjacent teeth are not in occlusal contact when it is known from the pre-operative occlusal assessment that they should be touching.
2. A cusp that occludes with the new restoration contacts prematurely.

Any contact area can be recognized on the amalgam by the depth of color imparted by the paper (and especially if the colored area has a silvery center). The deeper-colored or shiny-centered areas are reduced until all markings are uniformly of a light hue (and with no shiny centers), and contacts are noted on adjacent teeth (Fig. 14-23). Observing the space (short of touching) between surfaces of nearby teeth indicates how much to reduce when carving. If these opposing surfaces are 0.5 mm apart (by visual estimation), the high area should be reduced by approximately that amount. This expedites the occlusal adjustment compared with making an insufficient, shallower carving adjustment and then having to repeat closure and carving numerous times. The sequence of closure, observation, and carving is repeated until the appropriate surfaces of opposing teeth are touching. Carving should be accomplished so that opposing cusps contact on a surface that is perpendicular to the occlusal forces in maximum intercuspation. Occlusal contacts located on a cuspal incline or ridge slope are undesirable because they cause a deflective force on the tooth and should be adjusted until the resulting contact is stable (i.e., the force vector of the occlusal contacts should parallel the long axis of the tooth). The final anatomy of the restoration should be patterned after normal occlusal contours. The tip of an explorer should pass from the tooth surface to the restoration surface (and vice versa), without jumping or catching, thus verifying continuity of contour across the margin.

Up to this point, the patient has been instructed to close vertically into maximum intercuspation. After placing the articulating paper over the tooth, the patient is asked to occlude lightly and to slide the teeth lightly from side to side. Any additional occlusal marks are evaluated, and undesirable contact areas are eliminated. Appropriate caution is indicated, as amalgam restorations carved out of occlusion may result in undesirable tooth movement. Finally, the patient should be cautioned to protect the restoration from any heavy biting pressure for 24 hours.

Most amalgams do not require further finishing and polishing. These procedures are occasionally necessary, however, to (1) complete the carving; (2) refine the anatomy, contours, and marginal integrity; and (3) enhance the surface texture of the restoration. Additional finishing and polishing procedures for amalgam restorations are not attempted within 24 hours of insertion because crystallization is incomplete.[25] If used, these procedures are often delayed until all of the patient's amalgam restorations have been placed, rather than finishing and polishing periodically during the course of treatment. An amalgam restoration is less prone to tarnish and corrosion if a smooth, homogeneous surface is achieved.[25,31,54] Polishing of high-copper amalgams is less important than it is for low-copper amalgams because high-copper amalgams are less susceptible to tarnishing and marginal breakdown.[5,55-60]

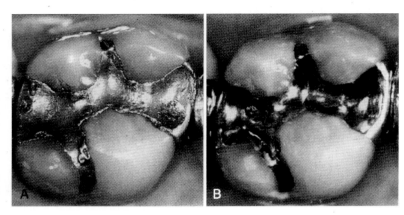

Fig. 14-25 **A,** Existing amalgam restoration exhibiting marginal deterioration and surface roughness. **B,** Same restoration after finishing and polishing.

As an alternative to rubber abrasive points, final polishing may be accomplished using a rubber cup with flour of pumice followed by a high-luster agent, such as precipitated chalk. Finishing and polishing of older, existing restorations may be performed to improve their contour, margins, surface, or anatomy, when indicated (Fig. 14-25).

Extensive Class I Amalgam Restorations

Caries is considered extensive if the distance between infected dentin and the pulp is judged to be less than 1 mm or when the faciolingual extent of the defect is up the cuspal inclines. Extensive caries requires a more extensive restoration (which is a more typical indication for amalgam). The use of amalgam in large Class I restorations provides good wear resistance and occlusal contact relationships. For very large Class I restorations, a bonding system may be used, although this book no longer promotes such use. The perceived benefits of bonded amalgams have not been substantiated.[58,61-63] Bonded amalgams have no advantages compared with the conventional technique, when done correctly.

Initial Clinical Procedures

The rubber dam should be used for isolation of the operating site when caries is extensive. If caries excavation exposes the pulp, pulp capping may be more successful if the site is isolated with a properly applied rubber dam. In addition, the dam prevents moisture contamination of the amalgam mix during insertion.[25]

Tooth Preparation
INITIAL TOOTH PREPARATION

In teeth with extensive caries, excavation of infected dentin and, if necessary, insertion of a liner may precede the establishment of the outline, resistance, and retention forms. This approach protects the pulp as early as possible from any additional insult of tooth preparation. Normally, however, the outline form and the primary resistance and retention forms are established through proper orientation of the No. 245 bur and preparation extension. An initial depth to reach the DEJ (measured approximately 1.5 mm at any pit or fissure and 2 mm on the prepared external walls) should be established and maintained. The preparation is extended laterally at the

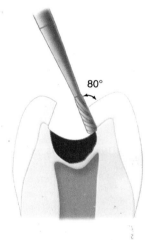

Fig. 14-26 Initial tooth preparation with extensive caries. When extending laterally to remove enamel undermined by caries, the bur's long axis is altered to prepare a 90- to 100-degree cavosurface angle. A 100-degree cavosurface angle on the cuspal incline results in an 80-degree marginal amalgam angle.

DEJ to remove all enamel undermined by caries by alternately cutting and examining the lateral extension of the caries. For caries extending up the cuspal inclines, it may be necessary to alter the bur's long axis to prepare a 90- to 100-degree cavosurface angle while maintaining the initial depth (Fig. 14-26). If not, a significantly obtuse cavosurface angle may remain (resulting in an acute, or weak, amalgam margin), or the pulpal floor may be prepared too deeply. The primary resistance form is obtained by extending the outline of the tooth preparation to include only undermined and defective tooth structure while preparing strong enamel walls and allowing strong cuspal areas to remain. Primary retention is obtained by the occlusal convergence of the enamel walls; the secondary retention form may result from undercut areas that are occasionally left in dentin (and that are not covered by a liner) after removal of infected dentin.

When extending the outline form, enameloplasty should be used, when possible (as described previously). When the defect extends to more than one-half the distance between the primary groove and a cusp tip, capping the cusp (i.e., reducing the cuspal tooth structure and restoring it with amalgam) may

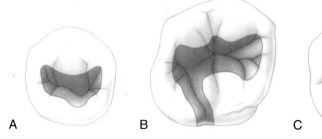

Fig. 14-27 Examples of Class I amalgam tooth preparation outline forms. **A,** Occlusal outline form in the mandibular second premolar. **B,** Occlusolingual outline form in the maxillary first molar. **C,** Occlusofacial outline form in the mandibular first molar.

A   B   C

be indicated. When that distance is two-thirds, cusp capping usually is required because of the risk of cusp fracture postoperatively. Figure 14-27 illustrates some examples of large Class I amalgam preparation outlines.

FINAL TOOTH PREPARATION

Removal of any remaining infected dentin is accomplished in the same manner as described previously for the conservative preparation. Pulp exposure will require a direct pulp cap with calcium hydroxide or endodontic treatment.

For pulpal protection in very deep caries excavations (where the remaining dentin thickness is judged to be <0.5 mm and a pulpal exposure is suspected), a thin layer (i.e., 0.5–0.75 mm) of a calcium hydroxide liner may be placed. The calcium hydroxide liner may stimulate secondary dentin formation in an area where a micro-exposure is suspected or may elicit tertiary dentin formation if the original odontoblasts were no longer vital. If the calcium hydroxide liner is used, it is placed by using the same instrument and the same technique as described for the RMGI liner. The calcium hydroxide liner should be placed only over the deepest portion of the excavation (nearest the pulp). An RMGI base should be used to cover the calcium hydroxide.[47] The entire dentin surface should not be covered (Fig. 14-28). The RMGI base is recommended to cover the calcium hydroxide to resist the forces of condensation and to prevent dissolution over time by sealing the deeply excavated area.[35] Usually, no secondary resistance or retention form features are necessary for extensive Class I amalgam preparations. The external walls of the preparation are finished as described previously.

Restorative Technique

After any indicated liner or base has been placed, regardless of the depth of the excavation, a dentin desensitizer is used. Trituration of the amalgam material is performed as described previously. The preparation is slightly overfilled, and final condensation is enhanced with precarve burnishing. Carving the extensive Class I restoration is often more complex because more cuspal inclines are included in the preparation. Appropriate contours, occlusal contacts, and groove and fossa anatomy must be provided. Finishing and polishing indications and techniques are as described previously.

Class I Occlusolingual Amalgam Restorations

Occlusolingual amalgam restorations may be used on maxillary molars when a lingual fissure connects with the distal

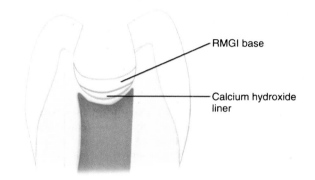

RMGI base

Calcium hydroxide liner

Fig. 14-28 Placement of calcium hydroxide liner and resin-modified glass ionomer (RMGI) base.

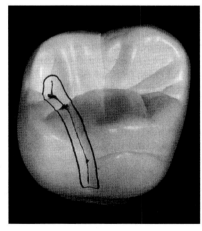

Fig. 14-29 Outline of margins for occlusolingual tooth preparation.

oblique fissure and distal pit on the occlusal surface (Fig. 14-29). Composite also may be used as the restorative material, especially in smaller restorations.

Initial Clinical Procedures

After local anesthesia and evaluation of the occlusal contacts, the use of a rubber dam is generally recommended for isolation of the operating field. In most cases, typical Class I preparations can be adequately isolated with cotton rolls.

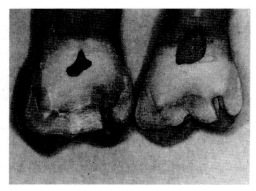

Fig. 14-30 Small distal inclination of the bur on smaller teeth may be indicated to conserve the dentinal support and the strength of the marginal ridge.

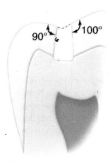

Fig. 14-31 Enamel cavosurface angles of 90 to 100 degrees are ideal.

Tooth Preparation

The initial tooth preparation involves the establishment of the outline, primary resistance, and primary retention forms, as well as initial preparation depth. The accepted principles of the outline form (previously presented) should be observed with special attention to the following:

- The tooth preparation should be no wider than necessary; ideally, the mesiodistal width of the lingual extension should not exceed 1 mm except for extension necessary to remove carious or undermined enamel or to include unusual fissuring.
- When indicated, the tooth preparation should be cut more at the expense of the oblique ridge, rather than centering over the fissure (weakening the small distolingual cusp).
- Especially on smaller teeth, the occlusal portion may have a slight distal tilt to conserve the dentin support of the distal marginal ridge (Fig. 14-30).
- The margins should extend as little as possible onto the oblique ridge, distolingual cusp, and distal marginal ridge.

These objectives help conserve the dentinal support and the strength of the tooth, and they aid in establishing an enamel cavosurface angle as close to 90 degrees as possible (Fig. 14-31). They also minimize deterioration of the restoration margins by locating the margins away from enamel eminences where occlusal forces may be concentrated.

The distal pit is identified with indirect vision and entered with the end of the No. 245 bur (Fig. 14-32, A). The long axis of the bur usually should be parallel to the long axis of the tooth crown. The dentinal support and strength of the distal marginal ridge and the distolingual cusp should be observed, and the bur positioned such that it cuts more of the tooth structure mesial to the pit rather than distal to the pit (e.g., 70:30 rather than 50:50), if needed. The initial cut is to the level of the DEJ (a depth of 1.5 to 2 mm) (see Fig. 14-32, B). At this depth, the pulpal floor is usually in dentin. When the entry cut is made (see Fig. 14-32, C), the bur (maintaining the initial established depth) is moved to include any remaining fissures facial to the point of entry (see Fig. 14-32, D). The bur is then moved along the fissure toward the lingual surface (see Fig. 14-32, E). As with Class I occlusal preparations, a slight distal inclination of the bur is indicated occasionally (e.g.,

smaller teeth) to conserve the dentinal support and strength of the marginal ridge and the distolingual cusp. To ensure adequate strength for the marginal ridge, the distopulpal line angle should not approach the distal surface of the tooth closer than 2 mm. On large molars, the bur position should remain parallel to the long axis of the tooth, particularly if the bur is offset slightly mesial to the center of the fissure. Keeping the bur parallel to the long axis of the tooth creates a distal wall with slight occlusal convergence, providing favorable enamel and amalgam angles. The bur is moved lingually along the fissure, maintaining a uniform depth until the preparation is extended onto the lingual surface (see Fig. 14-32, F). The pulpal floor should follow the contour of the occlusal surface and the DEJ, which usually rises occlusally as the bur moves lingually.

The mesial and distal walls of the occlusal portion of the preparation should converge occlusally because of the shape of the bur. This convergence provides a sufficient retention form to the occlusal portion of the preparation. If the slight distal bur tilt was required, the mesial and distal walls still should converge relative to each other (although the distal wall may be divergent occlusally, relative to the tooth's long axis). Occlusal retention form usually is adequate.

The lingual portion is prepared at this point by using one of two techniques. In one technique, the lingual surface is prepared with the bur's long axis parallel with the lingual surface (see Fig. 14-33, A and B). The tip of the bur should be located at the gingival extent of the lingual fissure. The bur should be controlled so that it does not "roll out" onto the lingual surface, which may "round over" or damage the cavosurface margin. The facial inclination of the bur must be altered as the cutting progresses to establish the axial wall of the lingual portion at a uniform depth of 0.5 mm inside the DEJ (see Fig. 14-33, C). The axial wall should follow the contour of the lingual surface of the tooth. An axial depth of 0.5 mm inside the DEJ is indicated if retentive grooves are required; an axial depth of 0.2 mm inside the DEJ is permissible if retentive grooves are not required.

The No. 245 bur may be used with its long axis perpendicular to the axial wall to accentuate (i.e., refine) the mesioaxial and distoaxial line angles; this also results in the mesial and distal walls converging lingually because of the shape of the bur (see Fig. 14-33, D and E). During this step, the axial wall depth is not altered (see Fig. 14-33, F). The occlusal and lingual convergences usually provide a sufficient preparation retention form; no retention grooves are needed.

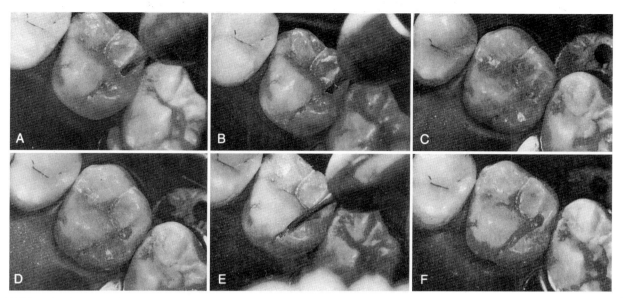

Fig. 14-32 Occlusolingual tooth preparation. **A,** No. 245 bur positioned for entry. **B,** Penetration to a minimal depth of 1.5 to 2 mm. **C,** Entry cut. **D,** The remaining fissures facial to the point of entry are removed with the same bur. **E** and **F,** A cut lingually along the fissure until the bur has extended the preparation onto the lingual surface.

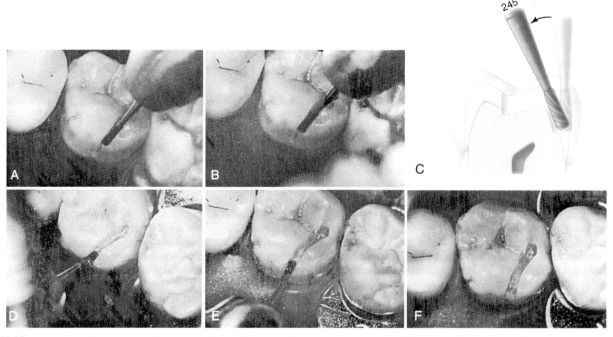

Fig. 14-33 Occlusolingual tooth preparation. **A,** Position of bur to cut the lingual portion. **B,** Initial entry of the bur for cutting the lingual portion. **C,** The inclination of the bur is altered to establish the correct axial wall depth. **D** and **E,** The bur is directed perpendicular to the axial wall to accentuate the mesioaxial and distoaxial line angles. **F,** The axial wall depth should be 0.2 to 0.5 mm inside the dentinoenamel junction (DEJ).

The axiopulpal line angle must be rounded to limit the areas of stress concentration and ensure adequate preparation depth and amalgam thickness (Fig. 14-34). Initial tooth preparation of the occlusolingual preparation is now complete. As mentioned previously, enameloplasty may be performed to conserve the tooth structure and limit extension.

The second technique is more difficult. In this case, the No. 245 bur is held perpendicular to the cusp ridge and the lingual surface, as it extends the preparation from the occlusal surface gingivally (to include the entire defect). This technique also results in opposing preparation walls that converge lingually.

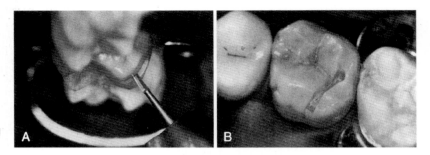

Fig. 14-34 **A,** Bur position for rounding the axiopulpal line angle. **B,** Axiopulpal line angle rounded.

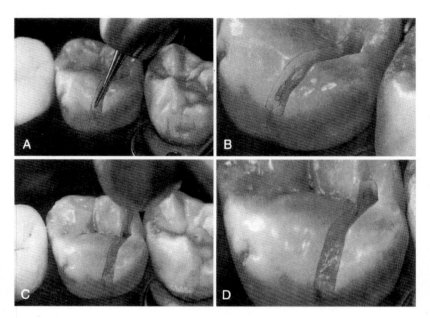

Fig. 14-35 Secondary retention form. **A,** Bur position for preparing groove in mesioaxial line angle. **B,** Completed groove. **C,** Bur position for the retention cove in the faciopulpal line angle. **D,** Completed cove.

Additional retention in the lingual extension may be required if the extension is wide mesiodistally or if it was prepared without a lingual convergence. If additional retention is required, the No. $\frac{1}{4}$ or No. 169 bur can be used to prepare grooves into the mesioaxial and distoaxial line angles (Fig. 14-35, *A*). If these angles are in enamel, the axial wall must be deepened to 0.5 mm axially of the DEJ (because the grooves must be in dentin so as to not undermine enamel). The depth of the grooves at the gingival floor is one-half the diameter of the No. $\frac{1}{4}$ bur. The cutting direction for each groove is the bisector of the respective line angle. The groove is slightly deeper pulpally than the correctly positioned axial wall and is 0.2 mm axial to the DEJ. The grooves should diminish in depth toward the occlusal surface, terminating midway along the axial wall (see Fig. 14-35, *B*). The adequacy of the groove should be tested by inserting the tine of an explorer into the groove and moving it lingually. The mesial or distal depth of the groove should prevent the explorer from being withdrawn lingually. (See the section on secondary resistance and retention forms for a description of placing retentive grooves in the proximal boxes of Class II amalgam preparations; the techniques are similar.)

Extension of a facial occlusal fissure may have required a slight divergence occlusally to the facial wall to conserve support of the facial ridge. If so and if deemed necessary, the $\frac{1}{4}$ round bur may be used to prepare a retention cove in the faciopulpal line angle (see Fig. 14-35, *C* and *D*). The tip of the No. 245 bur held parallel to the long axis of the tooth crown also might be used to prepare this cove. Care should be taken so as not to undermine the occlusal enamel (this retentive cove is recommended only if occlusal convergence of the mesial and distal walls of the occlusal portion is absent or inadequate).

The final tooth preparation is accomplished by removal of remaining caries on the pulpal and axial walls (Fig. 14-36) with an appropriate round bur, a discoid-type spoon excavator, or both. A liner or base (alone or together) is placed in the deep excavations for pulpal protection. The external walls are finished. Any irregularities at the margins may indicate weak enamel that may be removed by the side of the No. 245 bur rotating at slow speed.

Final Procedures: Cleaning and Inspecting

The usual procedure in cleaning is to free the preparation of visible debris with water from the syringe and then to remove the visible moisture with a few light bursts of air from the air syringe. In some instances, debris clings to walls and angles

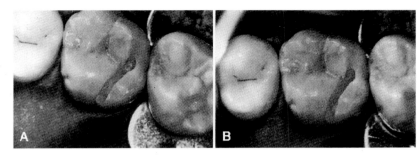

Fig. 14-36 **A,** Any remaining pit and fissure in enamel and infected dentin on established pulpal and axial walls are removed. **B,** Completed tooth preparation.

despite the aforementioned efforts, and it may be necessary to loosen this material with an explorer or small cotton pellet. After all of the visible debris has been removed, the excess moisture is removed. It is important not to dehydrate the tooth by overuse of air as this may damage the odontoblasts associated with the desiccated tubules. When the preparation has been cleaned adequately, it is visually inspected to confirm complete debridement and that the preparation does not require any additional modification.

Restorative Technique

DESENSITIZER PLACEMENT

After any indicated liner or base or both is placed, a dentin desensitizer is placed.

MATRIX PLACEMENT (IF NECESSARY)

Using a rigid matrix to support the lingual portion of the restoration during condensation is occasionally necessary. A matrix is helpful to prevent "landsliding" during condensation and to ensure marginal adaptation and strength of the restoration. The Tofflemire matrix retainer is used to secure a matrix band to the tooth (as described later). Because this type of matrix band does not intimately adapt to the lingual groove area of the tooth (Fig. 14-37, *A*), an additional step may be necessary to provide a matrix that is rigid on the lingual portion of the tooth preparation. If so, a piece of stainless steel matrix material (0.002 inch [0.05 mm] thick, $\frac{5}{16}$ inch [8 mm] wide) is cut to fit between the lingual surface of the tooth and the band already in place (see Fig. 14-37, *B*). The gingival edge of this segment of matrix material is placed slightly gingival to the gingival edge of the band to help secure the band segment. A quick setting rigid polyvinyl siloxane (PVS)–based material may be used, between the sectional matrix and the Tofflemire matrix band, to prevent lingual displacement of the sectional matrix during condensation of the amalgam. Alternatively, green stick compound may be used. In this case, the end of a toothpick wedge is covered with softened (heated) compound. The compound-coated wedge is then immediately inserted between the Tofflemire band and the cut piece of matrix material (see Fig. 14-37, *D*). While the compound is still soft, a suitable burnisher is used to press the compound gingivally, securing the matrix tightly against the gingival cavosurface margin and the lingual surface of the tooth to provide a rigid, lingual matrix (see Fig. 14-37, *E* and *F*). This matrix for the occlusolingual amalgam restoration is referred to as the *Barton matrix*. Occasionally, the piece of strip matrix can be positioned appropriately by using only the wedge (without the rigid PVS or compound matrix support).

INSERTION OF THE AMALGAM

The insertion of amalgam is accomplished as previously described for the Class I occlusal tooth preparation. Condensation is begun at the gingival wall. Care must be taken to ensure that landsliding of the amalgam does not occur because two adjoining surfaces of the tooth are being restored. For this technique, the last increments of amalgam may be condensed on the lingual surface with the side of a large condenser. Its long, broadly rounded contour conforms to the rectangular shape for the lingual groove preparation. Appropriate care should be taken (when condensing the occlusal surface) so as to not fracture the lingual amalgam. Another technique is to have the assistant secure the condensed lingual surface with a broad condenser nib, while the operator completes the condensation of the occlusal surface. Regardless of the technique used, the amalgam must be well condensed.

CONTOURING AND FINISHING OF THE AMALGAM RESTORATION

When the preparation is sufficiently overfilled, carving of the occlusal surface may begin immediately with a sharp discoid–cleoid instrument or a Hollenback carver. All carving should be done with the edge of the blade perpendicular to the margin and with the blade moving parallel to the margin. To prevent over-carving, the blade edge should be guided by the unprepared tooth surface adjacent to the margin. An explorer is used to remove excess amalgam adjacent to the lingual matrix before matrix removal (see Fig. 14-37, *G*). After carving is completed (see Fig. 14-37, *H*), the rubber dam is removed, and the restoration is adjusted to ensure proper occlusion. Most amalgams do not require finishing and polishing (the procedure is described in the section on conservative class I amalgam restorations). Figure 14-37, *I*, illustrates a polished occlusolingual restoration.

Class I Occlusofacial Amalgam Restorations

Occasionally, mandibular molars exhibit fissures that extend from the occlusal surface through the facial cusp ridge and onto the facial surface. The preparation and restoration of these defects are very similar to those described for Class I occlusolingual amalgam restorations. Although these may be restored with composite, an illustration of preparation and restoration with amalgam is provided in Figure 14-38. The amalgam restoration may be polished after it is completely set. The shape of abrasive points may need to be modified to allow optimal polishing (Fig. 14-38, *I* and *J*).

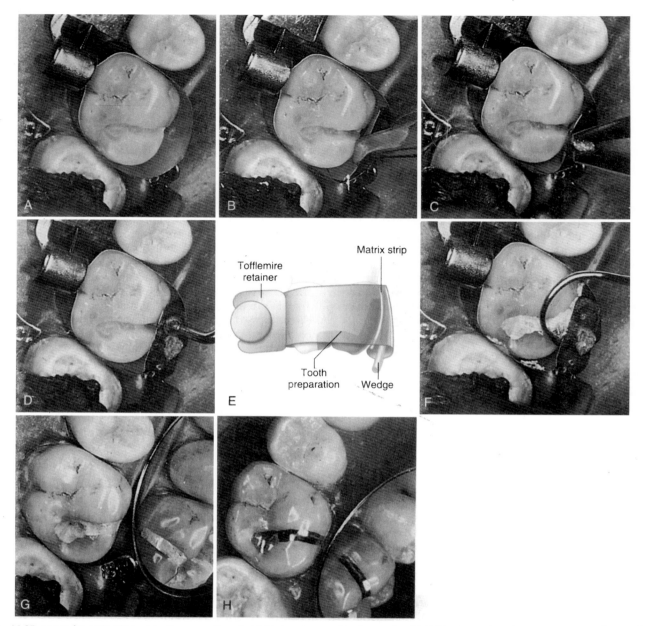

Fig. 14-37 Matrix for occlusolingual tooth preparation. **A,** Matrix band secured to the tooth with Tofflemire retainer. **B,** Positioning a small strip of stainless steel matrix material between the tooth and the band already in place. **C,** Inserting the wedge and the compound. **D,** Compressing the compound gingivally, which adapts the steel strip to the lingual surface. **E,** Cross-section of the tooth preparation and the matrix construction. **F,** Using the explorer to remove excess amalgam adjacent to the lingual matrix. **G,** Carving completed. **H,** Polished restoration.

Clinical Technique for Class II Amalgam Restorations

Amalgam restorations that restore one or both of the proximal surfaces of the tooth may provide years of service to the patient when (1) the tooth preparation is correct, (2) the matrix is suitable, (3) the operating field is isolated, and (4) the restorative material is manipulated properly. Inattention to these criteria may produce inferior restorations that are prone to early failure. This section discusses principles, techniques, and procedures using classic examples of Class II preparations. The outline forms should always conform to the restoration requirements of the tooth and not to the classic example of a Class II tooth preparation. Application of the principles discussed here will result in high-quality Class II amalgam restorations.

Initial Clinical Procedures

Occlusal contacts should be marked with articulating paper before tooth preparation. A mental image of these contacts will serve as a guide in tooth preparation and restoration. Any

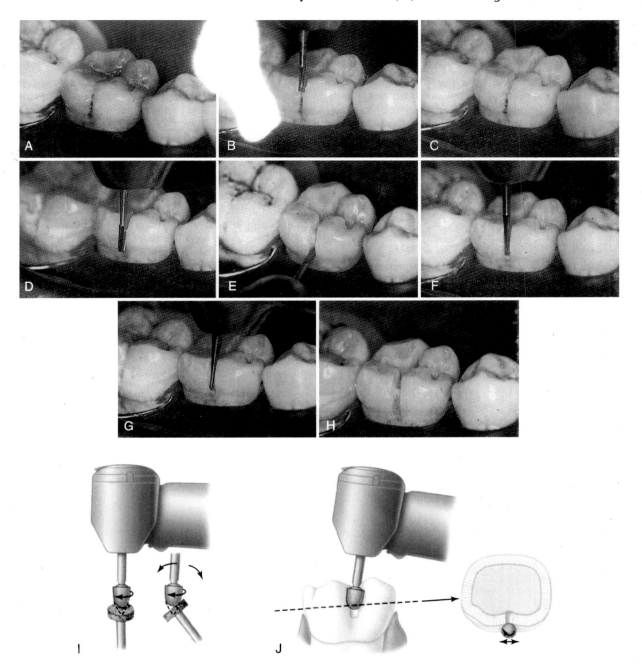

Fig. 14-38 Fissure extension. **A,** Facial occlusal fissure continuous with the fissure on the facial surface. **B,** Extension through the facial ridge onto the facial surface. **C,** Appearance of the tooth preparation after extension through the ridge. **D,** The facial surface portion of the extension is cut with the side of the bur. **E,** The line angles are sharpened by directing the bur from the facial aspect. **F,** Sharpening the line angles from the occlusal direction with a No. 169 L bur. **G,** Ensuring the retention form by preparing retention grooves with a No. ¼ round bur. **H,** Completed tooth preparation. **I,** The rubber polishing point may be trued up and blunted on a coarse diamond wheel. **J,** Proper orientation of the rubber point when polishing the facial surface groove area.

opposing "plunging cusp" or other pointed cusp may need to be recontoured to reduce the risk of fracture of the new restoration or the cusp from occlusal forces. Before tooth preparation for amalgam, the placement of a rubber dam is generally recommended. It is especially beneficial when the restoration is large, when the caries is extensive, and when quadrant dentistry is practiced. If the existing restoration has rough proximal contacts, the restoration may be removed before rubber

dam application. Infected dentin should be removed with the rubber dam in place, however, especially if a pulpal exposure is a possibility. Insertion of an interproximal wedge or wedges is the last step in rubber dam application when Class II tooth preparations are scheduled. The wedges depress and protect the rubber dam and underlying soft tissue, separate teeth slightly, and may serve as a guide to prevent gingival overextension of the proximal boxes.

Tooth Preparation
Class II Amalgam Restorations Involving Only One Proximal Surface

This section introduces the principles and techniques of a Class II tooth preparation for an amalgam restoration involving a carious lesion on one proximal surface. For illustration, a mesio-occlusal tooth preparation on the mandibular second premolar is presented. Although this restoration typically would use composite as the restorative material, the use of a small, conservative Class II amalgam restoration is presented to provide the basic concepts of Class II amalgam tooth preparation and restoration more clearly and simply.

INITIAL TOOTH PREPARATION
Occlusal Outline Form (Occlusal Step)

The occlusal outline form of a Class II tooth preparation for amalgam is similar to that for a Class I tooth preparation. Using high speed with air-water spray, the operator enters the pit nearest the involved proximal surface with a punch cut using a No. 245 bur oriented as illustrated in Figure 14-39, *A* and *B*. Entering the pit nearest the involved proximal surface

allows the mesial pit (in this case) not to be included if it is sound. The bur should be rotating when it is applied to the tooth and should not stop rotating until removed. Viewed from the proximal and lingual (facial) aspects, the long axis of the bur and the long axis of the tooth crown should remain parallel during the cutting procedures. Dentinal caries initially spreads at the DEJ, and therefore, the goal of the initial cut is to reach the DEJ. The DEJ location in posterior teeth is approximately 1.5 to 2.0 mm from the occlusal surface. As the bur enters the pit, a target depth of 0.1–0.2 mm into dentin should be established (i.e., one-half to two-thirds the length of the cutting portion of a No. 245 bur); 1.5 mm as measured at the central fissure, and approximately 2 mm on the prepared external walls such that the DEJ is identified. While maintaining the same depth and bur orientation, the bur is moved to extend the outline to include the central fissure and the opposite pit (the distal pit, in this example), if necessary (see Fig. 14-39, *C* and *D*). For the very conservative preparation, the isthmus width should be as narrow as possible, preferably no wider than one-quarter the intercuspal distance.[18,19,30,64,65] Ideally, it should be the width of the No. 245 bur. Narrow restorations provide a greater length of clinical service.[20,24] Generally, the amount of remaining tooth

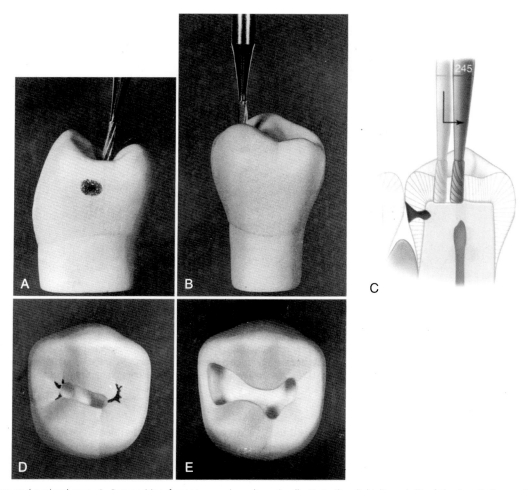

Fig. 14-39 Entry and occlusal step. **A,** Bur position for entry, as viewed proximally. Note the slight lingual tilt of the bur. **B,** Bur position as viewed lingually. **C,** The tooth is entered with a punch cut, and extension is done distally along central fissure at a uniform depth of 1.5 to 2 mm (1.5 mm at fissure; because of the inclination of the unprepared tooth surface, the corresponding measurement on the prepared wall is greater). **D,** Occlusal view of *C.* **E,** Completed occlusal step.

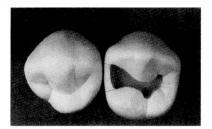

Fig. 14-40 Visualize final location of proximo-occlusal margins (*dotted lines*) before preparing the proximal box.

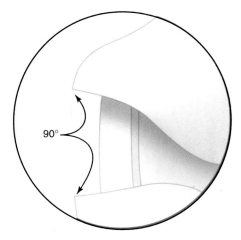

Fig. 14-41 The reverse curve in the occlusal outline usually is created when the mesiofacial enamel wall is parallel to the enamel rod direction. Lingually, the reverse curve is very slight, often unnecessary.

structure is more important to restoration longevity than is the restorative material used.[66] Ultimately, the extension of the caries at the DEJ will determine the amount of preparation extension and the resultant width. The pulpal floor of the preparation should follow the slight rise and fall of the DEJ along the central fissure in teeth with prominent triangular ridges.

Maintaining the bur parallel to the long axis of the tooth crown creates facial, lingual, and distal walls with a slight occlusal convergence, which provides favorable amalgam angles at the margins. The facial, lingual, and distal walls should be extended until a sound DEJ is reached. Proper extension will result in the formation of the peripheral seat which aids in the primary resistance form. It may be necessary to tilt the bur to diverge occlusally at the distal wall if further distal extension would undermine the marginal ridge of its dentinal support. During development of the distal pit area of the preparation, extension to include any distofacial and distolingual developmental fissures radiating from the pit may be indicated. The distal pit area (in this example) provides a dovetail retention form, which may prevent mesial displacement of the completed restoration. The dovetail feature is not required in the occlusal step of a single proximal surface preparation, unless a fissure emanating from an occlusal pit indicates it. Without a dovetail, however, the occlusal step should not be in a straight direction, which may reduce the retention form. This type of retention form also is provided by any extension of the central fissure preparation that is not in a straight direction from pit to pit (see Fig. 14-39, *E*). A dovetail outline form in the distal pit is not required if radiating fissures are not present.[67,68] Enameloplasty should be performed, where indicated, to conserve the tooth structure.

Before extending into the involved proximal marginal ridge (the mesial ridge, in this example), the final locations of the facial and lingual walls of the proximal box are visualized. This action prevents overextension of the occlusal outline form (i.e., occlusal step) where it joins the proximal outline form (i.e., proximal box). Figure 14-40 illustrates visualization of the final location of the proximo-occlusal margins before preparing the proximal box. Showing the view from the occlusal aspect, Figure 14-41 illustrates a reverse curve in the occlusal outline of a Class II preparation, which often results when developing the mesiofacial wall perpendicular to the enamel rod direction while, at the same time, conserving as much of the facial cusp structure as possible.[65] The extension into the mesiofacial cusp is limited to that amount required to permit a 90-degree mesiofacial margin which is indicated when using amalgam. Lingually, the reverse curve usually is minimal (if necessary at all) because the embrasure form is larger.

While maintaining the established pulpal depth and with the bur parallel to the long axis of the tooth crown, the preparation is extended mesially, stopping approximately 0.8 mm short of cutting through the marginal ridge into the contact area. The occlusal step in this region is made slightly wider faciolingually than in the Class I preparation because additional width is necessary for the proximal box. The proper depth of the occlusal portion of the preparation increases the strength of the restoration, however, more than does faciolingual width (see Fig. 14-39, *E*, for an illustration of the completed occlusal outline form). Although this extension includes part of the mesial marginal ridge, it also exposes the marginal ridge DEJ. The location of the DEJ is an important guide in the development of the proximal preparation.

Proximal Outline Form (Proximal Box)

The desired final location of the facial and lingual walls of the proximal box or the proximal outline form relative to the contact area is visualized. The objectives for the extension of the proximal margins are as follows:

- Include all caries, defects, or existing restorative material
- Create 90-degree cavosurface margins (i.e., butt-joint margins)
- Establish (ideally) not more than 0.5 mm clearance with the adjacent proximal surface facially, lingually, and gingivally

The initial procedure in preparing the outline form of the proximal box is the isolation of the proximal (i.e., mesial) enamel by the proximal ditch cut. While maintaining the same orientation of the bur, it is positioned over the DEJ in the pulpal floor next to the remaining mesial marginal ridge (Fig. 14-42, *A*). The end of the bur is allowed to cut a ditch gingivally along the exposed DEJ, two-thirds at the expense of enamel and one-third at the expense of dentin. The 0.8-mm diameter bur end cuts approximately 0.5 to 0.6 mm into enamel and 0.2 to 0.3 mm into dentin. Pressure is directed gingivally and lightly toward the mesial surface to keep the bur against the proximal enamel, while the bur is moved facially and lingually along the DEJ. The ditch is extended gingivally

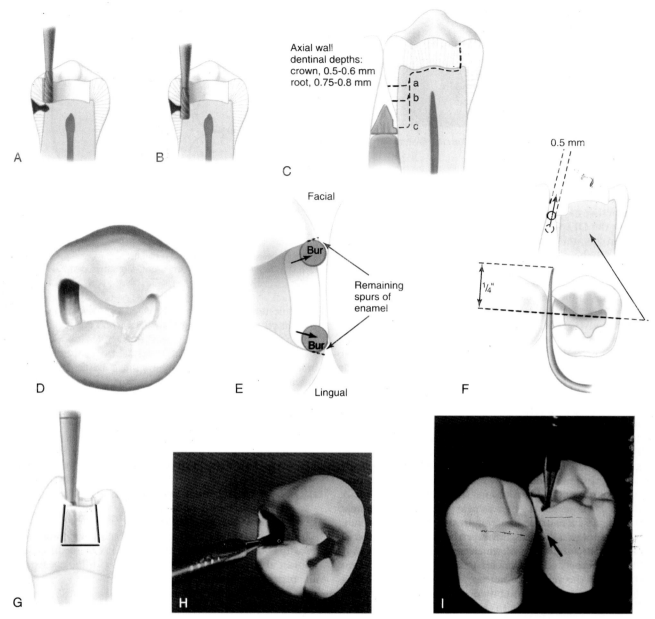

Fig. 14-42 Isolation of proximal enamel. **A,** Bur position to begin the proximal ditch cut. **B,** The proximal ditch is extended gingivally to the desired level of the gingival wall (i.e., floor). **C,** Variance in the pulpal depth of the axiogingival line angle as the extension of the gingival wall varies: *a,* at minimal gingival extension; *b,* at moderate extension; *c,* at extension that places gingival margin in cementum, whereupon the pulpal depth is 0.75 to 0.8 mm and the bur may shave the side of wedge. **D,** The proximal ditch cut results in the axial wall that follows the outside contour of the proximal surface. **E,** The position of the proximal walls (i.e., facial, lingual, gingival) should not be overextended with the No. 245 bur, considering additional extension will occur when the remaining spurs of enamel are removed. **F,** When a small lesion is prepared, the gingival margin should clear the adjacent tooth by only 0.5 mm. This clearance may be measured with the side of the explorer. The diameter of the tine of a No. 23 explorer is 0.5 mm, ¼ inch (6.3 mm) from its tip. **G,** The faciolingual dimension of the proximal ditch is greater at the gingival level than at the occlusal level. **H,** To isolate and weaken the proximal enamel further, the bur is moved toward and perpendicular to the proximal surface. **I,** The side of the bur may emerge slightly through the proximal surface at the level of the gingival floor (*arrow*).

just beyond the caries or the proximal contact, whichever is greater (see Fig. 14-42, *B*). Because dentin is softer and cuts more easily than enamel, the bur should be cutting away the dentin immediately supporting the enamel. Axial wall dentinal depths will vary based on the gingival extension of the preparation (see Fig. 14-42, *C*). The harder enamel acts to guide the bur, creating an axial wall that follows the

faciolingual contour of the proximal surface and the DEJ (see Fig. 14-42, *D*).

It is necessary to visualize the completed mesiofacial and mesiolingual margins as right-angle projections of the facial and lingual limits of the ditch to establish the proper faciolingual ditch extension (see Fig. 14-42, *E*). When preparing a tooth with a small lesion, these margins should clear the adjacent tooth by only 0.2 to 0.3 mm.[65] A guide for the gingival extension is the visualization that the finished gingival margin will be only slightly gingival to the gingival limit of the ditch. This gingival margin should clear the adjacent tooth by only 0.5 mm in a small tooth preparation (see Fig. 14-42, *F*).[67] Clearance of the proximal margins (i.e., mesiofacial, mesiolingual, gingival) greater than 0.5 mm is excessive, unless indicated to include any caries, undermined enamel, or existing restorative material. The location of the final proximal margins (i.e., facial, lingual, gingival) should be established with hand instruments (i.e., chisels, hatchets, trimmers) in conservative proximal box preparations. Otherwise, these margins may be overextended to achieve 90-degree cavosurface margins with the No. 245 bur (see Fig. 14-42, *E*). Extending gingival margins into the gingival sulcus should be avoided, where possible, because subgingival margins are more difficult to restore and may be a contributing factor to periodontal disease.[69-71]

The depth of the axial dentinal wall should be adjusted to approximately 0.5 mm if retention grooves are deemed necessary. This will allow the grooves to be prepared into the axiolingual and axiofacial line angles without undermining the proximal enamel. If the proximal ditch cut is entirely in dentin, the axial wall usually is too deep. Because the proximal enamel becomes thinner from the occlusal to the gingival aspect, the end of the bur comes closer to the external tooth surface as the cutting progresses gingivally (see Fig. 14-42, *B*). Premolars may have proximal boxes that are shallower pulpally than are molars because premolars typically have thinner enamel. In the tooth crown, the ideal dentinal depth of the axial wall of the proximal boxes of premolars and molars should be the same (two-thirds to three-fourths the diameter of the No. 245 bur [or 0.5–0.6 mm]).[65] When the extension places the gingival margin in cementum, the initial pulpal depth of the axiogingival line angle should be 0.7 to 0.8 mm (the diameter of the tip end of the No. 245 bur is 0.8 mm). The bur may shave the side of the wedge that is protecting the rubber dam and the underlying gingiva (see Fig. 14-42, *C*).

The gingival extension of the proximal ditch may be measured by first noting the depth of the nonrotating bur in the ditch. The dentist removes the bur from the preparation and holds it in the facial embrasure at the same level to observe the relationship of the end of the bur to the proximal contact. A periodontal probe also may be used.

The proximal ditch cut may diverge gingivally to ensure that the faciolingual dimension at the gingival aspect is greater than at the occlusal aspect (see Fig. 14-42, *G*). The shape of the No. 245 bur should provide this divergence. The gingival divergence contributes to the retention form and provides for the desirable extension of the facial and lingual proximal margins to include defective tooth structure or old restorative material at the gingival level, while conserving the marginal ridge and providing for 90-degree amalgam at the margins on this ridge.[19]

Occasionally, it is permissible not to extend the outline of the proximal box facially or lingually beyond the proximal contact to conserve the tooth structure.[67] An example of this modification is a narrow proximal lesion where broad proximal contact is present in a patient with low risk for caries. If it is necessary to extend 1 mm or more to break the contact arbitrarily, the proximal margin is left in the contact. Usually, the facial margin is affected by this rule, which may not extend beyond the proximal contact into the facial embrasure.

The proximal extensions are completed when two cuts, one starting at the facial limit of the proximal ditch and the other starting at the lingual limit, extending toward and perpendicular to the proximal surface (until the bur is nearly through enamel at the contact level), are made (see Fig. 14-42, *H*). The side of the bur may emerge slightly through the surface at the level of the gingival floor (see Fig. 14-42, *I*); this weakens the remaining enamel by which the isolated portion is held. If this level is judged to be insufficiently gingival, additional gingival extension should be accomplished using the isolated proximal enamel that is still in place to guide the bur. This prevents the bur from marring the proximal surface of the adjacent tooth. At this stage, however, the remaining wall of enamel often breaks away during cutting, especially when high speed is used. At such times, if additional use of the bur is indicated, a matrix band may be used around the adjacent tooth to prevent marring its proximal surface. The isolated enamel, if still in place, may be fractured with a spoon excavator (Fig. 14-43) or by additional movement of the bur.

To protect the gingiva and the rubber dam when extending the gingival wall gingivally, a wooden wedge should already be in place in the gingival embrasure to depress soft tissue and the rubber dam.[19] A round toothpick wedge is preferred unless a deep gingival extension is anticipated (Fig. 14-44, *A*). A triangular (i.e., anatomic) wedge is more appropriate for deep

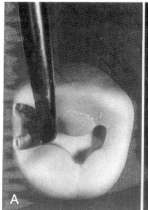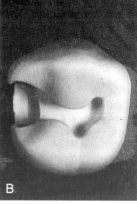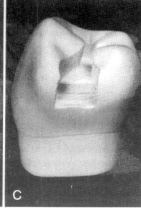

Fig. 14-43 Removing isolated enamel. **A,** Using a spoon excavator to fracture the weakened proximal enamel. **B,** Occlusal view with the proximal enamel removed. **C,** Proximal view with the proximal enamel removed.

gingival extensions because the greatest cross-sectional dimension of the wedge is at its base; as the gingival wall is cut, the bur's end corner may shave the wedge slightly (see Fig. 14-44, *B*). With the enamel hatchet (10-7-14), the bin-angle chisel (12-7-8), or both, the dentist cleaves away any remaining undermined proximal enamel (Fig. 14-45), establishing the proper direction to the mesiolingual and mesiofacial walls.

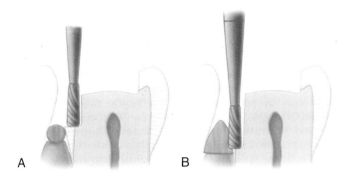

Fig. 14-44 Wedging. **A,** A round toothpick wedge placed in the gingival embrasure protects the gingiva and the rubber dam during preparation of the proximal box. **B,** A triangular wedge is indicated when a deep gingival extension of the proximal box is anticipated because the wedge's greatest cross-sectional dimension is at its base. Consequently, it more readily engages the remaining clinical tooth surface.

Proximal margins having cavosurface angles of 90 degrees are desired.[19] Cavosurface angles of 90 degrees ensure that no undermined enamel rods remain on the proximal margins and that the maximal edge strength of amalgam is maintained. The cutting edge of the instrument should not be aggressively forced against the gingival wall because this can cause a craze line (i.e., fracture) that extends gingivally in enamel, perhaps to the cervical line. Figure 14-46 shows the importance of the correct direction of the mesiofacial and mesiolingual walls, dictated by enamel rod direction and the physical properties of amalgam. If hand instruments were not used to remove the remaining spurs of enamel, the proximal margins would have undermined enamel. To create 90-degree facial and lingual proximal margins with the No. 245 bur, the proximal margins would have to be significantly overextended for an otherwise conservative preparation. The weakened enamel along the gingival wall is removed by using the enamel hatchet in a scraping motion (see Fig. 14-45, *C*).

When the isolation of the proximal enamel has been executed properly, the proximal box can be completed easily with hand-cutting instruments. Otherwise, more cutting with rotary instruments may be indicated. When a rotary instrument is used in a proximal box after the proximal enamel is removed, the instrument may either mar the adjacent proximal surface or "crawl out" of the box into the gingiva or across the proximal margins. The latter mishap produces a rounded cavosurface angle, which, if not corrected, results in a weak amalgam margin of less than 90 degrees. The risk of this

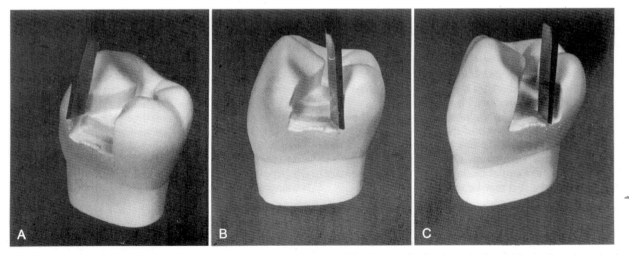

Fig. 14-45 Removing the remaining undermined proximal enamel with an enamel hatchet on the facial proximal wall (*A*), the lingual proximal wall (*B*), and the gingival wall (*C*).

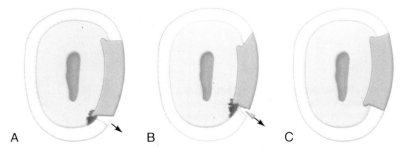

Fig. 14-46 Direction of mesiofacial and mesiolingual walls. **A,** Failure caused by a weak enamel margin. **B,** Failure caused by a weak amalgam margin. **C,** Proper direction to the proximal walls results in full-length enamel rods and 90-degree amalgam at the preparation margin. Retention grooves have been cut 0.2 mm inside the dentinoenamel junction (DEJ), and their direction of depth is parallel to the DEJ.

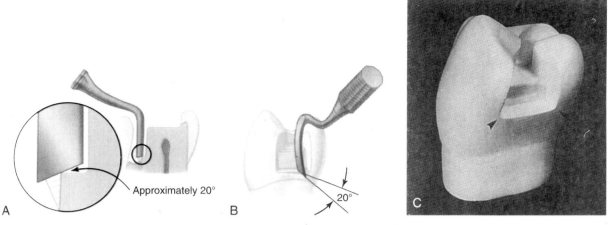

Fig. 14-54 A, The bevel of the enamel portion of the gingival wall is established with a gingival margin trimmer to ensure full-length enamel rods forming the gingival margin. **B** and **C,** The sharp angles at the linguogingival and faciogingival corners are rounded by rotational sweeping with a gingival margin trimmer.

indicated.[19] When beveling the gingival margin on the distal surface, the distal gingival margin trimmer (13-95-10-14, R and L) is used. Alternatively, the side of an explorer tine may be used to remove any friable enamel at the gingival margin. The tine is placed in the gingival embrasure apical to the gingival margin. With some pressure against the prepared tooth, the tine is moved occlusally across the gingival margin to "trim" the margin by removing enamel that is not supported.

Final Procedures: Cleaning and Inspecting

The reader is referred to the similar section earlier under conservative Class I amalgam restorations.

VARIATIONS OF PROXIMAL SURFACE TOOTH PREPARATIONS

The following sections describe variations in tooth preparation for some conservative Class II amalgam restorations. In most clinical situations, the restoration presented would be done with composite. If amalgam is used, the features presented should be considered in the tooth preparation portion of the procedure.

Mandibular First Premolar

For the conservative Class II tooth preparation for amalgam on the mandibular first premolar, the conventional approach and technique must be modified because the morphologic structure of this tooth is different from other posterior teeth (particularly because of the diminished size of the lingual cusp). For this tooth, as in all teeth, the principles of tooth preparation for amalgam must be correlated with the physical properties of the restorative material and the anatomic structure of the tooth. The relationship of the pulp chamber to the DEJ and the relatively small size of the lingual cusp are illustrated in Figure 14-55 (this figure also illustrates the correct position of the pulpal wall and how it differs in direction compared with the second premolar). Incorrect preparation of the central groove area could weaken the lingual cusp, and excessive extension in a facial direction could approach or expose the facial pulp horn. When preparing the occlusal

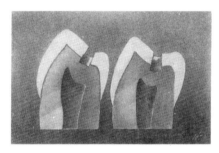

Fig. 14-55 The mandibular first and second premolars are compared. Note differences in the sizes of the pulp chambers, lingual cusps, and direction of pulpal walls.

portion, the bur is tilted slightly lingually to establish the correct pulpal wall direction (see Fig. 14-17, *B*).

In addition, the mandibular first premolar presents a variety of occlusal patterns, most of which exhibit a large transverse ridge of enamel. Often, such a ridge has no connecting fissure between the mesial and distal pits, dictating a Class II preparation with an outline form that does not extend to, or across, the ridge (Fig. 14-56, *A*). If the opposite pit or proximal surface is faulty, it is restored with a separate restoration.

For a preparation that does not cross the transverse ridge, the proximal box is prepared before the occlusal portion to prevent removing the tooth structure that will form the isthmus between the occlusal dovetail and the proximal box. The pit adjacent to the involved proximal surface is entered with the No. 245 bur. Immediately after the entry, the bur is directed into the proximal marginal ridge and then pulpally (if necessary) until the proximal DEJ is visible. The bur axis for the proximal ditch cut should be parallel to the tooth crown, which is tilted slightly lingually for mandibular posterior teeth. The proximal enamel is isolated and the proximal box completed as previously described for the mandibular second premolar. The bur is then returned to the area of entry, and the occlusal step is prepared with a dovetail, if needed. When preparing the occlusal portion, the bur is tilted slightly lingual to establish the correct pulpal wall direction (which maintains the dentin support for the small lingual

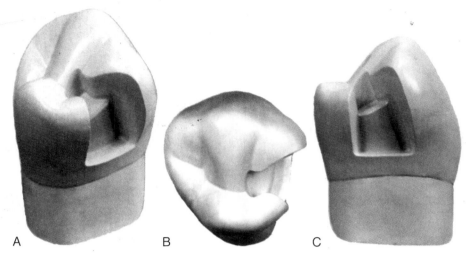

Fig. 14-56 The mandibular first premolar with a sound transverse ridge. **A,** A two-surface tooth preparation that does not include the opposite pit. **B,** Occlusal outline form. **C,** Proximal view of the completed preparation.

cusp and prevents encroachment on the facial pulp horn). The primary difference in tooth preparation on this tooth, compared with the preparation on other posterior teeth, is the facial inclination of the pulpal wall. The isthmus is broadened as necessary, but maintains the dovetail retention form, if required. Figure 14-56, *B,* illustrates the correct occlusal outline form. Removing any remaining caries (if present) and inserting necessary liners, bases, or both precede the placement of proximal grooves and the finishing of the enamel margins to complete the preparation (see Fig. 14-56, *C*).

Maxillary First Molar

When mesial and distal proximal surface amalgam restorations are indicated on the maxillary first molar that has an unaffected oblique ridge, separate two-surface tooth preparations are indicated (rather than a mesiooccluso-distal preparation) because the strength of the tooth crown is significantly greater when the oblique ridge is intact.[19] The mesio-occlusal tooth preparation is generally uncomplicated (Fig. 14-57, *A*). Occasionally, extension through the ridge and into the distal pit is necessary because of the extent of caries. The outline of this occlusolingual pit-and-fissure portion is similar to that of the Class I occlusolingual preparation. Figure 14-57, *B* and *C,* illustrates a mesio-occlusal preparation extended to include the distal pit and the outline form that includes the distal oblique and lingual fissures.

When the occlusal fissure extends into the facial cusp ridge and cannot be removed by enameloplasty, the defect should be eliminated by extension of the tooth preparation. Occasionally, this can be accomplished by tilting the bur to create an occlusal divergence of the facial wall while maintaining the dentin support of the ridge. If this fault cannot be eliminated without extending the margin to the height of the cusp ridge or undermining the enamel margin, the preparation should be extended facially through the ridge (see Fig. 14-57, *D*). The pulpal wall of this facial extension may have remaining enamel, but a depth of 1.5 to 2 mm is necessary to provide sufficient bulk of material for adequate strength. For the best esthetic results, minimal extension of the proximal mesiofacial margin is indicated.

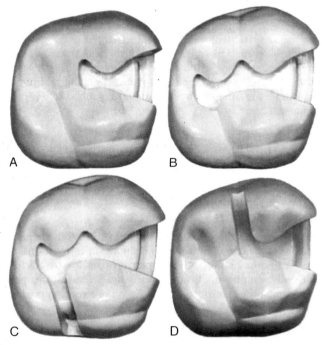

Fig. 14-57 Maxillary first molar. **A,** Conventional mesioocclusal preparation. **B,** Mesioocclusal preparation extended to include the distal pit. **C,** Mesiooccluso-lingual preparation, including the distal pit and the distal oblique and lingual fissures. **D,** Mesioocclusal preparation with facial fissure extension.

The disto-occlusal tooth preparation may take one of several outlines, depending on the occlusal anatomy. The occlusal outline is determined by the pit-and-fissure pattern and by the amount and extension of caries. An extension onto the lingual surface to include a lingual fissure should be prepared only after the distolingual proximal margin is established. This approach may allow conservation of more tooth structure between the distolingual wall and the lingual fissure extension, resulting in more strength of the distolingual cusp.

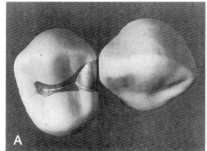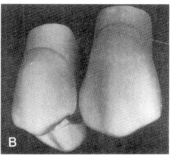

Fig. 14-58 To produce an inconspicuous margin on the maxillary first premolar, the mesiofacial wall does not diverge gingivally, and facial extension with a No. 245 bur should be minimal so that the mesiofacial proximal margin of the preparation minimally clears the contact as the margin is finished. **A,** Occlusal view. **B,** Facial view.

It is accomplished by preparing the lingual fissure extension more at the expense of the mesiolingual cusp than the distolingual cusp. Nevertheless, the distolingual cusp on many maxillary molars (particularly the maxillary second molars) may be weakened during such a disto-occluso-lingual tooth preparation because of the small cuspal portion remaining between the lingual fissure preparation and the distolingual proximal wall. In addition, caries excavation may weaken the cusp. Capping of the distolingual cusp is often necessary to provide the proper resistance form.

Maxillary First Premolar

A Class II amalgam tooth preparation involving the mesial surface of a maxillary first premolar requires special attention because the mesiofacial embrasure is esthetically prominent. The occlusogingival preparation of the facial wall of the mesial box should be parallel to the long axis of the tooth instead of converging occlusally to minimize an unesthetic display of amalgam in the faciogingival corner of the restoration. In addition, the facial extension of the mesiofacial proximal wall should be minimal so that the mesiofacial proximal margin of the preparation only minimally clears the contact as the margin is finished with an appropriate enamel hatchet or chisel (Fig. 14-58).

If the mesial proximal involvement (1) is limited to a fissure in the marginal ridge that is at risk for caries, (2) is not treatable by enameloplasty, and (3) does not involve the proximal contact, the proximal portion of the tooth preparation is prepared by extending through the fault with the No. 245 bur so that the margins are lingual to the contact. Often, this means that the proximal box is the faciolingual width of the bur, and the gingival floor may be at the same depth as the pulpal floor. The retention form for this extension is provided by the slight occlusal convergence of the facial and lingual walls (see Fig. 14-9).

If the proximal caries is limited to the mesiolingual embrasure, the mesial proximal contact should not be included in the tooth preparation. If only the lingual aspect of the mesial proximal contact is carious, the mesiofacial wall may be left in contact with the adjacent tooth (reducing the display of amalgam). A Class II tooth preparation involving the distal surface of the maxillary first premolar is similar to the preparation of the mandibular second premolar described earlier.

Box-Only Preparation

When restoring a small, cavitated proximal lesion in a tooth with neither occlusal fissures nor a previously inserted occlusal restoration, a proximal box preparation without an occlusal step has been recommended.[18,19] To maximize retention,

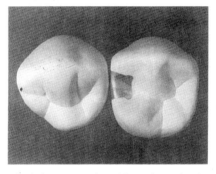

Fig. 14-59 A simple box restoration without the occlusal step is permissible when restoring a small proximal lesion in the tooth without either occlusal fissures or previously inserted occlusal restoration and when the involved marginal ridge does not support occlusal contact. The proximal grooves extend to the occlusal surface.

preparations with facial and lingual walls that almost oppose each other are recommended. This type of preparation should be limited to a proximal surface with a narrow proximal contact (allowing minimal facial and lingual extensions). As in the typical preparation, the facial and lingual proximal walls converge occlusally. Retention grooves are necessary in box-only preparations.[82] The proximal retention grooves should have a 0.5-mm depth at the gingival point angle, tapering to a depth of 0.3 mm at the occlusal surface (Fig. 14-59).

MODIFICATIONS IN TOOTH PREPARATION

Slot Preparation for Root Caries

Older patients who have gingival recession that exposes cementum may experience caries on the proximal root surface that is appreciably gingival to the proximal contact (Fig. 14-60, A). Assuming that the contact does not need restoring, the tooth preparation usually is approached from the facial direction and has the form of a slot (see Fig. 14-60, B). A lingual approach is used when the caries is limited to the linguoproximal surface. Amalgam is particularly indicated for slot preparations if isolation is difficult.[13]

The initial outline form is prepared from a facial approach with a No. 2 or No. 4 bur using high speed and air-water spray. Outline form extension to sound tooth structure is at a limited depth axially (i.e., 0.75–1 mm at the gingival aspect [if no enamel is present], increasing to 1–1.25 mm at the occlusal wall [if margin is in enamel]) (see Fig. 14-60, B). If the occlusal margin is in enamel, the axial depth should be 0.5 mm inside the DEJ. During this extension, the bur should not remove any infected carious dentin from the axial wall deeper than the

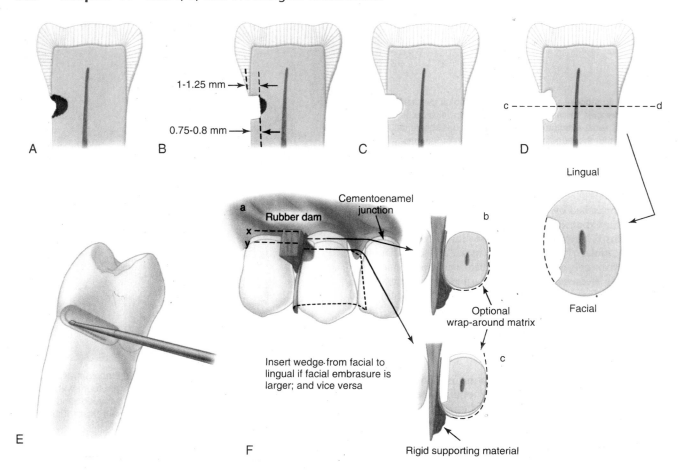

Fig. 14-60 Slot preparation. **A,** Mesiodistal longitudinal section illustrating a carious lesion. The proximal contact is not involved. **B,** Initial tooth preparation. **C,** Tooth preparation with infected carious dentin removed. **D,** The retention grooves are shown in longitudinal section, and the transverse section through plane *cd* illustrates the contour of the axial wall and the direction of the facial and lingual walls. **E,** Preparing the retention form to complete the tooth preparation. **F,** Matrix for slot preparation: *a,* facial view of wedged matrix; *b,* wedged matrix as viewed in transverse cross-section (*x*), gingival to gingival floor; *c,* wedged matrix as viewed in transverse cross-section (*y*), occlusal to gingival floor.

outline form initial depth. The remaining infected carious dentin (if any) is removed during final tooth preparation (see Fig. 14-60, *C*). The external walls should form a 90-degree cavosurface angle. With a facial approach, the lingual wall should face facially as much as possible; this aids condensation of amalgam during its insertion. The facial wall must be extended to provide access and visibility (convenience form) (see Fig. 14-60, *D*). In the final tooth preparation, the No. 2 or No. 4 bur should be used to remove any remaining infected carious dentin on the axial wall. A liner or base (or both) is applied, if indicated.

A No. $\frac{1}{4}$ bur is used to create retention grooves in the occlusoaxial and gingivoaxial line angles, 0.2 mm inside the DEJ or 0.3 to 0.5 mm inside the cemental cavosurface margin (see Fig. 14-60, *E*). The depth of these grooves is one-half the diameter of the bur head (i.e., 0.25 mm), and the bur is directed to bisect the angle formed by the junction of the occlusal (or gingival) and axial walls. Ideally, the direction of the occlusal groove is slightly more occlusal than axial, and the direction of the gingival groove would be slightly more gingival than axial (as in the Class III amalgam preparation). Before application of the matrix, a dentin desensitizer should be placed. The matrix for inserting amalgam in a slot

preparation for root caries is similar to that illustrated in Figure 14-60, *F*.

For instances in which root caries encircles the tooth, the proximal areas can be restored as described previously. Subsequently, Class V preparations are prepared and abutted with the proximal restorations. The amalgam used to restore the proximals should be fully set (to avoid dislocation during preparation and during insertion of the Class V restorations). Alternatively, the Class V portions can be restored first. When the proximals are restored first, the mesial and distal walls of the Class V preparations would be in amalgam. Doing a circumferential restoration in segments allows proper condensation of amalgam. A full-coverage restoration usually is preferred if caries encircles the tooth cervically.

Rotated Teeth

Tooth preparation for rotated teeth follows the same principles as for normally aligned teeth. The outline form for a mesio-occlusal tooth preparation on the rotated mandibular second premolar (Fig. 14-61, *A*) differs from normal in that its proximal box is displaced facially because the proximal caries involves the mesiofacial line angle of the tooth crown. When the tooth is rotated 90 degrees and the "proximal" lesion

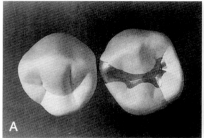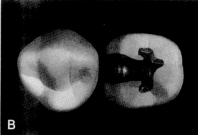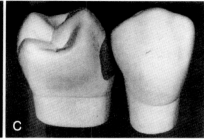

Fig. 14-61 Restoration outlines for rotated teeth. **A,** Mesio-occlusal outline for the mandibular premolar with 45-degree rotation. **B,** Mesio-occlusal outline for the mandibular premolar with 90-degree rotation. **C,** Slot preparation outline for the restoration of a small mesial lesion involving the proximal contact of the mandibular premolar with 90-degree rotation.

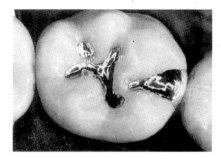

Fig. 14-62 Restoration of the mesio-occlusal tooth preparation, with the central fissure segmented by coalesced enamel.

is on the facial or lingual surface, or orthodontic correction is declined or ruled out, the preparation may require an isthmus that includes the cuspal eminence (see Fig. 14-61, *B*). If the lesion is small, consideration should be given to slot preparation. In this instance, the occlusal margin may be in the contact area or slightly occlusal to it (see Fig. 14-61, *C*).

Unusual Outline Forms

Outline forms should conform to the restoration requirements of the tooth and not to the classic example of a Class II tooth preparation. As mentioned earlier, a dovetail feature is not required in the occlusal step of a single proximal surface preparation unless a fissure emanating from the occlusal step is involved in the preparation. Another example is an occlusal fissure that is segmented by coalesced enamel (as illustrated previously for mandibular premolars and the maxillary first molars). This condition should be treated with individual amalgam restorations if the preparations are separated by approximately 0.5 mm or more of sound tooth structure (Fig. 14-62).[18,68]

Adjoining Restorations

It is permissible to repair or replace a defective portion of an existing amalgam restoration if the remaining portion of the original restoration retains adequate resistance and retention forms. Adjoining restorations on the occlusal surface occur more often in molars because the dovetail of the new restoration usually can be prepared without eliminating the dovetail of the existing restoration. Where the two restorations adjoin, care should be taken to ensure that the outline of the second restoration does not weaken the amalgam margin of the

first (Fig. 14-63, *A*). The intersecting margins of the two restorations should be at a 90-degree angle as much as possible. The decision to adjoin two restorations is based on the assumption that the first restoration, or a part of it, does not need to be replaced and that the procedure for the single proximal restoration (compared with a mesio-occluso-distal restoration) is less complicated, especially in matrix application.

Occasionally, preparing an amalgam restoration in two or more phases is indicated, such as for a Class II lesion that is contiguous with a Class V lesion. Preparing both lesions before placing amalgam introduces condensation problems that can be eliminated by preparing and restoring the Class II lesion before preparing and restoring the Class V lesion (see Fig. 14-63, *B*). It is better to condense amalgam against a carious wall of the first preparation than to attempt condensation where no wall exists.

Abutment Teeth for Removable Partial Denture

When the tooth is an abutment for a planned removable partial denture, the occlusoproximal outline form adjacent to the edentulous region may need additional extension if a rest seat is planned, such as for the tooth-borne partial denture. This additional extension must be sufficient facially, lingually, and axially to allow for preparing the rest seat in the restoration without jeopardizing its strength. The facial and lingual proximal walls and the respective occlusal margins must be extended so that the entire rest seat can be prepared in amalgam without encroaching on the occlusal margins. If the rest seat is to be within the amalgam margins, it is recommended that a minimum of 0.5 mm of amalgam be present between the rest seat and the margins (Fig. 14-64, *A*). The portion of the pulpal wall apical to the planned rest seat is deepened 0.5 mm so that the total depth of the axiopulpal line angle measured on the faciolingual wall is 2.5 mm (see Fig. 14-64, *B*). A rest seat used for a tissue-borne (i.e., distal extension) partial denture may involve amalgam and enamel (see Fig. 14-64, *C*). In this case, no modification of the outline form of the tooth preparation is indicated (see Fig. 14-64, *C*). Figure 14-64, *D*, illustrates the relationship of the tissue-borne removable partial denture with the abutment tooth (see Fig. 14-64, *C*).

Class II Amalgam Restorations Involving Both Proximal Surfaces

Perhaps the best indications for the use of amalgam restorations are moderate and large Class II defects that include both

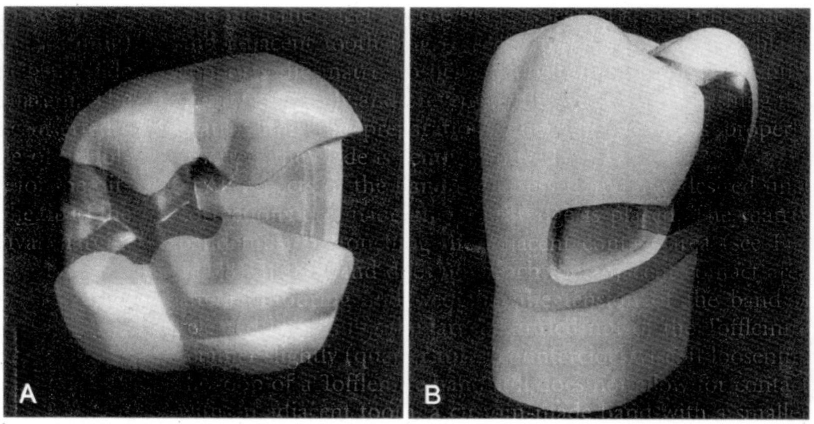

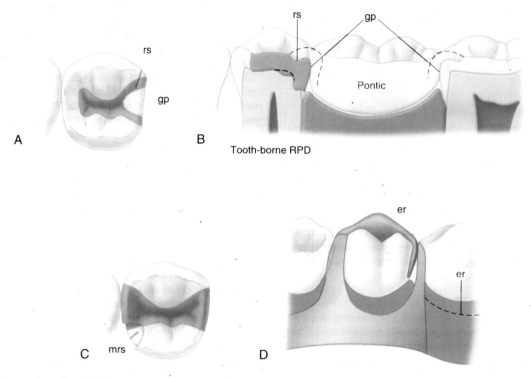

Fig. 14-63 Adjoining restorations. **A,** Adjoining mesio-occlusal tooth preparation with disto-occlusal restoration so that the new preparation does not weaken the amalgam margin of the existing restoration. **B,** Preparing and restoring a Class II lesion before preparing and restoring a Class V lesion contiguous with it eliminates condensation problems that occur when both lesions are prepared before either is restored.

Fig. 14-64 Abutment teeth with Class II restorations designed for a removable partial denture (RPD). **A,** Occlusal view showing the location of the rest seat (*rs*) and the guiding plane (*gp*) for a tooth-borne RPD. **B,** Cross-sectional view illustrating deepened pulpal wall in the area of the rest seat (*rs*) to provide adequate thickness of amalgam. Note the relationship of the guiding planes (*gp*) to the tooth-borne RPD. **C,** Occlusal view showing the mesial rest seat (*mrs*) for the tissue-borne (i.e., distal extension) RPD. **D,** Lingual view of the tissue-borne RPD showing the relationship of the RPD to the Class II restoration and the edentulous ridge (*er*).

proximal surfaces and much of the occlusal surface. This section describes factors to consider when amalgam is used for moderate and large Class II restorations. The principles of tooth preparation are the same for all amalgam restorations and are as follows:

- A cavosurface marginal design that results in an approximate 90-degree amalgam margin
- Appropriate removal of tooth structure to provide for adequate strength of the amalgam
- Appropriate retention features

The tooth preparation techniques presented for a two-surface Class II restoration apply to larger Class II restorations as well. When the defect is large, however, certain modifications in tooth preparation may be necessary.

Occlusal Extensions

Often, a larger Class II defect requires greater extension of the occlusal surface outline form. This may require extending the grooves that are fissured, capping the cusps that are undermined, or extending the outline form up the cuspal inclines. These alterations can be accomplished easily by following the principles presented previously. Groove extension occurs at the same initial pulpal floor depth (i.e., at the level of the DEJ), and follows the DEJ as the groove is extended in a facial or lingual direction. The pulpal floor of an extended groove usually rises slightly occlusally as it is extended toward the cusp ridge. If it is necessary to extend through the cusp ridge onto the facial or lingual surface, the preparation is accomplished as described for the occlusolingual Class I restoration.

If an occlusal outline form extends up a cuspal incline, the extension also should maintain the pulpal floor at the level of the DEJ. This extension (as well as the groove extension) usually requires some alteration in the orientation of the No. 245 bur—a slight lingual tilt when extending in a facial direction and a slight facial tilt when extending in a lingual direction. Maintaining the correct pulpal floor depth preserves tooth structure and reduces the potential for pulpal encroachment. The prepared facial (or lingual) cavosurface margin still should result in a 90-degree amalgam margin.

When the occlusal outline form extends from a primary groove to within two-thirds of the distance to a cusp tip, that cusp is usually sufficiently weakened so as to require replacement. Leaving the cusp in a weakened state may be acceptable if the cusp is very large or, occasionally, if the amalgam is to be bonded (which provides some reinforcement of the strength of the remaining cuspal structure). Routine preparations in some teeth may predispose some cusps for capping (i.e., reduction). The small distal cusp of the mandibular first molars, the distolingual cusp of maxillary molars, and the lingual cusp of some mandibular premolars (especially first premolars) may be weakened when normal preparations of surrounding areas of the tooth are included.

Cusp reduction for an amalgam restoration should result in a uniform amalgam thickness over the reduced cusp of 1.5 to 2 mm. The thicker amount is necessary for functional cusps. These dimensions provide adequate strength for amalgam by limiting flexure during loading. The cusp reduction should occur as early in the preparation as can be determined to provide better access and visibility for completing the preparation. To reduce the cusp, the dentist orients the No. 245 bur parallel to the cuspal incline (lingual incline for facial cusp reductions and facial inclines for lingual cusp reduction) and makes several depth cuts in the cusp (to a depth of 1.5 or 2 mm). The depth cuts provide guides for the correct amount of cusp reduction. Without depth cuts, after the beginning reduction of the cusp, the operator may no longer know how much more reduction is necessary. The operator uses the bur to reduce the cusp, following the mesiodistal inclines of the cusp; this results in a uniform reduction. If only one of two facial (or lingual) cusps is to be capped, the cusp reduction should extend slightly beyond the facial (or lingual) groove area, provide the correct amount of tooth structure removal, and meet the adjacent, unreduced cusp to create a 90-degree cavosurface margin. This approach results in adequate thickness and edge strength of the amalgam. Cusp capping reduces the amount of vertical preparation wall heights and increases the need for the use of secondary retention features. An increased retention form may be provided by the proximal box retention grooves but may require the use of pins or slots (as described in Chapter 16). If indicated, cusp capping increases the resistance form of the tooth.[83,84] It has been reported that the survival rate of cusp-covered amalgam restorations is 72% at 15 years.[85]

Proximal Extensions

Larger Class II restorations often require larger proximal box preparations. These may include not only increased faciolingual or gingival extensions but also extension around a facial or lingual line angle. Large proximal box preparations also need secondary retention features (i.e., retention grooves, pins, slots) for an adequate retention form. Extensive proximal boxes are usually prepared the same as a more conservative proximal box but may require modifications. For increased faciolingual extensions, it may be necessary to tilt the No. 245 bur to include proximal faults that are extensive gingival to the contact area. Tilting the bur lingually when extending a facial proximal wall, or facially when extending a lingual proximal wall, conserves more of the marginal ridge and cuspal tooth structure. Although this action enhances preservation of some tooth structure strength, it results in a more occlusally convergent wall, which increases the difficulty of amalgam condensation in the gingival corners of the preparation.

When proximal extension around a line angle is necessary, it usually is associated with a reduction of the involved cusp. Such proximal extension usually is necessitated by a severely defective (or fractured) cusp or a cervical lesion that extends from the facial (or lingual) surface into the proximal area. Often, these areas are included in the preparation by extending the gingival floor of the proximal box around the line angle, using the same criteria for preparation as the typical proximal box: (1) Facial (or lingual) extension results in an occlusogingival wall that has a 90-degree cavosurface margin, and (2) the axial depth is 0.5 mm inside the DEJ.

The increased dimensions of a large proximal box usually require the use of retention grooves or other secondary retention form features (i.e., pins or slots). Secondary retention form features better ensure the retention of amalgam within the preparation by resisting displacement of amalgam in a proximal direction (and occasionally in an occlusal direction). Placement of retention grooves may be more difficult because of the extent of the preparation and the amount of caries excavation that may be necessary. If the outline form is developed correctly, however, the axiofacial and axiolingual line angles are correctly positioned and can be used as the location for retention groove placement.

When the proximal defect is extensive gingivally, isolation of the area, tooth preparation, matrix placement, and condensation and carving of amalgam are more difficult. If the proximal box is extended onto the root surface, the axial wall depth is no longer dictated by the DEJ. Any root surface preparation for amalgam should result in an initial axial wall depth of approximately 0.8 mm. This axial depth provides appropriate strength for amalgam, preserves pulp integrity, and creates enough dimension for the placement of retention grooves of 0.5 mm depth while preserving the strength of the adjacent, remaining marginal dentin and cementum. The extent of the preparation onto the root surface, the contour of the tooth, or both may require that the bur be tilted toward the adjacent tooth when preparing the gingival floor of the proximal box. This tilting may result in an axial wall that has two planes, the more gingival plane angled slightly internally. It also may cause more difficulty in retention groove placement. The more occlusal part of the axial wall may be over-reduced if the bur is not tilted.

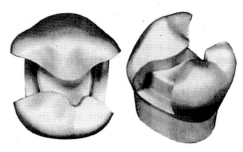

Fig. 14-65 Mesio-occluso-distal preparation on the mandibular second premolar.

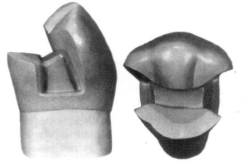

Fig. 14-66 Mandibular first premolar with the lingual cusp reduced for capping.

Caries Excavation and Pulp Protection

Larger Class II restorations often require more extensive caries excavation and pulp protection procedures during tooth preparation. Deep excavations indicate the increased need for pulp protection with a liner, a base, or both.

Matrix Placement

When a tooth preparation is extensive, matrix placement is more difficult. This is especially true for preparations that extend onto the root surface. Use of modified matrix bands and wedging techniques may be required. Different types of matrix systems are presented in Chapter 16.

Condensation and Carving of the Amalgam

Larger Class II preparations that extend around line angles or cap cusps or onto the root surface require careful amalgam condensation and carving techniques. Condensation of amalgam is more difficult in areas where cusps have been capped, where slots or pins have been placed, where vertical walls are more convergent occlusally, and where the root surface is involved. For larger restorations, lateral condensation is important to produce a properly condensed restoration in the gingival corners; also, carving cusps and gingival areas is more difficult.

EXAMPLES OF MODERATE CLASS II AMALGAM TOOTH PREPARATIONS THAT INVOLVE BOTH PROXIMAL SURFACES

Mandibular Second Premolar

A moderate mesio-occluso-distal tooth preparation in a mandibular second premolar is illustrated in Figure 14-65. Note the similarity with the two-surface mesio-occlusal preparation.

Mandibular First Premolar

When a mesio-occluso-distal amalgam tooth preparation is needed for the mandibular first premolar, the support of the small lingual cusp may be conserved by preparing the occlusal step more at the expense of tooth structure facial to the central groove than lingual. In addition, the bur is tilted slightly lingually to establish the correct pulpal wall direction. Despite these precautions, the lingual cusp may need to be reduced for capping if the lingual margin of the occlusal step extends more than two-thirds the distance from the central fissure to the cuspal eminence (Fig. 14-66). Special attention is given to such cusp reduction because retention is severely diminished when the cusp is reduced, eliminating the lingual wall of the occlusal

portion. Depth cuts of 1.5 mm aid the operator in establishing the correct amount of cusp reduction and in conserving a small portion of the lingual wall in the occlusal step. It is acceptable when restoring diminutive nonfunctional cusps, such as the lingual cusp of a mandibular first premolar, to reduce the cusp only 0.5 to 1 mm and restore the cusp to achieve an amalgam thickness of 1.5 mm. This procedure conserves more of the lingual wall of the isthmus for added retention form.

Maxillary First Molar

The mesio-occluso-distal tooth preparation of the maxillary first molar may require extending through the oblique ridge to unite the proximal preparations with the occlusal step. Cutting through the oblique ridge is indicated only if (1) the ridge is undermined by caries, (2) it is crossed by a deep fissure, or (3) occlusal portions of the separate mesio-occlusal and disto-occlusal outline forms leave less than 0.5 mm of the tooth structure between them. The remainder of the outline form is similar to the two-surface outline forms described previously in this chapter. Figure 14-67 illustrates typical three-surface and four-surface restorations for this tooth. The procedure for reducing the distolingual cusp of a maxillary first molar for capping is illustrated in Figure 14-68. Extending the facial or lingual wall of a proximal box to include the entire cusp is done (if necessary) to include weak or carious tooth structure or existing restorative material (Figs. 14-69 and 14-70).

Maxillary Second Molar with Caries on the Distal Portion of the Facial Surface

Close examination of the distal portion of the facial surface of the maxillary second molar may reveal decalcification or cavitation or both. When enamel is only slightly cavitated (i.e., softened and rough), polishing with sandpaper disks may eliminate the fault. Careful brushing technique, daily use of fluoride (i.e., rinses, toothpaste), and periodic applications of a fluoride varnish may prevent further breakdown. When decalcification is as deep as the DEJ and distal proximal caries is also present, however, the entire distofacial cusp may need to be included in a mesio-occluso-disto-facial tooth preparation. The facial lesion may be restored separately, if it is judged that the distofacial cusp would not be significantly weakened if left unrestored (i.e., uncapped) by amalgam. In that case, the mesio-occluso-distal preparation would be restored first, followed by preparation and restoration of the facial lesion. When such sequential preparations are contraindicated, the

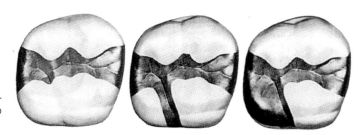

Fig. 14-67 Typical three- and four-surface restorations for the maxillary first molar. (See Fig. 14-68 for preparation of the distolingual cusp for capping.)

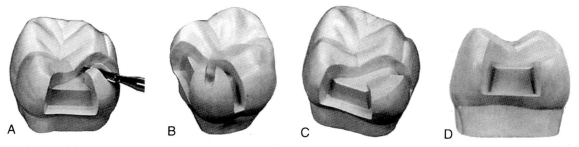

A   **B**   **C**   **D**

Fig. 14-68 Reduction of the distolingual cusp of the maxillary molar. **A,** Cutting a depth gauge groove with the side of the bur. **B,** Completed depth gauge groove. **C** and **D,** Completed cusp reduction.

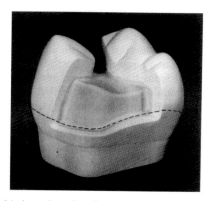

Fig. 14-69 Mesio-occluso-disto-facial preparation of the maxillary second molar showing extension to include moderate to extensive caries in the distal half of the facial surface. The outline includes the distofacial cusp and the facial groove. The dotted line represents the soft tissue level.

preparation outline is extended gingivally to include the distofacial cusp (just beyond the caries) and mesially to include the facial groove (see Fig. 14-69). The No. 245 bur should be used to create a gingival floor (i.e., shoulder) perpendicular to the occlusal force when extending the distal gingival floor to include the affected facial surface. Inclusion of distofacial caries often indicates a gingival margin that follows the gingival tissue level. The width of the shoulder should be approximately 1 or 0.5 mm inside the DEJ, whichever is greater. Some resistance form is provided by the shoulder. A retention groove should be placed in the axiofacial line angle of this distofacial extension, similar to the grooves placed in the proximal boxes. For additional retention, a slot may be placed (see Chapter 16).

Mandibular First Molar

The distal cusp on the mandibular first molar may be weakened when positioning the distofacial wall and margin. Facial extension of the distofacial margin to clear the distal contact often places the occlusal outline in the center of the cusp; this dictates relocation of the margin to provide a sound enamel wall and 90-degree amalgam that is not on a cuspal eminence. When the distal cusp is small or weakened or both, extension of the distal gingival floor and distofacial wall to include the distal cusp places the margin just mesial to the distofacial groove. Figure 14-70 illustrates the ideal distofacial extension and a preparation design that includes the distal cusp.

Capping the distal cusp is an alternative to extending the entire distofacial wall when the occlusal margin crosses the cuspal eminence (see Fig. 14-70, *C*). A minimal reduction of 2 mm should result in a 2-mm thickness of amalgam over the capped cusp (see Fig. 14-70, *D*). The cusp reduction should result in a butt joint between the tooth structure and amalgam. Whenever possible, capping the distal cusp is more desirable than extending the distofacial margin because this conserves the tooth structure, and the remaining portion of the cusp helps in applying the matrix for the development of proper embrasure form. The plane of the reduced cusp should parallel the facial (or lingual) outline of the unreduced cusp mesiodistally and the cuspal incline emanating from the central groove faciolingually.

Restorative Technique for Class II Amalgam Preparations
Desensitizer Placement

A dentin desensitizer is placed in the completed cavity preparation.

counterclockwise to obtain a larger loop to fit around the tooth. Care should be taken not to trap the rubber dam between the band and the gingival margin. If the dam material is trapped between the band and the tooth, the septum of the dam should be stretched and depressed gingivally to reposition the dam material. Next, the larger knurled nut is rotated clockwise to tighten the band slightly. Exploration along the gingival margin is accomplished to determine that the gingival edge of the band extends beyond the preparation margins. When the band is correctly positioned, the band is securely tightened around the tooth.

When one of the proximal margins is deeper gingivally, the Tofflemire mesio-occluso-distal band may be modified to prevent damage to the gingival tissue or attachment on the more shallow side. A band may be trimmed for the shallow gingival margin, permitting the matrix to extend farther gingivally for the deeper gingival margin (Fig. 14-77).

The mouth mirror is positioned to observe the proximal contours of the matrix through the interproximal space (Fig. 14-78). The occlusogingival contour should be convex, with the height of contour at proper contact level and contacting the adjacent tooth. The matrix is also observed from an occlusal aspect allowing evaluation of the position of the contact area in a faciolingual direction. It may be necessary to remove the retainer and reburnish the band for additional contouring. Minor alterations in contour and contact may be accomplished without removal from the tooth. The backside of the blade of the 15-8-14 spoon excavator (i.e., Black spoon) is an excellent instrument for improving contour and contact. If a smaller burnishing instrument is used, the dentist should take care not to create a grooved or bumpy surface that would result in a restoration with an irregular proximal surface. Ideally, the band should be positioned 1 mm apical to the gingival margin or deep enough to be engaged by the wedge

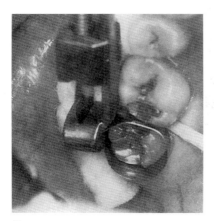

Fig. 14-74 Tofflemire retainer maintaining a cotton roll in the maxillary vestibule during condensation.

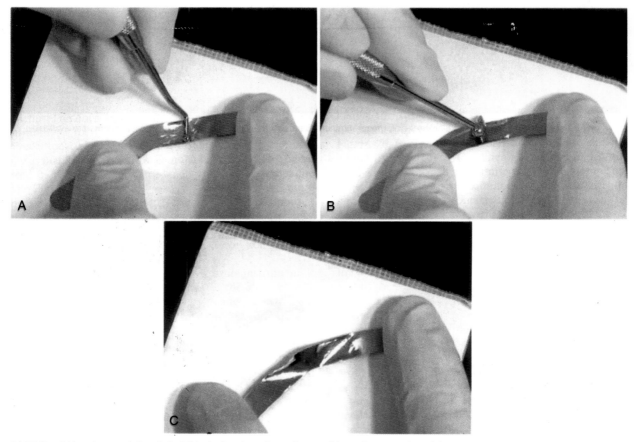

Fig. 14-75 Burnishing the matrix band. **A,** With the band on the pad, a small burnisher is used to deform the band. **B,** A large burnisher to smooth the band contour. **C,** Burnished matrix band for mesio-occluso-distal tooth preparation. *(Courtesy of Aldridge D. Wilder, DDS.)*

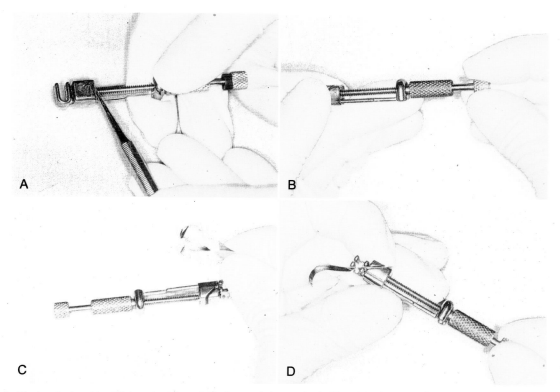

Fig. 14-76 Positioning the band in a Universal retainer. **A,** Explorer pointing to the locking vise. The gingival aspect of the vise is shown in this view. **B,** The pointed spindle is released from the locking vise when the small knurled nut is turned counterclockwise. **C,** The band is folded to form a loop and to be positioned in the retainer (occlusal edge of band first). **D,** The spindle is tightened against the band in the locking vise. *(From Daniel SJ, Harfst SA, Wilder RS: Mosby's dental hygiene: Concepts, cases, and competencies, ed 2, St. Louis, Mosby, 2008.)*

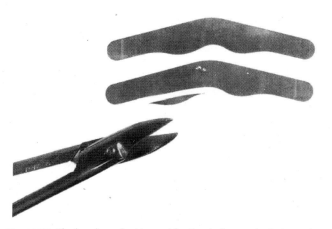

Fig. 14-77 The band may be trimmed for the shallower gingival margin, permitting the matrix to extend farther gingivally for the deeper gingival margin on the other proximal surface.

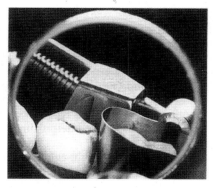

Fig. 14-78 Using a mirror from the facial or lingual position to evaluate the proximal contour of the matrix band.

(whichever is less) and 1 to 2 mm above the adjacent marginal ridge or ridges.

A minor modification of the matrix may be indicated for restoring the proximal surface that is planned for a guide plane for a removable partial denture. Abutment teeth for a tooth-supported removable partial denture must provide amalgam contour to allow defining (by carving or [later] disking) a guide plane extending from the marginal ridge 2.5 mm gingivally. Normal proximal contouring, rather than

over-contouring, is usually sufficient, however, and best for the development of a guide plane. Guide plane development results in a gingival embrasure between the natural tooth and denture teeth that is less open and less likely to trap food (see Fig. 14-64, *B*).

Abutment teeth adjacent to the residual ridge for a tissue-supported (i.e., distal extension) removable partial denture are carved to provide normal morphology. Sufficient gingival embrasure should be provided to allow for the difference between the compression under the load of the ridge soft tissue and that of the periodontal membrane (although a small area guide plane may be provided).

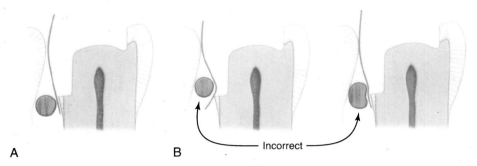

Fig. 14-79 **A,** Correct wedge position. **B,** Incorrect wedge positions.

After the matrix contour and extension are evaluated, a wedge is placed in the gingival embrasure or embrasures using the following technique: (1) Break off approximately 0.5 inch (1.2 cm) of a round toothpick. (2) Grasp the broken end of the wedge with the No. 110 pliers. (3) Insert the pointed tip from the lingual or facial embrasure (whichever is larger), slightly gingival to the gingival margin. (4) Wedge the band tightly against the tooth and margin (Fig. 14-79, *A*). If necessary, the gingival aspect of the wedge may be lightly moistened with lubricant to facilitate its placement. If the wedge is placed occlusal to the gingival margin, the band is pressed into the preparation, creating an abnormal concavity in the proximal surface of the restoration (see Fig. 14-79, *B*). The wedge should not be so far apical to the gingival margin that the band will not be held tightly against the gingival margin. This improper wedge placement results in gingival excess (i.e., "overhang") caused by the band moving slightly away from the margin during condensation of the amalgam. Such an overhang often goes undetected and may result in irritation of the gingiva or an area of plaque accumulation, which may increase the risk of secondary caries. To be effective, a wedge should be positioned as close to the gingival margin as possible without being occlusal to it. If the wedge is significantly apical of the gingival margin, a second (usually smaller) wedge may be placed on top of the first to wedge adequately the matrix against the margin (Fig. 14-80). This type of wedging is particularly useful for patients whose interproximal tissue level has receded.

The gingival wedge should be tight enough to prevent any possibility of an overhang of amalgam in at least the middle two-thirds of the gingival margin (see Fig. 14-80, *A* and *B*). Occasionally, double wedging is permitted (if access allows), securing the matrix when the proximal box is wide faciolingually. *Double wedging* refers to using two wedges: one from the lingual embrasure and one from the facial embrasure (see Fig. 14-80, *E* and *F*). Two wedges help ensure that the gingival corners of a wide proximal box can be properly condensed; they also help minimize gingival excess. Double wedging should be used only if the middle two-thirds of the proximal margins can be adequately wedged, however. Because the facial and lingual corners are accessible to carving, proper wedging is important to prevent gingival excess of amalgam in the middle two-thirds of the proximal box (see Fig. 14-80, *B*).

Occasionally, a concavity may be present on the proximal surface that is apparent in the gingival margin. This may occur on a surface with a fluted root, such as the mesial surface of the maxillary first premolar (see Fig. 14-80, *G1*). A gingival margin located in this area may be concave (see Fig. 14-80, *G2*). To wedge a matrix band tightly against such a margin, a second pointed wedge can be inserted between the first wedge and the band (see Fig. 14-80, *G3* and *G4*).

The wedging action between teeth should provide enough separation to compensate for the thickness of the matrix band. This ensures a positive contact relationship after the matrix is removed (after the condensation and initial carving of amalgam). If a Tofflemire retainer is used to restore a two-surface Class II preparation, the single wedge must provide enough separation to compensate for two thicknesses of band material. The tightness of the wedge is tested by pressing the tip of an explorer firmly at several points along the middle two-thirds of the gingival margin (against the matrix band) to verify that it cannot be moved away from the gingival margin (Fig. 14-81). As an additional test, the dentist attempts to remove the wedge (using the explorer with moderate pressure) after first having set the explorer tip into the wood near the broken end. Moderate pulling should not cause dislodgment. Often, the rubber dam has a tendency to loosen the wedge. Rebounding of the dam stretched during wedge placement may loosen the wedge. Stretching the interproximal dam septa before and during wedge placement in the direction opposite to the wedge (and lubricating the wedge) can prevent this. The stretched dam is released after the wedge is inserted.

Some situations may require a triangular wedge that can be modified (by knife or scalpel blade) to conform to the approximating tooth contours (Fig. 14-82). The round toothpick wedge is usually the wedge of choice with conservative proximal boxes, however, because its wedging action is more occlusal (i.e., nearer the gingival margin) than with the triangular wedge (Fig. 14-83, *A* and *B*).

The triangular (i.e., anatomic) wedge is recommended for a preparation with a deep gingival margin. The triangular wedge usually is indicated with the Tofflemire mesio-occlusodistal matrix band. The triangular wedge is positioned similarly to the round wedge, and the goal is the same. When the gingival margin is deep (cervically), the base of the triangular wedge more readily engages the tooth gingival to the margin without causing excessive soft tissue displacement. The anatomic wedge is preferred for deeply extended gingival margins because its greatest cross-sectional dimension is at its base (see Fig. 14-83, *C* and *D*).

To maintain gingival isolation attained by an anatomic wedge placed before the preparation of a deeply extended gingival margin, it may be appropriate to withdraw the wedge

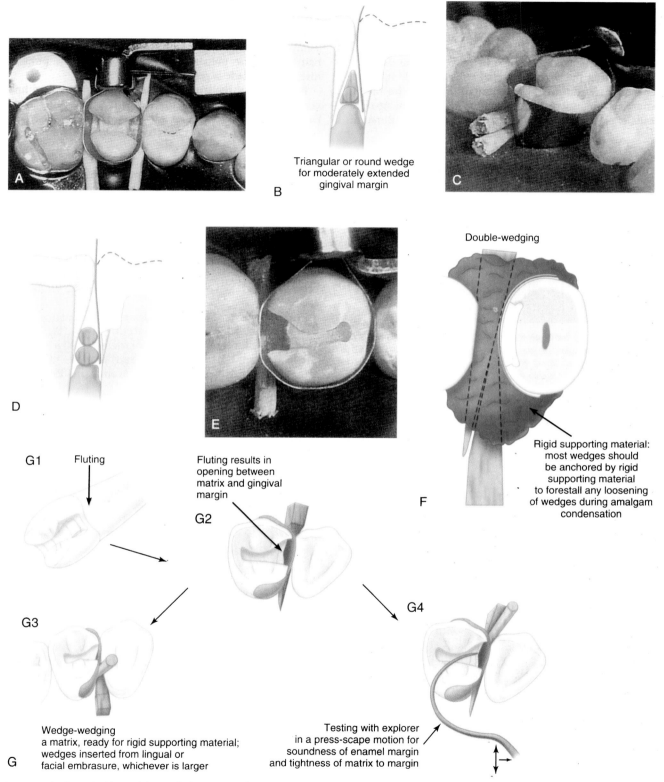

B Triangular or round wedge for moderately extended gingival margin

Double-wedging

F Rigid supporting material: most wedges should be anchored by rigid supporting material to forestall any loosening of wedges during amalgam condensation

G1 Fluting

G2 Fluting results in opening between matrix and gingival margin

G3 Wedge-wedging a matrix, ready for rigid supporting material; wedges inserted from lingual or facial embrasure, whichever is larger

G4 Testing with explorer in a press-scape motion for soundness of enamel margin and tightness of matrix to margin

Fig. 14-80 Various double-wedging techniques. **A** and **B,** Proper wedging for the matrix for a typical mesio-occluso-distal preparation. **C** and **D,** Technique to allow wedging near the gingival margin of the preparation when the proximal box is shallow gingivally, the interproximal tissue level has receded, or both. **E** and **F,** Double wedging may be used with faciolingually wide proximal boxes to provide maximal closure of the band along the gingival margin. **G,** Another technique may be used on the mesial aspect of the maxillary first premolars to adapt the matrix to the fluted (i.e., concave) area of the gingival margin (*G1, G2*); a second wedge inserted from the lingual embrasure (*G3*); testing the adaptation of the band after insertion of the wedges from the facial aspect (*G4*).

a small distance to allow passage of the band between the loosened wedge and the gingival margin. Tilting (i.e., canting) the matrix into place helps the gingival edge of the band slide between the loosened wedge and the gingival margin. The band is tightened, and the same wedge is firmly re-inserted.

Supporting the matrix material with the blade of a Hollenback carver during the insertion of the wedge for the difficult deep gingival restoration may be helpful.[19] The tip of the blade is placed between the matrix and the gingival margin,

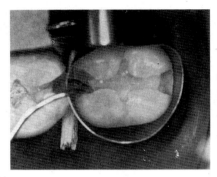

Fig. 14-81 Use of the explorer tip (with pressure) to ensure proper adaptation of the band to the gingival margin. In addition, the tip is pressed and dragged along the gingival margin in both directions to ensure removal of any friable enamel.

and then the "heel" of the blade is leaned against the matrix and adjacent tooth (Fig. 14-84). In this position, the blade supports the matrix to help in positioning the wedge sufficiently gingivally and preventing the wedge from pushing the matrix into the preparation. After the wedge is properly inserted, the blade is gently removed.

All aspects of the band are assessed and any desired final corrections are made after the wedge is placed. The matrix band must be touching the adjacent contact area (see Fig. 14-78). If the band does not reach the adjacent contact area after contouring and wedging, the tension of the band is released by turning the larger knurled nut of the Tofflemire retainer slightly (quarter turn) counterclockwise. If loosening the loop of a Tofflemire band still does not allow for contact with an adjacent tooth, a custom-made band with a smaller angle can be used. Reducing the angle of the band increases the difference in length (i.e., circumferences) of the gingival and occlusal edges. To reduce the angle of the band, the operator folds it as shown in Figure 14-85. Next, the operator burnishes for appropriate occlusogingival contour (in the contact areas) and inserts the band into the Tofflemire retainer.

A suitably trimmed tongue blade can wedge a matrix where the interproximal spacing between teeth is large (Fig. 14-86). Occasionally, however, it is impossible to use a wedge to secure the matrix band. In this case, the band must be sufficiently tight to minimize the gingival excess of amalgam. Because the

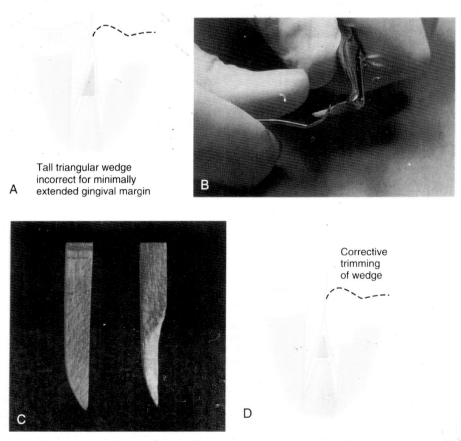

Tall triangular wedge incorrect for minimally extended gingival margin

A

B

Corrective trimming of wedge

C

D

Fig. 14-82 Modified triangular (i.e., anatomic) wedge. **A,** Depending on the proximal convexity, a triangular wedge may distort the matrix contour. **B,** A sharp-bladed instrument may be used to modify the triangular steepness of the wedge. **C,** Modified and unmodified wedges are compared. **D,** Properly modified triangular wedge prevents distortion of the matrix contour.

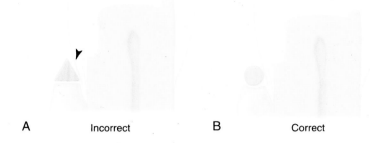

Fig. 14-83 Indications for the use of a round toothpick wedge versus a triangular (i.e., anatomic) wedge. **A,** As a rule, the triangular wedge does not firmly support the matrix band against the gingival margin in conservative Class II preparations (*arrowhead*). **B,** The round toothpick wedge is preferred for these preparations because its wedging action is nearer the gingival margin. **C,** In Class II preparations with deep gingival margins, the round toothpick wedge crimps the matrix band contour if it is placed occlusal to the gingival margin. **D,** The triangular wedge is preferred with these preparations because its greatest width is at its base.

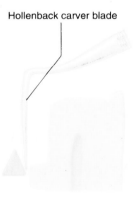

Fig. 14-84 Supporting the matrix with the blade of a Hollenback carver during wedge insertion.

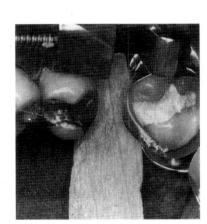

Fig. 14-86 A custom-made tongue blade wedge may be used when excessive space exists between adjacent teeth.

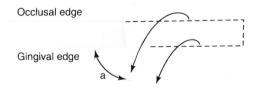

Fig. 14-85 The custom-made matrix strip is folded, as indicated by arrows. The smaller angle (*a*) compared with the angle of the commercial strip increases the difference between the lengths of the gingival and occlusal edges.

band is not wedged, special care must be exercised by placing small amounts of amalgam in the gingival floor and condensing the first 1 mm of amalgam lightly, but thoroughly, in a gingival direction. The condensation is then carefully continued in a gingival direction using a larger condenser with firm pressure. Condensation against an unwedged matrix may cause the amalgam to extrude grossly beyond the gingival margin. Without a wedge, some excess amalgam that is overcontoured remains at the proximal margins, requiring correction by a suitable carver immediately after matrix removal.

The matrix is removed after insertion of the amalgam, carving of the occlusal portion (including the occlusal embrasure or embrasures), and hardening of the amalgam to avoid fracture of the marginal ridge during band removal. The retainer is removed from the band after turning the small knurled nut counterclockwise to retract the pointed spindle.

The end of the index finger may be placed on the occlusal surface of the tooth to stabilize the band as the retainer is removed. Any rigid supporting material applied to support the matrix is then removed. The No. 110 pliers are used to tease the band free from one contact area at a time by pushing or pulling the band in a linguo-occlusal (or facio-occlusal) direction and, if possible, in the direction of wedge insertion (Fig. 14-87). The wedge may be left in place to provide separation of teeth while the matrix band is removed, and then it (the wedge) is removed. By maintaining slight interdental separation, the wedge reduces the risk of fracturing of amalgam. A straight occlusal direction should be avoided during matrix removal to prevent breaking of the marginal ridges.

RIGID-MATERIAL SUPPORTED SECTIONAL MATRIX

An alternative to the universal matrix is the use of a properly contoured sectional matrix that is wedged and supported by a material that is rigid enough to resist condensation pressure. The supporting material selected must be easy to place and to remove. Examples include light-cured, thermoplastic and quick-setting rigid polyvinyl siloxane (PVS) materials (Fig. 14-88). The gingival wedge is positioned interproximally to secure the band tightly at the gingival margin to prevent any excess of amalgam (i.e., overhang). The wedge also separates teeth slightly to compensate for the thickness of the band material.

The proximal surface contour of the matrix should allow the normal slight convexity between the occlusal and middle thirds of the proximal surface when viewed from the lingual (or facial) aspect. Proximal surface restorations often display an occlusogingival proximal contour that is too straight, thereby causing the contact relationship to be located too far

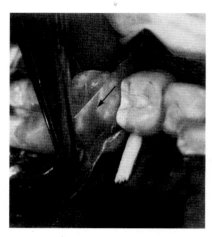

Fig. 14-87 Using No. 110 pliers, the matrix band should be removed in a linguo-occlusal (*arrow*) or facio-occlusal direction (not just in an occlusal direction).

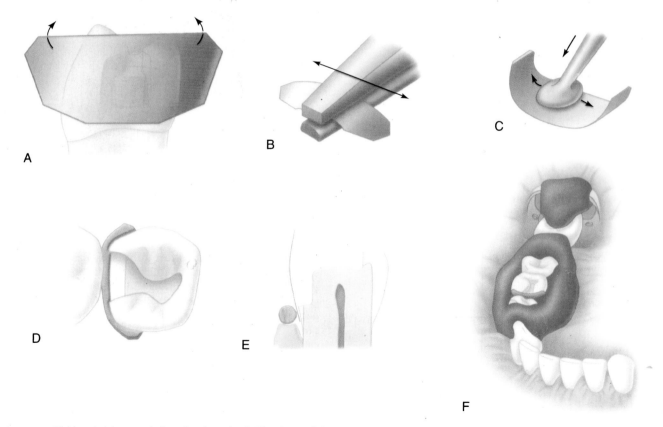

Fig. 14-88 Rigid material–supported sectional matrix. **A,** The shape of the stainless steel strip after trimming. **B,** The strip contoured to the circumferential contour of the tooth (fingers can be used). **C,** Burnishing the strip to produce occlusogingival contact contour (left and right arrows indicate the short, back-and-forth motion of the burnisher). **D,** Contoured strip in position. **E,** Matrix strip properly wedged. **F,** Completed rigid material–supported sectional matrix.

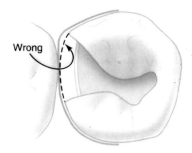

Fig. 14-89 Alteration of the matrix contour to provide the correct form to the proximofacial line angle region.

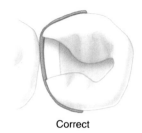

Correct

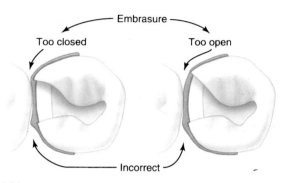

Fig. 14-90 Correct or incorrect facial and lingual embrasure form is determined by the shape of the matrix strip.

occlusally (with little or no occlusal embrasure). This condition allows food impaction between teeth, with resultant injury to the interproximal gingiva and supporting tissues, and invites caries. The proximal surface contour of the matrix should also provide the correct form to the proximofacial line angle region. If this contour is not present, the facial embrasure of the restoration is too open, inviting food impaction and injury to underlying supporting tissues. Correct and incorrect contours and matrix correction steps are illustrated in Figures 14-89 and 14-90.

The matrix should be tight against the facial and lingual margins on the proximal surface so that the amalgam can be well condensed at the preparation margins. In addition, when the matrix is tight against the tooth, minimal carving is necessary on the proximal margins after the matrix is removed. A matrix that is tight against the margins requires thorough condensation of the amalgam into the matrix and tooth corners to prevent amalgam voids at the proximal margins.

PRECONTOURED MATRIX STRIPS

Commercially available sectional metal strips (e.g., Palodent System; DENTSPLY Caulk, Milford, DE) are precontoured and ready for application to the tooth (Fig. 14-91). These strips have limited application when used for amalgam because of their rounded contour. They usually are most suitable for mandibular first premolars and the distal surface of maxillary canines. The contact area of the adjacent tooth occasionally is too close to allow placement of the contoured Palodent strip without causing a dent in the strip's contact area, making it unusable.

INSERTION AND CARVING OF THE AMALGAM

The principal objectives during the insertion of amalgam are as follows:

- Condensation to adapt the amalgam to the preparation walls and the matrix and to produce a restoration free of voids
- Keeping the mercury content in the restoration as low as possible to improve strength and decrease corrosion

Care should be taken to choose condensers that are best suited for use in each part of the tooth preparation and that can be used without binding.

The amount of amalgam initially transferred is the amount that (when condensed) will fill the gingival 1 mm (approximately) of the proximal box. It is condensed in a gingival

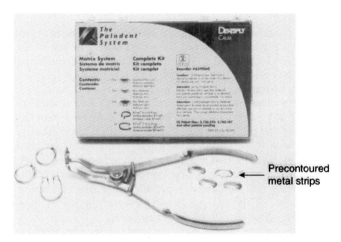

Fig. 14-91 Pre-contoured metal strips. *(The Palodent System; courtesy of DENTSPLY Caulk, Milford, DE.)*

direction with sufficient force to adapt amalgam to the gingival floor. Additional amalgam is carefully condensed against the proximal margins of the preparation and into the proximal retention grooves. Firm, facially and lingually directed pressure (i.e., lateral condensation) of the condenser accomplishes this at the same time as exertion of gingivally directed force (Fig. 14-92). Mesial (or distal) condensation of the amalgam in the proximal box is accomplished to ensure proximal contact with the adjacent tooth. Lateral condensation should be a routine step for Class II amalgams.[86] An advantage of amalgam over direct composite is that amalgam is condensed into place rather than being placed. Condensation strokes in a gingival direction help ensure that no voids occur internally or along the margins. Lateral condensation helps ensure that sufficient proximal contact and proximal contour

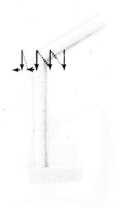

Fig. 14-92 Lateral and occlusogingival force is necessary to condense amalgam properly into the proximal grooves and into the angles at the junction of the matrix band and the margins of the preparation.

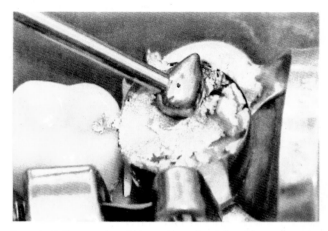

Fig. 14-93 Precarve burnishing with a large burnisher. *(Courtesy of Aldridge D. Wilder, DDS.)*

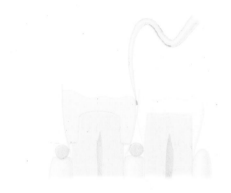

Fig. 14-94 Defining the marginal ridge and the occlusal embrasure with an explorer.

are achieved. Placement of composite resin materials will not allow distortion of the matrix band laterally into an optimal contact with the adjacent proximal surface. This results in a greater likelihood of restoration proximal undercontour and an open contact. Proximal contact and contour of the matrix band must be ensured prior to composite resin restoration placement.

The procedure of adding and condensing continues until amalgam reaches the level of the pulpal wall. The size of the condenser is changed (usually to a larger one), if indicated, and amalgam is condensed in the remaining proximal portion of the preparation concurrently with the occlusal portion. It may be necessary to return to a smaller condenser when condensing in a narrow extension of the preparation or near the proximal margins. A smaller condenser face is more effective at condensing, provided it does not significantly penetrate amalgam. The occlusal margins are covered and over-packed by at least 1 mm using a large condenser, ensuring that the margins are well condensed, especially in the area of the marginal ridge.[87] This step significantly reduces the risk of marginal ridge fracture during matrix removal.

Condensation should be completed within the working time for the alloy being used, as indicated by the manufacturer's recommendations. Condensation that occurs within this time frame will result in the following:

■ Proper coherence and homogeneity, with minimal voids in the restoration
■ Desired adaptation of the material to the walls of the preparation and matrix during condensation
■ Development of the maximal strength and minimal flow (i.e., creep) in the completed restoration
■ Proper intermingling of the adhesive and amalgam, if a bonding system is used

The plasticity and wetness of the amalgam mass should be monitored during condensation. Proper condensation requires that the mix should be neither wet (i.e., mercury-rich) nor dry and crumbly (i.e., mercury-poor). Amalgam that is beginning to set should be discarded and a new mix obtained to complete any condensation.

CARVING THE OCCLUSAL PORTION

Before carving procedures are initiated, precarve burnishing of the occlusal portion with a large egg-shaped or ball burnisher should be done (Fig. 14-93).[52]

With the matrix band still in place, careful carving of the occlusal portion should begin immediately after condensation and burnishing. Sharp discoid instruments of suitable size are the recommended carvers. The larger discoid is used first, followed by the smaller one in regions not accessible to the larger instrument.

While the matrix is in place, the marginal ridge is carved confluent with the tooth's anatomy such that it duplicates the height and shape of the adjacent marginal ridge (Fig. 14-94). An explorer or small Hollenback carver may be used to carefully define the occlusal embrasure. Occlusal contacts were evaluated before tooth preparation. Remembering the pattern of occlusal contacts, observing the height of the adjacent marginal ridge, and knowing where the preparation cavosurface margins are located all aid in completing the carving of the occlusal surface, including the marginal ridge and occlusal embrasure.

If the restoration has extensive axial involvement of the tooth, the occlusal carving should be accomplished quickly. The objectives would be to develop the general occlusal contour and, most importantly, to develop the correct marginal ridge height and occlusal embrasure form (see Fig.

14-94). Then, the matrix is removed, and access is gained to carve the axial portions of the restoration. This permits these areas (usually more inaccessible) to be carved while amalgam is carvable. When the axial carving is completed, the occlusal surface contouring is completed. Occasionally, this occlusal contouring may require the use of an abrasive stone or finishing bur if the setting of the amalgam is nearing completion.

REMOVAL OF THE MATRIX BAND AND COMPLETION OF CARVING

The matrix band (or sectional matrix) and any wedges are gently removed. The proximal surface should be nearly completed, with proper contact evident and minimal carving required except to remove a possible small amount of excess amalgam at the proximal facial and lingual margins, at the faciogingival and linguogingival corners, and along the gingival margin. Amalgam knives (scalers, No. 34 and No. 35) are ideal for removing gingival excess to prevent gingival overhangs (Fig. 14-95 and 14-96). They also are ideal for refining the embrasure form around the proximal contacts (Fig. 14-97). The secondary (or "back") edges on the blades of amalgam knives are occasionally helpful while either a pull stroke or a push stroke is used. The Hollenback carver No. 3 and (occasionally) the side of the explorer may be suitable instruments for carving these areas. The explorer cannot refine the margins and contour as accurately as amalgam knives can.

When carving the margins, the cutting surface of the carving instrument is held perpendicular to them. Carving should be parallel to the margins, however, with the adjacent tooth surface being used to guide the carver. The existence of the proximal contact is verified visually by using the mouth mirror. If an amalgam adhesive was used, any thin layers of set resin near the margin that formed between the matrix and the tooth should be removed. When carving is completed, the rubber dam is removed, and the occlusion is assessed and adjusted, as needed.

Before the patient is dismissed, thin unwaxed dental floss may be passed through the proximal contacts once to remove any amalgam shavings on the proximal surface of the restoration and to assess the gingival margin. Passing the floss through

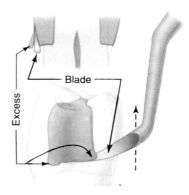

Fig. 14-95 Gingival excess may be removed with amalgam knives.

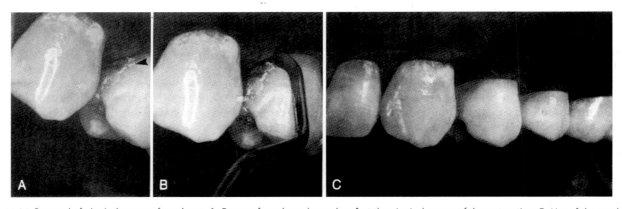

Fig. 14-96 Removal of gingival excess of amalgam. **A,** Excess of amalgam (*arrowhead*) at the gingival corner of the restoration. **B,** Use of the amalgam knife for removal of gingival excess. **C,** Gingival corner of restoration with excess removed.

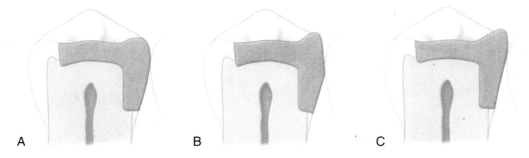

Fig. 14-97 Proximal contour. **A,** Correct proximal contour. **B,** Incorrect marginal ridge height and occlusal embrasure form. **C,** The occlusogingival proximal contour is too straight, the contact is too high, and the occlusal embrasure form is incorrect.

a contact more than once may weaken it. Wrapping the floss around the adjacent tooth when the floss is passed through the contact minimizes the pressure exerted on amalgam. When positioned in the gingival embrasure, the floss is wrapped around the restored tooth and positioned apical to the gingival margin of the restoration. The floss is moved in a faciolingual direction while extended occlusally. The floss not only removes amalgam shavings but also smooths the proximal amalgam and detects any gingival overhang of amalgam. If an overhang is detected, further use of an amalgam knife is necessary.[88] Floss also can be used to verify that the weight of the contact is similar to that of neighboring teeth. Final rinsing of the oral cavity is then accomplished. The patient is advised to avoid chewing with the restored tooth for 24 hours.

Finishing and Polishing of the Amalgam

Finishing of amalgam restorations may be necessary to correct a marginal discrepancy or to improve the contour. Polishing of high-copper amalgams is unnecessary.[57] Although they are less prone to corrosion and marginal deterioration than are their low-copper predecessors, some operators still prefer to polish amalgam restorations. Finishing (and polishing) usually is delayed until all proposed restorations have been placed, rather than being done periodically during the course of treatment. Polishing an amalgam restoration is not attempted within 24 hours after insertion because crystallization is incomplete.

Finishing and polishing the occlusal portion is similar to the procedures described for Class I amalgam restoration. Finishing and polishing of the proximal surface is indicated where the proximal amalgam is accessible. This area usually includes the facial and lingual margins and amalgam that is occlusal to the contact. The remainder of the proximal surface is often inaccessible; however, the matrix band should have imparted sufficient smoothness to it.

If amalgam along the facial and lingual proximal margins was slightly over-carved, the enamel margin can be felt as the explorer tip passes from amalgam across the margin onto the external enamel surface. Finishing burs or sandpaper disks, rotating at slow speed, may be used to smooth the enamel–amalgam margin. Sandpaper disks also can be used to smooth and contour the marginal ridge. Inappropriate use of sandpaper disks may "ledge" the restoration around the contact, however, resulting in inappropriate proximal contours.

In conservative preparations, the facial and lingual proximal margins are generally inaccessible for finishing and polishing. Fine abrasive disks or the tip of a sharpened rubber polishing point should be used to polish the proximal portion that is accessible. When proximal margins are inaccessible to finishing and polishing with disks or rubber polishing points, and some excess amalgam remains (e.g., at the gingival corners and margins), amalgam knives occasionally may be used to trim amalgam back to the margin and to improve the contour. Accessible facial and lingual proximal margins also may be polished using the edge of an abrasive rubber polishing cup.

Final polishing of the occlusal surface and the accessible areas of the proximal surface may be accomplished with a fine-grit rubber polishing point or by the rubber cup with flour of pumice followed by a high-luster agent such as precipitated chalk. Figure 14-98 provides examples of properly finished and polished amalgam restorations.

Quadrant Dentistry

When several teeth are to be restored, they are usually treated by quadrants rather than individually. Quadrant dentistry increases efficiency and reduces chairtime for the patient. The use of the rubber dam is particularly important in quadrant dentistry. For maximal efficiency, when a quadrant of amalgam tooth preparations is planned, each rotary or hand instrument should be used on every tooth where it is needed before being exchanged.

When restoring a quadrant of Class II amalgam tooth preparations, it is permissible to apply matrix bands on alternate preparations in the quadrant and restore teeth two at a time. Banding adjacent preparations requires excessive wedging to compensate for a double thickness of band material and makes the control of proximal contours and interproximal contacts difficult. Extensive tooth preparations may need to be restored one at a time. If proximal boxes differ in size, teeth with smaller boxes should be restored first because often the proximal margins are inaccessible to carving if the larger adjacent box is restored first. In addition, smaller boxes can be

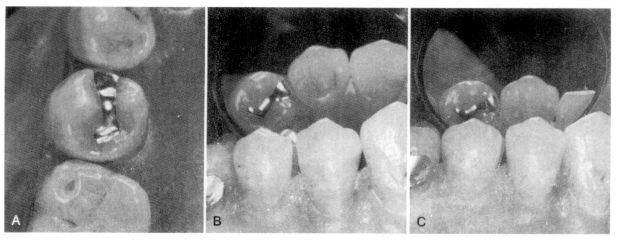

Fig. 14-98 Polished mesio-occlusal amalgam restoration. Note the conservative extension. **A,** Occlusal view. **B,** Mesiofacial and occlusal views of the mesiofacial margin. **C,** Facial and occlusal views of the proximal surface contour and the location of the proximal contact.

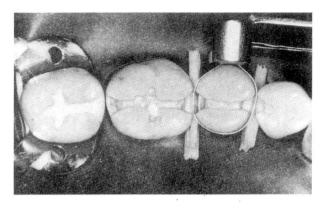

Fig. 14-99 Quadrant dentistry. Unless otherwise indicated, a quadrant of Class II preparations with similarly sized proximal boxes can be restored using two bands simultaneously if they are placed on every other prepared tooth. It is recommended that the posterior most tooth be restored first.

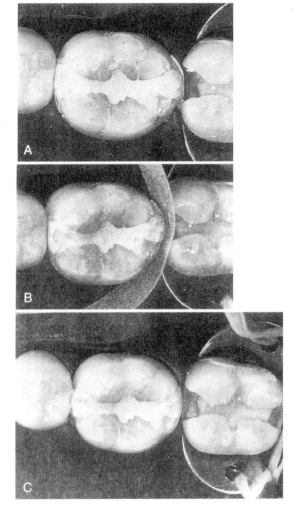

Fig. 14-100 When the first of two adjacent Class II preparations is restored, proper contour can be established by using a finishing and contouring strip before the second is restored. **A,** Before using the strip. **B,** Applying the strip. **C,** Verification of proper contouring can be done by viewing the restoration with a mirror from the occlusal, facial, and lingual positions. The proximal contour also can be evaluated after matrix placement by noting the symmetry between the restored surface and the burnished matrix band.

restored more quickly and accurately because more tooth structure remains to guide the carver. If the larger proximal box is restored first, the gingival contour of the restoration could be damaged when the wedge is inserted to secure the matrix band for the second, smaller restoration. If the adjacent proximal boxes are similar in size, the banding of alternate preparations should be started with the most posterior preparation because this allows the patient to close slightly as subsequent restorations are inserted (Fig. 14-99).

Before restoring the second of two adjacent teeth, the proximal contour of the first restoration should be carefully established. Its anatomy serves as the guide to establish proper contact size and location of the second restoration; it also serves as good embrasure form. If necessary, a finishing strip can be used to refine the contour of the first proximal amalgam (Fig. 14-100). The finishing strip is indicated, however, only where the proximal contact is open. Using a finishing strip between contacting amalgam restorations may lighten or eliminate the proximal contact.

Class VI Amalgam Restorations

The Class VI tooth preparation is used to restore the incisal edge of anterior teeth or the cusp tip regions of posterior teeth.

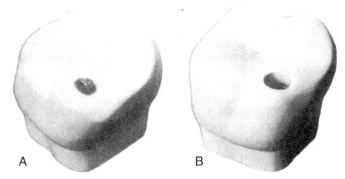

Fig. 14-101 Class VI preparation. **A,** Exposed dentin on the mesiofacial cusp. **B,** Tooth preparation necessary to restore the involved area.

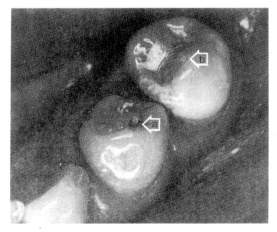

Fig. 14-102 Class VI lesions. Carious cusp tip fault on the first premolar (*a*). Noncarious fault on the second premolar (*b*).

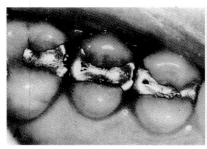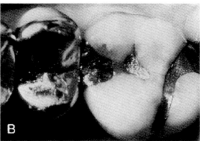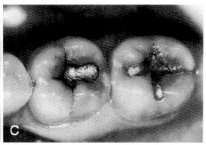

Fig. 14-103 Clinical examples of long-term amalgam restorations. **A,** 44-year-old amalgams. **B,** 58-year-old amalgams in the first molar. **C,** 65-year-old amalgams in molars. (**A** and **B,** courtesy of Drs. John Osborne and James Summitt.)

Such tooth preparations are frequently indicated where attrition (loss of tooth substance from the occluding of food, abrasives, and opposing teeth) has removed enamel to expose the underlying dentin on those areas (Fig. 14-101). This occurs more frequently in older patients. When the softer dentin is exposed, it wears faster than the surrounding enamel, resulting in "cupped-out" areas. As the dentin support is lost, enamel begins to fracture away, exposing more dentin and often causing sensitivity. Sensitivity to hot and cold is a frequent complaint with Class VI lesions, and some patients are bothered by food impaction in the deeper depressions. Enamel edges may become jagged and sharp to the tongue, lips, or cheek. Lip, tongue, or cheek biting is occasionally a complaint. Rounding and smoothing such incisoaxial (or occlusoaxial) edges is an excellent service to the patient. Early recognition and restoration of these lesions is recommended to limit the loss of dentin and the subsequent loss of enamel supported by this dentin.

The Class VI tooth preparation also is indicated to restore the hypoplastic pit occasionally found on cusp tips (Fig. 14-102). Such developmental faults are vulnerable to caries, especially in high-risk patients, and should be restored as soon as they are detected. Caries are rarely found in dentin where attritional wear has removed the overlying enamel.

Composite is generally used to restore Class VI preparations. Amalgam may be selected for posterior class VI preparations because of its wear resistance and longevity. Moisture control for Class VI restorations is usually achieved with cotton roll isolation. Class VI amalgam preparations may be accomplished with a small tapered fissure bur (e.g., No. 169 L or 271) and involves extension to place the cavosurface margin on enamel that has sound dentin support (see Fig. 14-101). The preparation walls may need to diverge occlusally to ensure a 90-degree cavosurface margin. A depth of 1.5 mm is sufficient to provide bulk of material for strength. Retention of the restoration is ensured by the creation of small undercuts along the internal line angles. Do not remove dentin that is immediately supporting enamel. Conservative tooth preparation is particularly important with Class VI preparations because it is easy to undermine the enamel on incisal edges and cusp tips. Inserting, carving, and polishing are similar to procedures described for Class I tooth preparations for amalgam.

Some older patients have excessive occlusal wear of most of their teeth in the form of large concave areas with much exposed dentin. Teeth with excessive wear may require indirect restorations.

Summary

Class I and II amalgam restorations are still common procedures performed by general dentists. Class VI amalgam restorations are done infrequently. It is important for practitioners to understand the indications, advantages, techniques, and limitations of these restorations. When used correctly and in properly selected cases, these restorations have the potential to serve for many years (Fig. 14-103).

References

1. Bjertness E, Sonju T: Survival analysis of amalgam restorations in long-term recall patients, *Acta Odontol Scand* 48:93, 1990.
2. Downer MC, Azli NA, Bedi R, et al: How long do routine restorations last? A systematic review, *Br Dent J* 187:432, 1999.
3. Letzel H, van 't Hof MA, Marshall GW, et al: The influence of the amalgam alloy on the survival of amalgam restorations: A secondary analysis of multiple controlled clinical trials, *J Dent Res* 76:1787, 1997.
4. Mjör IA, Jokstad A, Qvist V: Longevity of posterior restorations, *Int Dent J* 40:11, 1990.
5. Osborne JW, Norman RD: 13-year clinical assessment of 10 amalgam alloys, *Dent Mater* 6:189, 1990.
6. Osborne JW, Norman RD, Gale EN: A 14-year clinical assessment of 12 amalgam alloys, *Quintessence Int* 22:857, 1991.
7. Maryniuk GA: In search of treatment longevity—a 30-year perspective, *J Am Dent Assoc* 109:739, 1984.
8. Maryniuk GA, Kaplan SH: Longevity of restorations: survey results of dentists' estimates and attitudes, *J Am Dent Assoc* 112:39, 1986.
9. Jokstad A, Mjor IA: The quality of routine class II cavity preparations for amalgam, *Acta Odontol Scand* 47:53, 1989.
10. Kreulen CM, Tobi H, Gruythuysen RJ, et al: Replacement risk of amalgam treatment modalities: 15-year results, *J Dent* 26:627, 1998.
11. Smales RJ: Longevity of low- and high-copper amalgams analyzed by preparation class, tooth site, patient age, and operator, *Oper Dent* 16:162, 1991.
12. Bader JD, Shugars DA: Variations in dentists' clinical decisions, *J Public Health Dent* 55:181, 1995.
13. Burgess JO: Dental materials for the restorations of root surface caries, *Am J Dent* 8:342, 1995.
14. Gottlieb EW, Retief DH, Bradley EL: Microleakage of conventional and high-copper amalgam restorations, *J Prosthet Dent* 53:355, 1985.
15. Hilton TJ: Can modern restorative procedures and materials reliably seal cavities? In vitro investigations: Part 2, *Am J Dent* 15:279, 2002.
16. Dilley DC, Vann WF Jr, Oldenburg TR, et al: Time required for placement of composite versus amalgam restorations, *J Dent Child* 57:177, 1990.
17. Gilmore HW: Pulpal considerations for operative dentistry, *J Prosthet Dent* 14:752, 1964.
18. Almquist TC, Cowan RD, Lambert RL: Conservative amalgam restorations, *J Prosthet Dent* 29:524, 1973.
19. Markley MR: Restorations of silver amalgam, *J Am Dent Assoc* 43:133, 1951.
20. Berry TG, Laswell HR, Osborne JW, et al: Width of isthmus and marginal failure of restorations of amalgam, *Oper Dent* 6:55, 1981.

21. Osborne JW, Gale EN: Relationship of restoration width, tooth position and alloy to fracture at the margins of 13- to 14-year-old amalgams, *J Dent Res* 69:1599, 1990.
22. Goel VK, Khera SC, Gurusami S, et al: Effect of cavity depth on stresses in a restored tooth, *J Prosthet Dent* 67:174, 1992.
23. Lagouvardos P, Sourai P, Douvitsas G: Coronal fractures in posterior teeth, *Oper Dent* 14:28, 1989.
24. Osborne JW, Gale EN: Failure at the margin of amalgams as affected by cavity width, tooth position, and alloy selection, *J Dent Res* 60:681, 1981.
25. Anusavice KJ, editor: *Phillips' science of dental materials*, ed 11, St. Louis, 2003, Mosby.
26. Council on Dental Materials, Instruments, and Equipment: Dental mercury hygiene: summary of recommendations in 1990, *J Am Dent Assoc* 122:112, 1991.
27. Sockwell CL: Dental handpieces and rotary cutting instruments, *Dent Clin North Am* 15:219, 1971.
28. Goho C, Aaron GR: Enhancement of anti-microbial properties of cavity varnish: A preliminary report, *J Prosthet Dent* 68:623, 1992.
29. Blaser PK, Lund MR, Cochran MA, et al: Effect of designs of Class 2 preparations on resistance of teeth to fracture, *Oper Dent* 8:6, 1983.
30. Vale WA: Tooth preparation and further thoughts on high speed, *Br Dent J* 107:333, 1959.
31. Gilmore HW: Restorative materials and tooth preparation design, *Dent Clin North Am* 15:99, 1971.
32. Fusayama T: Two layers of carious dentin: Diagnosis and treatment, *Oper Dent* 4:63, 1979.
33. Hebling J, Giro EM, Costa CA: Human pulp response after an adhesive system application in deep cavities, *J Dent* 27:557, 1999.
34. Hilton TJ: Cavity sealers, liners, and bases: Current philosophies and indications for use, *Oper Dent* 21:134, 1996.
35. Eliades G, Palaghias G: In-vitro characterization of visible-light-cured glass-ionomer liners, *Dent Mater* 9:198, 1993.
36. Wieczkowski G Jr, Yu XY, Joynt RB, et al: Microleakage evaluation in amalgam restorations used with bases, *J Esthet Dent* 4:37, 1992.
37. Robbins JW: The placement of bases beneath amalgam restorations: Review of literature and recommendations for use, *J Am Dent Assoc* 113:910, 1986.
38. Mahler DB, Terkla LG: Analysis of stress in dental structures, *Dent Clin North Am* 2:789, 1958.
39. Vlietstra JR, Sidaway DA, Plant CG: Cavity cleansers, *Br Dent J* 149:293, 1980.
40. Berry FA, Parker SD, Rice D, et al: Microleakage of amalgam restorations using dentin bonding system primers, *Am J Dent* 9:174, 1996.
41. Schüpbach P, Lutz F, Finger WJ: Closing of dentinal tubules by Gluma desensitizer, *Eur J Oral Sci* 105:414, 1997.
42. Mahler DB, Nelson LW: Sensitivity answers sought in amalgam alloy microleakage study, *J Am Dent Assoc* 125:282, 1994.
43. Ziskind D, Venezia E, Kreisman I, et al: Amalgam type, adhesive system, and storage period as influencing factors on microleakage of amalgam restorations, *J Prosthet Dent* 90:255, 2003.
44. Lindemuth JS, Hagge MS, Broome JS: Effect of restoration size on fracture resistance of bonded amalgam restorations, *Oper Dent* 25:177, 2000.
45. Mahler DB: The amalgam-tooth interface, *Oper Dent* 21:230, 1996.
46. Symons AL, Wing G, Hewitt GH: Adaptation of eight modern dental amalgams to walls of Class I cavity preparations, *J Oral Rehabil* 14:55, 1987.
47. Hilton TJ: Sealers, liners, and bases, *J Esthet Restor Dent* 15:141, 2003.
48. Bauer JG: A study of procedures for burnishing amalgam restorations, *J Prosthet Dent* 57:669, 1987.
49. Lovadino JR, Ruhnke LA, Consani S: Influence of burnishing on amalgam adaptation to cavity walls, *J Prosthet Dent* 58:284, 1987.
50. Restoration of tooth preparations with amalgam and tooth-colored materials: Project ACCORDE student syllabus, Washington, D.C., 1974, US Department of Health, Education, and Welfare.
51. Kanai S: Structure studies of amalgam II: Effect of burnishing on the margins of occlusal amalgam fillings, *Acta Odontol Scand* 24:47, 1966.
52. May KN, Wilder AD, Leinfelder KF: Clinical evaluation of various burnishing techniques on high-copper amalgam [abstract], *J Prosthet Dent* 61:213, 1982.
53. May KN Jr, Wilder AD Jr, Leinfelder KF: Burnished amalgam restorations: a two-year evaluation, *J Prosthet Dent* 49:193, 1983.
54. Straffon LH, Corpron RE, Dennison JB, et al: A clinical evaluation of polished and unpolished amalgams: 36-month results, *Pediatr Dent* 6:220, 1984.
55. Collins CJ, Bryant RW: Finishing of amalgam restorations: a three-year clinical study, *J Dent* 20:202, 1992.
56. Drummond JL, Jung H, Savers EE, et al: Surface roughness of polished amalgams, *Oper Dent* 17:129, 1992.
57. Moffa JP: The longevity and reasons for replacement of amalgam alloys [abstract], *J Dent Res* 68:188, 1989.
58. Summitt JB, Burgess JO, Berry TG, et al: Six-year clinical evaluation of bonded and pin-retained complex amalgam restorations, *Oper Dent* 29:261, 2004.
59. Mayhew RB, Schmeltzer LD, Pierson WP: Effect of polishing on the marginal integrity of high-copper amalgams, *Oper Dent* 11:8, 1986.
60. Osborne JW, Leinfelder KF, Gale EN, et al: Two independent evaluations of ten amalgam alloys, *J Prosthet Dent* 43:622, 1980.
61. Dias de Souza GM, Pereira GD, Dias CT, et al: Fracture resistance of teeth restored with the bonded amalgam technique, *Oper Dent* 26:511, 2001.
62. Mahler DB, Engle JH: Clinical evaluation of amalgam bonding in class I and II restorations, *J Am Dent Assoc* 131:43, 2000.
63. Smales RJ, Wetherell JD: Review of bonded amalgam restorations and assessment in a general practice over five years, *Oper Dent* 25:374, 2000.
64. Larson TD, Douglas WH, Geistfeld RE: Effect of prepared cavities on the strength of teeth, *Oper Dent* 6:2, 1981.
65. Rodda JC: Modern class II amalgam tooth preparations, *N Z Dent J* 68:132, 1972.
66. Joynt RB, Davis EL, Wieczkowski G Jr, et al: Fracture resistance of posterior teeth with glass ionomer-composite resin systems, *J Prosthet Dent* 62:28, 1989.
67. Osborne JW, Summitt JB: Extension for prevention: is it relevant today? *Am J Dent* 11:189, 1998.
68. Summitt JB, Osborne JW: Initial preparations for amalgam restorations: Extending the longevity of the tooth-restoration unit, *J Am Dent Assoc* 123:67, 1992.
69. Leon AR: The periodontium and restorative procedures: A critical review, *J Oral Rehabil* 4:105, 1977.
70. Loe H: Reactions of marginal periodontal tissues to restorative procedures, *Int Dent J* 18:759, 1968.
71. Waerhaug J: Histologic considerations which govern where the margins of restorations should be located in relation to the gingivae, *Dent Clin North Am* 4:161, 1960.
72. Della Bona A, Summitt JB: The effect of amalgam bonding on resistance form of class II amalgam restorations, *Quintessence Int* 29:95, 1998.
73. Görücü J, et al: Effects of preparation designs and adhesive systems on retention of class II amalgam restorations, *J Prosthet Dent* 78:250, 1997.
74. Mondelli J, Ishikiriama A, de Lima Navarro MF, et al: Fracture strength of amalgam restorations in modern Class II preparations with proximal retentive grooves, *J Prosthet Dent* 32:564, 1974.
75. Mondelli J, Francischone CE, Steagall L, et al: Influence of proximal retention on the fracture strength of Class II amalgam restorations, *J Prosthet Dent* 46:420, 1981.
76. Summitt JB, Howell ML, Burgess JO, et al: Effect of grooves on resistance form of conservative class 2 amalgams, *Oper Dent* 17:50, 1992.
77. Moore DL: Retentive grooves for the Class 2 amalgam restoration: Necessity or hazard? *Oper Dent* 17:29, 1992.
78. Sturdevant JR, Taylor DF, Leonard RH, et al: Conservative preparation designs for Class II amalgam restorations, *Dent Mater* 3:144, 1987.
79. Crockett WD, Shepard FE, Moon PC, et al: The influence of proximal retention grooves on the retention and resistance of class II preparations for amalgam, *J Am Dent Assoc* 91:1053, 1975.
80. Summitt JB, Osborne JW, Burgess JO, et al: Effect of grooves on resistance form of Class 2 amalgams with wide occlusal preparations, *Oper Dent* 18:42, 1993.
81. Khera SC, Chan KC: Microleakage and enamel finish, *J Prosthet Dent* 39:414, 1978.
82. Summitt JB, Osborne JW, Burgess JO: Effect of grooves on resistance/retention form of Class 2 approximal slot amalgam restorations, *Oper Dent* 18:209, 1993.
83. Gwinnett AJ, Baratieri LN, Monteiro S Jr, et al: Adhesive restorations with amalgam: guidelines for the clinician, *Quintessence Int* 25:687, 1994.
84. Mondelli RF, Barbosa WF, Mondelli J, et al: Fracture strength of weakened human premolars restored with amalgam with and without cusp coverage, *Am J Dent* 11:181, 1998.
85. Smales RJ: Longevity of cusp-covered amalgams: Survival after 15 years, *Oper Dent* 16:17, 1991.
86. Duncalf WV, Wilson NHF: Adaptation and condensation of amalgam restorations in Class II preparations of conventional and conservative design, *Quintessence Int* 23:499, 1992.
87. Jokstad A, Mjor IA: Cavity design and marginal degradation of the occlusal part of Class II amalgam restorations, *Acta Odontol Scand* 48:389, 1990.
88. Pack AR: The amalgam overhang dilemma: A review of causes and effects, prevention, and removal, *N Z Dent J* 85:55, 1989.

Chapter 15

Class III and V Amalgam Restorations

Lee W. Boushell, Theodore M. Roberson, Aldridge D. Wilder, Jr.

This chapter presents information about Class III and V amalgam restorations. Class III restorations are indicated for defects located on the proximal surface of anterior teeth that do not affect the incisal edge. Part of the facial or the lingual surfaces also may be involved in Class III restorations. Class V restorations are indicated to restore defects on the facial or lingual cervical one third of any tooth.

The Class III amalgam restoration is rarely used. Its use has been supplanted by tooth-colored restorations (primarily composite), which have become increasingly wear-resistant and color-stable. Because indications exist for Class III amalgam restorations, however, practitioners should be familiar with this restorative technique.

The Class V amalgam restoration can be especially technique-sensitive because of location, extent of caries, and limited access and visibility. Cervical caries usually develops because of the chronic presence of acidogenic plaque located in the non–self-cleansing area just beneath the coronal height of contour. Patients with gingival recession are predisposed to cervical caries because dentin is more susceptible to demineralization than enamel. Patients with a reduced salivary flow caused by certain medical conditions (e.g., Sjögren's syndrome), medications, or head and neck radiation therapy also also are predisposed to cervical caries. These patients usually have less saliva to buffer the acids produced by oral bacteria. Patients with gingival recession that has exposed the root surface have a predisposition to *root caries* because dentin is more susceptible to demineralization than enamel. Class V restorations may be used to treat both cervical and root caries lesions.

Incipient, smooth-surface enamel caries appears as a chalky white line just occlusal or incisal to the crest of the marginal gingiva (usually on the facial surface) (Fig. 15-1). These areas often are overlooked in the oral examination, unless teeth are free of debris, isolated with cotton rolls, and dried gently with the air syringe. When incipient cervical caries has not decalcified the enamel sufficiently to result in cavitation (i.e., a break in the continuity of the surface), the lesion may be remineralized by appropriate techniques, including patient motivation

toward proper diet and hygiene. Occasionally, an enamel surface that is only slightly cavitated may be treated successfully by smoothing with sandpaper disks, polishing, and treating with a fluoride varnish or a dentin adhesive in an attempt to prevent further caries that may require treatment. This prophylactic, preventive treatment cannot be instituted if caries has progressed to decalcify and soften enamel to an appreciable depth. In this instance, a Class V tooth preparation and restoration is indicated, particularly if caries has penetrated to the dentinoenamel junction (DEJ) (Fig. 15-2, *A*). When numerous cervical lesions are present (see Fig. 15-2, *B*), a relatively high caries index is obvious. In addition to the restorative treatment, the patient should be instructed and encouraged to implement an aggressive prevention program to avoid recurrent decay.

Pertinent Material Qualities and Properties

Material qualities and properties important for Class III and V amalgam restorations are strength, longevity, ease of use, and past success. See Chapter 13 for a discussion of the pertinent material qualities and properties of amalgam.

Indications

Few indications exist for a Class III amalgam restoration. It is generally reserved for the distal surface of maxillary and mandibular canines if (1) the preparation is extensive with only minimal facial involvement, (2) the gingival margin primarily involves cementum, or (3) moisture control is difficult. For esthetic reasons, amalgam rarely is indicated for the proximal surfaces of incisors and the mesial surface of canines.

Class V amalgam restorations may be used anywhere in the mouth. As with Class III amalgam restorations, they generally are reserved for non-esthetic areas, for areas where access and visibility are limited and where moisture control is difficult, and for areas that are significantly deep gingivally. Because of limited access and visibility, many Class V restorations are difficult and present special problems during the preparation and restorative procedures.

One measure of clinical success of cervical amalgam restorations is the length of time the restoration serves without failing (Fig. 15-3). Properly placed Class V amalgams have the

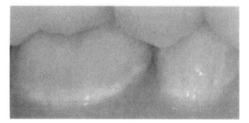

Fig. 15-1 Incipient caries lesions of enamel appear as white spots. The affected surface may be smooth (i.e., non-cavitated). White spots are more visible when dried. *(From Cobourne MT, DiBiase AT:* Handbook of orthodontics, *Edinburgh, 2010, Mosby.)*

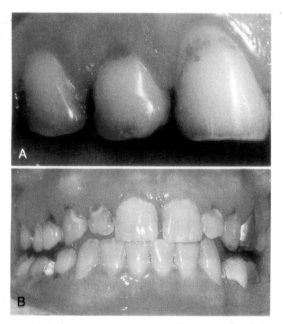

Fig. 15-2 Cervical caries. **A,** Cavitation involving enamel and dentin in several teeth. **B,** Relatively high caries index is obvious when numerous cervical lesions are present. *(From Perry DA, Beemsterboer PL:* Periodontology for the dental hygienist, *ed 3, St. Louis, 2007, Saunders.)*

potential to be clinically acceptable for many years. Some cervical amalgam restorations show evidence of failure, however, even after a short period. Inattention to tooth preparation principles, improper manipulation of the restorative material, and moisture contamination contribute to early failure. Extended service depends on the operator's care in following accepted treatment techniques and proper care by the patient.

Amalgam may be used on partial denture abutment teeth because amalgam resists wear as clasps move over the restoration. Contours prepared in the restoration to retentive areas for the clasp tips may be achieved relatively easily and maintained when an amalgam restoration is used. Occasionally, amalgam is preferred when the caries lesion extends gingivally enough that a mucoperiosteal flap must be reflected for adequate access and visibility (Fig. 15-4). Proper surgical procedures must be followed, including sterile technique, careful soft tissue management, and complete debridement of the surgical and operative site before closure.

Contraindications

Class III and V amalgam restorations usually are contraindicated in esthetically important areas because many patients object to metal restorations that are visible (Fig. 15-5). Generally, Class V amalgams placed on the facial surface of mandibular canines, premolars, and molars are not readily visible. Amalgams placed on maxillary premolars and first molars may be visible. The patient's esthetic demands should be considered when planning treatment.

Advantages

Amalgam restorations are stronger than other Class III and V direct restorations. In addition, they are generally easier to place and may be less expensive to the patient. Because of its metallic color, amalgam is easily distinguished from the surrounding tooth structure. Amalgam restorations are usually easier to finish and polish without damage to the adjacent surfaces.

Disadvantages

The primary disadvantage of Class III and V amalgam restorations is that they are metallic and unesthetic. In addition, the preparation for an amalgam restoration typically requires

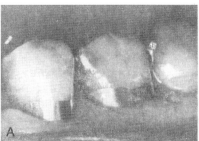
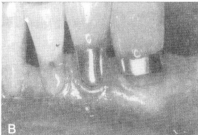
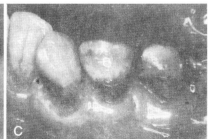

Fig. 15-3 **A,** 6-year-old cervical amalgam restorations. **B,** After 16 years, some abrasion and erosion are evident at the gingival margin of the lateral incisor and canine restorations. **C,** 20-year-old cervical amalgam restorations.

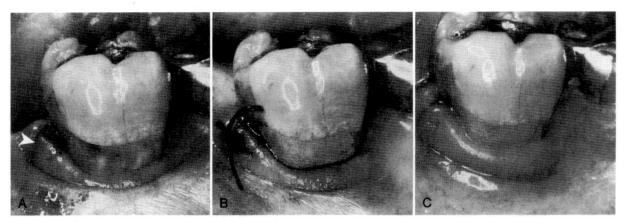

Fig. 15-4 Surgical access. **A,** Class V preparation requiring mucoperiosteal flap reflection with a releasing incision (*arrowhead*). **B,** Completed restoration with suture in place. **C,** Suture removed 1-week after the procedure.

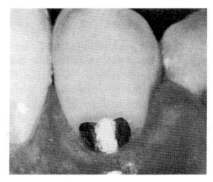

Fig. 15-5 Patients may object to metal restorations that are visible during conversation.

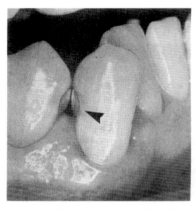

Fig. 15-6 Restoration for Class III tooth preparation using facial approach on mandibular canine. Restoration is 5 years old. *(Courtesy of Dr. C. L. Sockwell.)*

90-degree cavosurface margins and specific axial depths that allow incorporation of secondary retentive features. These features result in a less conservative preparation than that required for most esthetic restorative materials.

Clinical Technique for Class III Amalgam Restorations

Initial Procedures

After appropriate review of the patient records (including medical history), treatment plan, and radiographs, the gingival extension of the preparation should be anticipated. Anesthesia is usually necessary when a vital tooth is to be restored. Pre-wedging in the gingival embrasure of the proximal site to be restored provides (1) better protection of soft tissue and the rubber dam, (2) better access because of the slight separation of teeth, and (3) better re-establishment of the proximal contact. The use of a rubber dam is generally recommended; however, cotton roll isolation is acceptable if moisture can be adequately controlled.

Tooth Preparation

A lingual access preparation on the distal surface of the maxillary canine is described here because the use of amalgam in

that location is more likely. For esthetic reasons, use of amalgam is best suited for caries that can be accessed from the lingual rather from the facial. A facial approach for a mandibular canine may be indicated, however, if the lesion is more facial than lingual. The mandibular restoration is often not visible at conversational distance (Fig. 15-6).

The outline form of the Class III amalgam preparation may include only the proximal surface. A lingual dovetail may be indicated if one existed previously or if additional retention is needed for a larger restoration.

Initial Tooth Preparation

Bur size selection depends on the anticipated size of the lesion. Bur options may include a No. 2 (or smaller) round bur or No. 330 bur. The bur is positioned so that the entry cut penetrates into the caries lesion, which is usually apical to (and slightly into) the contact area. Ideally, the bur is positioned so that its long axis is perpendicular to the lingual surface of the tooth, but directed at a mesial angle as close to the adjacent tooth as possible. (The bur position may be described as perpendicular to the distolingual line angle of the tooth.) This position conserves the marginal ridge enamel (Fig. 15-7, *A*

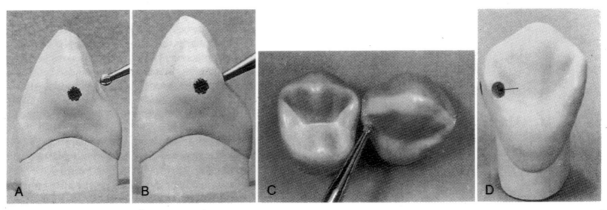

Fig. 15-7 Entry for Class III tooth preparation on maxillary canine. **A,** Bur position is perpendicular to the enamel surface at the point of entry. **B,** Initial penetration through enamel is directed toward cavitated, caries lesion. **C,** Initial entry should isolate the proximal enamel, while preserving as much of the marginal ridge as possible. **D,** Initial cutting reveals the dentinoenamel junction (DEJ) *(arrow)*.

through *C*). Penetration through enamel positions the bur so that additional cutting isolates the proximal enamel affected by caries and removes some or all of the infected dentin. In addition, penetration should be at a limited initial axial depth (i.e., 0.5–0.6 mm) inside the DEJ (see Fig. 15-7, *C* and *D*) or at a 0.75-0.8-mm axial depth when the gingival margin is on the root surface (in cementum) (Fig. 15-8). This 0.75-mm axial depth on the root surface allows a 0.25-mm distance (the diameter of the No. ¼ bur is 0.5 mm) between the retention groove (which is placed later) and the gingival cavosurface margin. Infected dentin that is deeper than this limited initial axial depth is removed later during final tooth preparation.

For a small lesion, the facial margin is extended 0.2-0.3 mm into the facial embrasure (if necessary), with a curved outline from the incisal to the gingival margin (resulting in a less visible margin). The lingual outline blends with the incisal and gingival margins in a smooth curve, creating a preparation with little or no lingual wall. The cavosurface angle should be 90 degrees at all margins. The facial, incisal, and gingival walls should meet the axial wall at approximately right angles (although the lingual wall meets the axial wall at an obtuse angle or may be continuous with the axial wall) (Fig. 15-9). If a large round bur is used, the internal angles are more rounded. The axial wall should be uniformly deep into dentin and follow the faciolingual contour of the external tooth surface (Fig. 15-10). The initial axial wall depth may be in sound dentin (i.e., shallow lesion), in infected dentin (i.e., moderate to deep lesion), or in existing restorative material, if a restoration is being replaced.

Incisal extension to remove carious tooth structure may eliminate the proximal contact (Fig. 15-11). It is important to conserve as much of the distoincisal tooth structure as possible to reduce the risk for subsequent fracture. When possible, it is best to leave the incisal margin in contact with the adjacent tooth.

When preparing a gingival wall that is near the level of the rubber dam or apical to it, it is beneficial to place a wedge in the gingival embrasure earlier to depress and protect soft tissue and the rubber dam. As the bur is preparing the gingival wall, it may lightly shave the wedge. A triangular (i.e., anatomic) wedge, rather than a round wedge, is used for a deep gingival margin.

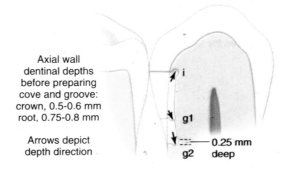

Axial wall dentinal depths before preparing cove and groove: crown, 0.5-0.6 mm root, 0.75-0.8 mm

Arrows depict depth direction

i
g1
0.25 mm
g2 deep

Fig. 15-8 Mesiodistal vertical section showing location, depth direction *(arrows)*, and direction depth of the retention form in Class III tooth preparations of different gingival depths. *i,* incisal cove; *g1,* gingival groove, enamel margin; *g2,* gingival groove, root surface margin. Distance from outer aspect of *g2* groove to margin is approximately 0.3 mm; bur head diameter is 0.5 mm; direction depth of groove is half this diameter (or approximately 0.3 mm [0.25 mm]).

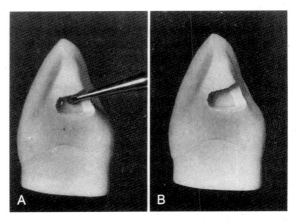

Fig. 15-9 Class III tooth preparation on maxillary canine. **A,** Round bur shaping the incisal area. The incisal angle remains. **B,** Initial shape of the preparation accomplished with a round bur.

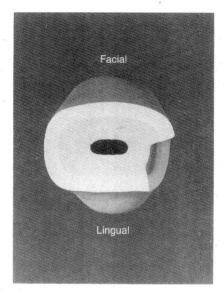

Fig. 15-10 Transverse section of mandibular lateral incisor illustrating that the lingual wall of a Class III tooth preparation may meet the axial wall at an obtuse angle and that the axial wall is a uniform depth into dentin and follows the faciolingual contour of the external tooth surface.

The initial tooth preparation is completed by using a No. ½ round bur to accentuate the axial line angles (Fig. 15-12, A and B), particularly the axiogingival angle. This facilitates the subsequent placement of retention grooves and leaves the internal line angles slightly rounded. Rounded internal preparation angles permit more complete condensation of the amalgam. The No. ½ round bur also may be used to smooth any roughened, undermined enamel produced at the gingival and facial cavosurface margins (see Fig. 15-12, C). The incisal margin of the minimally extended preparation is often not accessible to the larger round bur without marring the adjacent tooth (see Fig. 15-12, D). Further finishing of the incisal margin is presented later. At this point, the initial tooth preparation is completed.

Final Tooth Preparation

Final tooth preparation involves removing any remaining infected dentin; protecting the pulp; developing secondary resistance and retention forms; finishing external walls; and cleaning, inspecting, and desensitizing or bonding. Any remaining infected carious dentin on the axial wall is removed by using a slowly revolving round bur (No. 2 or No. 4),

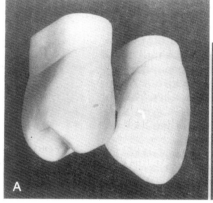

Fig. 15-11 Distofacial (A) and incisal (B) views of the canine to show the curved proximal outline necessary to preserve the distoincisal corner of the tooth. The incisal margin of this preparation example is located slightly incisally of the proximal contact (but whenever possible, the margin may be in the contact area).

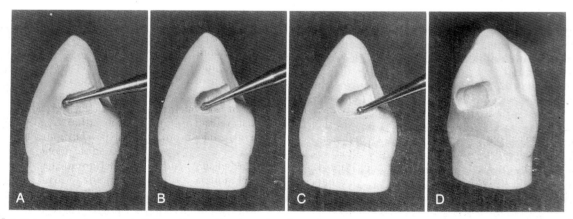

Fig. 15-12 Refining proximal portion. **A–C,** A small, round bur is used to shape the preparation walls, define line angles, and initiate removal of any undermined enamel along the gingival and facial margins. **D,** Tooth preparation completed, except for the final finishing of the enamel margins and placing the retention form.

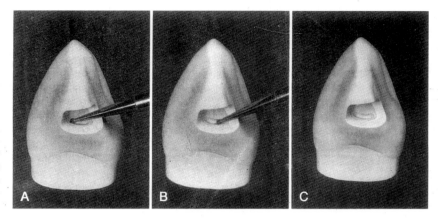

Fig. 15-13 Preparing the gingival retention form. **A,** Position of No. ¼ round bur in axio-facio-gingival point angle. **B,** Advancing the bur lingually to prepare the groove along the axiogingival line angle. (See Fig. 15-8 regarding location, depth direction, and direction depth of groove.) **C,** Completed gingival retention groove.

appropriate spoon excavators, or both. (See Chapter 5 for the indications and technique for placing a liner.)

For the Class III amalgam restoration, resistance form against post-restorative fracture is provided by (1) cavosurface and amalgam margins of 90 degrees, (2) enamel walls supported by sound dentin, (3) sufficient bulk of amalgam (minimal 1-mm thickness), and (4) no sharp preparation internal angles. The box-like preparation form provides primary retention form. Secondary retention form is provided by a gingival groove, an incisal cove, and sometimes a lingual dovetail.

The gingival retention groove is prepared by placing a No. ¼ round bur (rotating at low speed) in the axio-facio-gingival point angle. It is positioned in the dentin to maintain 0.2 mm of dentin between the groove and the DEJ. The rotating bur is moved lingually along the axiogingival line angle, with the angle of cutting generally bisecting the angle between the gingival and axial walls. Ideally, the direction of the gingival groove is slightly more gingival than axial (and the direction of an incisal [i.e., occlusal] groove would be slightly more incisal [i.e., occlusal] than axial) (Fig. 15-13; see also Fig. 15-8).

Alternatively, if less retention form is needed, two gingival coves may be used, as opposed to a continuous groove. One each may be placed in the axio-gingivo-facial and axio-gingivo-lingual point angles. The diameter of the ¼ round bur is 0.5 mm, and the depth of the groove should be half this diameter (0.25 mm). (See the location and depthwise direction of the groove, where the gingival wall remains in enamel, in Fig. 15-18.) When preparing a retention groove on the root surface (gingival wall in cementum or dentin), the angle of cutting is more gingival, resulting in the distance from the gingival cavosurface margin to the groove being approximately 0.3 mm (see Fig. 15-8). Careful technique is necessary in preparing the gingival retention groove. If the dentin that supports gingival enamel is removed, enamel is subject to fracture. In addition, if the groove is placed only in the axial wall, no effective retention form is developed, and a risk of pulpal involvement is possible.

An incisal retention cove is prepared at the axio-facio-incisal point angle with a No. ¼ round bur in dentin, being careful not to undermine enamel. It is directed similarly into the incisal point angle and prepared to half the diameter of the bur (Fig. 15-14). Undermining the incisal enamel should

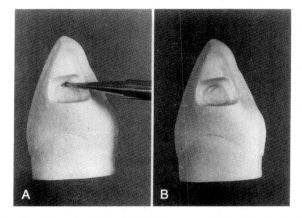

Fig. 15-14 Preparing the incisal retention cove. **A,** Position of No. ¼ round bur in the axioincisal point angle. **B,** Completed incisal cove.

be avoided. For the maxillary canine, the palm-and-thumb grasp may be used to direct the bur incisally (Fig. 15-15). This completes the typical Class III amalgam tooth preparation (Fig. 15-16). Similar to Class I and II amalgams, it is recommended that the clinician prepare mechanical retention.

A lingual dovetail is not required in small or moderately sized Class III amalgam restorations. It may be used in large preparations, especially preparations with excessive incisal extension in which additional retention form is needed. The dovetail may not be necessary (even in large preparations), however, if an incisal secondary retention form can be accomplished (Fig. 15-17).

If a lingual dovetail is needed, it is prepared only after initial preparation of the proximal portion has been completed. Otherwise, the tooth structure needed for the isthmus between the proximal portion and the dovetail may be removed when the proximal outline form is prepared. The lingual dovetail should be conservative, generally not extending beyond the mesiodistal midpoint of the lingual surface; this varies according to the extent of the proximal caries. The axial depth of the dovetail should approximate 1 mm, and the axial wall should be parallel to the lingual surface of the tooth. This wall may or may not be in dentin. The No. 245 bur is positioned in the proximal portion at the correct depth and angulation and moved in a mesial direction (Fig. 15-18, *A* and *B*). The correct angulation places the long axis of the bur perpendicular to the lingual surface. The bur is moved to the point that corresponds to the most mesial extent of the dovetail (see Fig. 15-18, *C* and *D*). The bur is then moved incisally and gingivally to create sufficient incisogingival dimension to the dovetail (approximately 2.5 mm) (see Fig. 15-18, *E* and *F*). The incisal and gingival walls of the isthmus are prepared in smooth curves connecting the dovetail to the proximal outline form (see Fig. 15-18, *G* and *H*).

The gingival margin trimmer can be used to bevel (or round) the axiopulpal line angle (i.e., the junction of the proximal and dovetail preparation). This increases the strength of the restoration at the junction of the proximal and lingual portions by providing bulk and reducing stress concentration. The lingual convergence of the dovetail's external walls (prepared with the No. 245 bur) usually provides a sufficient retention form. Retention coves, one in the incisal corner and one in the gingival corner (Fig. 15-19), may be placed in the dovetail to enhance retention if the axial wall of the dovetail is in dentin. The coves are prepared with the No. ¼ round bur in dentin that does not immediately support the lingual enamel. This preparation may require deepening of the axial wall. Unsupported enamel is removed, the walls or margins are smoothed, and the cavosurface angles are refined, where indicated. The 8-3-22 hoe is recommended for finishing minimally extended margins (Fig. 15-20). If the gingival margin is in enamel, a slight bevel (approximately 20 degrees) is necessary to ensure full-length enamel rods forming the cavosurface margin. All the walls of the preparation should meet the external tooth surface to form a right angle (i.e., butt joint) (Fig. 15-21; see also Fig. 15-16). The various steps involved in the clinical procedure with the dovetail are shown in Figure 15-22. The completed tooth

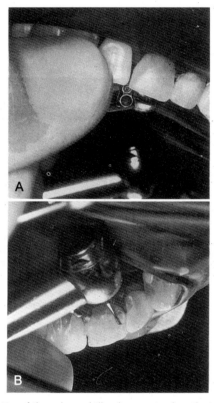

Fig. 15-15 Use of the palm-and-thumb grasp to place the incisal retention cove. **A,** Hand position showing thumb rest. **B,** Handpiece position for preparing the incisal retention.

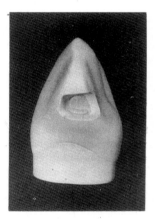

Fig. 15-16 Completed Class III tooth preparation for amalgam restoration.

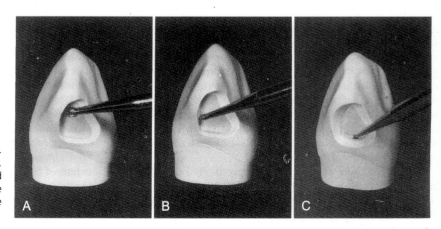

Fig. 15-17 Extensive Class III tooth preparation. **A,** Initial tooth preparation with No. 2 round bur. **B,** Defining line angles and removing undermined enamel with No. ½ round bur. **C,** Placing the retention groove using No. ¼ round bur. Note the completed incisal cove.

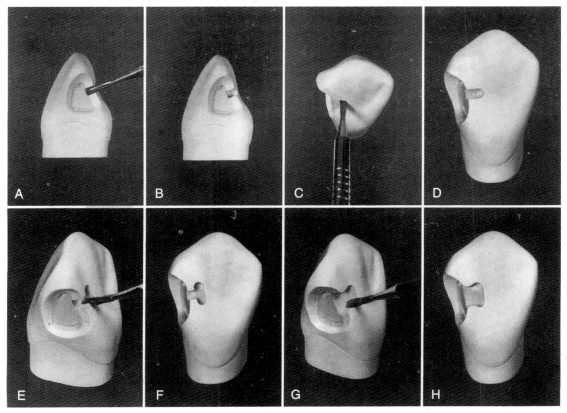

Fig. 15-18 Lingual dovetail providing additional retention for extensive amalgam restoration. **A,** Bur position at correct depth and angulation to begin cutting. **B,** Initial cut in beginning dovetail. **C,** Bur moved to most mesial extent of dovetail. **D,** If possible, cutting should not extend beyond the midlingual position. **E,** Bur cutting gingival extension of the dovetail. **F,** Incisal and gingival extensions of the dovetail. **G,** Completing the isthmus. The proximal and lingual portions are connected by the incisal and gingival walls in smooth curves. **H,** Completed lingual dovetail.

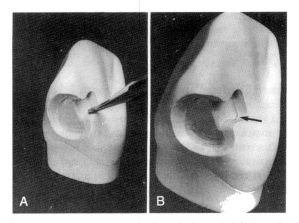

Fig. 15-19 Ensuring retention in lingual dovetail (often optional). **A,** Position of No. 33½ bur for cutting the retention cove. **B,** Preparation of the cove should not remove the dentinal support of the lingual enamel (*arrow*).

preparation should be cleaned of any residual debris and inspected. Careful assessment should be made to see that all of the caries has been removed, that the depth and retention are appropriate, and that cavosurface margins provide for the amalgam bulk.

Restorative Technique
Desensitizer Placement

The use of a dentin desensitizer over the prepared tooth structure before placing amalgam is generally recommended. The dentin desensitizer is rubbed onto the prepared tooth surface for 30 seconds and excess moisture is removed without desiccating the dentin.

Matrix Placement

The wedged, rigid material–supported sectional matrix may be used for the Class III amalgam restoration. Insertion of amalgam into the Class III tooth preparation is usually from the lingual aspect. It is essential to trim the lingual portion of the sectional matrix material correctly to avoid covering the preparation and blocking access for insertion of the amalgam. A length of ⁵⁄₁₆ inch (8 mm) wide, 0.002 inch (0.05 mm) thick stainless steel matrix material that covers one-third of the facial surface and extends through the proximal to the lingual surface is obtained. The lingual portion is trimmed at an angle that corresponds approximately to the slope of the lingual surface of the tooth (Fig. 15-23). The section of matrix is burnished on a resilient paper pad to create the desired contact and contour form. The sectional matrix is placed in position and wedged from the facial or lingual embrasure, whichever

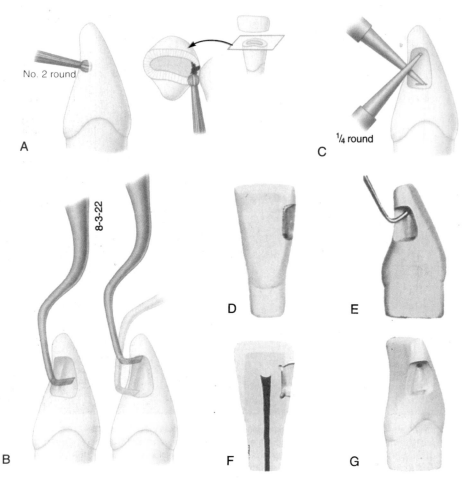

Fig. 15-20 Class III tooth preparation for amalgam restoration on the mandibular incisor. **A,** Entering the tooth from the lingual approach. **B,** Finishing the facial, incisal, and gingival enamel margins with an 8-3-22 triple angle hoe. Note how the reverse bevel blade is used on the gingival enamel. **C,** Placing incisal and gingival retention forms with No. ¼ round bur. **D,** Dotted line indicates the outline of the additional extension that is sometimes necessary for access in placing the incisal retention cove. **E,** Position of a bi-beveled hatchet to place the incisal retention cove. **F,** The axial wall forms a convex surface over the pulp. **G,** Completed tooth preparation. Note the gingival retention groove.

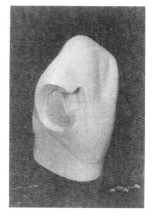

Fig. 15-21 Completed distolingual Class III tooth preparation for amalgam.

is greater. The facial and lingual portions of the matrix are stabilized with a rigid material (see Fig. 15-22, *G*). Precontoured metallic matrices may be used (instead of custom-made matrices) if the contour of the precontoured matrix coincides with that of the proximal surface being restored. If the preparation is small and the matrix is sufficiently rigid, additional rigid material to support the matrix may not be required.

Condensation and Carving

Insertion of the amalgam, initial carving, matrix removal, wedge removal, and final carving are similar to the techniques for posterior teeth (see Chapter 14). When properly placed, conservative restorations in incisors and canines are relatively inconspicuous (Fig. 15-24). Figure 15-25 illustrates a Class III amalgam restoration in a mandibular incisor.

Finishing and Polishing

The finishing and polishing techniques and procedures are the same as those presented in Chapters 13 and 14.

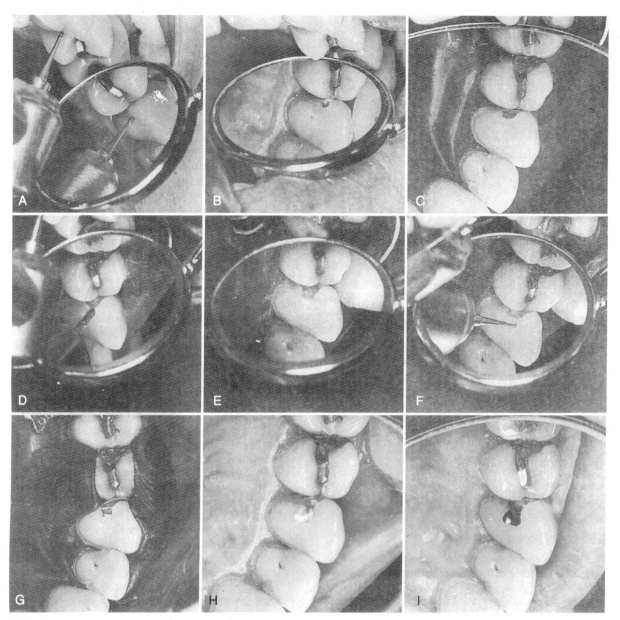

Fig. 15-22 Distolingual tooth preparation and restoration. **A,** Bur position for entry. **B,** Penetration made through the lingual enamel to the caries. **C,** Proximal portion completed, except for the retention form. **D,** Preparing the dovetail. **E,** Completed preparation, except for the retention groove and the coves. **F,** Bur position for the incisal cove in the dovetail. **G,** Rigid material–supported matrix ready for the insertion of amalgam. **H,** Carving completed and rubber dam removed. **I,** Polished restoration.

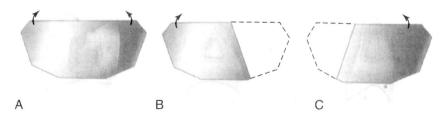

Fig. 15-23 Matrix strip design. **A,** Design required for rigid material–supported matrix for Class II tooth preparations. **B,** Alteration necessary for Class III preparation on the maxillary canine. **C,** Alteration necessary for the mandibular incisor. The strip material is cut to approximate the slope of the lingual surface.

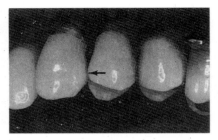

Fig. 15-24 Inconspicuous facial margin (*arrow*) of Class III amalgam restoration on the maxillary canine.

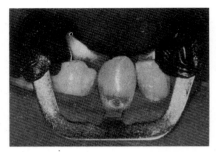

Fig. 15-26 A rubber dam and a No. 212 retainer may be required to isolate the carious area properly.

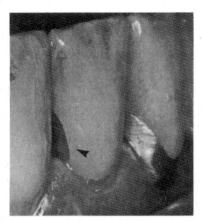

Fig. 15-25 Class III amalgam restoration on the mandibular incisor (*arrowhead*).

Clinical Technique for Class V Amalgam Restorations

Initial Procedures

Proper isolation prevents moisture contamination of the operating site, enhances asepsis, and facilitates access and visibility. Moisture in the form of saliva, gingival sulcular fluid, or gingival hemorrhage must be excluded during caries removal, liner application, and insertion and carving of amalgam. Moisture impairs visual assessment, may contaminate the pulp during caries removal (especially with a pulpal exposure), and negatively affects the physical properties of restorative materials. The gingival margin of Class V tooth preparations is often apical to the gingival crest. Such a gingival margin necessitates retraction of the free gingiva with a retraction cord or appropriate rubber dam and retainer to protect it and to provide access, while eliminating seepage of sulcular fluid into the tooth preparation or restorative materials.

These isolation objectives are met by local anesthesia and isolation by (1) a cotton roll and a retraction cord or (2) a rubber dam and a suitable cervical retainer (Fig. 15-26). Isolation with a cotton roll and a retraction cord is satisfactory when properly performed. This type of isolation is practical and probably the approach most often used. The retraction cord should be placed in the sulcus before initial tooth preparation to reduce the possibility of cutting instruments damaging the free gingiva. The cord should produce a temporary,

adequate, atraumatic apical retraction and lateral deflection of the free gingiva. The cord may be treated with hemostatic preparations containing aluminum chloride or ferrous sulfate. Alternatively, the cord may be treated with epinephrine. However, caution must be used as epinephrine on abraded gingiva can be absorbed rapidly into the circulatory system, causing an increase in blood pressure, elevated heart rate, and possible dysrhythmia. The retraction cord may be braided, twisted, or woven. The diameter of the cord should be easily accommodated in the gingival sulcus. An appropriate amount is cut to a length $\frac{1}{4}$ inch (6 mm) longer than the gingival margin. Some operators prefer to place the cord in a Dappen dish, wet it with a drop of hemostatic solution and blot it with a 2×2 inch (5×5 cm) gauze to remove excess liquid. A braided or woven cord is usually easier to use because it does not unravel during placement. A larger cord can be inserted over the first cord if the sulcus is large enough to accommodate two cords. A thin, blunt-edged instrument blade or the side of an explorer tine may be used to gently insert the cord progressively into place. A slight backward direction of the instrument as it steps along the cord helps prevent dislodgment of previously inserted cord (Fig. 15-27). In addition, using a second instrument stepping along behind the first instrument can help prevent dislodgment of cord. Additionally, using the air syringe or cotton pellets to reduce or absorb the sulcular fluid in the cord already placed is helpful during cord placement. The cord results in adequate retraction in a short time. If significant blanching of the free gingiva is observed (or if too much pressure has to be applied to place the cord), it means that an oversized cord has been selected, and it should therefore be exchanged with a cord of smaller diameter. The cord can be moistened before or after placement with the hemostatic solution if slight hemorrhage is anticipated or observed. Alternatively, the cord can be used dry.

The cord usually remains in place throughout tooth preparation as well as insertion and initial carving of amalgam. While carving amalgam at the gingival margin, the presence of the cord may cause difficulty in feeling the unprepared tooth surface apical to the margin to prevent under-carving of the margin; this results in over-contouring and marginal excess. In this instance, after carving gross excess, the cord can be teased from its place before the carving is completed.

Tooth Preparation

Proper outline form for Class V amalgam tooth preparations results in extending the cavosurface margins to sound tooth structure while maintaining a limited axial depth of 0.5 mm

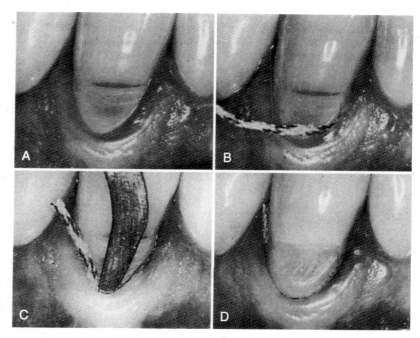

Fig. 15-27 Use of the retraction cord for isolation of a Class V lesion. **A,** Pre-operative view. **B,** Cord placement initiated. **C,** Cord placement using a thin, flat-bladed instrument. **D,** Cord placement completed.

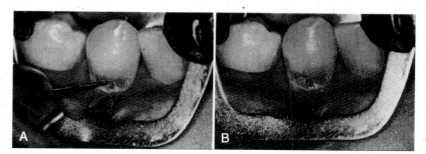

Fig. 15-28 Starting Class V tooth preparation. **A,** Bur positioned for entry into caries lesion. **B,** The entry cut is the beginning of the outline form having a limited axial depth. (The end of the bur in the center of the lesion may be in the carious tooth structure or in the air.)

inside the DEJ and 0.75 mm inside cementum (when on the root surface). The outline form for the Class V amalgam tooth preparation is determined primarily by the location and size of the caries or old restorative material. Clinical judgment determines final preparation outline, especially when the cavosurface margins approach or extend into areas of enamel decalcification. The operator must observe the prepared enamel wall to evaluate the depth of the decalcified enamel and to determine if cavitation exists peripheral to the wall. When no cavitation has occurred and when the decalcification does not extend appreciably into the enamel, extension of the outline form often should cease. In some cases, if all decalcification were included in the outline form, the preparation would extend into the proximal cervical areas (if not circumferentially around the tooth). Such a preparation would be difficult and perhaps unrestorable. A full-coverage restoration should be considered for teeth with extensive cervical decalcification.

Initial Tooth Preparation

A Class V amalgam restoration is not used often in a mandibular canine, but it is presented here for illustration. The same general principles for tooth preparation apply for all other tooth locations. A tapered fissure bur of suitable size (e.g., No. 271) is used to enter the caries lesion (or existing restoration) to a limited initial axial depth of 0.5 mm inside the DEJ (Fig. 15-28). This depth is usually 1 to 1.25 mm total axial depth, depending on the incisogingival (i.e., occlusogingival) location. The enamel is considerably thicker occlusally and incisally than cervically. If the preparation is on the root surface, however, the axial depth is approximately 0.75 mm. The end of the bur at the initial depth is in dentin, in infected carious dentin, or in old restorative material. The edge of the end of the bur can be used to penetrate the area; this is more efficient than using the flat end of the bur, reducing the possibility of the bur's "crawling." When the entry is made, the bur orientation is adjusted to ensure that all external walls are perpendicular to the external tooth surface and parallel to the enamel rods (Fig. 15-29). Often, this requires changing the orientation of the handpiece to accommodate the cervical mesiodistal and incisogingival (i.e., occlusogingival) convexity of the tooth. The preparation is extended incisally, gingivally, mesially, and distally until the cavosurface margins are positioned in sound tooth structure such that an initial axial depth of 0.5 mm inside the DEJ (if on the root surface, the axial

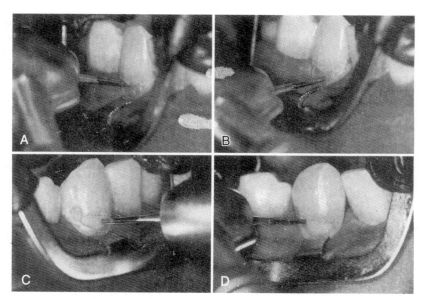

Fig. 15-29 When extending incisally (*A*), gingivally (*B*), mesially (*C*), and distally (*D*), the bur is positioned to prepare these walls perpendicular to the external tooth surface.

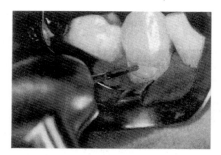

Fig. 15-30 The flat-bladed instrument protects the rubber dam from the bur.

depth is 0.75 mm) is established. When extending mesially and distally, it may be necessary to protect the rubber dam from the bur by placing a flat-bladed instrument over the dam (Fig. 15-30). Because the axial wall follows the mesiodistal and incisogingival (i.e., occlusogingival) contours of the facial surface of the tooth, it usually is convex in both directions. In addition, the axial wall usually is slightly deeper at the incisal wall, where more enamel (i.e., approximately 1-1.25 mm in depth) is present than at the gingival wall, where little or no enamel (i.e., approximately 0.75-1 mm in depth) may be present. A depth of 0.5 mm inside the DEJ permits placement of necessary retention grooves without undermining enamel. This subtle difference in depth serves also to increase the thickness of the remaining dentin (between the axial wall and the pulp) in the gingival aspect of the preparation to aid in protecting the pulp. For the tooth preparation that is extended incisogingivally, the axial wall should be more convex (because it follows the contour of the DEJ).

Alternatively, an appropriate carbide bur (usually No. 2 or No. 4) may be used for the initial tooth preparation. Round burs are indicated in areas inaccessible to a fissure bur that is held perpendicular to the tooth surface. If needed, smaller round burs may also be used to define the internal angles in these preparations, enhancing proper placement of the retention grooves.

Final Tooth Preparation

Final tooth preparation involves removing any remaining infected dentin; pulp protection; retention form; finishing external walls; and cleaning, inspecting, and desensitizing. Any remaining infected axial wall dentin is removed with a No. 2 or No. 4 round bur. Any old restorative material (including base and liner) remaining may be left if (1) no clinical or radiographic evidence of recurrent caries exists, (2) the periphery of the base and liner is intact, and (3) the tooth is asymptomatic. With proper outline form, the axial line angles are already in sound dentin. If needed, an appropriate liner or base is applied.

Because the mesial, distal, gingival, and incisal walls of the tooth preparation are perpendicular to the external tooth surface, they usually diverge facially. Consequently, this form provides no inherent retention, and retention form must be provided because the primary retention form for an amalgam restoration is macromechanical. A No. ¼ round bur is used to prepare two retention grooves, one along the incisoaxial line angle and the other along the gingivoaxial line angle (Fig. 15-31). The handpiece is positioned so that the No. ¼ round bur is directed generally to bisect the angle formed at the junction of the axial wall and the incisal (i.e., occlusal) wall. Ideally, the direction of the incisal (i.e., occlusal) groove is slightly more incisal (i.e., occlusal) than axial, and the direction of the gingival groove is slightly more gingival than axial. Alternatively, four retention coves may be prepared, one in each of the four axial point angles of the preparation (Fig. 15-32).

Using four coves instead of two full-length grooves conserves the dentin near the pulp, reducing the possibility of a mechanical pulp exposure. The depth of the grooves should be approximately 0.25 mm, which is half the diameter of the bur. It is important that the retention grooves be adequate because they provide the only retention form to the preparation. Regardless, the grooves should not remove dentin immediately supporting enamel. In a large Class V amalgam preparation, extending the retention groove circumferentially

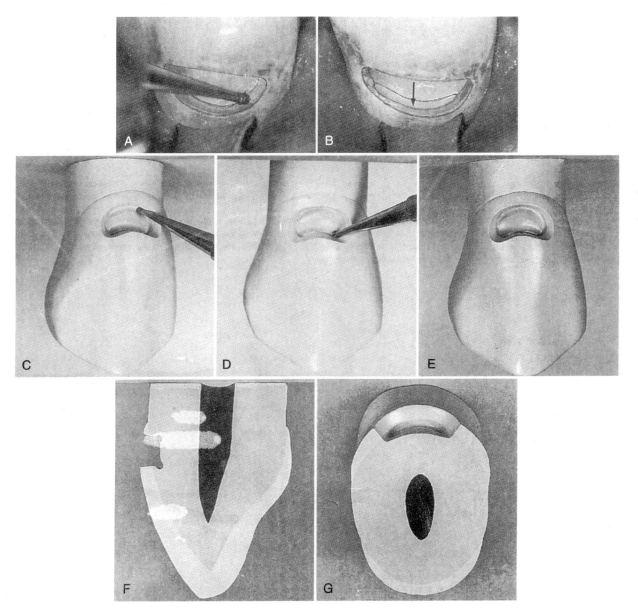

Fig. 15-31 Retention form. **A,** A No. ¼ round bur positioned to prepare the gingival retention groove. **B,** Gingival retention groove (*arrow*) prepared along the gingivoaxial line angle generally to bisect the angle formed by the gingival and axial walls. Ideally, the direction of preparation is slightly more gingival than pulpal. An incisal retention groove is prepared along the incisoaxial line angle and directed similarly. **C** and **D,** A groove is placed with a No. ¼ round bur along the gingivoaxial and incisoaxial line angles 0.2 mm inside the dentinoenamel junction (DEJ) and 0.25 mm deep. Note the slight pulpal inclination of the shank of the No. ¼ round bur. **E,** Facial view. **F,** Incisogingival section. Grooves depthwise are directed mostly incisally (gingivally) and slightly pulpally. **G,** Mesiodistal section.

around all the internal line angles of the tooth preparation may enhance the retention form.

If access is inadequate for use of the No. ¼ round bur, an angle-former chisel may be used to prepare the retention form. In addition, a No. 33½ bur can be used. Both methods result in retention grooves that are angular, but positioned in the same location and approximately to the same depth as when the No. ¼ round bur is used. The rounded retention form placed with the No. ¼ round bur is generally preferred, however, because amalgam can be condensed into rounded areas better than into sharp areas, resulting in better

adaptation of amalgam into the retention grooves. If necessary, suitable hand instruments (e.g., chisels, margin trimmers) are used to plane the enamel margins, verifying soundness and 90-degree cavosurface angles. Finally, the preparation is cleaned and inspected for completeness. A desensitizer is then applied.

Large Preparations That Include Line Angles

Caries on the facial (or lingual) surface may extend beyond the line angles of the tooth. Maxillary molars, particularly the

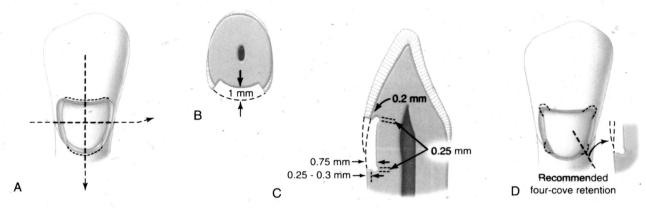

Fig. 15-32 A–C, Extended Class V tooth preparation (*A*) with the axial wall contoured parallel to the dentinoenamel junction (DEJ) mesiodistally (*B*) and incisogingivally (*C*). The axial wall pulpal depth is 1 mm in the crown and 0.75 mm in the root. In addition, note location and direction depth (0.25 mm) of the retention grooves and the dimension of the gingival wall (0.25 mm) from the root surface to the retention groove. **D,** Large Class V preparation with retention coves prepared in the four axial point angles.

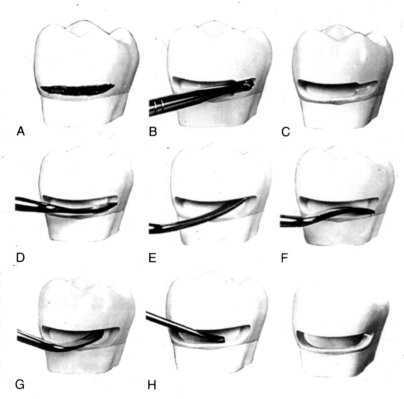

Fig. 15-33 Tooth preparation on maxillary molar. **A,** Caries extending around distofacial corner of the tooth. **B** and **C,** Distal extension is accomplished with round bur. **D–F,** A gingival margin trimmer may be useful in completing the distal half of the preparation when handpiece access is limited. **G,** A gingival margin trimmer may be used to provide the retention grooves. **H,** An angle-former chisel may be used to prepare the retention grooves in the distal portion of the preparation. **I,** Completed tooth preparation.

second molars, are most commonly affected by these extensive defects (Fig. 15-33, *A*). In this example, if the remainder of the distal surface is sound and the distal caries is accessible facially, the facial restoration should extend around the line angle. This prevents the need for a Class II proximal restoration to restore the distal surface. As much of the preparation as possible should be completed with a fissure bur. A round bur, approximately the same diameter as the fissure bur, is then used to initiate the distal portion of the preparation (see Fig. 15-33, *B* and *C*). Smaller round burs should be used to accentuate the internal line angles of the distal portion. Preparing the facial portion first provides better access and visibility to the distal

portion. Occasionally, hand instruments may be useful for completing the distal half of the preparation when space for the handpiece is limited (see Fig. 15-33, *D* through *F*).

Grooves placed along the entire length of the occlusoaxial and gingivoaxial line angles help ensure retention of the restoration. The No. ¼ round bur is used as previously described to prepare the retention grooves. A gingival margin trimmer or a 7-85- 2½ -6 angle-former chisel can be used in the distal half of the preparation to provide retention form when access for the handpiece is limited (see Fig. 15-33, *G* and *H*).

Because of the proximity of the coronoid process, access to the facial surfaces of maxillary molars, particularly the second

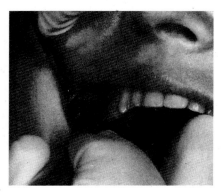

Fig. 15-34 The mandible shifted laterally for improved access and visibility.

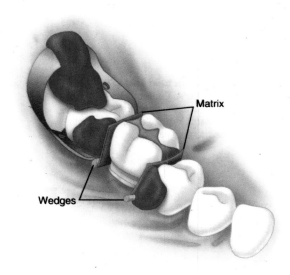

Fig. 15-36 Application of the matrix to confine amalgam in the mesial and distal extensions of the preparation.

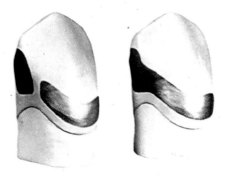

Fig. 15-35 When a Class V outline form closely approaches an existing restoration, the preparation should be extended to remove the remaining thin enamel wall to achieve adjoining restorations.

molars, is often limited. Having the patient partially close and shift the mandible toward the tooth being restored improves access and visibility (Fig. 15-34).

If the Class V outline form approaches an existing proximal restoration, it is better to extend slightly into the bulk of the proximal restoration, rather than to leave a thin section of the tooth structure between the two restorations (Fig. 15-35). In this illustration, the previously placed amalgam served as the distal wall of the preparation. When proper treatment requires Class II and V amalgam restorations on the same tooth, the Class II preparation and restoration is completed before initiating the Class V restoration. If the Class V restoration were done first, it might be damaged by the matrix band and wedge needed for the Class II restoration.

Restorative Technique
Desensitizer Placement

The same considerations presented earlier apply for the Class V amalgam restoration.

Matrix Placement

Most Class V amalgam restorations are placed without the use of any type of matrix. The most difficult condensation occurs in a tooth preparation with an axial wall that is convex mesiodistally. Two alternative methods for insertion may be used.

The preferred method is the application of a matrix that confines amalgam in the mesial and distal portions of the preparation (Fig. 15-36). Short lengths of stainless steel matrix material, one each for the mesial and distal surfaces, are passed through the proximal contacts, carefully guided into the gingival sulcus, and wedged. The strips must be wide enough to extend occlusally through the respective proximal contacts and long enough to extend slightly past the facial line angles. The strip usually requires rigid material support for stability. The strips offer resistance against condensing the mesial and distal portions, which provides support for condensing the center of the restoration. The gingival edge of the steel strip often must be trimmed to conform to the circumferential contour (level) of the base of the gingival sulcus to prevent soft tissue damage. Rather than using two short pieces, the operator can use a longer length that may be passed through one proximal contact, extended around the lingual surface, and passed through the other contact, forming a U-shaped matrix. Trimming the gingival edge to conform to the interproximal soft tissue anatomy usually is more difficult with one matrix strip than when two strips are used.

A conventional Tofflemire band and retainer may be used with a window cut into the band allowing access to the preparation for condensation (Fig. 15-37). Alternatively, the tooth may be prepared and restored in sections without using a matrix. Each successive section of the preparation should be extended slightly into the previously condensed portion to ensure caries removal. This procedure is time-consuming but effective.

Insertion and Carving of the Amalgam

The amalgam carrier is used to insert the mixed amalgam into the preparation in small increments (Fig. 15-38, *A*). Amalgam is condensed into the retention areas first by using an appropriate condenser (see Fig. 15-38, *B*). Next, amalgam

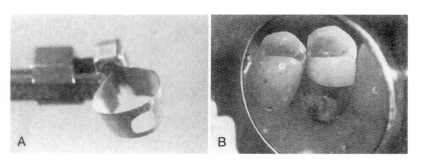

Fig. 15-37 Customized matrix band used to restore an area of proximal root caries. **A,** Conventional Tofflemire matrix with window cut into the band to allow access for condensation. **B,** Matrix in place around the tooth, allowing lingual access to preparation.

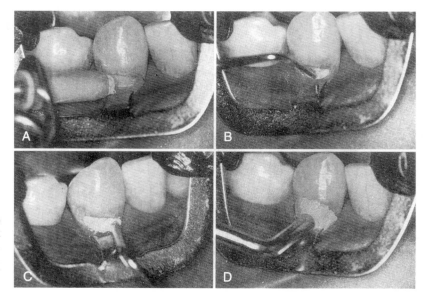

Fig. 15-38 Inserting amalgam. **A,** Place amalgam into the preparation in small increments. **B,** Condense first into the retention grooves with a small condenser. **C,** Condense against the mesial and distal walls. **D,** Overfill and provide sufficient bulk to allow for carving.

is condensed against the mesial and distal walls of the preparation (see Fig. 15-38, *C*). Finally, a sufficient bulk of amalgam is placed in the central portion to allow for carving the correct contour (see Fig. 15-38, *D*). As the surface of the restoration becomes more convex, condensation becomes increasingly difficult. It is important to guard against the "landsliding" of amalgam during over-packing. A large condenser or flat-bladed instrument held against amalgam may help resist pressure applied elsewhere on the restoration (Fig. 15-39).

Carving may begin immediately after the insertion of amalgam (Fig. 15-40). All carving should be done using the side of the explorer tine or a Hollenback No. 3 carver held parallel to the margins. The side of the carving instrument always should rest on the unprepared tooth surface adjacent to the prepared cavosurface margin; this prevents over-carving. The carving procedure is begun by removing excess amalgam to expose the incisal (or occlusal) margin. Removal of excess material continues until the mesial and distal margins are exposed. Finally, material excess at the gingival margin is carved away. Carving the marginal areas should result in developing the desired convex contours in the completed restoration. Improper use of the carving instruments results in a poorly contoured restoration. Note in Figure 15-41 how carving instruments are positioned to provide the desired contours. No amalgam excess should remain at the margins

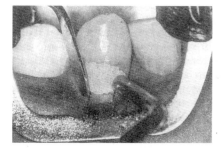

Fig. 15-39 Use a large condenser or a flat-bladed instrument to offer resistance to condensation pressure applied elsewhere on the restoration.

because amalgam may break away, creating a defect at the margin, or cause gingival irritation.

In some instances, it is appropriate to change facial contours because of altered soft tissue levels (e.g., cervical lesions in periodontally treated patients). Facial contours may be increased (or relocated) only enough to prevent food impaction into the gingival sulcus and to provide access for the patient to clean the area. Over-contouring must be avoided because it results in reduced stimulation and cleansing of the gingiva during mastication.

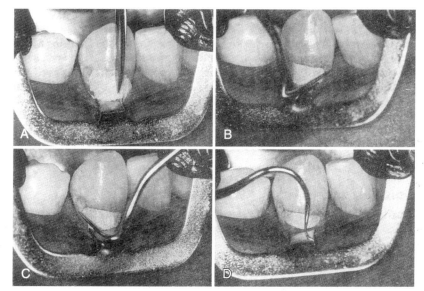

Fig. 15-40 Carving and contouring the restoration. **A,** Begin the carving procedure by removing any excess and locating the incisal margin. **B** and **C,** An explorer may be used to remove the excess and locate the mesial and distal margins. **D,** Remove the excess and locate the gingival margin.

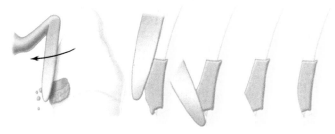

Fig. 15-41 Positioning of the carving instrument to prevent over-carving amalgam and to develop the desired gingival contours.

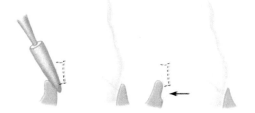

Fig. 15-42 Incorrect use of a pointed stone at the gingival margin results in the removal of cementum, notching of the tooth structure gingival to the margin, or both.

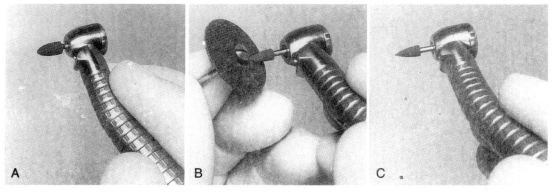

Fig. 15-43 Reshaping a rubber abrasive point against a mounted carborundum disk.

When a rubber dam and the No. 212 cervical retainer have been used for isolation, the retainer is removed using care to open the jaws of the retainer wide enough to prevent marring the surface of the restoration. The rubber dam is removed, and the area is examined carefully to ensure that no amalgam particles remain in the sulcus.

When a retraction cord is used for isolation, it may interfere with carving any excess amalgam at the gingival margin. If so, removal of the gross excess of amalgam is followed by careful removal of the cord, followed by completion of the carving along the margin.

Finishing and Polishing of the Amalgam

If carving procedures were performed correctly, no finishing of the restoration should be required. A slightly moistened cotton pellet held in cotton pliers may be used to further smooth the carved restoration. Additional finishing and polishing of amalgam restorations may be necessary, however, to correct a marginal discrepancy or to improve contour. Care is required when using stones or any rotating cutting instruments on margins positioned below the cementoenamel junction (CEJ) because of the possibility of removing cementum, notching the tooth structure gingival to the margin, or both (Fig. 15-42). Figure 15-43 illustrates re-shaping a rubber abrasive point to allow optimal access to the gingival portion of a Class V amalgam restoration.

indirect restoration is placed. Occasionally, when providing a temporary or control restoration, sufficient retention and resistance forms are included in the preparation to meet the requirements of a foundation.

As a rule, foundations are placed in anticipation of a full-coverage indirect restoration. Not all teeth with foundations, however, need to be immediately restored with full-coverage crowns. For example, amalgam can be used as a definitive partial-coverage restoration if only minimal coronal damage has occurred in endodontically treated teeth.[19] The greatest influence on fracture resistance is the amount of remaining tooth structure.[20]

The restorative materials used for foundations include amalgam, composite, and occasionally resin-modified glass ionomers (RMGIs). Of the direct filling materials, amalgam may be preferred by some clinicians because it is easy to use and is strong. Threaded pins and slots can be used for retention in vital teeth. Prefabricated posts and cast post and cores also may be used to provide additional retention for the foundation material in endodontically treated teeth receiving foundations. The use of prefabricated posts and cast post and cores is limited to endodontically treated teeth and is used generally on anterior teeth or single-canal premolars with little or no remaining coronal tooth structure. On endodontically treated molars, the pulp chamber or canals typically provide retention for the foundation, and it is not necessary to use any form of intra-radicular retention.

Tooth Preparation
Tooth Preparation for Pin-Retained Amalgam Restorations

INITIAL TOOTH PREPARATION

The general concept of the initial tooth preparation is presented in Chapter 14, and it applies to the pin-retained complex amalgam restorations described here. When caries is extensive, reduction of one or more of the cusps for capping may be indicated. For cusps prone to fracture, capping of cusps reduces the risk of cusp fracture and extends the life of the restoration.[21,22] Complex amalgam restorations with one or more capped cusps have documented longevity of 72% after 15 years and show no differences in the survival rate of cusp-covered and non–cusp-covered amalgam restorations, whether or not pins were used.[4,23]

When the facial or lingual extension exceeds two-thirds the distance from a primary groove toward the cusp tip (or when the faciolingual extension of the occlusal preparation exceeds two-thirds the distance between the facial and lingual cusp tips), reduction of the cusp for amalgam usually is required for the development of adequate resistance form (Fig. 16-9, A). Reduction should be accomplished during the initial tooth preparation because it improves access and visibility for subsequent steps. If the cusp to be capped is located at the correct occlusal height before preparation, depth cuts should be made on the remaining occlusal surface of each cusp to be capped, using the side of a carbide fissure bur or a suitable diamond instrument (see Fig. 16-9, B). The depth cuts should be a minimum of 2 mm for functional cusps and 1.5 mm for nonfunctional cusps.[24] To correct an occlusal relationship, if the unreduced cusp height is located at less than the correct occlusal height, the depth cuts may be less. Likewise, if the

unreduced cusp height is located at more than the correct occlusal height, the depth cuts may be deeper. The goal is to ensure that the final restoration has restored cusps with a minimal thickness of 2 mm of amalgam for functional cusps and 1.5 mm of amalgam for nonfunctional cusps (see Fig. 16-9, C), while developing an appropriate occlusal relationship.

Using the depth cuts as a guide, the reduction is completed to provide for a uniform reduction of tooth structure (see Fig. 16-9, D). The occlusal contour of the reduced cusp should be similar to the normal contour of the unreduced cusp. Any sharp internal corners of the tooth preparation formed at the junction of prepared surfaces should be rounded to reduce stress concentration in the amalgam and improve its resistance to fracture from occlusal forces (see Fig. 16-9, E). When reducing only one of two facial or lingual cusps, the cusp reduction should be extended just past the facial or lingual groove, creating a vertical wall against the adjacent unreduced cusp. Figure 16-9, F and G, illustrates a final restoration. The procedure for capping the distolingual cusp of a maxillary first molar is illustrated in Figure 14-68. Extending the facial or lingual wall of a proximal box to include the entire cusp is indicated only when necessary to include carious or unsupported tooth structure or existing restorative material. The typical extension of the proximal box for restoring an entire cusp is illustrated in Figures 14-69 and 14-70, B.

When possible, opposing vertical walls should be formed to converge occlusally, to enhance the primary retention form. Also, a facial or lingual groove can be extended arbitrarily to increase the retention form. The pulpal and gingival walls should be relatively flat and perpendicular to the long axis of the tooth.

FINAL TOOTH PREPARATION

After the initial tooth preparation of a severely involved tooth, removal of any remaining infected carious dentin or remaining old restorative material is usually necessary and is accomplished as described previously. An RMGI base can be applied, if needed; if used, a liner or base should not extend closer than 1 mm to a slot or a pin.

Pins placed into prepared pinholes (also referred to as *pin channels*) provide auxiliary resistance and retention forms. Coves and retention locks should be prepared when possible (Figs. 16-10, and 16-11). Coves are prepared in a horizontal plane, and locks are prepared in a vertical plane. These locks and coves should be prepared before preparing the pinholes and inserting the pins. Cusp reduction significantly diminishes the retention form by decreasing the height of the vertical walls. When additional retention is indicated, pins may be inserted in carefully positioned pinholes, thus increasing retention. Slots may be prepared along the gingival floor, axial to the dentinoenamel junction (DEJ) instead of, or in addition to, pinholes (see Fig. 16-10, B). Slot preparation is discussed later in this chapter.

TYPES OF PINS

The most frequently used pin type is the self-threading pin. Friction-locked and cemented pins, although still available, are rarely used (Fig. 16-12). The pin-retained amalgam restoration using self-threading pins originally was described by Going in 1966.[25] The diameter of the prepared pinhole is

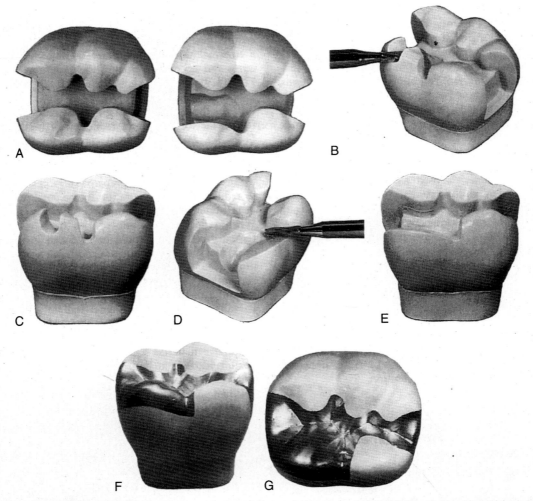

Fig. 16-9 Capping the cusp with amalgam. **A,** Comparison of the mesial aspects of normally extended (*left*) and extensive (*right*) mesio-occluso-distal tooth preparation. The resistance form of the mesiolingual cusp of extensive preparation is compromised and indicated for capping with amalgam. **B,** Preparing depth cuts. **C,** Depth cuts prepared. **D,** Reducing the cusp. **E,** Cusp reduced. **F** and **G,** Final restoration.

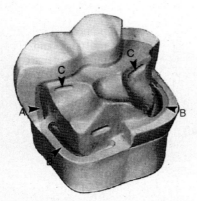

Fig. 16-10 Lock (*A*), slots (*B*), and coves (*C*).

0.0015 to 0.004 inch smaller than the diameter of the pin (Table 16-1). The threads engage dentin as the pin is inserted, thus retaining it. The elasticity (resiliency) of dentin permits insertion of a threaded pin into a hole of smaller diameter.[26] Although the threads of self-threading pins do not engage dentin for their entire width, self-threading pins are the most retentive of the three types of pins (Fig. 16-13), being three to six times more retentive than cemented pins.[27-29]

Vertical and horizontal stresses can be generated in dentin when a self-threading pin is inserted. Craze lines in dentin may be related to the size of the pin. The insertion of 0.031-inch self-threading pins produces more dentinal craze lines than does the insertion of 0.021-inch self-threading pins.[30] Some evidence suggests, however, that self-threading pins may not cause dentinal crazing.[26] Pulpal stress is maximal when the self-threading pin is inserted perpendicular to the pulp.[31] The depth of the pinhole varies from 1.3 to 2 mm, depending on the diameter of the pin used.[32] A general guideline for pinhole depth is 2 mm.

Several styles of self-threading pins are available. The Thread Mate System (TMS) (Coltène/Whaledent Inc., Mahwah, NJ) is the most widely used self-threading pin because of its (1) versatility, (2) wide range of pin sizes, (3) color-coding system, and (4) greater retentiveness.[33,34] TMS pins are available in gold-plated stainless steel or in titanium. Other titanium alloy pins (Max system, Coltène/Whaledent Inc.) are available.

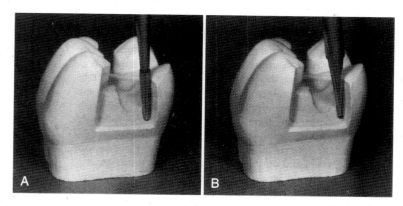

Fig. 16-11 Placement of retention locks. **A,** Position of No. 169L bur to prepare the retention lock. **B,** Lock prepared with No. ¼ bur.

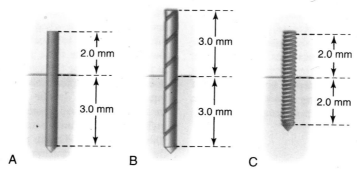

Fig. 16-12 Three types of pins. **A,** Cemented. **B,** Friction-locked. **C,** Self-threading.

Table 16-1 The Thread Mate System (TMS) Pins

Name	Illustration (not to scale)	Color Code	Pin Diameter (inches/mm)*	Drill Diameter (inches/mm)*	Total Pin Length (mm)	Pin Length Extending from Dentin (mm)
Regular (standard)		Gold	0.031/0.78	0.027/0.68	7.1	5.1
Regular (self-shearing)		Gold	0.031/0.78	0.027/0.68	8.2	3.2
Regular (two-in-one)		Gold	0.031/0.78	0.027/0.68	9.5	2.8
Minim (standard)		Silver	0.024/0.61	0.021/0.53	6.7	4.7
Minim (two-in-one)		Silver	0.024/0.61	0.021/0.53	9.5	2.8
Minikin (self-shearing)		Red	0.019/0.48	0.017/0.43	7.1	1.5
Minuta (self-shearing)		Pink	0.015/0.38	0.0135/0.34	6.2	1

*1 mm = 0.03937 inch.

FACTORS AFFECTING RETENTION OF THE PIN IN DENTIN AND AMALGAM

Type

With regard to the retentiveness of the pin in dentin, the self-threading pin is the most retentive, the friction-locked pin is intermediate, and the cemented pin is the least retentive.[27]

Surface Characteristics

The number and depth of the elevations (serrations or threads) on the pin influence the retention of the pin in the amalgam restoration. The shape of the self-threading pin gives it the greatest retention value.

Orientation, Number, and Diameter

Placing pins in a non-parallel manner increases their retention. Bending pins to improve their retention in amalgam is not advisable because the bends may interfere with adequate condensation of amalgam around the pin and decrease amalgam retention. Bending also may weaken the pin and risk fracturing dentin. Pins should be bent only to provide for an adequate amount of amalgam (approximately 1 mm) between the pin and the external surface of the finished restoration (on the tip of the pin and on its lateral surface). Only the specific bending tool should be used to bend a pin, not other hand instruments.

In general, increasing the number of pins increases their retention in dentin and amalgam. The benefits of increasing the number of pins must be compared with the potential problems. As the number of pins increases, (1) the crazing of dentin and the potential for fracture increase, (2) the amount of available dentin between the pins decreases, and (3) the strength of the amalgam restoration decreases.[35,36] Also, as the diameter of the pin increases, retention in dentin and amalgam generally increases. As the number, depth, and diameter of pins increase, the danger of perforating into the pulp or the external tooth surface increases. Numerous long pins also can

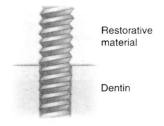

Fig. 16-13 The complete width of the threads of self-threading pins does not engage dentin.

severely compromise condensation of amalgam and amalgam's adaptation to the pins. A pin technique that permits optimal retention with minimal danger to the remaining tooth structure should be used.[37]

Extension into Dentin and Amalgam

Self-threading pin extension into dentin and amalgam should be approximately 1.5 to 2 mm to preserve the strength of dentin and amalgam.[27] Extension greater than this is unnecessary for pin retention and is contraindicated.

PIN PLACEMENT FACTORS AND TECHNIQUES
Pin Size

Four sizes of TMS pins are available (Fig. 16-14), each with a corresponding color-coded drill (see Table 16-1). Familiarity with drill sizes and their corresponding colors is necessary to ensure that a proper-sized pinhole is prepared for the desired pin. It is difficult to specify a particular size of pin that is always appropriate for a particular tooth. Two determining factors for selecting the appropriate-sized pin are the amount of dentin available to receive the pin safely and the amount of retention desired. In the TMS system, the pins of choice for severely involved posterior teeth are the Minikin (0.019 inch [0.48 mm]) and, occasionally, the Minim (0.024 inch [0.61 mm]). The Minikin pins usually are selected to reduce the risk of dentin crazing, pulpal penetration, and potential perforation. The Minim pins usually are used as a backup in case the pinhole for the Minikin is over-prepared or the pin threads strip dentin during placement and the Minikin pin lacks retention. Larger-diameter pins have the greatest retention.[38] The Minuta (0.015 inch [0.38 mm]) pin is approximately half as retentive as the Minim and one-third as retentive as the Minim pin.[33,34] It is usually too small to provide adequate retention in posterior teeth. The Regular (0.031 inch [0.78 mm]), or largest-diameter, pin is rarely used because a significant amount of stress and crazing, or cracking, in the

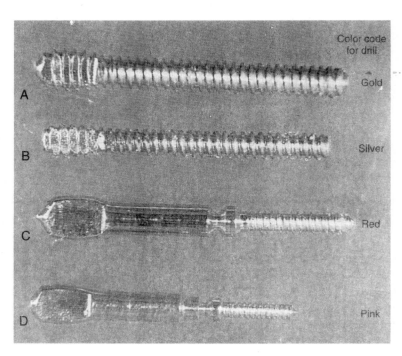

Fig. 16-14 Four sizes of the Thread Mate System (TMS) pins. **A,** Regular (0.031 inch [0.78 mm]). **B,** Minim (0.024 inch [0.61 mm]). **C,** Minikin (0.019 inch [0.48 mm]). **D,** Minuta (0.015 inch [0.38 mm]).

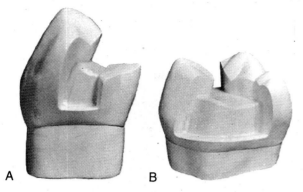

Fig. 16-15 Examples illustrating reduction of cusps without need for pins. **A,** Mandibular first premolar with lingual cusp reduced for capping. **B,** Maxillary second molar prepared for restoration of mesial and distal surfaces and distofacial cusp.

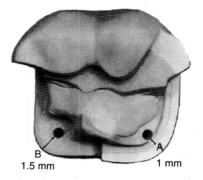

Fig. 16-16 Pinhole position. **A,** Position relative to the dentinoenamel junction (DEJ). **B,** Position relative to external tooth surface.

tooth (dentin and enamel) may be created during its insertion.[30,39] Of the four types of pins, the Regular pin is associated with the highest incidence of dentinal cracking communicating with the pulp chamber.[10]

Number of Pins

Several factors must be considered when deciding how many pins are required: (1) the amount of missing tooth structure, (2) the amount of dentin available to receive the pins safely, (3) the amount of retention required, and (4) the size of the pins. As a rule, one pin per missing axial line angle should be used. Certain factors may cause the operator to alter this rule. The fewest pins possible should be used to achieve the desired retention for a given restoration. If only 2 to 3 mm of the occlusogingival height of a cusp has been removed, no pin is required because enough tooth structure remains to use conventional retention features (Fig. 16-15; see also Fig. 16-9). Although the retention of the restoration increases as the number of pins increases, an excessive number of pins can fracture the tooth and significantly weaken the amalgam restoration.

Location

Several factors aid in determining the pinhole locations: (1) knowledge of normal pulp anatomy and external tooth contours, (2) a current radiograph of the tooth, (3) a periodontal probe, and (4) the patient's age. Although the radiograph is only a two-dimensional image of the tooth, it can give an indication of the position of the pulp chamber and the contour of the mesial and distal surfaces of the tooth. Consideration also must be given to the placement of pins in areas where the greatest bulk of amalgam would occur to minimize the weakening effect of the pins on the tooth structure.[40] Areas of occlusal contacts on the restoration must be anticipated because a pin oriented vertically and positioned directly below an occlusal load weakens amalgam significantly.[41] Occlusal clearance should be sufficient to provide 2 mm of amalgam over the pin.[42,43]

Several attempts have been made to identify the ideal location of the pinhole.[9,14,30,44] The following principles of pin placement are recommended. In the cervical third of molars and premolars (where most pins are located), pinholes should be located near the line angles of the tooth except as described

later.[37,45] The pinhole should be positioned no closer than 0.5 to 1 mm to the DEJ or no closer than 1 to 1.5 mm to the external surface of the tooth, whichever distance is greater (Fig. 16-16). Before the final decision is made about the location of the pinhole, the operator should probe the gingival crevice carefully to determine if any abnormal contours exist that would predispose the tooth to an external perforation. The pinhole should be parallel to the adjacent external surface of the tooth.

The position of a pinhole must not result in the pin being so close to a vertical wall of tooth structure that condensation of amalgam against the pin or wall is jeopardized (Fig. 16-17, A). It may be necessary to first prepare a recess in the vertical wall with the No. 245 bur to permit proper pinhole preparation and to provide a minimum of 0.5 mm clearance around the circumference of the pin for adequate condensation of amalgam (see Fig. 16-17, B and C).[46] If necessary, after a pin is inappropriately placed, the operator should provide clearance around the pin to provide sufficient space for the smallest condenser nib to ensure that amalgam can be condensed adequately around the pin. A No. 169L bur can be used, taking care not to damage or weaken the pin. Pinholes should be prepared on a flat surface that is perpendicular to the proposed direction of the pinhole. Otherwise, the drill tip may slip or "crawl," and a depth-limiting drill (discussed later) cannot prepare the hole as deeply as intended (Fig. 16-18).

Whenever three or more pinholes are placed, they should be located at different vertical levels on the tooth, if possible; this reduces stresses resulting from pin placement in the same horizontal plane of the tooth. Spacing between pins, or the inter-pin distance, must be considered when two or more pinholes are prepared. The optimal inter-pin distance depends on the size of pin to be used. The minimal inter-pin distance is 3 mm for the Minikin pin and 5 mm for the Minim pin.[35] Maximal inter-pin distance results in lower levels of stress in dentin.[47]

Several posterior teeth have anatomic features that may preclude safe pinhole placement. Fluted and furcal areas should be avoided.[46] Specifically, external perforation may result from pinhole placement (1) over the prominent mesial concavity of the maxillary first premolar; (2) at the mid-lingual and mid-facial bifurcations of the mandibular first and second molars; and (3) at the mid-facial, mid-mesial, and mid-distal furcations of the maxillary first and second molars. Pulpal penetration may result from pin placement at the mesiofacial corner of the maxillary first molar and the mandibular first molar.

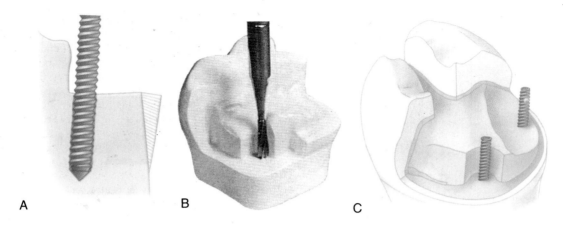

Fig. 16-17 **A,** Pin placed too close to the vertical wall such that adequate condensation of amalgam is jeopardized. **B** and **C,** Recessed area prepared in the vertical wall of the mandibular molar with a No. 245 bur to provide adequate space for amalgam condensation around the pin.

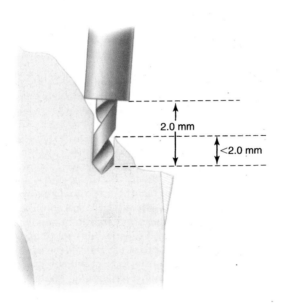

Fig. 16-18 Use of a depth-limiting drill to prepare a pinhole in the surface that is not perpendicular to the direction of the pinhole results in a pinhole of inadequate depth.

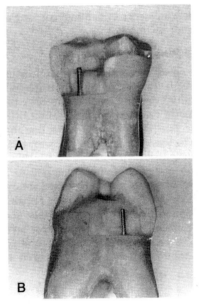

Fig. 16-19 Distal flaring of the mandibular molar (A) and palatal root flaring of the maxillary molar (B). Root angulation should be considered before pinhole placement.

When possible, the location of pinholes on the distal surface of mandibular molars and lingual surface of maxillary molars should be avoided. Obtaining the proper direction for preparing a pinhole in these locations is difficult because of the abrupt flaring of the roots just apical to the cementoenamel junction (CEJ) (Fig. 16-19). If the pinhole is placed parallel to the external surface of the tooth crown in these areas, penetration into the pulp is likely.[45]

When the pinhole locations have been determined, a No. ¼ round bur is first used to prepare a pilot hole (dimple) approximately one half the diameter of the bur at each location (Fig. 16-20). The purpose of this hole is to permit more accurate placement of the twist drill and to prevent the drill from "crawling" when it has begun to rotate.

Pinhole Preparation

The Kodex drill (a twist drill) should be used for preparing pinholes (Fig. 16-21). The aluminum shank of this drill, which acts as a heat absorber, is color coded so that it can be matched easily with the appropriate pin size (see Tables 16-1 and 16-2). The drill shanks for the Minuta and Minikin pins are tapered to provide a built-in "wobble" when placed in a latch-type contra-angle handpiece. This wobble allows the drill to be "free-floating" and to align itself as the pinhole is prepared to minimize dentinal crazing or the breakage of small drills.

Because the optimal depth of the pinhole into the dentin is 2 mm (only 1.5 mm for the Minikin pin), a depth-limiting

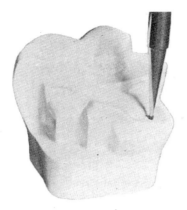

Fig. 16-20   Pilot hole (dimple) prepared with a No. ¼ bur.

drill should be used to prepare the hole (see Fig. 16-21). This type of drill can prepare the pinhole to the correct depth only when used on a flat surface that is perpendicular to the drill (see Fig. 16-18). When the location for starting a pinhole is not perpendicular to the desired pinhole direction, the location area should be flattened, or the standard twist drill should be used (see Fig. 16-21). The standard twist drill has blades that are 4 to 5 mm in length, which would allow preparation of a pinhole with an effective depth. Creation of a flat area and use of the depth-limiting drill is recommended.

With the drill in the latch-type contra-angle handpiece, the drill is placed in the gingival crevice beside the location for the pinhole and positioned such that it lies flat against the external surface of the tooth; without changing the angulation obtained from the crevice position, the handpiece is moved occlusally and the drill placed in the previously prepared pilot hole (Fig. 16-22, *A*). The drill is then viewed from a 90-degree angle to the previous viewing position to ascertain that the drill also is angled correctly in this plane (see Fig. 16-22, *B*). Incorrect angulation of the drill may result in pulpal exposure or external perforation. If the proximity of an adjacent tooth interferes

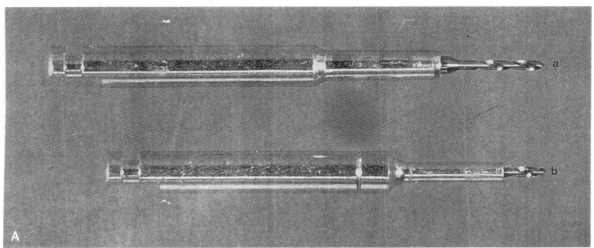

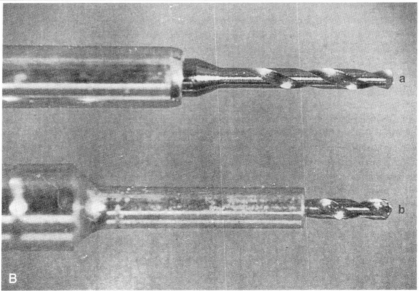

Fig. 16-21   **A,** Two types of Kodex twist drills: standard (*a*) and depth-limiting (*b*). **B,** Drills enlarged: standard (*a*) and depth-limiting (*b*).

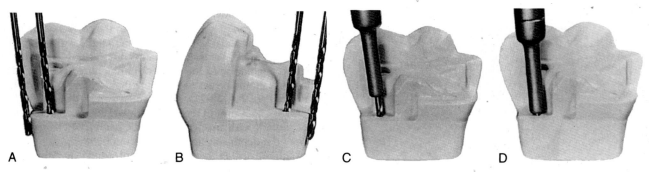

Fig. 16-22 Determining the angulation for the twist drill. **A,** Drill placed in the gingival crevice, positioned flat against the tooth, and moved occlusally into position without changing the angulation obtained. **B,** A repeated while viewing the drill from position 90 degrees left or right of that viewed in A. **C** and **D,** With twist drill at correct angulation, the pinhole is prepared in one or two thrusts until the depth-limiting portion of drill is reached.

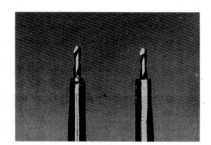

Fig. 16-23 Minikin self-limiting drill with worn shank shoulder (*left*) compared with a new drill with an unworn shoulder (*right*).

with placement of the drill into the gingival crevice, a flat, thin-bladed hand instrument is placed into the crevice and against the external surface of the tooth to indicate the proper angulation for the drill.[48] With the drill tip in its proper position and with the handpiece rotating at very low speed (300–500 revolutions per minute [rpm]), pressure is applied to the drill. The pinhole is prepared, in one or two movements, until the depth-limiting portion of the drill is reached. The drill is immediately removed from the pinhole (see Fig. 16-22, *C* and *D*). Using more than one or two movements, tilting the handpiece during the drilling procedure, or allowing the drill to rotate more than briefly at the bottom of the pinhole will result in a pinhole that is too large. The drill should never stop rotating (from insertion to removal from the pinhole) to prevent the drill from binding and breaking while in the pinhole.

Dull drills used to prepare pinholes can cause increased frictional heat and cracks in the dentin. Standlee et al. showed that a twist drill becomes too dull for use after cutting 20 pinholes or less, and the signal for discarding the drill is the need for increased pressure on the handpiece.[49] Using a drill when its self-limiting shank shoulder has become rounded is contraindicated (Fig. 16-23). A worn and rounded shoulder may not properly limit pinhole depth and may permit pins to be placed too deeply.

Certain clinical locations require extra care in determining pinhole angulation. The distal aspect of mandibular molars and the lingual aspect of maxillary molars have been mentioned previously as areas of potential problems because of the abrupt flaring of the roots just apical to the CEJ (see Fig. 16-19). Mandibular posterior teeth (with their lingual crown tilt), teeth that are rotated in the arch, and teeth that are

abnormally tilted in the arch warrant careful attention before and during pinhole placement. For mandibular second molars that are severely tilted mesially, care must be exercised to orient the drill properly to prevent external perforation on the mesial surface and pulpal penetration on the distal surface (Fig. 16-24). Because of limited interarch space, it is sometimes difficult to orient the twist drill correctly when placing pinholes at the distofacial or distolingual line angles of the mandibular second and third molars (Fig. 16-25).

Pin Design

For each of the four sizes of TMS pins, several designs are available: standard, self-shearing, two-in-one, Link Series, and Link Plus (Fig. 16-26).

The pin is free floating in the plastic sleeve, and this allows it to align itself as it is threaded into the pinhole (Fig. 16-27). When the pin reaches the bottom of the hole, the top portion of the pin shears off, leaving a length of pin extending from dentin. The plastic sleeve is then discarded. The Minuta, Minikin, Minim, and Regular pins are available in the Link Series. The Link Series pins are recommended because of their versatility, self-aligning ability, and retentiveness.[33]

The Link Plus pins are self-shearing and are available as single and two-in-one pins contained in color-coded plastic sleeves (Fig. 16-28). This design has a sharper thread, a shoulder stop at 2 mm, and a tapered tip to fit the bottom of the pinhole more readily as prepared by the twist drill. It also provides a 2.7-mm length of pin to extend out of dentin, which usually needs to be shortened. Theoretically, and as suggested by Standlee et al, these innovations should reduce the stress created in the surrounding dentin as the pin is inserted and reduce the apical stress at the bottom of the pinhole.[50] Kelsey et al showed for the two-in-one Link Plus pin that the first and second pins seat completely into the pinhole before shearing.[51] The Link Series pin is contained in a color-coded plastic sleeve that fits a latch-type contra-angle handpiece or the specially designed plastic hand wrench (Fig. 16-29, *D*).

The self-shearing pin has a total length that varies according to the diameter of the pin (see Table 16-1). It also consists of a flattened head to engage the hand wrench or the appropriate handpiece chuck for threading into the pinhole. When the pin approaches the bottom of the pinhole, the head of the pin shears off, leaving a length of pin extending from dentin.

The two-in-one pin is actually two pins in one, with each one being shorter than the standard pin. The two-in-one pin

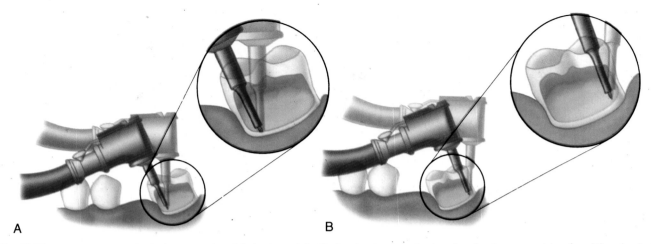

Fig. 16-24 Care must be exercised when preparing pinholes in mesially tilted molars to prevent external perforation on mesial surface (*A*) and pulpal penetration on the distal surface (*B*). Broken line indicates incorrect angulation of the twist drill.

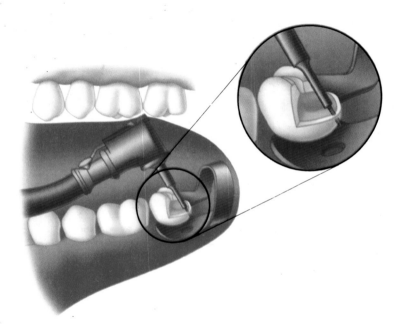

Fig. 16-25 When placing pinholes in molars and interarch space is limited care must be exercised to prevent external perforation on distal surface.

is approximately 9.5 mm in length and has a flattened head to aid in its insertion. When the pin reaches the bottom of the pinhole, it shears approximately in half, leaving a length of pin extending from dentin with the other half remaining in the hand wrench or the handpiece chuck. This second pin may be positioned in another pinhole and threaded to place in the same manner as the standard pin. The designs available with each size of pin are shown in Table 16-1 and Table 16-2.

Selection of a particular pin design is influenced by the size of the pin being used, the amount of interarch space available, and operator preference. The Minuta and Minikin pins are available only in the self-shearing and Link (also self-shearing) designs. With minimal interarch space, the two-in-one design is undesirable because of its length. The two-in-one pin and the self-shearing pin sometimes may fail to reach the bottom of the pinhole, whereas 93% of Link Series and Link Plus two-in-one pins extended to the optimal depth of 2 mm.[52-55]

Pin Insertion

Two instruments for the insertion of threaded pins are available: (1) conventional latch-type contra-angle handpieces (Figs. 16-30 and 16-31) and (2) TMS hand wrenches (see Fig. 16-29). The results of studies are conflicting as to which method of pin insertion produces the best results. The latch-type handpiece is recommended for the insertion of the Link Series and the Link Plus pins. The hand wrench is recommended for the insertion of standard pins.

When using the latch-type handpiece, a Link Series or a Link Plus pin is inserted into the handpiece and positioned over the pinhole. The handpiece is activated at low speed until the plastic sleeve shears from the pin. The pin sleeve is discarded. For low-speed handpieces with a low gear, the low gear should be used. Using the low gear increases the torque and increases the tactile sense of the operator. It also reduces the risk of stripping the threads in dentin when the pin is in place.

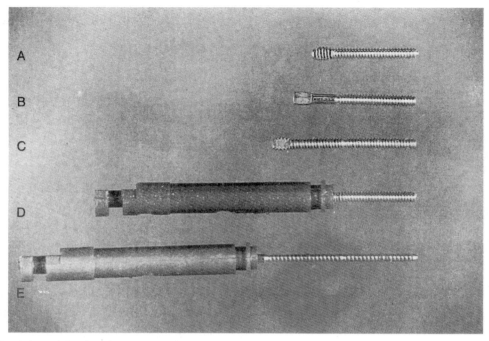

Fig. 16-26 Five designs of the Thread Mate System (TMS) pins. **A,** Standard. **B,** Self-shearing. **C,** Two-in-one. **D,** Link Series. **E,** Link Plus.

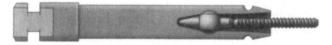

Fig. 16-27 Cross-sectional view of Link Series pin.

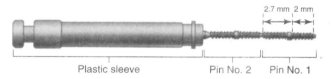

2.7 mm 2 mm

Plastic sleeve   Pin No. 2   Pin No. 1

Fig. 16-28 Link Plus pin.

A standard design pin is placed in the appropriate wrench (Fig. 16-32, *A*) and slowly threaded clockwise into the pinhole until a definite resistance is felt when the pin reaches the bottom of the hole (see Fig. 16-32, *B*). The pin should be rotated one-quarter to one half-turn counterclockwise to reduce the dentinal stress created by the end of the pin that is pressing on dentin.[56] The hand wrench should be removed from the pin carefully. If the hand wrench is used without rubber dam isolation, a gauze throat shield must be in place, and a strand of dental tape approximately 12 to 15 inches (30–38 cm) in length should be tied securely to the end of the wrench (Fig. 16-33) to prevent accidental swallowing or aspiration by the patient.

After the pins are placed, their lengths are evaluated (see Fig. 16-32, *C*). Any length of pin greater than 2 mm should be removed. A sharp No. ¼, No. ½, or No. 169L bur, at high speed and oriented perpendicular to the pin, is used to remove the excess length (Fig. 16-34, *A*). If oriented otherwise, the rotation of the bur may loosen the pin by rotating it

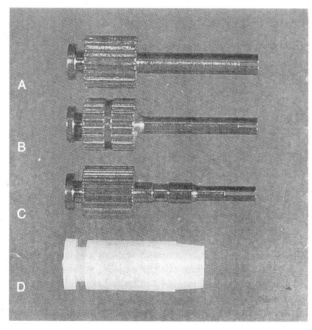

Fig. 16-29 Hand wrenches for the Thread Mate System (TMS) pins. **A,** Regular and Minikin. **B,** Minim. **C,** Minuta. **D,** Link Series and Link Plus.

counterclockwise. During removal of excess pin length, the assistant may apply a steady stream of air to the pin and have the evacuator tip positioned to remove the pin segment. Also, during removal, the pin may be stabilized with a small hemostat or cotton pliers. After placement, the pin should be tight, immobile, and not easily withdrawn.

Using a mirror, the preparation is viewed from all directions (particularly from the occlusal direction) to determine if any

Table 16-2 The Thread Mate System (TMS) Link Series and Link Plus Pins

Name	Illustration (not to scale)	Color Code	Pin Diameter (inches/mm)*	Drill Diameter (inches/mm)*	Pin Length Extending from Sleeve (mm)	Pin Length Extending from Dentin (mm)
LINK SERIES						
Regular		Gold	0.031/0.78	0.027/0.68	5.5	3.2 (single shear)
Regular		Gold	0.031/0.78	0.027/0.68	7.8	2.6 (double shear)
Minim		Silver	0.024/0.61	0.021/0.53	5.4	3.2 (single shear)
Minim		Silver	0.024/0.61	0.021/0.53	7.6	2.6 (double shear)
Minikin		Red	0.019/0.48	0.017/0.43	6.9	1.5 (single shear)
Minuta		Pink	0.015/0.38	0.0135/0.34	6.3	1 (single shear)
LINK PLUS						
Minim		Silver	0.024/0.61	0.021/0.53	10.8	2.7 (double shear)

*1 mm = 0.03937 inch.

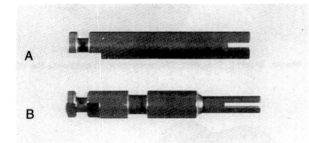

Fig. 16-30 Handpiece chucks for the Thread Mate System (TMS) regular self-shearing and Minikin pins (*A*) and TMS Minuta pins (*B*).

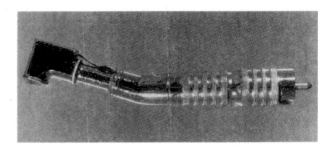

Fig. 16-31 Conventional latch-type contra-angle handpiece.

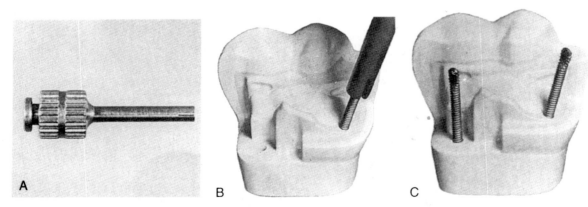

Fig. 16-32 A, Use of a hand wrench to place a pin. **B,** Threading the pin to the bottom of the pinhole and reversing the wrench one-quarter to one-half turn. **C,** Evaluating the length of the pin extending from dentin.

pins need to be bent to be positioned within the anticipated contour of the final restoration and to provide adequate bulk of amalgam between the pin and the external surface of the final restoration (see Fig. 16-34, *B* and *C*). Pins should not be bent to make them parallel or to increase their retentiveness. Occasionally, bending a pin may be necessary to allow for

condensation of amalgam occlusogingivally. When pins require bending, the TMS bending tool (Fig. 16-35, *A*) must be used. The bending tool should be placed on the pin where the pin is to be bent, and with firm controlled pressure, the bending tool should be rotated until the desired amount of bend is achieved (see Fig. 16-35, *B* through *D*). Use of the

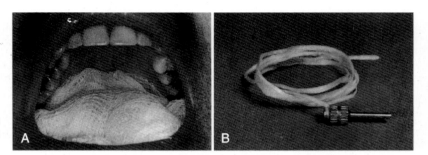

Fig. 16-33 Precautions to be taken if a rubber dam is not used. **A,** Gauze throat shield. **B,** Hand wrench with 12 to 15 inches (30–38 cm) of dental tape attached.

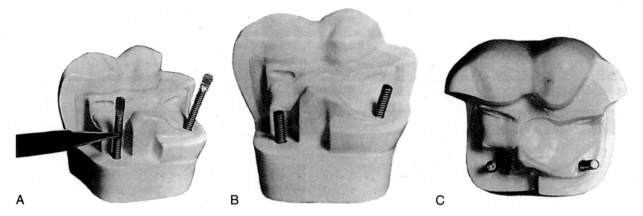

Fig. 16-34 **A,** Use of sharp No. ¼ bur held perpendicular to the pin to shorten the pin. **B** and **C,** Evaluating the preparation to determine the need for bending the pins.

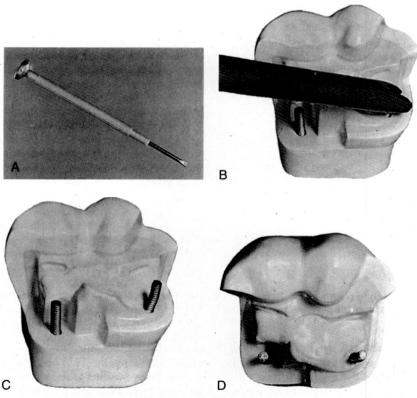

Fig. 16-35 **A,** The Thread Mate System (TMS) bending tool. **B,** Use of the bending tool to bend the pin. **C** and **D,** The pin is bent to a position that provides adequate bulk of amalgam between the pin and the external surface of the final restoration.

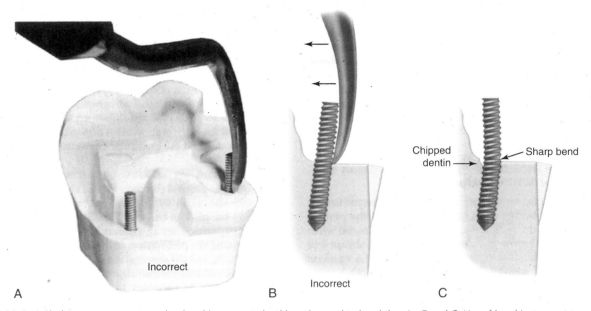

Fig. 16-36 A, A Black spoon excavator or other hand instrument should not be used to bend the pin. **B** and **C,** Use of hand instruments may create a sharp bend in the pin and fracture dentin.

bending tool allows placement of the fulcrum at some point along the length of the exposed pin. Other instruments should not be used to bend a pin because the location of the fulcrum would be at the orifice of the pinhole. These hand instruments may cause crazing or fracture of dentin, and the abrupt or sharp bend that usually results increases the chances of breaking the pin (Fig. 16-36). Also, the operator has less control when pressure is applied with a hand instrument, and the risk of slipping is increased.

POSSIBLE PROBLEMS WITH PINS

Failure of Pin-Retained Restorations

The failure of pin-retained restorations might occur at any of five different locations (Fig. 16-37). Failure can occur (1) within the restoration (restoration fracture), (2) at the interface between the pin and the restorative material (pin–restoration separation), (3) within the pin (pin fracture), (4) at the interface between the pin and dentin, and (5) within dentin (dentin fracture). Failure is more likely to occur at the pin–dentin interface than at the pin–restoration interface. The operator must keep these areas of potential failure in mind at all times and apply the necessary principles to minimize the possibility of an inadequate restoration.

Broken Drills and Broken Pins

Occasionally, a twist drill breaks if it is stressed laterally or allowed to stop rotating before it is removed from the pinhole. Use of sharp twist drills helps eliminate the possibility of drill breakage. Pins also can break during bending if care is not exercised. The treatment for broken drills and broken pins is to choose an alternative location, at least 1.5 mm remote from the broken item, and prepare another pinhole. Removal of a broken pin or drill is difficult, if not impossible, and usually should not be attempted. The best solution for these two problems is prevention.

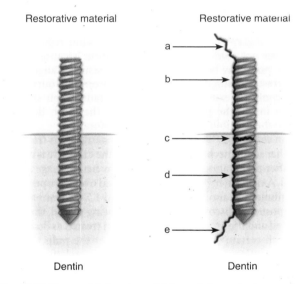

Fig. 16-37 Five possible locations of failure of pin-retained restorations: fracture of restorative material (a), separation of pin from restorative material (b), fracture of pin (c), separation of pin from dentin (d), fracture of dentin (e).

Loose Pins

Self-threading pins sometimes do not engage dentin properly because the pinhole was inadvertently prepared too large or a self-shearing pin failed to shear, resulting in stripped-out dentin. The pin should be removed from the tooth and the pinhole re-prepared with the next largest size drill, and the appropriate pin should be inserted. Preparing another pinhole of the same size 1.5 mm from the original pinhole also is acceptable.

As described earlier, a properly placed pin can be loosened while being shortened with a bur, if the bur is not held perpendicularly to the pin and the pin is stabilized. A loose pin should be removed from the pinhole by holding a rotating bur parallel to the pin and lightly contacting the surface of the pin; this causes the pin to rotate counterclockwise out of the pinhole. A second attempt should be made with the same-size pin. If the second pin fails to engage dentin tightly, a larger hole is prepared, and the appropriate pin is inserted. Preparing another pinhole of the same size 1.5 mm from the original pinhole also is acceptable.

Penetration into the Pulp and Perforation of the External Tooth Surface

Penetration into the pulp or perforation of the external surface of the tooth is obvious if hemorrhage occurs in the pinhole after removal of the drill. Usually, the operator can tell when a penetration or perforation has occurred by an abrupt loss of resistance of the drill to hand pressure. Also, if a standard or Link Series pin continues to thread into the tooth beyond the 2 mm depth of the pinhole, this is an indication of a penetration or perforation. A pulpal penetration might be suspected if the patient is anesthetized and has had no sensitivity to tooth preparation until the pinhole is being completed or the pin is being placed. With profound anesthesia, however, some patients may not feel pulpal penetration.

Radiographs can confirm that a pulpal penetration has not occurred if the view shows dentin between the pulp and the pin. A radiograph projecting the pin in the same region as the pulp does not confirm a pulpal penetration because the pin and the pulp may be superimposed as a result of angulation. In contrast, a radiograph showing a pin projecting outside the tooth confirms external perforation. A radiograph showing the pin inside the projected outline of the tooth does not exclude the possibility of an external perforation.

In an asymptomatic tooth, a pulpal penetration is treated as any other small mechanical exposure. If the exposure is discovered after preparation of the pinhole, any hemorrhage is controlled. A calcium hydroxide liner is placed over the opening of the pinhole, and another hole is prepared 1.5 to 2 mm away. If the exposure is discovered as the pin is being placed, the pin is removed and the area of pulp penetration treated as described. Although certain studies have shown that the pulp tolerates pin penetration when the pin is placed in a relatively sterile environment, it is not recommended that pins be left in place when a pulpal penetration has occurred.[43,57] If the pin were left in the pulp, (1) the depth of the pin into pulpal tissue would be difficult to determine, (2) considerable postoperative sensitivity might ensue, and (3) the pin location might complicate subsequent endodontic therapy. Regardless of the method of treatment rendered, the patient must be informed of the perforation or pulpal penetration at the completion of the appointment. The affected tooth should be evaluated periodically using appropriate radiographs. The patient should be instructed to inform the dentist if any discomfort develops.

Because most teeth receiving pins have had extensive caries, restorations, or both, the health of the pulp probably has already been compromised to some extent. The ideal treatment of a pulpal penetration for such a compromised tooth generally is endodontic therapy. Endodontic treatment should be strongly considered when such a tooth is to receive an indirect restoration.

An external perforation might be suspected if an unanesthetized patient senses pain when a pinhole is being prepared or a pin is being placed in a tooth that has had endodontic therapy. Observation of the angulation of the twist drill or the pin should indicate whether a pulpal penetration or external perforation has occurred. Perforation of the external surface of the tooth can occur occlusal or apical to the gingival attachment. Careful probing and radiographic examination must diagnose the location of a perforation accurately. The method of treatment for a perforation often depends on the experience of the operator and the particular circumstances of the tooth being treated.

Three options are available for perforations that occur occlusal to the gingival attachment: (1) The pin can be cut off flush with the tooth surface and no further treatment rendered; (2) the pin can be cut off flush with the tooth surface and the preparation for an indirect restoration extended gingivally beyond the perforation; or (3) the pin can be removed, if still present, and the external aspect of the pinhole enlarged slightly and restored with amalgam. Surgical reflection of gingival tissue may be necessary to render adequate treatment. The location of perforations occlusal to the attachment often determines the option to be pursued.

Two options are available for perforations that occur apical to the attachment: (1) Reflect the tissue surgically, remove the necessary bone, enlarge the pinhole slightly, and restore with amalgam, or (2) perform a crown-extension procedure, and place the margin of a cast restoration gingival to the perforation (Fig. 16-38). As with perforations located occlusal to the gingival attachment, the location of the perforation and the design of the present or planned restoration help determine which option to pursue. As with pulpal penetration, the patient must be informed of the perforation and the proposed treatment. The prognosis of external perforations is favorable when they are recognized early and treated properly.

Tooth Preparation for Slot-Retained Amalgam Restorations

Slot length depends on the extent of the tooth preparation. A slot may be continuous or segmented, depending on the amount of missing tooth structure and whether pins were used. Shorter slots provide as much resistance to horizontal force as do longer slots.[58] Preparations with shorter slots fail less frequently than do preparations with longer slots.[58]

A No. 330 bur is used to place a slot in the gingival floor 0.5 mm axial of the DEJ (see Fig. 16-5). The slot is 1 mm in depth and 1 mm or more in length, depending on the distance between the vertical walls.

Tooth Preparation for Amalgam Foundations

The technique of tooth preparation for a foundation depends on the type of retention that is selected—pin retention; slot retention; or, in the case of endodontically treated teeth, pulp chamber retention. The techniques have in common the axial location of the retention. As stated previously, the retention for a foundation must be sufficiently deep axially so that the final preparation for the subsequent indirect restoration does not compromise the resistance and retention forms of the foundation. The technique for each type of retention is discussed below.

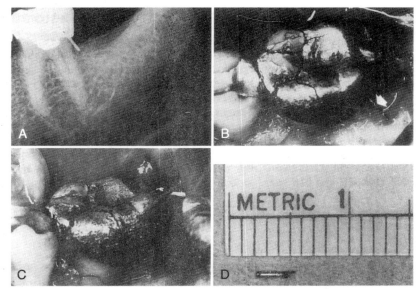

Fig. 16-38 External perforation of a pin. **A,** Radiograph showing the external perforation of a pin. **B,** Surgical access to extruding pin (*arrow*). **C,** Pin cut flush with the tooth structure and crown-lengthening procedure performed. **D,** Length of pin removed.

PIN RETENTION

Severely broken teeth with few or no vertical walls, in which an indirect restoration is indicated, may require a pin-retained foundation. The main difference between the use of pins for foundations and the use of pins in definitive restorations is the distance of the pinholes from the external surface of the tooth.[59] For foundations, the pinholes must be located farther from the external surface of the tooth (farther internally from the DEJ), and more bending of the pins may be necessary to allow for adequate axial reduction of the foundation without exposing the pins during the cast metal tooth preparation. Any removal of the restorative material from the circumference of the pin would compromise its retentive effect. If the material is removed from more than half the diameter of the pin, any retentive effect of the pin probably has been eliminated.

The location of the pinhole from the external surface of the tooth for foundations depends on (1) the occlusogingival location of the pin (external morphology of the tooth), (2) the type of restoration to be placed (a porcelain-fused-to-metal [PFM] or all-ceramic preparation requires more reduction than a full gold crown), and (3) the type of margin to be prepared. Preparations with heavily chamfered margins at a normal occlusogingival location require pin (and slot) placement at a greater axial depth. Proximal retention locks still should be used, wherever possible. The length of the pins also must be considered to permit adequate occlusal reduction without exposing the pins.

SLOT RETENTION

Slots are placed in the gingival floor of a preparation with a No. 330 bur (see Fig. 16-5). Foundation slots, as with pins, are placed slightly more axial (farther inside the DEJ) than indicated for conventional amalgam preparations. This more pulpal positioning depends on the type of preparation for a casting that is planned. The preparation for an indirect restoration should not eliminate or cut into the foundation's retentive features. The number of remaining vertical walls determines the indication for slots. Slots are used to oppose

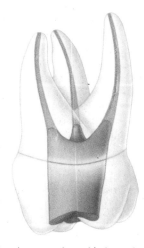

Fig. 16-39 Pulp chamber retention with 2- to 4-mm extension of the foundation into the canal spaces.

retention locks in vertical walls or to provide retention where no vertical walls remain. Slots are generally 1 mm in depth and the width of the No. 330 bur. Their length is usually 2 to 4 mm, depending on the distance between the remaining vertical walls. Increasing the width and depth of the slot does not increase the retentive strength of the amalgam restoration.[24] Retention locks are placed in the remaining vertical walls with a No. 169L or No. ¼ bur as illustrated in Fig. 16-7.

PULP CHAMBER RETENTION

For developing foundations in multi-rooted, endodontically treated teeth, an alternative technique has been recommended only when (1) dimension of the pulp chamber is adequate to provide retention and bulk of amalgam, and (2) dentin thickness in the region of the pulp chamber is adequate to provide rigidity and strength to the tooth.[60] Extension into the root canal space 2 to 4 mm is recommended when the pulp chamber height is 2 mm or less (Fig. 16-39).[61] When the pulp chamber height is 4 to 6 mm in depth, no advantage is gained from extension into the root canal space. After matrix application, amalgam is thoroughly condensed into the pulp canals, the pulp chamber, and the coronal portion of the tooth. Natural undercuts in the pulp chamber and the divergent canals provide the necessary retention form. The resistance form against forces that otherwise may cause tooth fracture is improved by gingival extension of the crown preparation approximately 2 mm beyond the foundation onto sound tooth structure. This extension should have a total taper of opposing walls of less than 10 degrees.[62] If the pulp chamber height is less than 2 mm, the use of a prefabricated post, cast post and core, pins, or slots should be considered.

Restorative Technique
Desensitizer Placement

The completed preparation is treated with a desensitizer to reduce dentin permeability.

Matrix Placement

One of the most difficult steps in restoring a severely carious posterior tooth is development of a satisfactory matrix. Fulfilling the objectives of a matrix is complicated by possible gingival extensions, missing line angles, and capped cusps typical of complex tooth preparations.

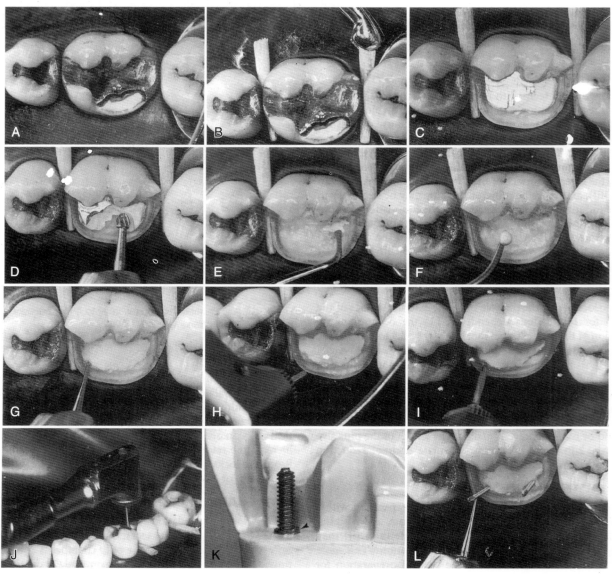

Fig. 16-40 A, Mandibular first molar with fractured distolingual cusp. **B,** Insertion of wedges. **C,** Initial tooth preparation. **D** and **E,** Excavation of any infected dentin; if indicated, any remaining old restorative material is removed. **F,** Application of a liner and a base (if necessary). **G,** Preparation of pilot holes. **H,** Alignment of the twist drill with the external surface of the tooth. **I,** Preparation of pinholes. **J,** Insertion of Link pins with a slow-speed handpiece. **K,** Depth-limiting shoulder (*arrowhead*) of inserted Link Plus pin. **L,** Use of a No. ¼ bur to shorten pins.

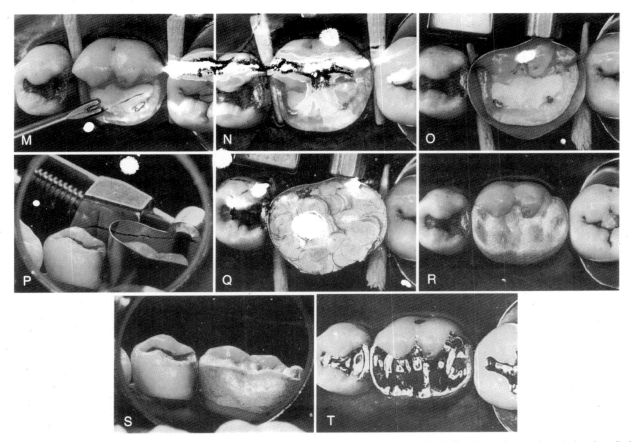

Fig. 16-40, cont'd M, Bending pins (if necessary) with a bending tool. **N,** Final tooth preparation. **O,** Tofflemire retainer and matrix band applied to the prepared tooth. **P,** Reflecting light to evaluate the proximal area of the matrix band. **Q,** Preparation overfilled. **R,** Restoration carved. **S,** Reflecting light to evaluate the adequacy of the proximal contact and contour. **T,** Restoration polished.

UNIVERSAL MATRIX

The Tofflemire retainer and band can be used successfully for most amalgam restorations (Fig. 16-40). Use of the Tofflemire retainer requires sufficient tooth structure to retain the band after it is applied. When the Tofflemire retainer is placed appropriately, but an opening remains next to prepared tooth structure, a closed system can be developed as illustrated in Figure 16-41. A strip of matrix material that is long enough to extend from the mesial to the distal corners of the tooth is cut. The strip must extend into these corners sufficiently that the band, when tight, holds the strip in position. Also, it must not extend into the proximal areas, or a ledge would result in the restoration contour when the matrix is removed. The Tofflemire retainer is loosened one-half turn, and the strip of matrix material is inserted next to the opening between the matrix band and the tooth. The retainer is then tightened and the matrix is completed. Sometimes, it is helpful to place a small amount of rigid material (hard-setting polyvinyl siloxane [PVS] or compound) between the strip and the open aspect of the band retainer to stabilize and support the strip (see Fig. 16-41, *G* and *H*).

When little tooth structure remains and deep gingival margins are present, the Tofflemire matrix may not function successfully, and the Automatrix system (DETNSPLY Caulk, Milford, DE) may be an alternative method (Fig. 16-42).

AUTOMATRIX

The Automatrix is a retainerless matrix system designed for any tooth regardless of its circumference and height. The Automatrix bands are supplied in three widths: (1) 3/16 inch, (2) 1/4 inch, and (3) 5/16 inch (4.8 mm, 6.35 mm, and 7.79 mm). The medium band is available in two thicknesses (0.0015 inch and 0.002 inch [0.038 mm and 0.05 mm]). The 3/16-inch and the 5/16-inch band widths are available in the 0.002-inch thickness only. Advantages of this system include (1) convenience, (2) improved visibility because of absence of a retainer, and (3) ability to place the auto-lock loop on the facial or lingual surface of the tooth. Disadvantages of this system are that (1) the band is flat and difficult to burnish and is sometimes unstable even when wedges are in place, and (2) development of proper proximal contours and contacts can be difficult with the Automatrix bands. Use of the Automatrix system is illustrated in Figure 16-43.

Regardless of the type of matrix system used, the matrix must be stable. If the matrix for a complex amalgam restoration is not stable during condensation, a homogeneous restoration will not be developed. The restoration might be improperly condensed, disintegrate when the matrix is removed, or eventually fail because of lack of sufficient strength. In addition to providing stability, the matrix should extend beyond the gingival margins of the preparation enough

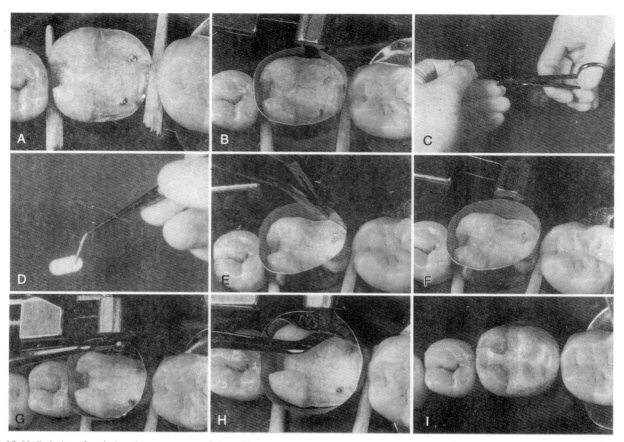

Fig. 16-41 Technique for closing the open space of the Tofflemire matrix system. **A,** Tooth preparation with wedges in place. **B,** Open aspect of the matrix band next to the prepared tooth structure. **C** and **D,** Cutting an appropriate length of the matrix material. **E,** Insertion of a strip of the matrix material. **F,** Closed matrix system. **G** and **H,** Placement of the rigid supporting material between the strip and the matrix band, and contouring, if necessary. **I,** Restoration carved.

to provide support for the matrix and to permit appropriate wedge stabilization. The matrix should extend occlusally beyond the marginal ridge of the adjacent tooth by 1 to 2 mm. Matrix stability during condensation is especially important for slot-retained amalgam restorations. If the matrix is not secure during condensation, it may slip out of position causing loss of the restoration. Clinical experience determines whether the pin-retained amalgam or slot-retained amalgam is more appropriate.

Insertion, Contouring, and Finishing of Amalgam

A high-copper alloy is strongly recommended for the complex amalgam restoration because of excellent clinical performance and high early compressive strengths.[63-65] Spherical alloys have a higher early strength than admixed alloys, and spherical alloys can be condensed more quickly with less pressure to ensure good adaptation around the pins. Proximal contacts can be easier to achieve with admixed alloys because of their condensability, however, and their extended working time might allow more adequate time for condensation, removal of the matrix band, and final carving. Because complex amalgam restorations usually are quite large, a slow-set or medium-set amalgam may be selected to provide more time for the carving and adjustment of the restoration.

Regardless of the insertion technique, care must be taken to condense amalgam thoroughly in and around the retentive features of the preparation, such as slots, grooves, and pins. If a mix of amalgam becomes dry or crumbly, a new mix is triturated immediately. Condensation is continued until the preparation is overfilled.

With a complex (or any large) amalgam, carving time must be properly allocated. The time spent on occlusal carving must be shortened to allow adequate time for carving the more inaccessible gingival margins and the proximal and axial contours. The bulk of excess amalgam on the occlusal surface is removed and the anatomy grossly developed, especially the marginal ridge heights, with a discoid carver. The occlusal embrasures are defined by running the tine of an explorer against the internal aspect of the matrix band. Appropriate marginal ridge heights and embrasures reduce the potential of fracturing the marginal ridge when the matrix is removed.

Matrix removal is crucial when placing complex amalgam restorations, especially slot-retained restorations.[13] If the matrix is removed prematurely, the newly placed restoration may fracture immediately adjacent to the areas where amalgam has been condensed into the slot(s). Any rigid material supporting the matrix is removed with an explorer or a Black spoon. Tofflemire matrices are removed first by loosening and removing the retainer while the wedges are still in place. Leaving the wedges in place may help prevent fracturing the

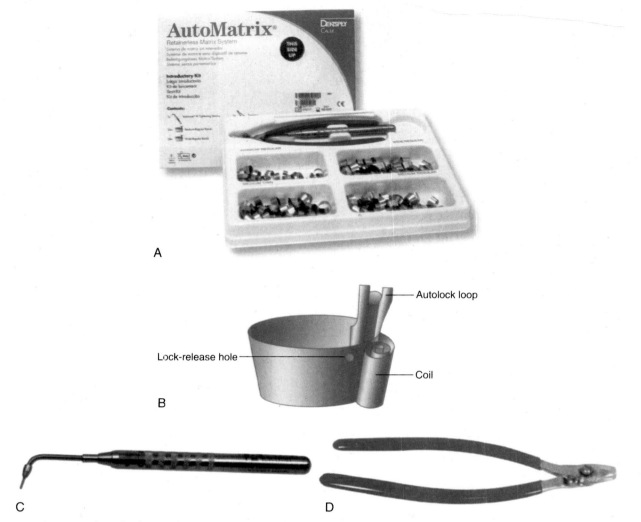

Fig. 16-42 **A,** Automatrix retainerless matrix system. **B,** Automatrix band. **C,** Automate II tightening device. **D,** Shielded nippers. (**A,** courtesy of Dentsply Caulk, Milford, DE.)

marginal ridge amalgam. It may be beneficial to place a fingertip on the occlusal surface of the restored tooth to stabilize the matrix while loosening and removing the retainer from the band. Otherwise, the torqued force of loosening the retainer may fracture the inserted amalgam. The matrix is removed by sliding each end of the band in an oblique direction (i.e., moving the band facially or lingually while simultaneously moving it in an occlusal direction). Moving the band obliquely toward the occlusal surface minimizes the possibility of fracturing the marginal ridge. Preferably, the matrix band should be removed in the same direction as the wedge placement to prevent dislodging the wedges. Automatrix bands are removed by using the system's instruments and, after the band is open, by the same technique described for the Tofflemire-retained matrices. The carving of the restoration is then continued (see Figs. 16-40, R, and 16-43, N).

The wedges are then removed, and the interproximal gingival excess of amalgam is removed with an amalgam knife or an explorer. Facial and lingual contours are developed with a Hollenback carver, an amalgam knife, or an explorer to complete the carving (see Fig. 16-40, R). Appropriately shaped

rotary instruments are used to complete the occlusal carving if amalgam has become so hard that the force needed to carve with hand instruments might fracture portions of the restoration.

Each proximal contact is evaluated by using a mirror occlusally and lingually to ensure that no light can be reflected between the restoration and the adjacent tooth at the level of the proximal contact (see Fig. 16-40, S). When the proper proximal contour or contact cannot be achieved in a large, complex restoration, it may be possible to prepare a conservative two-surface tooth preparation within the initial amalgam to restore the proper proximal surface. Amalgam forming the walls of this "ideal" preparation must have sufficient bulk to prevent future fracture.

The rubber dam is removed, and the occlusal surface of the amalgam is adjusted to obtain appropriate occlusal contacts. Thin, unwaxed dental floss may be passed through the proximal contacts once to remove amalgam shavings and smooth the proximal surface of amalgam. The floss is wrapped around the proximal aspect of the adjacent tooth when being inserted to reduce the force applied to the newly condensed amalgam.

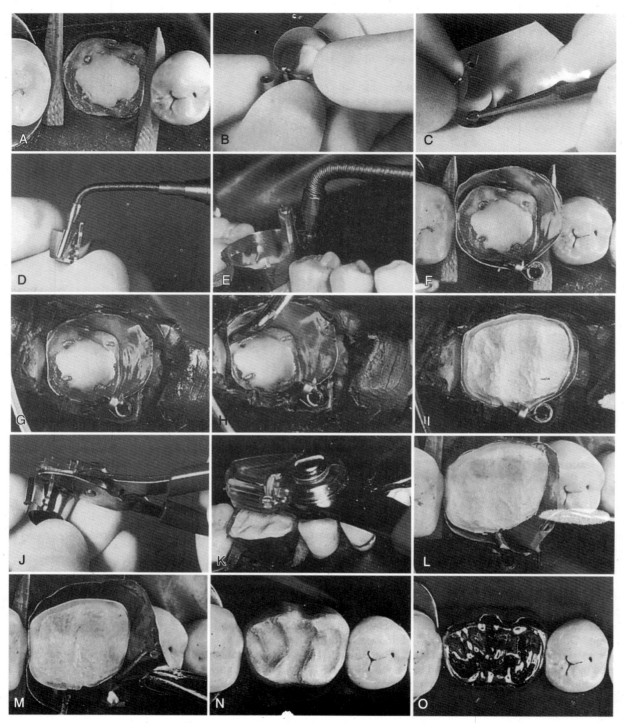

Fig. 16-43 Application of Automatrix for developing a pin-retained amalgam crown on the mandibular first molar. **A,** Tooth preparation with wedges in place. **B,** Enlargement of the circumference of the band, if necessary. **C,** Burnishing the band with an egg-shaped burnisher. **D–F,** Placement of the band around the tooth, tightening with an Automate II tightening device, and setting wedges firmly in place. **G,** Application of the green compound. **H,** Contouring of the band with the back of a warm Black spoon excavator. **I,** Overfilling the preparation and carving the occlusal aspect. **J** and **K,** Use of shielded nippers to cut an auto-lock loop. **L,** Separating the band with an explorer. **M,** Removing the band in an oblique direction (facially with some occlusal vector). **N,** Restoration carved. **O,** Restoration polished.

Amalgam excess and loose particles are removed from the gingival sulcus by moving the floss occlusogingivally and faciolingually. The patient should be cautioned not to apply biting forces to the restoration for several hours. Fast-setting high-copper amalgam can be prepared within 30 to 45 minutes after insertion of the foundation. Further finishing and polishing of the complex amalgam may be accomplished, if desired, as early as 24 hours after placement.

Summary

The complex amalgam remains a predictable, cost-effective, and safe means for the restoration of posterior teeth that are missing large amounts of structure. The design of the tooth preparation must be based on the material properties of dental amalgam for success. Restoration of normal anatomic contours can be readily accomplished with dental amalgam through the use of slots, pins, and customized matrix designs.

References

1. Van Nieuwenhuysen JP, D'Hoore W, Carvalho J, et al: Long-term evaluation of extensive restorations in permanent teeth, *J Dent* 31:395–405, 2003.
2. Mondelli RF, Barbosa WF, Mondelli J, et al: Fracture strength of weakened human premolars restored with amalgam with and without cusp coverage, *Am J Dent* 11:181–184, 1998.
3. Martin JA, Bader JD: Five-year treatment outcomes for teeth with large amalgams and crowns, *Oper Dent* 22:72–78, 1997.
4. Smales RJ: Longevity of cusp-covered amalgams: Survivals after 15 years, *Oper Dent* 16:17–20, 1991.
5. Christensen GJ: Achieving optimum retention for restorations, *J Am Dent Assoc* 135:1143–1145, 2004.
6. Mozer JE, Watson RW: The pin-retained amalgam, *Oper Dent* 4:149–155, 1979.
7. Fischer GM, Stewart GP, Panelli J: Amalgam retention using pins, boxes, and Amalgambond, *Am J Dent* 6:173–175, 1993.
8. Boyde A, Lester KS: Scanning electron microscopy of self-threading pins in dentin, *Oper Dent* 4:56–62, 1979.
9. Standlee JP, Caputo AA, Collard EW, et al: Analysis of stress distribution by endodontic posts, *Oral Surg* 33:952–960, 1972.
10. Webb EL, Straka WF, Phillips CL: Tooth crazing associated with threaded pins: A three-dimensional model, *J Prosthet Dent* 61:624–628, 1989.
11. Going RE, Moffa JP, Nostrant GW, et al: The strength of dental amalgam as influenced by pins, *J Am Dent Assoc* 77:1331–1334, 1968.
12. Welk DA, Dilts WE: Influence of pins on the compressive and horizontal strength of dental amalgam and retention of pins in amalgam, *J Am Dent Assoc* 78:101–104, 1969.
13. Robbins JW, Burgess JO, Summitt JB: Retention and resistance features for complex amalgam restorations, *J Am Dent Assoc* 118:437–442, 1989.
14. Felton DA, Webb EL, Kanoy BE, et al: Pulpal response to threaded pin and retentive slot techniques: A pilot investigation, *J Prosthet Dent* 66:597–602, 1991.
15. Bailey JH: Retention design for amalgam restorations: Pins versus slots, *J Prosthet Dent* 65:71-74, 1991.
16. Garman TA, Outhwaite WC, Hawkins IK, et al: A clinical comparison of dentinal slot retention with metallic pin retention, *J Am Dent Assoc* 107:762–763, 1983.
17. Outhwaite WC, Garman TA, Pashley DH: Pin vs. slot retention in extensive amalgam restorations, *J Prosthet Dent* 41:396–400, 1979.
18. Outhwaite WC, Twiggs SW, Fairhurst CW, et al: Slots vs. pins: A comparison of retention under simulated chewing stresses, *J Dent Res* 61:400–402, 1982.
19. Smith CT, Schuman N: Restoration of endodontically treated teeth: A guide for the restorative dentist, *Quintessence Int* 28:457–462, 1997.
20. Oliveira F, de C, Denehy GE, et al: Fracture resistance of endodontically prepared teeth using various restorative materials, *J Am Dent Assoc* 115:57–60, 1987.
21. Davis R, Overton JD: Efficacy of bonded and nonbonded amalgam in the treatment of teeth with incomplete fractures, *J Am Dent Assoc* 131:469–478, 2000.
22. McDaniel RJ, Davis RD, Murchison DF, et al: Causes of failure among cuspal-coverage amalgam restorations: A clinical survey, *J Am Dent Assoc* 131:173–177, 2000.
23. Robbins JW, Summitt JB: Longevity of complex amalgam restorations, *Oper Dent* 13:54–57, 1988.
24. Chan CC, Chan KC: The retentive strength of slots with different width and depth versus pins, *J Prosthet Dent* 58:552–557, 1987.
25. Going RE: Pin-retained amalgam, *J Am Dent Assoc* 73:619–624, 1966.
26. Pameijer CH, Stallard RE: Effect of self-threading pins, *J Am Dent Assoc* 85:895–899, 1972.
27. Moffa JP, Razzano MR, Doyle MG: Pins—a comparison of their retentive properties, *J Am Dent Assoc* 78:529–535, 1969.
28. Perez E, Schoeneck G, Yanahara H: The adaptation of noncemented pins, *J Prosthet Dent* 26:631–639, 1971.
29. Vitsentzos SI: Study of the retention of pins, *J Prosthet Dent* 60:447–451, 1988.
30. Dilts WE, Welk DA, Laswell HR, et al: Crazing of tooth structure associated with placement of pins for amalgam restorations, *J Am Dent Assoc* 81:387–391, 1970.
31. Trabert KC, Caputo AA, Collard EW, et al: Stress transfer to the dental pulp by retentive pins, *J Prosthet Dent* 30:808–815, 1973.
32. Dilts WE, Welk DA, Stovall J: Retentive properties of pin materials in pin-retained silver amalgam restorations, *J Am Dent Assoc* 77:1085–1089, 1968.
33. Eames WB, Solly MJ: Five threaded pins compared for insertion and retention, *Oper Dent* 5:66–71, 1980.
34. Hembree JH: Dentinal retention of pin-retained devices, *Gen Dent* 29:420–422, 1981.
35. Khera SC, Chan KC, Rittman BR: Dentinal crazing and interpin distance, *J Prosthet Dent* 40:538–543, 1978.
36. Wing G: Pin retention amalgam restorations, *Aust Dent J* 10:6–10, 1965.
37. Courtade GL, Timmermans JJ, editors: *Pins in restorative dentistry*, St. Louis, 1971, Mosby.
38. Dilts WE, Duncanson MG Jr, Collard EW, et al: Retention of self-threading pins, *J Can Dent Assoc* 47:119–120, 1981.
39. Durkowski JS, Harris RK, Pelleu GB, et al: Effect of diameters of self-threading pins and channel locations on enamel crazing, *Oper Dent* 7:86–91, 1982.
40. Mondelli J, Vieira DF: The strength of Class II amalgam restorations with and without pins, *J Prosthet Dent* 28:179–188, 1972.
41. Cecconi BT, Asgar K: Pins in amalgam: A study of reinforcement, *J Prosthet Dent* 26:159–169, 1971.
42. Dilts WE, Mullaney TP: Relationship of pinhole location and tooth morphology in pin-retained silver amalgam restorations, *J Am Dent Assoc* 76:1011–1015, 1968.
43. Dolph R: Intentional implanting of pins into the dental pulp, *Dent Clin North Am* 14:73–80, 1970.
44. Caputo AA, Standlee JP: Pins and posts—why, when, and how, *Dent Clin North Am* 20:299–311, 1976.
45. Gourley JV: Favorable locations for pins in molars, *Oper Dent* 5:2–6, 1980.
46. Wacker DR, Baum L: Retentive pins: their use and misuse, *Dent Clin North Am* 29:327–340, 1985.
47. Caputo AA, Standlee JP, Collard EW: The mechanics of load transfer by retentive pins, *J Prosthet Dent* 29:442–449, 1973.
48. Dilts WE, Coury TL: Conservative approach to the placement of retentive pins, *Dent Clin North Am* 20:397–402, 1976.
49. Standlee JP, Collard EW, Caputo AA: Dentinal defects caused by some twist drills and retentive pins, *J Prosthet Dent* 24:185–192, 1970.
50. Standlee JP, Caputo AA, Collard EW: Retentive pin installation stresses, *Dent Pract Dent Rec* 21:417–422, 1971.
51. Kelsey WP III, Blankenau RJ, Cavel WT: Depth of seating of pins of the Link Series and Link Plus Series, *Oper Dent* 8:18–22, 1983.
52. Barkmeier WW, Cooley RL: Self-shearing retentive pins: A laboratory evaluation of pin channel penetration before shearing, *J Am Dent Assoc* 99:476–479, 1979.
53. Barkmeier WW, Frost DE, Cooley RL: The two-in-one, self-threading, self-shearing pin: Efficacy of insertion technique, *J Am Dent Assoc* 97:51–53, 1978.
54. Garman TA, Binon PP, Averette D, et al: Self-threading pin penetration into dentin, *J Prosthet Dent* 43:298–302, 1980.
55. May KN, Heymann HO: Depth of penetration of Link Series and Link Plus pins, *Gen Dent* 34:359–361, 1986.
56. Irvin AW, Webb EL, Holland GA, et al: Photoelastic analysis of stress induced from insertion of self-threading retentive pins, *J Prosthet Dent* 53:311–316, 1985.

57. Abraham G, Baum L: Intentional implantation of pins into the dental pulp, *J South Cal Dent Assoc* 40:914–920, 1972.

58. McMaster DR, House RC, Anderson MH, et al: The effect of slot preparation length on the transverse strength of slot-retained restorations, *J Prosthet Dent* 67:472–477, 1992.

59. Lambert RL, Goldfogel MH: Pin amalgam restoration and pin amalgam foundation, *J Prosthet Dent* 54:10–12, 1985.

60. Nayyar A, Walton RE, Leonard LA: An amalgam coronal-radicular dowel and core technique for endodontically treated posterior teeth, *J Prosthet Dent* 43:511–515, 1980.

61. Kane JJ, Burgess JO, Summitt JB: Fracture resistance of amalgam coronal-radicular restorations, *J Prosthet Dent* 63:607–613, 1990.

62. Shillingburg HT, Jr, editor: *Fundamentals of fixed prosthodontics*, ed 3, Chicago, 1997, Quintessence.

63. Leinfelder KF: Clinical performance of amalgams with high content of copper, *Gen Dent* 29:52–55, 1981.

64. Osborne JW, Binon PP, Gale EN: Dental amalgam: Clinical behavior up to eight years, *Oper Dent* 5:24–28, 1980.

65. Eames WB, MacNamara JF: Eight high copper amalgam alloys and six conventional alloys compared, *Oper Dent* 1:98–107, 1976.

Chapter 17

Class II Cast Metal Restorations

John R. Sturdevant

The cast metal restoration is versatile and is especially applicable to Class II onlay preparations. The process has many steps, involves numerous dental materials, and requires meticulous attention to detail. Typically, a dental laboratory is involved, and the dentist and the laboratory technician must be devoted to perfection. The high degree of satisfaction and service derived from a properly made cast metal restoration is a reward for the painstaking application required.[1] The Class II *inlay* involves the occlusal surface and one or more proximal surfaces of a posterior tooth. When cusp tips are restored, the term *onlay* is used. The procedure requires two appointments: the first for preparing the tooth and making an impression, and the second for delivering the restoration to the patient. The fabrication process is referred to as an *indirect procedure* because the casting is made on a replica of the prepared tooth in a dental laboratory.

Material Qualities

Cast metal restorations can be made from a variety of casting alloys. Although the physical properties of these alloys vary, their major advantages are their high compressive and tensile strengths. These high strengths are especially valuable in restorations that rebuild most or all of the occlusal surface.

The American Dental Association (ADA) Specification No. 5 for Dental Casting Gold Alloys requires a minimum total gold-plus-platinum-metals content of 75 weight percent (wt%). Such traditional high-gold alloys are unreactive in the oral environment and are some of the most biocompatible materials available to the restorative dentist.[2] At present, four distinct groups of alloys are in use for cast restorations: (1) traditional high-gold alloys, (2) low-gold alloys, (3) palladium–silver alloys, and (4) base metal alloys. Each of the alternatives to high-gold alloys has required some modification of technique or acceptance of reduced performance, most commonly related to decreased tarnish resistance and decreased burnishability.[3] Also, they have been associated with higher incidences of post-restorative allergy, most often exhibited by irritated soft tissue adjacent to the restoration.[2]

Indications

Large Restorations

The cast metal inlay is an alternative to amalgam or composite when the higher strength of a casting alloy is needed or when the superior control of contours and contacts that the indirect procedure provides is desired. The cast metal onlay is often an excellent alternative to a crown for teeth that have been greatly weakened by caries or by large, failing restorations but where the facial and lingual tooth surfaces are relatively unaffected by disease or injury. For such weakened teeth, the superior physical properties of a casting alloy are desirable to withstand the occlusal loads placed on the restoration; also, the onlay can be designed to distribute occlusal loads over the tooth in a manner that decreases the chance of tooth fracture in the future. Preserving intact facial and lingual enamel (or cementum) is conducive to maintaining the health of contiguous soft tissue. When proximal surface caries is extensive, favorable consideration should be given to the cast inlay or onlay. The indirect procedure used to develop the cast restoration allows more control of contours and contacts (proximal and occlusal).

Endontically Treated Teeth

A molar or premolar with endodontic treatment can be restored with a cast metal onlay, provided that the onlay has been thoughtfully designed to distribute occlusal loads in such a manner as to reduce the chance of tooth fracture.

Teeth at Risk for Fracture

Fracture lines in enamel and dentin, especially in teeth having extensive restorations, should be recognized as cleavage planes for possible future fracture of the tooth. Restoring these teeth with a restoration that braces the tooth against fracture injury may be warranted sometimes. Such restorations are cast onlays (with skirting) and crowns.

Dental Rehabilitation with Cast Metal Alloys

When cast metal restorations have been used to restore adjacent or opposing teeth, the continued use of the same material may be considered to eliminate electrical and corrosive activity that sometimes occurs between dissimilar metals in the mouth, particularly when they come in contact with each other.

Diastema Closure and Occlusal Plane Correction

Often, the cast inlay or onlay is indicated when extension of the mesiodistal dimension of the tooth is necessary to form a contact with an adjacent tooth. Cast onlays also can be used to correct the occlusal plane of a slightly tilted tooth.

Removable Prosthodontic Abutment

Teeth that are to serve as abutments for a removable partial denture can be restored with a cast metal restoration. The major advantages of a cast restoration are as follows: (1) The superior physical properties of the cast metal alloy allow it to better withstand the forces imparted by the partial denture, and (2) the rest seats, guiding planes, and other aspects of contour relating to the partial denture are better controlled when the indirect technique is used.

Contraindications

High Caries Rate

Facial and lingual (especially lingual) smooth-surface caries indicates a high caries activity that should be brought under control before expensive cast metal restorations are used. Full crown restorations are usually indicated if caries is under control, but defects exist on the facial and lingual surfaces, as well as on the occlusal and proximal surfaces.

Young Patients

With younger patients, direct restorative materials (e.g., composite or amalgam) are indicated, unless the tooth is severely broken or endodontically treated. An indirect procedure requires longer and more numerous appointments, access is more difficult, the clinical crowns are shorter, and younger patients may neglect oral hygiene, resulting in additional caries.

Esthetics

The dentist must consider the esthetic impact (display of metal) of the cast metal restoration. This factor usually limits the use of cast metal restorations to tooth surfaces that are invisible at a conversational distance. Composite and porcelain restorations are alternatives in esthetically sensitive areas.

Small Restorations

Because of the success of amalgam and composite, few cast metal inlays are done in small Class I and II restorations.

Advantages

Strength

The inherent strength of dental casting alloys allows them to restore large damaged or missing areas and be used in ways that protect the tooth from future fracture injury. Such restorations include onlays and crowns.

Biocompatibility

As previously mentioned, high-gold dental casting alloys are unreactive in the oral environment. This biocompatibility can be helpful for many patients who have allergies or sensitivities to other restorative materials.

Low Wear

Although individual casting alloys vary in their wear resistance, castings are able to withstand occlusal loads with minimal changes. This is especially important in large restorations that restore a large percentage of occlusal contacts.

Control of Contours and Contacts

Through the use of the indirect technique, the dentist has great control over contours and contacts. This control becomes especially important when the restoration is larger and more complex.

Disadvantages

Number of Appointments and Higher Chair Time

The cast inlay or onlay requires at least two appointments and much more time than a direct restoration, such as amalgam or composite.

Temporary Restorations

Patients must have temporary restorations between the preparation and delivery appointments. Temporaries occasionally loosen or break, requiring additional visits.

Cost

In some instances, cost to the patient becomes a major consideration in the decision to restore teeth with cast metal restorations. The cost of materials, laboratory bills, and the time involved make indirect cast restorations more expensive than direct restorations.

Technique Sensitivity

Every step of the indirect procedure requires diligence and attention to detail. Errors at any part of the long, multi-step process tend to be compounded, resulting in less than ideal fits.

Splitting Forces

Small inlays may produce a wedging effect on facial or lingual tooth structure and increase the potential for splitting the tooth. Onlays do not have this disadvantage.

Initial Procedures

Occlusion

Before the anesthetic is administered and before preparation of any tooth, the occlusal contacts of teeth should be

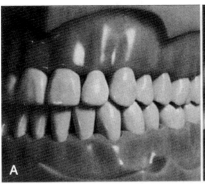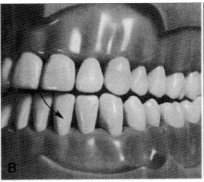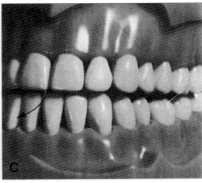

Fig. 17-1 **A–C,** Evaluate occlusal relationships in maximum intercuspation (*A*) and during mandibular movements (*B* and *C*). Be alert for problems with tooth alignment and contact position. Note the amount of posterior separation provided by the guidance of anterior teeth (working side) and articular eminence (nonworking side).

evaluated. As part of this evaluation, the dentist must decide if the existing occlusal relationships can be improved with the cast metal restoration. An evaluation should include (1) the occlusal contacts in maximum intercuspation where teeth are brought into full interdigitation and (2) the occlusal contacts that occur during mandibular movements (Fig. 17-1). The pattern of occlusal contacts influences the preparation design, selection of interocclusal records, and type of articulator or cast development needed.

Anesthesia

Local anesthesia of the tooth to be operated on and of adjacent soft tissue usually is recommended. Anesthesia in these areas eliminates pain and reduces salivation, resulting in a more pleasant procedure for the patient and the operator.

Considerations for Temporary Restorations

Before preparation of the tooth, consideration must be given to the method that will be used to fabricate the temporary restoration. Most temporary restoration techniques require the use of a preoperative impression to reproduce the occlusal, facial, and lingual surfaces of the temporary restoration to the preoperative contours.

The technique involves making a preoperative impression with an elastic impression material. Alginate impression materials may be used and are relatively inexpensive. The preoperative impression may be made with a polyvinyl siloxane (PVS) impression material if additional accuracy, stability, and durability are required. If the tooth to be restored has any large defects such as a missing cusp, either of two methods may be used to reproduce the missing cusp in the temporary. First, an instrument can be used to remove the impression material in the area of the missing cusp or tooth structure, to simulate the desired form for the temporary restoration. Second, wax can be added to the tooth before the impression, as follows: The tooth is dried and large defects filled with utility wax. The wax is smoothed, and an impression is made by using a quadrant tray if no more than two teeth are to be prepared (Fig. 17-2, *A*). A full-arch tray may be used for greater stability. The tray filled with impression material is then seated (see Fig. 17-2, *B*). After the impression has set, the impression is removed

and examined for completeness (see Fig. 17-2, *C*). Alginate impressions can distort quickly if they are allowed to gain or lose moisture, so the impression is wrapped in wet paper towels to serve as a humidor (see Fig. 17-2, *D*). Pre-operative polyvinyl impressions do not need to be wrapped. The preoperative impression is set aside for later use in forming the temporary restoration.

Tooth Preparations for Class II Cast Metal Restorations

A small, distal, cavitated caries lesion in the maxillary right first premolar is used to illustrate the classic two-surface preparation for an inlay (Fig. 17-3, *A*). Treatment principles for other defects are presented later. As indicated previously, few small one-surface or two-surface inlays are done. Because the description of a small tooth preparation presents the basic concepts, it is used to illustrate the technique. More extensive tooth preparations are presented later.

Tooth Preparation for Class II Cast Metal Inlays
Initial Preparation

Carbide burs used to develop the vertical internal walls of the preparation for cast metal inlays and onlays are plane cut, tapered fissure burs. These burs are plane cut so that the vertical walls are smooth. The side and end surfaces of the bur should be straight to aid in the development of uniformly tapered walls and smooth pulpal and gingival walls. Recommended dimensions and configurations of the burs to be used are shown in Figure 17-3, *B*. Suggested burs are the No. 271 and the No. 169L burs (Brasseler USA, Inc., Savannah, GA). Before using unfamiliar burs, the operator is cautioned to verify measurements to judge the depth into the tooth during preparation. The sides and end surface of the No. 271 bur meet in a slightly rounded manner so that sharp, stress-inducing internal angles are not formed in the preparation.[4] The marginal bevels are placed with a slender, fine-grit, flame-shaped diamond instrument such as the No. 8862 bur (Brasseler USA, Inc.).

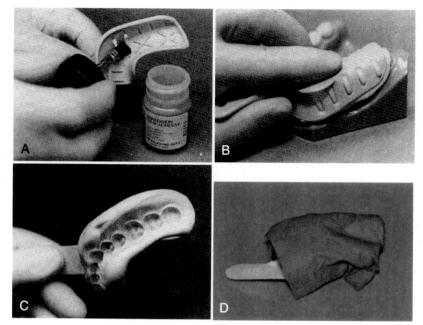

Fig. 17-2 **A,** Applying tray adhesive to stock quadrant tray. **B,** Making pre-operative impression. **C,** Inspecting pre-operative impression for completeness. **D,** When using alginate, wrap the impression with wet paper towels to serve as a humidor.

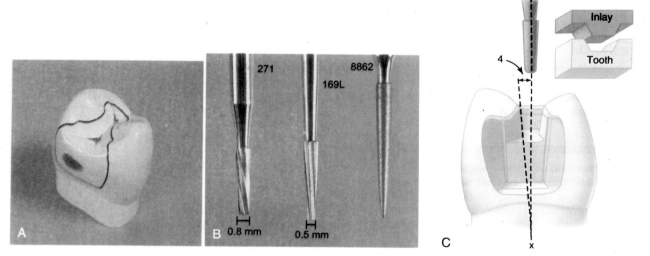

Fig. 17-3 **A,** Proposed outline form for disto-occlusal preparation. **B,** Dimensions and configuration of No. 271, No. 169L, and No. 8862 instruments. **C,** Conventional 4-degree divergence from line of draw (line *xy*).

Throughout the preparation for a cast inlay, the cutting instruments used to develop the vertical walls are oriented to a single "draw" path, usually the long axis of the tooth crown, so that the completed preparation has draft (no undercuts) (see Fig. 17-3, *C*). The gingival-to-occlusal divergence of these preparation walls may range from 2 to 5 degrees per wall from the line of draw. If the vertical walls are unusually short, a maximum of 2 degrees occlusal divergence is desirable to increase retention potential. As the occlusogingival height increases, the occlusal divergence should increase because lengthy preparations with minimal divergence (more parallel) may present difficulties during the seating and withdrawal of the restoration.

OCCLUSAL STEP

With the No. 271 carbide bur held parallel to the long axis of the tooth crown, the dentist enters the fossa or pit closest to the involved marginal ridge, using a punch cut to a depth of 1.5 mm to establish the depth of the pulpal wall (Fig. 17-4, *A* and *B*). In the initial preparation, this specified depth should not be exceeded, regardless of whether the bur end is in dentin, caries, old restorative material, or air. The bur should be rotating at high speed (with air-water spray) before application to the tooth and should not stop rotating until it is removed; this minimizes perceptible vibration and prevents breakage or chipping of the bur blades. A general rule is to maintain the long axis of the bur parallel to the long axis of the tooth crown

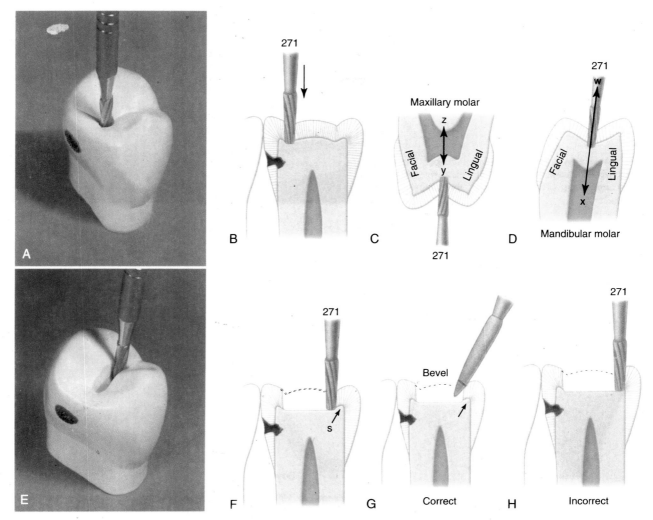

Fig. 17-4 **A** and **B,** Bur after punch cut to a depth of 1.5 mm. **C,** For maxillary posterior teeth, the long axis of the bur should parallel the long axis of the tooth crown (line *yz*). **D,** For molar and second premolar teeth of mandibular dentition, the long axis of the bur should tilt slightly lingually to parallel the long axis of the tooth crown (line *wx*). **E** and **F,** Extending the mesial wall, taking care to conserve dentin that supports marginal ridge (*s*). **G,** The marginal bevel can provide additional extension. **H,** Improper extension that has weakened the marginal ridge.

at all times (see Fig. 17-4, *B* and *C*). For mandibular molars and second premolars whose crowns tilt slightly lingually, this rule dictates that the bur should also be tilted slightly (5–10 degrees) lingually to conserve the strength of the lingual cusps (see Fig. 17-4, *D*). When the operator is cutting at high speeds, a properly directed air-water spray is used to provide the necessary cooling and cleansing effects.[5]

Maintaining the 1.5-mm initial depth and the same bur orientation, the dentist extends the preparation outline mesially along the central groove or fissure to include the mesial fossa or pit (see Fig. 17-4, *E* and *F*). Ideally, the faciolingual dimension of this cut should be minimal. The dentist takes care to keep the mesial marginal ridge strong by not removing the dentin support of the ridge (see Fig. 17-4, *F* and *H*). The use of light intermittent pressure minimizes heat production on the tooth surface and reduces the incidence of enamel crazing ahead of the bur. Occasionally, a fissure extends onto the mesial marginal ridge. This defect, if shallow, may be treated with enameloplasty, or it may be included in the

outline form with the cavosurface bevel, which is applied in a later step in the tooth preparation (see Fig. 17-4, *G*).

Enameloplasty, as presented in earlier chapters, occasionally reduces extension along the fissures, conserving the tooth structure vital for pulp protection and the strength of the remaining tooth crown. The extent to which enameloplasty can be used usually cannot be determined until the operator is in the process of extending the preparation wall, when the depth of the fissure in the enamel wall can be observed (Fig. 17-5). When enameloplasty shows a fissure in a marginal ridge to be deeper than one third the thickness of enamel, the procedures described in the later section should be used.

Extend to include faulty facial and lingual fissures radiating from the mesial pit. During this extension cutting, the operator is cautioned again not to remove the dentin support of the proximal marginal ridge. To conserve the tooth structure and the strength of the remaining tooth, the final extension up these fissures can be accomplished with the slender No. 169L carbide bur (Fig. 17-6, *A*). The tooth structure and strength

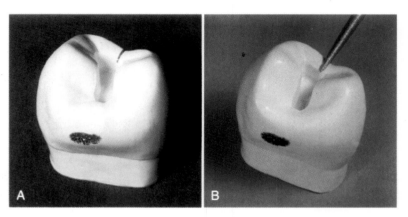

Fig. 17-5 A, Shallow enamel fault that is no deeper than one third the thickness of enamel. **B,** Using fine-grit diamond instrument to remove enamel that contains shallow fault.

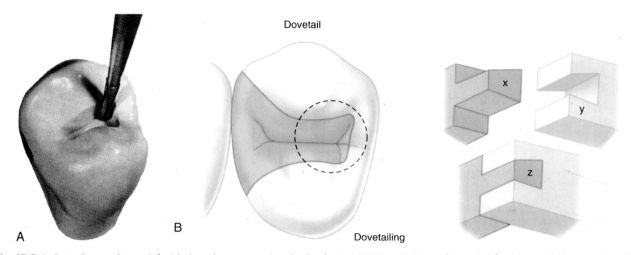

Dovetail

Dovetailing

Fig. 17-6 A, Extending up the mesiofacial triangular groove using the slender No. 169L bur. **B,** Dovetail retention form is created by extension shown in *A*. As *x* fits into *y* only in one direction resulting in *z*, similarly dovetail portion of inlay fits into the dovetail portion of the preparation only in an occlusal-to-gingival direction.

can be conserved further by using (1) enameloplasty of the fissure ends, when possible, and (2) the marginal bevel of the final preparation to include (eliminate) the terminal ends of these fissures in the outline form. The facial and lingual extensions in the mesial pit region should provide the desired dovetail retention form, which resists distal displacement of the inlay (see Fig. 17-6, *B*). When these facial and lingual grooves are not faulty, sufficient facial extension in the mesial pit region should be made to provide this dovetail retention form against distal displacement. Minor extension in the transverse ridge area to include any remaining facial or lingual caries may necessitate additional facial or lingual extension in the mesial pit to provide this dovetail feature. (During such facial or lingual extensions to sound tooth structure, the bur depth is maintained at 1.5 mm.) If major facial or lingual extension is required to remove undermined occlusal enamel, capping the weak remaining cuspal structure and additional features in the preparation to provide adequate retention and resistance forms may be indicated. These considerations are discussed in subsequent sections.

Continuing at the initial depth, the occlusal step is extended distally into the distal marginal ridge sufficiently to expose the junction of the proximal enamel and dentin (Fig. 17-7, *A* and

B). While extending distally, the dentist progressively widens the preparation to the desired faciolingual width in anticipation of the proximal box preparation. The increased faciolingual width enables the facial and lingual walls of the box to project (visually) perpendicularly to the proximal surface at positions that clear the adjacent tooth by 0.2 to 0.5 mm (see Fig. 17-7, *F*). The facial and lingual walls of the occlusal step should go around the cusps in graceful curves, and the prepared isthmus in the transverse ridge ideally should be only slightly wider than the bur, thus conserving the dentinal protection for the pulp and maintaining the strength of the cusps. If the occlusal step has been prepared correctly, any caries on the pulpal floor should be uncovered by facial and lingual extensions to sound enamel (supported by dentin).

PROXIMAL BOX

Continuing with the No. 271 carbide bur, the distal enamel is isolated by cutting a proximal ditch (see Fig. 17-7, *C* through *F*). The harder enamel should guide the bur. Slight pressure toward enamel is necessary to prevent the bur from cutting only dentin. If the bur is allowed to cut only dentin, the resulting axial wall would be too deep. The mesiodistal width of the ditch should be 0.8 mm (the tip diameter of the bur) and

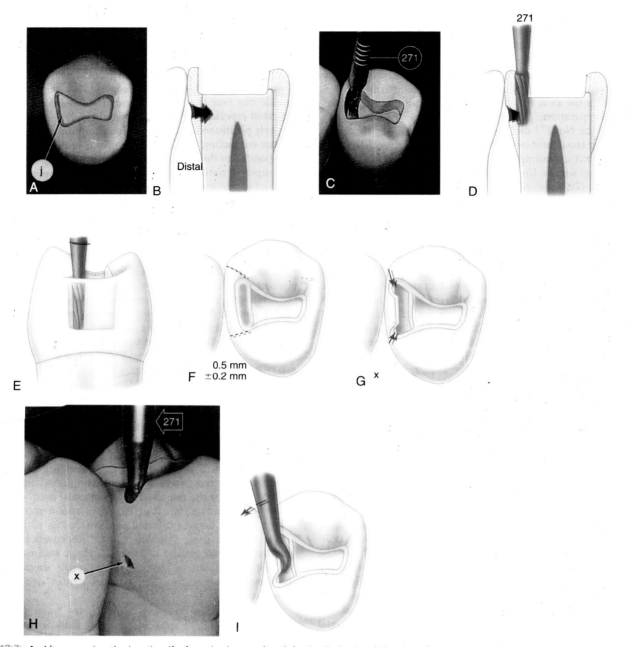

Fig. 17-7 **A,** After exposing the junction (*j*) of proximal enamel and dentin. **B,** Sectional drawing of *A*. **C,** Cutting the proximal ditch. **D,** Sectional drawing of *C*. **E,** Proximal view of *D*. **F,** Occlusal view of the proximal ditch with proposed ideal clearance with the adjacent tooth. **G** and **H,** Proximal ditch extended distally. *x,* penetration of enamel by side of bur at its gingival end. **I,** Breaking away isolated enamel.

prepared approximately two thirds (0.5 mm) at the expense of dentin and one third (0.3 mm) at the expense of enamel. The gingival extension of this cut may be checked with the length of the bur by first measuring the depth from the height of the marginal ridge and then removing the bur and holding it beside the tooth. A periodontal probe also may be used for this measurement. While penetrating gingivally, the dentist extends the proximal ditch facially and lingually beyond the caries to the desired position of the facioaxial and linguoaxial line angles. If the caries lesion is minimal, the ideal extension facially and lingually is performed as previously described (see Fig. 17-7, *F*). Ideal gingival extension of a minimal, cavitated

lesion eliminates caries on the gingival floor and provides a 0.5-mm clearance of the unbeveled gingival margin with the adjacent tooth. Moderate to extensive caries on the proximal surface dictates continued extension of the proximal ditch to the extent of the caries at the dentinoenamel junction (DEJ), but not pulpally (see Fig. 17-11, *D*). When preparing the proximal portion of the preparation, the dentist maintains the side of the bur at the specified axial wall depth regardless of whether it is in dentin, caries, old restorative material, or air. The operator should guard against overcutting the facial, lingual, and gingival walls, which would not conserve the tooth structure and could result in (1) overextension of the margins in the completed preparation, (2) a weakened tooth, and (3) possible injury of soft tissue. Because the proximal enamel diminishes in thickness from the occlusal to gingival level, the end of the bur is closer to the external tooth surface as the cutting progresses gingivally. The axial wall should follow the contour of the tooth faciolingually. Any carious dentin on the axial wall should not be removed at this stage of the preparation.

With the No. 271 carbide bur, the dentist makes two cuts, one at the facial limit of the proximal ditch and the other at the lingual limit, extending from the ditch perpendicularly toward the enamel surface (in the direction of the enamel rods) (see Fig. 17-7, G). These cuts are extended until the bur is nearly through the marginal ridge enamel (the side of the bur may emerge slightly through the surface at the level of the gingival floor) as shown in Figure 17-7, H. This weakens the enamel by which the remaining isolated portion is held. Also, the level of the gingival floor is verified by observing where the end of the bur emerged through the proximal surface. If indicated, additional gingival extension can be accomplished while the remaining enamel still serves to guide the bur and to prevent it from marring the proximal surface of the adjacent tooth. At this time, however, the remaining wall of enamel often breaks away during cutting, especially when high speeds are employed. If the isolated wall of enamel is still present, it can be fractured out with a spoon excavator (see Fig. 17-7, I). At this stage, the ragged enamel edges left from breaking away the proximal surface may be touching the adjacent tooth.

Planing the distofacial, distolingual, and gingival walls by hand instruments to remove all undermined enamel may be indicated if minimal extension is needed to fulfill an esthetic objective. Depending on access, the operator can use a No. 15 (width) straight chisel, bin-angle chisel (Fig. 17-8), or enamel hatchet. For a right-handed operator, the distal beveled bin-angle chisel is used on the distofacial wall of a disto-occlusal preparation for the maxillary right premolar. The dentist planes the wall by holding the instrument in the modified palm-and-thumb grasp and uses a chisel-like motion in an occlusal-to-gingival direction (see Fig. 17-8, A and B). The dentist planes the gingival wall by using the same instrument as a hoe, scraping in a lingual-to-facial direction (see Fig. 17-8, C). In this latter action, the axial wall may be planed with the side edge (secondary edge) of the blade. The distolingual wall is planed smooth by using the bin-angle chisel with the mesial bevel (see Fig. 17-8, D). When proximal caries is minimal, ideal facial and lingual extensions at this step in the preparation result in margins that clear the adjacent tooth by 0.2 to 0.5 mm.

The experienced operator usually does not use chisel hand instruments during the preparation for inlays, considering that the narrow, flame-shaped, fine-grit diamond instrument, when artfully used, removes ragged, weak enamel during application of the cavosurface bevel and flares and causes the patient to be less apprehensive (see Figs. 17-12 and 17-13). If the diamond instrument is to be used exclusively in finishing the enamel walls and margins, this procedure is postponed until after the removal of any remaining infected dentin, old restorative material, or both and the application of any necessary base. Waiting prevents any hemorrhage (which occasionally follows the beveling of the gingival margin) from hindering (1) the suitable removal of remaining infected dentin and old restorative material and (2) the proper application of a

necessary base. Hand instruments are more useful on the mesiofacial surfaces of maxillary premolars and first molars, where minimal extension is desired to prevent an unsightly display of metal.

Shallow (0.3-mm deep) retention grooves may be cut in the facioaxial and linguoaxial line angles with the No. 169L carbide bur (see Fig. 17-8, E through I). These grooves are indicated especially when the prepared tooth is short. When properly positioned, the grooves are in sound dentin, close to but not contacting, the DEJ. The long axis of the bur must be held parallel to the line of draw. Preparing these grooves may be postponed until after any required bases are applied during the final preparation.

Final Preparation
REMOVAL OF INFECTED CARIOUS DENTIN AND PULP PROTECTION

After the initial preparation has been completed, the dentist evaluates the internal walls of the preparation visually and tactilely (with an explorer) for indications of any remaining carious dentin. If carious dentin remains, and if it is judged to be infected, but shallow or moderate (≥1 mm of remaining dentin between the caries and the pulp), satisfactory isolation for the removal of such caries and the application of any necessary base may be attained by reducing salivation through anesthesia and the use of cotton rolls, a saliva ejector, and gingival retraction cord. The retraction cord also serves to widen the gingival sulcus and slightly retract the gingiva in preparation for beveling and flaring the proximal margins (Fig. 17-9; see also Fig. 17-12, A and B). For insertion of the cord, see the sections on preparation of bevels and flares and tissue retraction. The removal of the remaining caries and placement of a necessary base can be accomplished during the time required for the full effect of the inserted cord. A slowly revolving round bur (No. 2 or No. 4) or spoon excavator is used to remove carious infected dentin (see Fig. 17-9, F and G). If a bur is used, visibility can be improved by using air alone. This excavation is done just above stall-out speed with light, intermittent cutting. The operator should avoid unnecessarily desiccating the exposed dentin during this procedure.

Light-cured glass ionomer cement may be mixed and applied with a suitable applicator to these shallow (or moderately deep) excavated regions to the depth and form of the ideally prepared surface. Placing a base takes little time and should be considered because it results in working dies (subsequently in the laboratory phase) that have preparation walls with no undercuts and "ideal" position and contour. Also, applying a base at this time minimizes additional irritation of the pulp during subsequent procedures necessary for the completion of the restoration. The light-cured glass ionomer adheres to the tooth structure and does not require retentive undercuts when the base is small to moderate. The material is applied by conveying small portions on the end of a periodontal probe and is light-cured when the correct form has been achieved (see Fig. 17-9, H and I). Any excess cement can be trimmed back to the ideal form with the No. 271 carbide bur after the cement has hardened.

If the caries lesion is judged to approach the pulp closely, a rubber dam should be applied before the removal of infected dentin. Rubber dam provides the optimal environment for

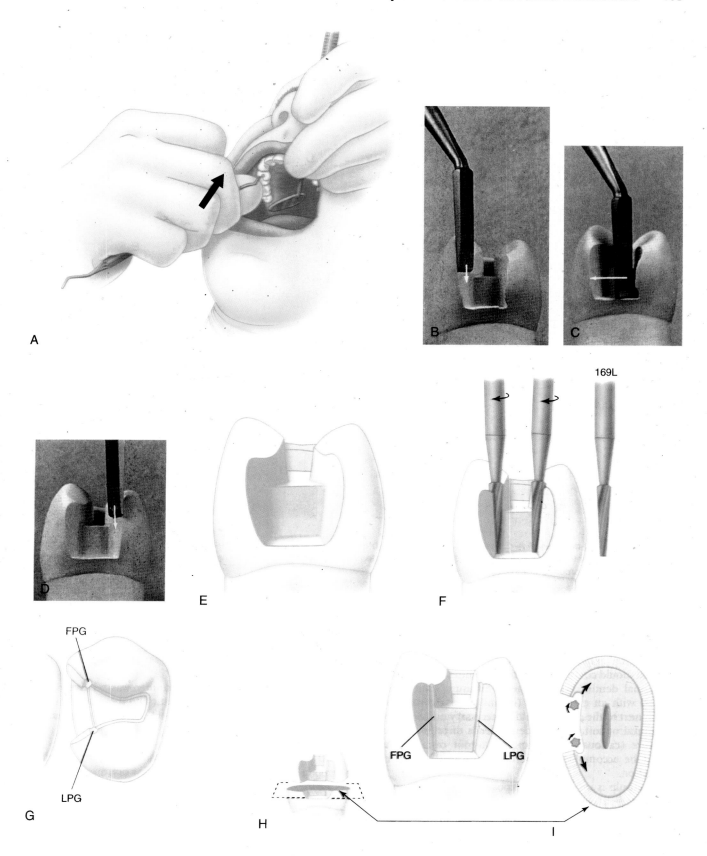

Fig. 17-8 **A–D,** Using modified palm-and-thumb grasp (*A*) to plane distofacial and distolingual walls (*B* and *D*) and to scrape gingival wall (*C*). **E,** Before cutting retention grooves. **F,** Cutting retention grooves. **G** and **H,** Facial proximal groove (*FPG*) and lingual proximal groove (*LPG*). **I,** Section in plane *x*. Large arrows depict the direction of translation of the rotating bur.

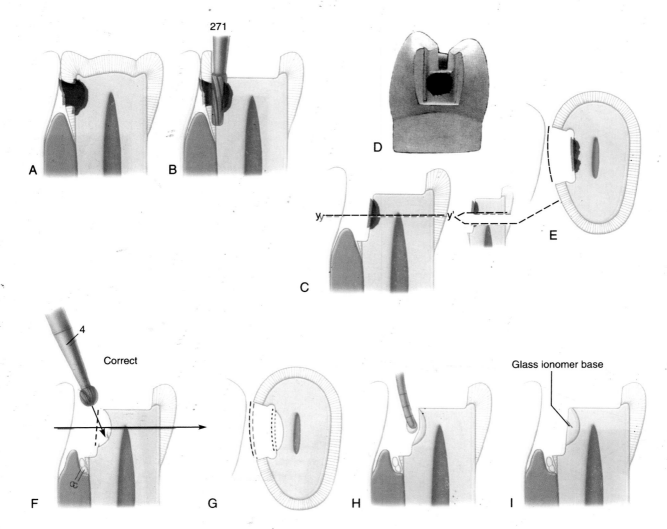

Fig. 17-9 Moderately deep caries. **A–C,** Extending the proximal ditch gingivally (*B*) to a sound floor free from caries (*C*). **D,** Remaining caries on the axial wall. **E,** Section of *C* in plane *yy*. **F,** Removing the remaining infected dentin. *c*, inserted retraction cord. **G,** Section of *F*. **H,** Inserting glass ionomer base with periodontal probe. **I,** Completed base.

successfully treating a pulp exposure should it occur. When excavating extensive caries, the dentist attempts to remove only infected dentin and not affected dentin because removal of the latter might expose a healthy pulp. Ideally, caries removal should continue until the remaining dentin is as hard as normal dentin; however, heavy pressure should not be applied with an explorer tip (or any other instrument) on dentin next to the pulp to avoid unnecessary pulpal exposure. If removal of soft, infected dentin leads directly to a pulpal exposure (carious pulpal exposure), root canal treatment should be accomplished before completing the cast metal restoration.

If the pulp is inadvertently exposed as a result of operator error or misjudgment (mechanical pulpal exposure), the operator must decide whether to proceed with the root canal treatment or to attempt a direct pulp capping procedure. A clinical evaluation should be made to determine the health of the pulp. A favorable prognosis for the pulp after direct pulp capping may be expected if the following criteria are met:

- The exposure is small (<0.5 mm in diameter).
- The tooth has been asymptomatic, showing no signs of pulpitis.
- Any hemorrhage from the exposure site is easily controlled.
- The invasion of the pulp chamber was relatively atraumatic with little physical irritation to the pulp tissue.
- A clean, uncontaminated operating field is maintained (i.e., by using a rubber dam).

If the excavation closely approaches the pulp or if a direct pulp cap is indicated, the dentist should first apply a lining of calcium hydroxide using a flow technique (without pressure). This calcium hydroxide liner should cover and protect any possible near or actual exposure and extend over a major portion of the excavated dentinal surface (Fig. 17-10, *A*). Although undetected, an exposed recessional tract of a pulp horn may exist in any deep excavation. Calcium hydroxide treatment of an exposed, healthy pulp promotes the formation of a dentin bridge, which would close the exposure.[3] The

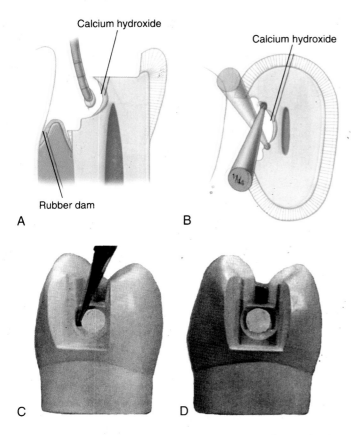

Calcium hydroxide

Rubber dam

A

Calcium hydroxide

B

C

D

Fig. 17-10 A, Deep caries excavations near the pulp are first lined with calcium hydroxide. Note the rubber dam. **B–D,** Cutting retention coves for retaining glass ionomer cement.

peripheral 0.5 to 1 mm of the dentin excavation should be left available for bonding the subsequently applied light-cured glass ionomer cement base.

Although the light-cured glass ionomer cement is adhesive to dentin, large cement bases can be subjected to considerable stresses during fabrication of the temporary and try-in and cementation of the cast metal restoration. Also, if a calcium hydroxide liner has been applied, less dentin is available for adhesive bonding. In these circumstances, small mechanical undercuts can increase the retention of the glass ionomer base. If suitable undercuts are not present after the removal of infected dentin, retention coves are placed with the No. $\frac{1}{4}$ carbide bur (see Fig. 17-10, B through D). These coves are placed in the peripheral dentin of the excavation and are as remote from the pulp as possible. Light-cured glass ionomer cement should be applied without pressure. It should completely cover the calcium hydroxide lining and some peripheral dentin for good adhesion (Fig. 17-11). The cement base should be sufficiently thick in dimension to protect the thin underlying dentin and the calcium hydroxide liner from subsequent stresses. Usually, good resistance form dictates that the pulpal wall should not be formed entirely by a cement base; rather, in at least two regions, one diametrically across the excavation from the other, the pulpal wall should be in normal position, flat, and formed by sound dentin (see region S in Fig. 17-11, E, which depicts basing in a mandibular molar). The dentist should consider the addition of other

retention features such as proximal grooves if a major portion of a proximal axial wall is composed mostly of cement base because this base should not be relied on for contributing to retention of the cast restoration (see Fig. 17-8, F).

Any remaining old restorative material on the internal walls should be removed if any of the following conditions are present: (1) The old material is judged to be thin, nonretentive, or both, (2) radiographic evidence of caries under the old material is present, (3) the pulp was symptomatic preoperatively, or (4) the periphery of the remaining restorative material is not intact (i.e., some breach exists in the junction of the material with the adjacent tooth structure that may indicate caries under the material). If none of these conditions is present, the operator may elect to leave the remaining restorative material to serve as a base, rather than risk unnecessary removal of sound dentin or irritation or exposure of the pulp. The same isolation conditions described previously for the removal of infected dentin also apply for the removal of old restorative material.

Future root canal therapy is a possibility for any tooth treated for deep caries that approximates or exposes the pulp. When treating a tooth that has had such extensive caries, the following should be considered: (1) reducing all cusps to cover the occlusal surface with metal, for better distribution of occlusal loads, and (2) adding skirts to the preparation to augment the resistance form because teeth are more prone to fracture after root canal therapy.

PREPARATION OF BEVELS AND FLARES

After the cement base (where indicated) is completed, the slender, flame-shaped, fine-grit diamond instrument is used to bevel the occlusal and gingival margins and to apply the secondary flare on the distolingual and distofacial walls. This should result in 30- to 40-degree marginal metal on the inlay (see Figs. 17-12, H, 17-13, J, and 17-14, B). This cavosurface design helps seal and protect the margins and results in a strong enamel margin with an angle of 140 to 150 degrees. A cavosurface enamel angle of more than 150 degrees is incorrect because it results in a less defined enamel margin (finish line), and the marginal cast metal alloy is too thin and weak if its angle is less than 30 degrees. Conversely, if the enamel margin is 140 degrees or less, the metal is too bulky and difficult to burnish when its angle is greater than 40 degrees (see Fig. 17-14, F).

Usually, it is helpful to insert a gingival retraction cord of suitable diameter into the gingival sulcus adjacent to the gingival margin and leave it in place for several minutes just before the use of the flame-shaped diamond instrument on the proximal margins (Fig. 17-12, A through C). The cord should be small enough in diameter to permit relatively easy insertion and to preclude excessive pressure against the gingival tissue, and yet it should be large enough to widen the sulcus to about 0.5 mm. Immediately before the flame-shaped diamond instrument is used, the cord may be removed to create an open sulcus that improves visibility for beveling the gingival margin and helps prevent injury and subsequent hemorrhage of gingival tissue. Some operators prefer to leave the cord in the sulcus while placing the gingival bevel.

Using the flame-shaped diamond instrument that is rotating at high speed, the dentist prepares the lingual secondary flare (see Fig. 17-12, D through F; Fig. 17-13, A). The dentist approaches from the lingual embrasure (see Fig. 17-12, F),

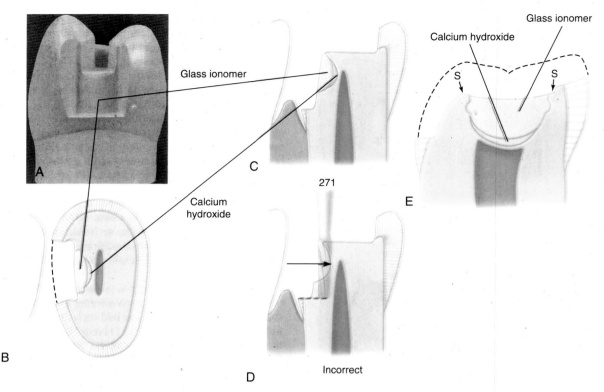

Fig. 17-11 **A–C,** Completed base for the treatment of deep caries. **D,** *Never* deepen entire axial wall with the side of a fissure bur to remove caries because the pulp would be greatly irritated from the resulting closeness of the gingivoaxial region of the preparation. **E,** Cement base placed deep in the excavation on the mandibular molar. Note the flat seats in sound dentin (*S*) that are required for adequate resistance form.

moving the instrument mesiofacially. The direction of the distolingual wall and the position of the distolingual margin are compared before and after this extension (see Figs. 17-8, *G,* and 17-13, *A*). The distolingual wall extends from the linguoaxial line angle into the lingual embrasure in two planes (see Fig. 17-13, *A*). The first is termed *lingual primary flare;* the second is termed *lingual secondary flare.* During this (secondary) flaring operation, the long axis of the instrument is held nearly parallel to the line of draw, with only a slight tilting mesially and lingually for assurance of draft (see Fig. 17-12, *D* and *E*), and the direction of translation of the instrument is that which results in a marginal metal angle of 40 degrees (see Figs. 17-12, *F,* and 17-13, *J*).

The dentist bevels the gingival margin by moving the instrument facially along the gingival margin (see Figs. 17-12, *G,* and 17-13, *A*). While cutting the gingival bevel, the rotational speed should be reduced to increase the sense of touch; otherwise, over-beveling may result. The instrument should be tilted slightly mesially to produce a gingival bevel with the correct steepness to result in 30-degree marginal metal (see Fig. 17-12, *C, H,* and *J*). If the instrument is not tilted in this manner, the bevel is too steep, resulting in gingival bevel metal that is too thin (<30-degree metal) and too weak. Although the instrument is tilted mesially, its long axis must not tilt facially or lingually (see Fig. 17-12, *G*). The gingival bevel should be 0.5 to 1 mm wide and should blend with the lingual secondary flare.

The operator completes the gingival bevel and prepares the facial secondary flare (see Fig. 17-13, *A* through *F*). The long

axis of the instrument during this secondary flare is again returned nearly to the line of draw, with only a small tilting mesially and facially, and the direction of translation of the instrument is that which results in 40-degree marginal metal (see Fig. 17-13, *E* and *J*). When the adjacent proximal surface (mesial of the second premolar) is not being prepared, care must be exercised to avoid abrading the adjacent tooth and overextending the distofacial margin. To prevent such abrasion or overextension, the instrument may be raised occlusally (using the narrower portion at its tip end) to complete the most facial portion of the wall and margin (see Fig. 17-13, *D*). Also, the more slender No. 169L carbide bur may be used, rather than the flame-shaped diamond instrument (see Fig. 17-13, *H*). The No. 169L bur produces an extremely smooth surface to the secondary flare and a smooth, straight distofacial margin. When access permits, a fine-grit sandpaper disk may be used on the facial and lingual walls and on the margins of the proximal preparation, especially when minimal extension of the facial margin is desired (see Fig. 17-13, *I*). This produces smooth walls and helps create respective margins that are straight (not ragged) and sound.

In the flaring and beveling of the proximal margins, as described in the previous paragraphs, the procedure began at the lingual surface and proceeded to the facial surface. The direction may be reversed, however, starting at the facial surface and moving toward the lingual surface. On the mesiofacial surface of maxillary premolars and first molars where extension of the facial margin should be minimal, it is usually desirable to use the lingual-to-facial direction.

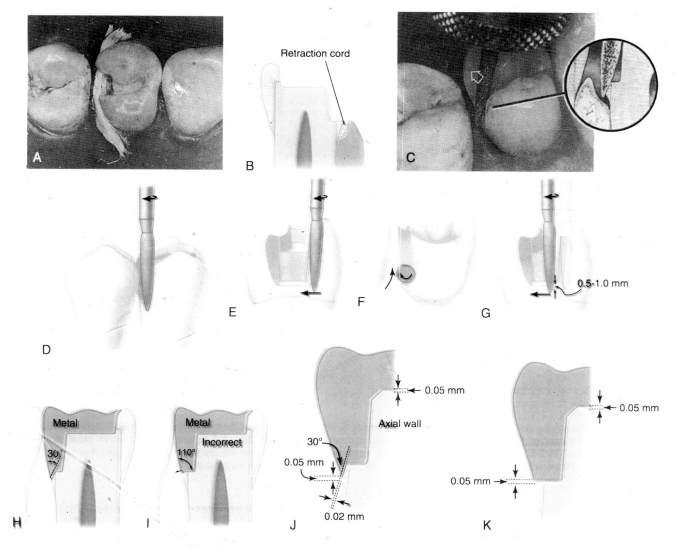

Fig. 17-12 **A** and **B,** The retraction cord is inserted in the gingival sulcus and left for several minutes. **C,** An open gingival sulcus after the cord shown in *A* is removed facilitates beveling the gingival margin with a diamond instrument. **D–F,** Diamond instrument preparing lingual secondary flare. Large arrow in *F* indicates the direction of the translation. **G,** Beveling the gingival margin. Note in *C* the mesial tilting of diamond instrument to produce a bevel that is properly directed to result in 30-degree marginal metal as shown in *H.* **H,** Properly directed gingival bevel resulting in 30-degree marginal metal. **I,** Failure to bevel the gingival margin results in a weak margin formed by undermined rods (note the easily displaced wedge of enamel) and 110-degree marginal metal, an angular design unsuitable for burnishing. **J,** Lap, sliding fit of prescribed bevel metal decreases the 50-μm error of seating to 20 μm. **K,** A 50-μm error of seating produces an equal cement line of 50 μm along the unbeveled gingival margin.

The gingival bevel serves the following purposes:

- Weak enamel is removed. If the gingival margin is in the enamel, it would be weak if not beveled because of the gingival declination of the enamel rods (see Fig. 17-12, *I*).
- The bevel results in 30-degree metal that is burnishable (on the die) because of its angular design (see Fig. 17-12, *H*). Bulky 110-degree metal along an unbeveled margin is not burnishable (see Fig. 17-12, *I*).
- A lap, sliding fit is produced at the gingival margin (see Fig. 17-12, *J*). This helps improve the fit of the casting in this region. With the prescribed gingival bevel, if the inlay fails to seat by 50 μm, the void between the bevel metal and the gingival bevel on the tooth may be 20 μm; however, failure to apply such a bevel would result in a void

(and a cement line) as great as in the failure to seat (see Fig. 17-12, *K*).

Uninterrupted blending of the gingival bevel into the secondary flares of the distolingual and distofacial walls results in the distolingual and distofacial margins joining the gingival margin in a desirable arc of a small circle; also, the gingivofacial and gingivolingual line angles no longer extend to the marginal outline. If such line angles are allowed to extend to the preparation outline, early failure may follow because of an "open" margin, dissolution of exposed cement, and eventual leakage, all potentially resulting in caries.

The secondary flare is necessary for several reasons: (1) The secondary flaring of the proximal walls extends the margins into the embrasures, making these margins more self-cleaning

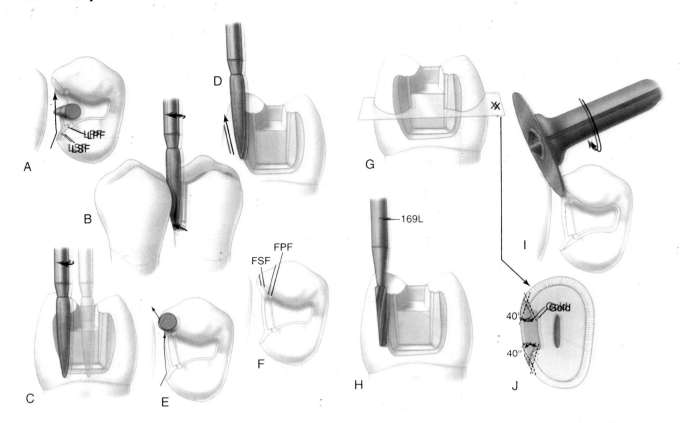

Fig. 17-13 **A,** Occlusal view of Figure 17-12, *G. LSF,* lingual secondary flare; *LPF,* lingual primary flare. **B–E,** Preparing the facial secondary flare. Large arrows in *B, D,* and *E* indicate the direction of the translation. **F,** Completed facial secondary flare. *FSF,* facial secondary flare; *FPF,* facial primary flare. **G,** Distal view of *F. x,* Plane of cross-section shown in *J.* **H** and **I,** Preparing the secondary flare with the No. 169L carbide bur (*H*) or with paper disk (*I*). **J,** The secondary flares are directed to result in 40-degree marginal metal and 140-degree marginal enamel.

and more accessible to finishing procedures during the inlay insertion appointment, and does so with conservation of dentin. (2) The direction of the flare results in 40-degree marginal metal (see Fig. 17-13, *J*). Metal with this angular design is burnishable; however, metal shaped at a larger angle is unsatisfactory for burnishing; metal with an angle less than 30 degrees is too thin and weak, with a corresponding enamel margin that is too indefinite and ragged. (3) A more blunted and stronger enamel margin is produced because of the secondary flare.

In a later section, the secondary flare is omitted for esthetic reasons on the mesiofacial proximal wall of preparations on premolars and first molars of the maxillary dentition. In this location, the wall is completed with minimal extension by using either hand instruments (straight bin-angle chisel) followed by a fine-grit sandpaper disk or very thin rotary instruments.

The flame-shaped, fine-grit diamond instrument also is used for occlusal bevels. The width of the cavosurface bevel on the occlusal margin should be approximately one-fourth the depth of the respective wall (Fig. 17-14, *A* and *B*). The exception to the rule is when a wider bevel is desired to include an enamel defect (see Fig. 17-14, *G* and *H*). The resulting occlusal marginal metal of the inlay should be 40-degree metal; the occlusal marginal enamel is 140-degree enamel (see Fig. 17-14, *B* and *E*). Beveling the occlusal margins

in this manner increases the strength of the marginal enamel and helps seal and protect the margins. While beveling the occlusal margins, a guide to diamond positioning is to maintain an approximate 40-degree angle between the side of the instrument and the external enamel surface; this also indicates when an occlusal bevel is necessary (see Fig. 17-14, *A*). If the cusp inclines are so steep that the diamond instrument, when positioned at a 40-degree angle to the external enamel surface, is parallel with the enamel preparation wall, no bevel is indicated (see Fig. 17-14, *C*). By using this technique, it can be seen that margins on the proximal marginal ridges always require a cavosurface bevel (see Fig. 17-14, *D* and *I*). Failure to apply a bevel in these regions leaves the enamel margin weak and subject to injury by fracture before the inlay insertion appointment and during the try-in of the inlay when burnishing the marginal metal. Also, failure to bevel the margins on the marginal ridges results in metal alloy that is difficult to burnish because it is too bulky (see Fig. 17-14, *F*). Similarly, the importance of extending the occlusal bevel to include the portions of the occlusal margin that cross over the marginal ridge cannot be overemphasized (see Fig. 17-14, *H* and *I*). These margins are beveled to result in 40-degree marginal metal. Otherwise, fracture of the enamel margin in such stress-vulnerable regions may occur in the interim between the preparation and the cementation appointment.

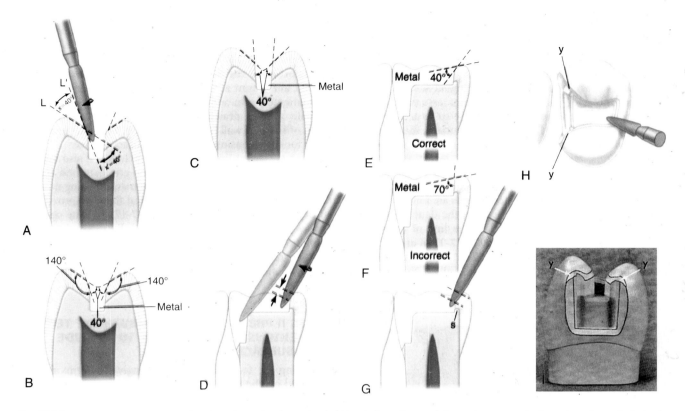

Fig. 17-14 **A,** The diamond instrument beveling the occlusal margin when it is indicated to result in 40-degree marginal metal, as shown in *B*. Angles *x* and *x* are equal because the opposite angles are equal when two lines (*L* and *L*) intersect. The diamond instrument is always directed such that an angle of 40 degrees is made by the side of the instrument and the external enamel surface. **B,** Occlusal marginal metal is approximately 40 degrees in cross-section, making the enamel angle 140 degrees. **C,** When the cuspal inclines are steep, no beveling is indicated considering that 40-degree metal would result without beveling. **D,** Beveling the mesial margin and the axiopulpal line angle. **E,** The mesial bevel is directed correctly to result in 40-degree marginal metal. **F,** An unbeveled mesial margin is incorrect because it results in a weak enamel margin and unburnishable marginal metal. **G,** To conserve dentinal support (*s*), occlusal defects on the marginal ridge are included in the outline form by applying a cavosurface bevel, which may be wider than usual, when necessary. **H,** Occlusal view of *G*. Preparing a 140-degree cavosurface enamel angle at regions labeled *y* usually dictates that the occlusal bevel be extended over the marginal ridges into the secondary flares. **I,** Distal view of *H*.

The diamond instrument also is used to bevel the axiopulpal line angle lightly (see Fig. 17-14, *D*). Such a bevel provides a thicker and stronger wax pattern at this critical region. The desirable metal angle at the margins of inlays is 40 degrees except at the gingival margins, where the metal angle should be 30 degrees. The completed preparation is illustrated in Figure 17-15, *A*.

Modifications in Inlay Tooth Preparations

Because the indications for small inlays are rare, the following sections provide procedural information that may promote better understanding of their applications in more complex and larger inlay or onlay restorations.

MESIO-OCCLUSO-DISTAL PREPARATION

If a marginal ridge is severely weakened because of excessive extension, the preparation outline often should be altered to include the proximal surface. The disto-occlusal preparation illustrated in the previous section would be extended to a mesio-occluso-distal preparation (Fig. 17-16, *A* through *C*; see also Fig. 17-15, *B* through *D*). The decision to extend the

preparation in this manner calls for clinical judgment as to whether the remaining marginal ridge would withstand occlusal forces without fracture. A fortunate factor in favor of not extending the preparation is that such ridge enamel usually is composed of gnarled enamel and is stronger than it appears. Caries present on both proximal surfaces would result in a mesio-occluso-distal preparation and restoration. The only difference in technique as described previously is the inclusion of the other proximal surface.

MODIFICATIONS OF CLASS II PREPARATION FOR ESTHETICS

For esthetic reasons, minimal flare is desired for the mesiofacial proximal wall in maxillary premolars and first molars in Class II cast metal preparations (see Fig. 17-15, *D*). The mesiofacial margin is minimally extended facially of the contact to such a position that the margin is barely visible from a facial viewing position. To accomplish this, the secondary flare is omitted, and the wall and margin are developed with (1) a chisel or enamel hatchet and final smoothing with a fine-grit paper disk or (2) a narrow diamond or bur when access permits.

FACIAL OR LINGUAL SURFACE GROOVE EXTENSION

Sometimes, a faulty facial groove (fissure) on the occlusal surface is continuous with a faulty facial surface groove (mandibular molars), or a faulty distal oblique groove on the occlusal surface is continuous with a faulty lingual surface groove (maxillary molar). This situation requires extension of the preparation outline to include the fissure to its termination (Fig. 17-17; see also Fig. 17-19, *C*). Occasionally, the operator may extend further gingivally than the fissure length to improve retention form. Such groove extensions, when sufficiently long, are effective for increasing retention. Likewise, this extension may be indicated to provide sufficient retention form even though the facial or lingual surface grooves are not fissured.

For extension onto the facial surface, the dentist uses the No. 271 carbide bur held parallel to the line of draw and extends through the facial ridge (see Fig. 17-17, *A* and *B*). The depth of the cut should be 1.5 mm. The floor (pulpal wall) should be continuous with the pulpal wall of the occlusal portion of the preparation (see Fig. 17-17, *D*).

With the bur still aligned with the path of draw, the dentist uses the side of the bur to cut the facial surface portion of this extension (see Fig. 17-17, *C*). The diameter of the bur serves as a depth gauge for the axial wall, which is in dentin. The blade portion of the No. 271 bur is 0.8 mm in diameter at its tip end and 1 mm at the neck; the axial wall depth should approximate 1 mm or slightly more. The bur should be tilted lingually as it is drawn occlusally, to develop the uniform depth of the axial wall (see Fig. 17-17, *D*). The same principles apply for the extension of a lingual surface groove.

When a facial or lingual groove is included, it also must be beveled. With the flame-shaped, fine-grit diamond instrument, the operator bevels the gingival margin (using no more than one third the depth of the gingival floor) to provide for 30-degree marginal metal (see Fig. 17-17, *E*). The operator applies a light bevel on the mesial and distal margins that is continuous with the occlusal and gingival bevels and results in 40-degree metal at these margins (see Fig. 17-17, *F* and *G*). The bevel width around the extended groove is approximately 0.5 mm.

CLASS II PREPARATION FOR ABUTMENT TEETH AND EXTENSION GINGIVALLY TO INCLUDE ROOT-SURFACE LESIONS

Extending the facial, lingual, and gingival margins may be indicated on the proximal surfaces of abutments for removable partial dentures to increase the surface area for the development of guiding planes. In addition, the occlusal outline form must be wide enough faciolingually to accommodate any contemplated rest preparation without involving the margins of the restoration. These extensions may be accomplished by simply increasing the width of the bevels.

The following modified preparation is recommended when further gingival extension is indicated to include a root lesion on the proximal surface. The gingival extension should be accomplished primarily by lengthening the gingival bevel, especially when preparing a tooth that has a longer clinical crown than normal as a result of gingival recession. It is necessary to extend (gingivally) the gingival floor only slightly, and although the axial wall consequently must be moved pulpally, this should be minimal. If additional extension of the gingival floor is necessary, it should not be as wide pulpally as when the floor level is at a normal position (Fig. 17-18, *A*). These considerations are necessary because of the draft requirement and because the tooth is smaller apically. Extending the preparation gingivally without these modifications would result in a dangerous encroachment of the axial wall on the pulp (see Fig. 17-18, *B*).

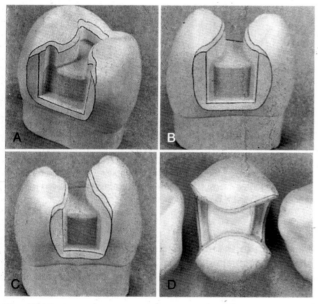

Fig. 17-15 **A,** Completed disto-occlusal preparation for the inlay. **B,** Mesio-occluso-distal preparation for the inlay on the maxillary right first premolar, disto-occlusal view. **C,** Same preparation as in *B*, mesio-occlusal view. **D,** Same preparation as in *B*, occlusal view. Note the absence, for esthetic reasons, of secondary flare on the mesiofacial aspect and minimal extension of the mesiofacial margin.

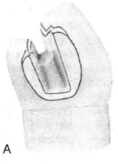
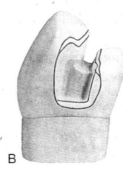
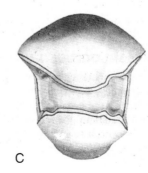

Fig. 17-16 Mandibular first premolar prepared for the mesio-occluso-distal inlay. Distal view (*A*), mesial view (*B*), and occlusal view (*C*).

A   B   C

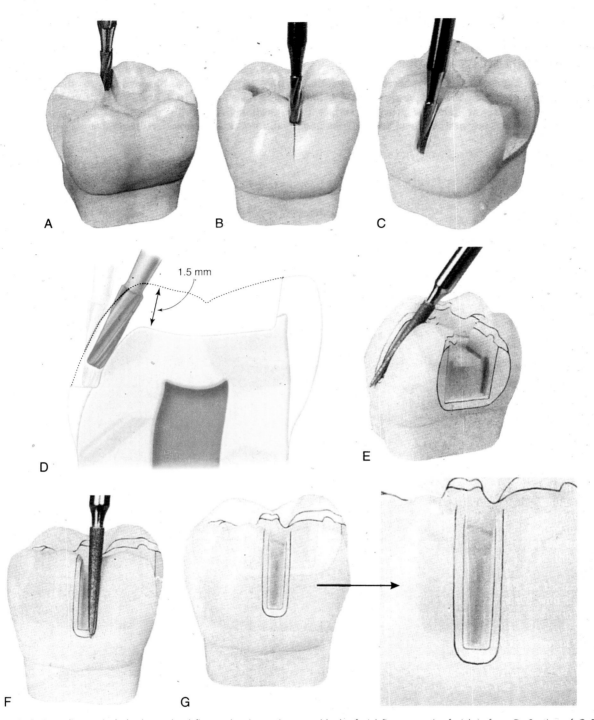

Fig. 17-17 **A–C,** Extending to include the occlusal fissure that is continuous with the facial fissure on the facial surface. **D,** Section of *C*. **E** and **F,** Beveling the gingival margin (*E*) and the mesial and distal margins (*F*) of fissure extension. **G,** Beveling completed.

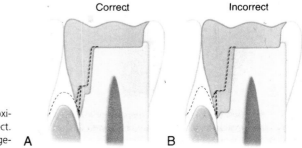

Correct   Incorrect

Fig. 17-18 Modifications of the preparation when extending to include the proximal root-surface lesions after moderate gingival recession. **A,** Correct. **B,** Incorrect. Note the decreased dentinal protection of the pulp compared with the management depicted in *A*.

MAXILLARY FIRST MOLAR WITH UNAFFECTED, STRONG OBLIQUE RIDGE

When a maxillary first molar is to be restored, consideration should be given to preserving the oblique ridge if it is strong and unaffected, especially if only one proximal surface is carious. A mesio-occlusal preparation for an inlay is illustrated in Figure 17-19, *A* and *B*. If a distal surface lesion appears subsequent to the insertion of a mesio-occlusal restoration, the tooth may be prepared for a disto-occluso-lingual inlay (see Fig. 17-19, *H* and *I*). The disto-occluso-lingual restoration that caps the distolingual cusp is preferable to the disto-occlusal restoration because it protects the miniature

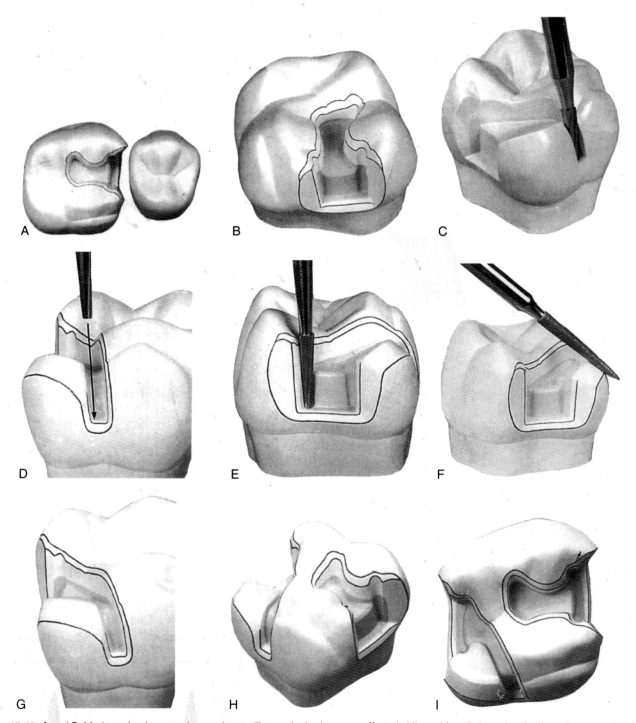

Fig. 17-19 **A** and **B,** Mesio-occlusal preparation on the maxillary molar having an unaffected oblique ridge. **C,** Preparing the lingual groove extension of the disto-occluso-lingual preparation. **D** and **E,** Cutting retention grooves in the lingual surface extension (*D*) and the distal box (*E*). **F** and **G,** Completed disto-occluso-lingual preparation on the maxillary molar having an unaffected oblique ridge. **H** and **I,** Preparations for treating both proximal surfaces of the maxillary molar having a strong, unaffected oblique ridge.

distolingual cusp from subsequent fracture. The disto-occluso-lingual preparation requires diligent application to develop satisfactory retention and resistance forms. Retention form is attained by (1) creating a maximum of 2-degree occlusal divergence of the vertical walls, (2) accentuating some line angles, and (3) extending the lingual surface groove to create an axial wall height in this extension of at least 2.5 mm occlusogingivally. The proper resistance form dictates (1) routine capping of the distolingual cusp and (2) maintaining sound tooth structure between the lingual surface groove extension and the distolingual wall of the proximal boxing.

To prepare the disto-occluso-lingual preparation, the operator first reduces the distolingual cusp with the side of the No. 271 carbide bur. The cusp should be reduced a uniform 1.5 mm. Next, the operator completes the remaining occlusal step of the preparation with the No. 271 carbide bur. The operator prepares the proximal box portion of the preparation. The lingual groove extension is prepared only after the position of the distolingual wall of the proximal boxing is established. This permits the operator to judge the best position of the lingual surface groove extension to maintain a minimum of 3 mm of sound tooth structure between this extension and the distolingual wall; if this is not possible because of extensive caries, a more extensive type of preparation may be indicated (one that crosses the oblique ridge). One can use the side of the No. 271 carbide bur to produce the lingual surface groove extension (see Fig. 17-19, C). The diameter of the bur is the gauge for the depth (pulpally) of the axial wall in this extension, and the occlusogingival dimension of this axial wall is a minimum of 2.5 mm. With the end of this bur, the operator also establishes a 2-mm depth to the portion of the pulpal floor that connects the proximal boxing to the lingual surface groove extension. This additional depth to the pulpal floor helps strengthen the wax pattern and casting in later steps of fabrication. This should create a definite 0.5-mm step from the reduced distolingual cusp to the pulpal floor. Using the No. 169L carbide bur, the operator increases retention form in the disto-occluso-lingual preparation by (1) creating mesioaxial and distoaxial grooves in the lingual surface groove extension (see Fig. 17-19, D) and (2) preparing facial and lingual retention grooves in the distal boxing (see Fig. 17-19, E).

The dentist uses the flame-shaped, fine-grit diamond instrument to bevel the proximal gingival margin and to prepare the secondary flares on the proximal enamel walls and to bevel the lingual margins. A lingual counterbevel is prepared on the distolingual cusp that is generous in width and results in 30-degree metal at the margin (see Fig. 17-19, F). Occlusion should be checked at this point because the counterbevel should be sufficiently wide to extend beyond any occlusal contacts, either in maximum intercuspation or during mandibular movements. The bevel on the gingival margin of the lingual extension should be 0.5 mm wide and should provide for a 30-degree metal angle. The bevels on the mesial and distal margins of the lingual extension also are approximately 0.5 mm wide and result in 40-degree marginal metal.

FISSURES IN THE FACIAL AND LINGUAL CUSP RIDGES OR MARGINAL RIDGES

In the preparation of Class II preparations for inlays, facial and lingual occlusal fissures may extend nearly to, or through, the respective facial and lingual cusp ridges, but not onto the facial or lingual surface. The proper outline form dictates that the preparation margin should not cross such fissures but should be extended to include them. For the occlusal step portion of the preparation, the dentist initially extends along the lingual fissure with the No. 271 carbide bur until only 2 mm of tooth structure remains between the bur and the lingual surface of the tooth. Additional lingual extension at this time is incorrect because it may remove the supporting dentin unnecessarily (Fig. 17-20, A and B). If this extension almost includes the length of the fissure, additional extension is achieved later by using the occlusal bevel; this bevel may be wider than conventional if the remaining fissure can be eliminated by such a wider bevel (see Fig. 17-20, C). Enameloplasty sometimes may eliminate the end portion of the fissure and provide a smooth enamel surface where previously a fault was present, thus reducing the extent of the required extension (see Fig. 17-20, D). If possible, the fissure should be included in the preparation outline without extending the margin to the height of the ridge. If the occlusal bevel places the margin on the height of the ridge, however, the marginal enamel likely is weak because of its sharpness and because of the inclination of the enamel rods in this region. The preparation outline should be extended just onto the facial or lingual surface (see Fig. 17-20, I and J). Such extension onto the facial or lingual surface also would be indicated if the fissure still remains through the ridge after enameloplasty (see Fig. 17-20, E).

When necessary, extension through a cusp ridge is accomplished by cutting through the ridge at a depth of 1 mm with the No. 271 carbide bur (see Fig. 17-20, F and G). The dentist bevels the margins of the extension with the flame-shaped, fine-grit diamond instrument to provide for the desired 40-degree marginal metal on the occlusal, mesial, and distal margins and for 30-degree marginal metal on the gingival margin (see Fig. 17-20, C, D, I, and J). In the same manner, the operator should manage the fissures that may extend into or through a proximal marginal ridge, assuming that the proximal surface otherwise was not to be included in the outline form and that such fissure management does not extend the preparation outline near the adjacent tooth contact. This treatment particularly applies to a mesial fissure of the maxillary first premolar (Fig. 17-21). If this procedure extends the margin near or into the contact, the outline form on the affected proximal surface must be extended to include the contact, as for a conventional proximal surface preparation.

CUSP-CAPPING PARTIAL ONLAY

The term *partial onlay* is used when a cast metal restoration covers and restores at least one but not all of the cusp tips of a posterior tooth. The facial and lingual margins on the occlusal surface frequently must be extended toward the cusp tips to the extent of the existing restorative materials and to uncover caries (Fig. 17-22, B and C). Undermined occlusal enamel should be removed because it is weak; removing such enamel provides access for the proper excavation of caries. When the occlusal outline is extended up the cusp slopes more than half the distance from any primary occlusal groove (central, facial, or lingual) to the cusp tip, covering (capping) the cusp should be considered. If the preparation outline is extended two thirds of this distance or more, capping the cusp is usually necessary to (1) protect the weak, underlying cuspal structure from fracture caused by masticatory force and

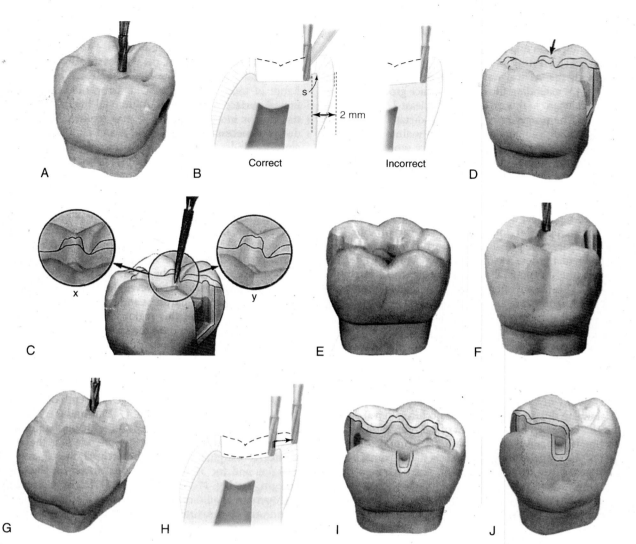

Fig. 17-20 A, Extending to include the lingual (occlusal) fissure. **B,** Section of A. The dentinal support (s) of the lingual cusp ridge should not be removed. A bevel can provide additional extension to include the fissure that does not extend to the crest of the ridge. **C,** Completed preparations with standard width bevel (x) and with wider bevel to include a groove defect that nearly extends to the ridge height (y). **D,** Completed preparation illustrating enameloplasty for the elimination of a shallow fissure extending to or through the lingual ridge height. (Compare the smooth, saucer-shaped lingual ridge contour with C, in which no enameloplasty has been performed.) **E,** Fissure remaining through the lingual ridge after unsuccessful enameloplasty. This indicates procedures subsequently illustrated. **F** and **G,** Extending the preparation if enameloplasty has not eliminated the fissure in the lingual ridge (F) or the facial ridge (G). **H,** Section of F. **I** and **J,** Completed preparations after beveling the margins of the extensions through the lingual ridge (I) and the facial ridge (J).

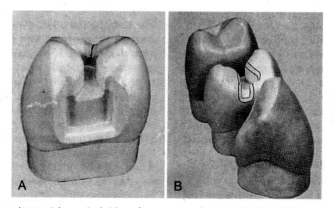

Fig. 17-21 The fissure that remains on the mesial marginal ridge after unsuccessful enameloplasty (A) is treated (B) in the same manner as lingual or facial ridge fissures (see Fig. 17-20, I and J).

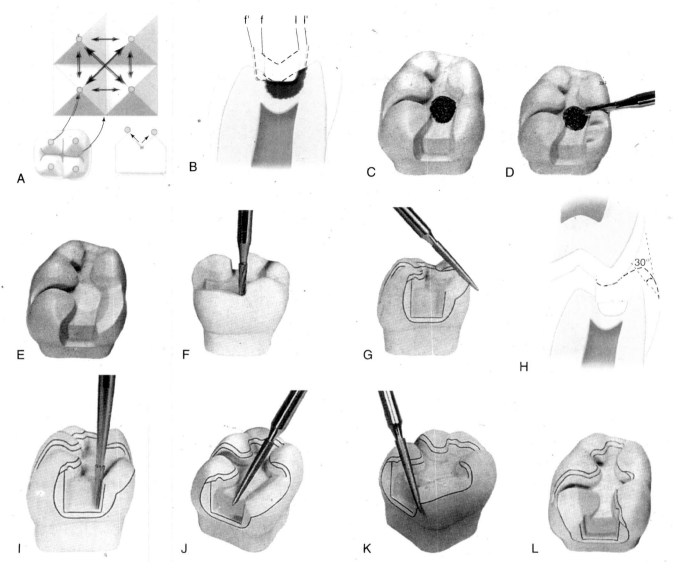

Fig. 17-22 **A,** When the extension of the occlusal margin is one half the distance from any point on the primary grooves (*cross*) toward the cusp tip (*dot*), capping of the cusp should be considered; when this distance is two thirds or more, capping of the cusp is usually indicated. **B,** *l* is midway between the central groove and the lingual cusp tip; *f* is midway between the central groove and the facial cusp tip. When enamel at *l* and *f* is undermined by caries, the respective walls must be extended to the dotted lines *l* and *f* to uncover caries. Cusps should be reduced for capping. **C,** Extension to uncover caries indicates that the mesiolingual cusp should be reduced for capping. **D,** Depth cuts. **E,** Reduced mesiolingual cusp. Caries has been removed, and the cement base has been placed. **F,** Applying the bur vertically helps establish the vertical wall that barely includes the lingual groove. **G,** Counterbeveling reduced cusp. **H,** Section of the counterbevel. **I,** Improving the retention form by cutting the proximal retention grooves. **J** and **K,** The preparation is complete except for the rounding of the axiopulpal line angle (*J*) and the rounding of the junction of the counterbevel and the secondary flare (*K*). Facial surface groove extension improves the retention and resistance forms. **L,** Preparation when reducing one of two facial cusps on the mandibular molar.

(2) remove the occlusal margin from a region subjected to heavy stress and wear (see Fig. 17-22, *A* and *B*). At this point in the preparation of the pulpal floor, depth can be increased from 1.5 mm to 2 mm. This additional pulpal depth ensures sufficient reduction in an area that is often under-reduced and results in imparting greater strength and rigidity to the wax pattern and cast restoration.

Reduce the cusps for capping as soon as the indication for such capping is determined because this improves access and visibility for the subsequent steps in the preparation. If a cusp is in infraocclusion of the desired occlusal plane before

reduction, the amount of cusp reduction is less and needs to be only that which provides the required clearance with the desired occlusal plane. Before reducing the surface, the operator prepares depth gauge grooves (depth cuts) with the side of the No. 271 carbide bur (see Fig. 17-22, *D*). Such depth cuts should help to prevent thin spots in the restoration. With the depth cuts serving as guides, the operator completes the cusp reduction with the side of the carbide bur (see Fig. 17-22, *E*). The reduction should provide for a uniform 1.5 mm of metal thickness over the reduced cusp. On maxillary premolars and first molars, the reduction should be minimal (i.e.,

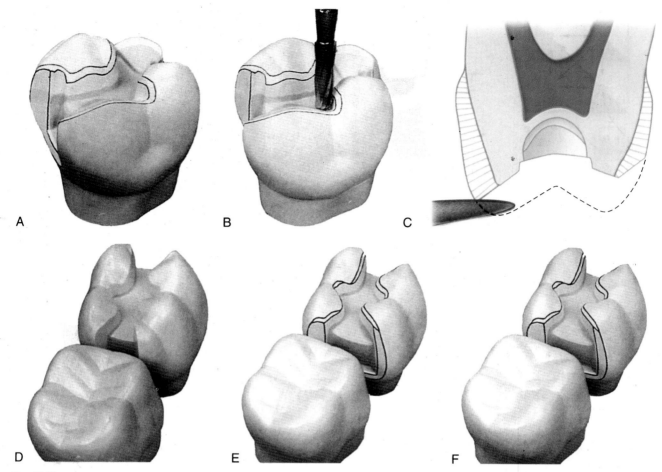

Fig. 17-23 **A** and **B,** Capping one of two facial cusps on the maxillary molar. **C,** Blunting the margin of the reduced cusp when esthetics is a major consideration. **D–F,** The margin shown crossing the distal cusp in *D* indicates treatment illustrated in *E* or *F*.

0.75–1 mm) on the facial cusp ridge to decrease the display of metal. This reduction should increase progressively to 1.5 mm toward the center of the tooth to help impart rigidity to the capping metal (Fig. 17-23, *A* and *C*).

If only one of the two lingual cusps of a molar is reduced for capping, the reduction must extend to include just the lingual groove between the reduced and unreduced cusps. This reduction should terminate with a distinct vertical wall that has a height that is the same as the prescribed cusp reduction. Applying the bur vertically (see Fig. 17-22, *F*) should help establish a vertical wall of proper depth and direction. Similar principles apply when only one of the facial cusps is to be reduced (see Figs. 17-22, *L,* and 17-23, *B*).

A bevel of generous width is prepared on the facial (lingual) margin of a reduced cusp with the flame-shaped, fine-grit diamond instrument (with the exception of esthetically prominent areas). This bevel is referred to as *reverse bevel* or *counterbevel*. The width varies because it usually should extend beyond any occlusal contact with opposing teeth, either in maximum intercuspation or during mandibular movements (see Fig. 17-24, *C*). It should be at an angle that results in 30-degree marginal metal (see Fig. 17-22, *G* and *H*). The exception is the facial margin on maxillary premolars and the first molar, where esthetic requirements dictate only a

blunting and smoothening of the enamel margin (a stub margin) by the light application of a fine-grit sandpaper disk or the fine-grit diamond instrument (flame-shaped) held at a right angle to the facial surface (see Fig. 17-23, *C*). Any sharp external corners should be rounded slightly to strengthen them and reduce the problems they may generate in future steps (see Fig. 17-22, *J* and *K*).

Cusp reduction appreciably decreases the retention form because it decreases the height of the vertical walls. Therefore, proximal retention grooves usually are recommended (see Fig. 17-22, *I*). It may be necessary to increase the retention form by extending facial and lingual groove regions of the respective surfaces or by collar and skirt features (see later). These additional retention features also provide the desired resistance form against forces tending to split the tooth (see Figs. 17-22, *K,* and 17-28).

The principles stated in the preceding paragraphs may be applied in the treatment of the distal cusp of the mandibular first molar when preparing a mesio-occluso-distal preparation (see Fig. 17-23, *D*). Proper extension of the distofacial margin usually places the occlusal margin in a region subjected to heavy masticatory forces and wear. Satisfactory treatment usually dictates either extending the distofacial margin (and wall) slightly mesial of the distofacial groove (see Fig. 17-23,

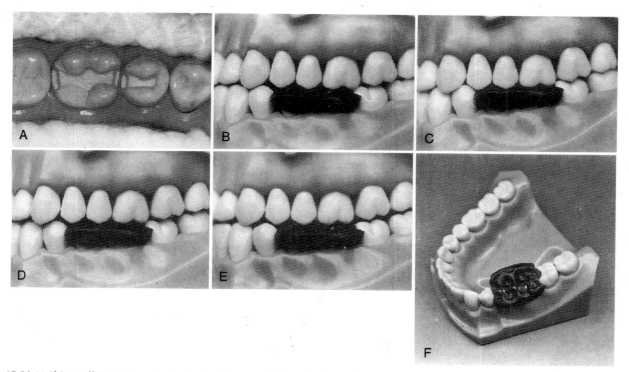

Fig. 17-24 Verifying sufficient cusp reduction by forming a wax interocclusal record. **A,** The walls of the preparations (disto-occlusal for the second premolar, and mesio-occluso-distal for the first molar) are air-dried of visible moisture. The low-fusing inlay wax that is the same length as the mesio-distal length of the inlay preparations is softened and pressed over the prepared teeth. **B–E,** The patient moves the mandible into all occlusal positions, left lateral (*B*), through maximum intercuspation (*C*), to right lateral (*D*), and protrusive (*E*). **F,** Completed interocclusal record.

E) or capping the remaining portion of the distal cusp (see Fig. 17-23, *F*).

After cusp reduction, the dentist visually verifies that the occlusal clearances are sufficient. A wax interocclusal record is helpful when checking the occlusal clearances, especially in areas that are difficult to visualize, for example, in the central groove and lingual cusp regions. To make a wax "bite," the dentist first dries the preparation free of any visible moisture; however, dentin should not be desiccated (Fig. 17-24, *A*). Next, the dentist lightly presses a portion of softened, low-fusing inlay wax over the prepared tooth; the dentist immediately requests the patient to close into the soft wax and slide the teeth in all directions (see Fig. 17-24, *B* through *F*). During the mandibular movements, the dentist observes to verify that (1) the patient performs right lateral, left lateral, and protrusive movements; (2) the adjacent unprepared teeth are in contact with the opposing teeth; (3) the wax in the preparation is stable (not loose and rocking); and (4) the wax is not in infraocclusion. The dentist cools the wax and carefully removes it, holds it up to a light, and notes the degree of light transmitted through it. With experience, this is a good indicator of the thickness of the wax. An alternative method is to use wax calipers or to section the wax to verify its thickness. Insufficient thickness calls for more reduction in the indicated area before proceeding. As an alternative to wax, an interocclusal record can be made in maximum intercuspation with a quick-setting polyvinyl impression material. Once set, this interocclusal record can be measured with wax calipers to evaluate the reduction. If wax calipers are not available, the interocclusal record can be sectioned with a knife to see the

thickness in cross-section. However, a polyvinyl interocclusal record will not offer as much information as would the softened inlay wax technique, since the lateral and protrusive paths are not registered in the former.

INCLUDING PORTIONS OF THE FACIAL AND LINGUAL SMOOTH SURFACES AFFECTED BY CARIES OR OTHER INJURY

When portions of a facial (lingual) smooth surface and a proximal surface are affected by caries or some other factor (e.g., fracture) (Fig. 17-25, *A* and *I*), the treatment may be a large inlay, an onlay, a three-quarter crown, a full crown, or multiple amalgam or composite restorations. Generally, if carious portions are extensive, the choice between the previously listed cast metal restorations is determined by the degree of tooth circumference involved. A full crown is indicated if the lingual and the facial smooth surfaces are defective, especially if the tooth is a second or third molar. When only a portion of the facial smooth surface is carious, and the lingual surfaces of the teeth are conspicuously free of caries, a mesio-occlusal, distofacial, and distolingual inlay or onlay with a lingual groove extension is chosen over the crown because the former is more favorable to the health of the gingival tissues and more conservative in the removal of tooth structure. Often, this is the treatment choice for the maxillary second molar, which may exhibit caries or decalcification on the distofacial surface as a result of poor oral hygiene (owing to poor access) in this region.

In the preparation of the maxillary molar referred to in the preceding paragraph, the mesiofacial and distolingual cusps

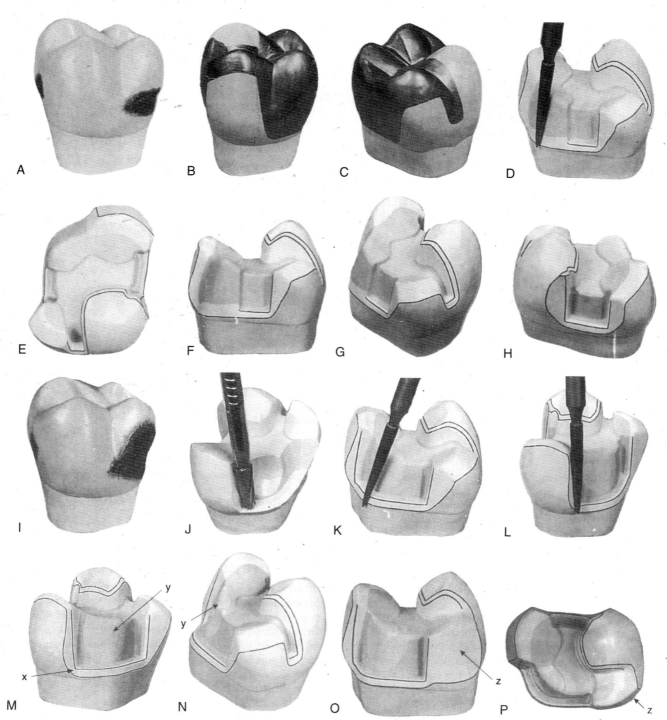

Fig. 17-25 A, Maxillary molar with caries on the distofacial corner and the mesial surface. **B** and **C,** Completed mesio-occlusal, distofacial, and distolingual inlay for treating caries shown in *A,* facio-occlusal view (*B*) and disto-linguo-occlusal view (*C*). **D–H,** Preparation for treating caries illustrated in *A,* disto-occlusal view with diamond instrument being applied (*D*), occlusal view (*E*), distal view (*F*), disto-linguo-occlusal view (*G*), and mesio-occlusal view (*H*). **I,** Maxillary molar with deeper caries on the distofacial corner and with mesial caries. **J,** Preparation (minus bevels and flares) for mesio-occlusal, distofacial, and distolingual inlay to restore the carious molar shown in *I.* A No. 271 carbide bur is used to prepare the gingival shoulder and the vertical wall. **K** and **L,** Beveling margins. **M** and **N,** Completed preparation for treating the caries shown in *I.* Gingival and facial bevels blend at *x,* and *y* is the cement base. **O** and **P,** When the lingual surface groove has not been prepared and when the facial wall of the proximal box is mostly or totally missing, forces directed to displace the inlay facially can be opposed by lingual skirt extension (*z*).

and the distofacial cusp are usually reduced for capping. If the distofacial cusp defect is primarily shallow decalcification, the flame-shaped diamond instrument is used to reduce the involved facial surface and distofacial corner approximately to the depth of enamel and to establish the gingival margin of this reduction apical to the affected area (see Fig. 17-25, D). This instrument also is used to terminate the facial surface reduction in a definite facial margin running gingivo-occlusally and in a manner to provide for 40-degree metal at this margin (see Fig. 17-25, E).

If the distofacial defect is more extensive and deeper into the tooth (see Fig. 17-25, I), eliminating the opportunity for an effective distal box or groove (no facial wall possible), the No. 271 carbide bur should be used to cut a gingival shoulder extending from the distal gingival floor around to include the affected facial surface. This shoulder partially provides the desired resistance form. (A gingival floor, perpendicular to occlusal force, has been provided in lieu of the missing pulpal wall in the distofacial cusp region.) The No. 271 bur is used to create a nearly vertical wall in the remaining facial enamel (see Fig. 17-25, J). The width of the shoulder should be the diameter of the end of the cutting instrument. The vertical walls should have the appropriate degree of draft to contribute to retention form. Then, the faciogingival and facial margins are beveled with the flame-shaped, fine-grit diamond instrument to provide 30-degree metal at the gingival margin (see Fig. 17-25, K) and 40-degree metal along the facial margin (see Fig. 17-25, L). These two bevels should blend together (see x in Fig. 17-25, M), and the faciogingival bevel should be continuous with the gingival bevel on the distal surface. Additional retention and resistance forms are indicated for this preparation and can be developed by an arbitrary lingual groove extension (see Fig. 17-25, N) or a distolingual skirt extension (see Fig. 17-25, O and P). These preparation features resist forces normally opposed by the missing distofacial wall and help protect the restored tooth from fracture injury.

Tooth Preparation for Full Cast Metal Onlays

The preceding sections have presented basic tooth preparation principles and techniques for small, simple cast metal inlays and for partial onlays that cap less than all the cusps. This section presents the tooth preparation principles and techniques for *full onlay* restorations that cover the entire occlusal surface. Onlay restorations have many clinical applications and may be desired by many patients. These restorations have a well-deserved reputation for providing excellent service.

The cast metal onlay restoration spans the gap between the inlay, which is primarily an intracoronal restoration, and the full crown, which is a totally extracoronal restoration. The full onlay by definition caps all of the cusps of a posterior tooth and can be designed to help strengthen a tooth that has been weakened by caries or previous restorative experiences. It can be designed to distribute occlusal loads over the tooth in a manner that greatly decreases the chance of future fracture.[4,6] It is more conservative of the tooth structure than the full crown preparation, and its supragingival margins, when possible, are less irritating to the gingiva. Usually, an onlay diagnosis is made pre-operatively because of the tooth's status. Sometimes, the diagnosis is deferred until the extension of the occlusal step of an inlay preparation facially and lingually to

the limits of the caries lesion shows that cusp reduction is mandatory. The mandibular first molar is used to illustrate one mesio-occluso-distal preparation for a full cast metal onlay.

Initial Preparation
OCCLUSAL REDUCTION

As soon as the decision is made to restore the tooth with a full cast metal onlay, the cusps should be reduced because this improves the access and the visibility for subsequent steps in tooth preparation. With the cusps reduced, the efficiency of the cutting instrument and the air-water cooling spray is improved. Also, when the cusps are reduced, it is easier to assess the height of the remaining clinical crown of the tooth, which determines the degree of occlusal divergence necessary for adequate retention form. Using the No. 271 carbide bur held parallel to the long axis of the tooth crown, a 2-mm deep pulpal floor is prepared along the central groove (Fig. 17-26, A). To verify the pre-operative diagnosis for cusp reduction, this occlusal preparation is extended facially and lingually just beyond the caries to sound tooth structure (see Fig. 17-26, B). The groove should not be extended farther, however, than two thirds the distance from the central groove to the cusp tips because the need for cusp reduction is verified at this point. With the side of the No. 271 carbide bur, uniform 1.5-mm deep depth cuts are prepared on the remaining occlusal surface (see Fig. 17-26, C and D). Depth cuts usually are placed on the crest of the triangular ridges and in the facial and lingual groove regions. These depth cuts help prevent thin spots in the final restoration. If a cusp is in infraocclusion of the desired occlusal plane before reduction, the amount of cusp reduction is less and needs only that which provides the required clearance with the desired occlusal plane. Caries and old restorative material that is deeper in the tooth than the desired clearance are not removed at this step in preparation.

With the depth cuts serving as guides for the amount of reduction, the cusp reduction is completed with the side of the No. 271 bur. When completed, this reduction should reflect the general topography of the original occlusal surface (see Fig. 17-26, E). The operator should not attempt to reduce the mesial and distal marginal ridges completely at this time to avoid hitting an adjacent tooth. The remainder of the ridges are reduced in a later step when the proximal boxes are prepared.

Throughout the next steps in the initial preparation, the cutting instruments used to develop the vertical walls are oriented continually to a single draw path, usually the long axis of the tooth crown, so that the completed preparation has draft (i.e., no undercuts). For mandibular molars and second premolars whose crowns tilt slightly lingually, the bur should be tilted slightly (5–10 degrees) lingually to help preserve the strength of the lingual cusps (see Fig. 17-4, D). The gingival-to-occlusal divergence of these preparation walls may range from 2 to 5 degrees from the line of draw, depending on their heights. If the vertical walls are unusually short, a minimum of 2 degrees occlusal divergence is desirable for retentive purposes. Cusp reduction appreciably decreases the retention form because it decreases the height of the vertical walls, so this minimal amount of divergence is often indicated in the preparation of a tooth for a cast metal onlay. As the

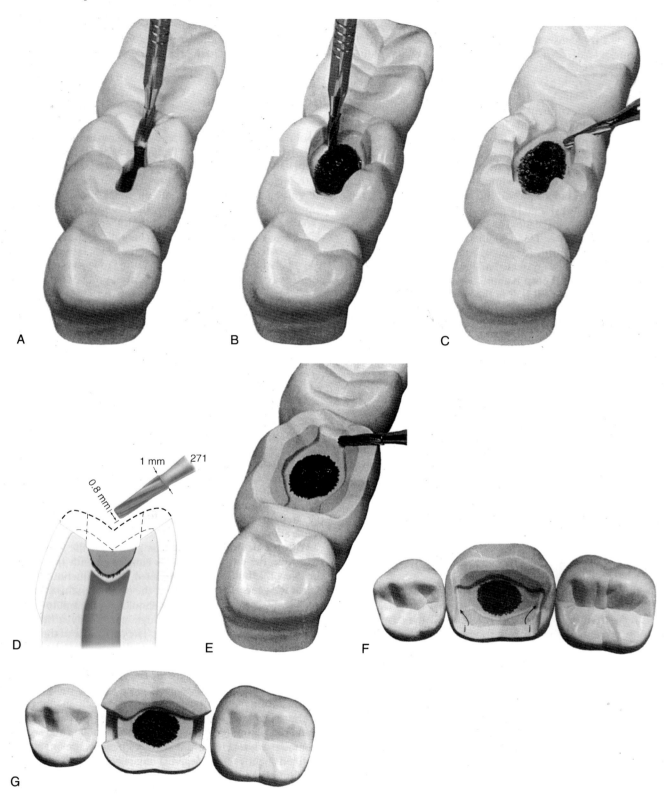

Fig. 17-26 **A,** Cutting a 2-mm deep central groove. **B,** Extending the central groove cut facially and lingually to verify any need for cusp capping. **C,** Depth cuts. **D,** Section of C. **E,** Completion of cusp reduction. Small portions of the mesial and distal marginal ridges are left unreduced to avoid scarring the adjacent teeth. **F,** The occlusal step is extended facially and lingually past any carious areas and is extended to expose the proximal dentinoenamel junction (DEJ) (*j*) in anticipation of proximal boxing. **G,** Preparation with proximal boxes prepared. Note the clearances with the adjacent teeth.

gingivo-occlusal height of the vertical walls increases, the occlusal divergence should increase, allowing 5 degrees in the preparation of the greatest gingivo-occlusal length. The latter preparations present difficulties during pattern withdrawal, trial seating and withdrawal of the casting, and cementing, unless this maximal divergence is provided.

OCCLUSAL STEP

After cusp reduction, a 0.5-mm deep occlusal step should be present in the central groove region between the reduced cuspal inclines and the pulpal floor. Maintaining the pulpal depth (0.5 mm) of the step, it is extended facially and lingually just beyond any carious areas, to sound tooth structure (or to sound base or restorative material if certain conditions, discussed subsequently, have been met). Next, the operator extends the step mesially and distally far enough to expose the proximal DEJ (see Fig. 17-26, F). The step is extended along any remaining facial (and lingual) occlusal fissures as far as they are faulty (fissured). The facial and lingual walls of the occlusal step should go around the cusps in graceful curves, and the isthmus should be only as wide as necessary to be in sound tooth structure or sound base or restorative material. Old restorative material or caries that is deeper pulpally than this 0.5-mm step is not removed at this stage of tooth preparation.

As the occlusal step approaches the mesial and distal surfaces, it should widen faciolingually in anticipation of the proximal box extensions (see Fig. 17-26, F). This 0.5-mm occlusal step contributes to the retention of the restoration and provides the wax pattern and cast metal onlay with additional bulk for rigidity.[7]

PROXIMAL BOX

Continuing with the No. 271 carbide bur held parallel to the long axis of the tooth crown, the proximal boxes are prepared as described in the inlay section. Figure 17-26, G, illustrates the preparation after the proximal boxes are prepared.

Final Preparation
REMOVAL OF INFECTED CARIOUS DENTIN AND DEFECTIVE RESTORATIVE MATERIALS AND PULP PROTECTION

If the occlusal step and the proximal boxes have been extended properly, any caries or previous restorative materials remaining on the pulpal and axial walls should be visible. They should be removed as described previously.

PREPARATION OF BEVELS AND FLARES

After the cement base (when indicated) is completed (Fig. 17-27, A), the slender, flame-shaped, fine-grit diamond instrument is used to place counterbevels on the reduced cusps, to apply the gingival bevels, and to create secondary flares on the facial and lingual walls of the proximal boxes. First, a gingival retraction cord is inserted, as described in the previous inlay section. During the few minutes required for the cord's effect on the gingival tissues, the diamond instrument is used to prepare the counterbevels on the facial and lingual margins of the reduced cusps. The bevel should be of generous width and should result in 30-degree marginal metal. The best way to judge this is to always maintain a 30-degree angle between the

side of the instrument and the external enamel surface beyond the counterbevel (see Fig. 17-27, B and C). The counterbevel usually should be wide enough so that the cavosurface margin is beyond (gingival to) any contact with the opposing dentition. If a facial (lingual) surface fissure extends slightly beyond the normal position of the counterbevel, it may be included (removed) by deepening the counterbevel in the region of the fissure (see Fig. 17-27, D). If the fissure extends gingivally more than 0.5 mm, however, the fissure is managed as described later.

A counterbevel is not placed on the facial cusps of maxillary premolars and first molars where esthetic considerations may dictate using a stubbed margin by blunting and smoothing the enamel margin by the light application of a fine-grit sandpaper disk or the fine-grit diamond instrument (flame-shaped) held at a right angle to the facial surface (see Fig. 17-23, C). The surface created by this blunting should be approximately 0.5 mm in width. For beveling the gingival margins and flaring (secondary) the proximal enamel walls, refer to the inlay section.

After beveling and flaring, any sharp junctions between the counterbevels and the secondary flares are rounded slightly (see Fig. 17-27, E). The fine-grit diamond instrument also is used to bevel the axiopulpal line angles lightly (see Fig. 17-27, F). Such a bevel produces a stronger wax pattern at this critical region by increasing its thickness. Any sharp projecting corners in the preparation are rounded slightly because these projections are difficult to reproduce without voids when developing the working cast and often cause difficulties when seating the casting. The desirable metal angle at the margins of onlays is 40 degrees except at the gingivally directed margins, where the metal angle should be 30 degrees.

When deemed necessary, shallow (0.3 mm deep) retention grooves may be cut in the facioaxial and the linguoaxial line angles with the No. 169L carbide bur (see Fig. 17-27, G). These grooves are especially important for retention when the prepared tooth is short, which is often the case after reducing all the cusps. When properly positioned, the grooves are entirely in dentin near the DEJ and do not undermine enamel. The direction of cutting (translation of the bur) is parallel to the DEJ. The long axis of the No. 169L bur must be held parallel to the line of draw, and the tip of the bur must be positioned in the gingival box internal point angles. If the axial walls are deeper than ideal, however, the correct reference for placing retention grooves is just inside the DEJ to minimize pulpal impacts but avoids undermining enamel. The model showing the completed preparation is illustrated in Figure 17-27, H.

Modifications in Full Onlay Tooth Preparations
FACIAL OR LINGUAL SURFACE GROOVE EXTENSION

A facial surface fissure (mandibular molar) or a lingual surface fissure (maxillary molar) is included in the outline in the same manner as described in the section on inlays. This extension sometimes is indicated to provide additional retention form, even though the groove is not faulty. A completed mesio-occluso-disto-facial onlay preparation on a mandibular first molar is illustrated in Figure 17-27, I.

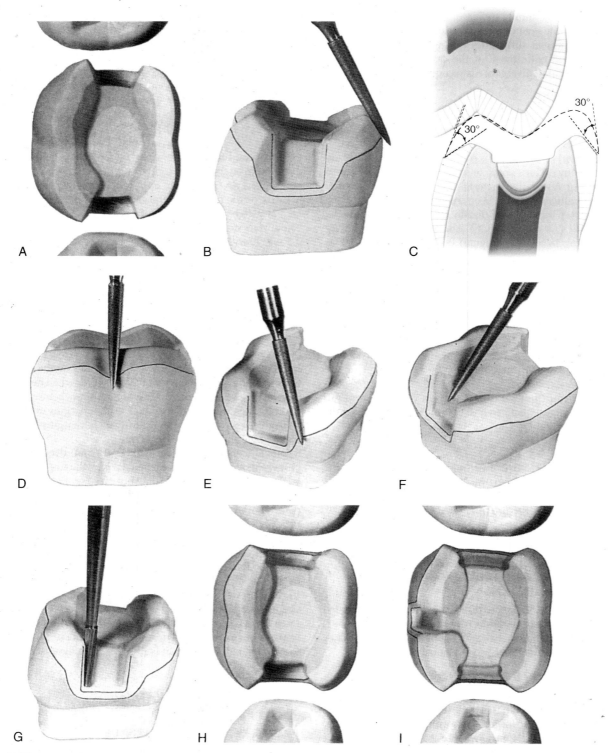

Fig. 17-27 A, Caries has been removed, and the cement base has been inserted. **B,** Counterbeveling facial and lingual margins of reduced cusps. **C,** Section of *B*. **D,** The fissure that extends slightly gingival to the normal position of the counterbevel may be included by slightly deepening the counterbevel in the fissured area. **E,** The junctions between the counterbevels and the secondary flares are slightly rounded. **F,** The axiopulpal line angle is lightly beveled. **G,** Improving the retention form by cutting proximal grooves. **H,** Completed mesio-occluso-distal onlay preparation. **I,** Completed mesio-occluso-disto-facial onlay preparation showing the extension to include the facial surface groove or fissure.

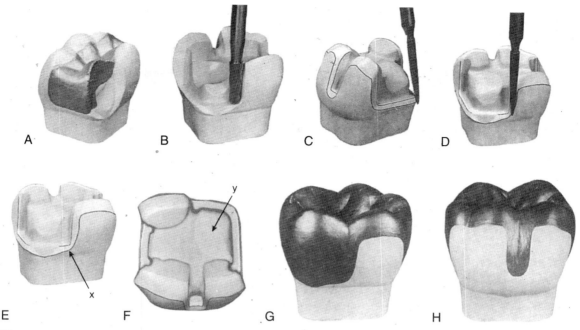

Fig. 17-28 A, Mandibular first molar with large mesio-occluso-distal amalgam and fractured mesiolingual cusp. **B,** Preparation (minus bevels and flares) for mesio-occlusal, distofacial, and distolingual onlay to restore the fractured molar shown in *A*. A No. 271 carbide bur is used to prepare the gingival shoulder and the vertical lingual wall. Reducing cusps for capping and extending out the facial groove improve the retention and resistance forms. **C** and **D,** Beveling of margins. **E** and **F,** Completed preparation. The gingival and lingual bevels blend at *x,* and *y* is the cement base. **G** and **H,** Completed onlay.

INCLUSION OF PORTIONS OF THE FACIAL AND LINGUAL SMOOTH SURFACES AFFECTED BY CARIES, FRACTURED CUSPS, OR OTHER INJURY

For inclusion of shallow to moderate lesions on the facial and lingual smooth surfaces, refer to the section on inlays. A mandibular molar with a fractured mesiolingual cusp is used to illustrate the treatment of a fractured cusp of a molar (Fig. 17-28, *A*). The dentist uses a No. 271 carbide bur to cut a shoulder perpendicular to occlusal force by extending the proximal gingival floor (adjacent to the fracture) to include the affected surface. This shoulder partially provides the desired resistance form by being perpendicular to gingivally directed occlusal force. This instrument also is used to create a vertical wall in the remaining lingual enamel (see Fig. 17-28, *B*). The width of the gingival floor should be the diameter of the end of the cutting instrument. The vertical walls should have the degree of draft necessary for the retention form. If the clinical crown of the tooth is short, it is advisable to cut proximal grooves for additional retention with the No. 169L bur. The linguogingival and lingual margins are beveled with the flame-shaped, fine-grit diamond instrument to provide 30-degree metal at the gingival margin (see Fig. 17-28, *C*) and 40-degree metal along the lingual margin (see Fig. 17-28, *D*).

These two bevels should blend together (see *x* in Fig. 17-28, *E*), and the linguogingival bevel is continuous with the gingival bevel on the mesial surface. Additional features to improve the retention and resistance forms are indicated and can be developed by a mesiofacial skirt extension or by a facial groove extension. These preparation features (discussed in the following section) improve the retention form, resist forces normally opposed by the missing mesiolingual wall, and help protect the restored tooth from further fracture injury.

ENHANCEMENT OF RESISTANCE AND RETENTION FORMS

When the tooth crown is short (which is often the case when all cusps are reduced), the operator must strive to maximize the retention form in the preparation. Retention features that already have been presented are as follows:

1. Minimal amount of taper (2 degrees per wall) on the vertical walls of the preparation
2. Addition of proximal retention grooves
3. Preparation of facial (or lingual) surface groove extensions

In the preparation of a tooth that has been grossly weakened by caries or previous filling material and is judged to be prone to fracture under occlusal loads, the resistance form that cusp capping provides should be augmented by the use of skirts, collars, or facial (lingual) surface groove extensions. When properly placed, these features result in onlays that distribute the occlusal forces over most or all of the tooth and not just a portion of it, reducing the likelihood of fractures of teeth (Fig. 17-29, *A* and *B*). The lingual "skirt" extension (see Fig. 17-29, *C* through *E*), the lingual "collar" preparation (see Fig. 17-29, *F*), or the lingual surface groove extension on a maxillary molar protects the facial cusps from fracture. The facial skirt extension, the facial collar preparation, or the facial surface groove extension on a mandibular molar protects the lingual cusp from fracture.

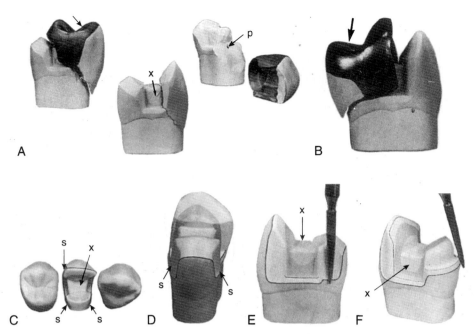

Fig. 17-29 The large cement base *x* indicates severely weakened tooth crown. Occlusal force (*thick arrow*) may fracture the facial cusp (*A*) or the lingual cusp (*B*), which may expose the pulp (*p*). *C* and *D,* Skirt extensions (*s*) on the mesiolingual, distolingual, and distofacial transitional line angles prevent the fractures shown in *A* and *B.* Esthetic consideration contraindicates skirting the mesiofacial line angle. *E,* Distal view of the preparation shown in *D.* Skirt extensions are prepared with a fine-grit diamond instrument. *F,* A collar preparation around the lingual cusp prevents the fracture shown in *A.*

SKIRT PREPARATION

Skirts are thin extensions of the facial or lingual proximal margins of the cast metal onlay that extend from the primary flare to a termination just past the transitional line angle of the tooth. A skirt extension is a conservative method of improving the retention and resistance forms of the preparation. It is relatively atraumatic to the tooth because it involves removing very little (if any) dentin. Usually, the skirt extensions are prepared entirely in enamel.

When the proximal portion of a Class II preparation for an onlay is being prepared and the lingual wall is partially or totally missing, the retention form normally provided by this wall can be developed with a skirt extension of the facial margin (Fig. 17-30, *A* through *C*). Similarly, if the facial wall is not retentive, a skirt extension of the lingual margin supplies the desired retention form (see Fig. 17-25, *O* and *P*). When the lingual and facial walls of a proximal box are inadequate, skirt extensions on the respective lingual and facial margins can satisfy the retention and resistance form requirements. The addition of properly prepared skirts to three of four line angles of the tooth virtually eliminates the chance of post-restorative fracture of the tooth because the skirting onlay is primarily an extracoronal restoration that encompasses and braces the tooth against forces that might otherwise split the tooth. The skirting onlay is often used successfully for many teeth that exhibit split-tooth syndrome.

The addition of skirt extensions also is recommended when the proximal surface contour and contact are to be extended more than the normal dimension to develop a proximal contact. Extending these proximal margins onto the respective facial and lingual surfaces aids in recontouring the proximal surface to this increased dimension. Also, when improving the

occlusal plane of a mesially tilted molar by a cusp-capping onlay, reshaping the mesial surface to a satisfactory contour and contact is facilitated when the mesiofacial and mesiolingual margins are extended generously.

Skirting also is recommended when splinting posterior teeth together with onlays. The added retention and resistance forms are desirable because of the increased stress on each unit. Because the facial and lingual proximal margins are extended generously, the ease of soldering the connector and finishing of the proximal margins is increased.

A disadvantage of skirting is that it increases the display of metal on the facial and lingual surfaces of the tooth. For this reason, skirts are not placed on the mesiofacial margin of maxillary premolars and first molars. Skirting the remaining three line angles of the tooth provides ample retention and resistance forms.

The preparation of a skirt is done entirely with the slender, flame-shaped, fine-grit diamond instrument. Skirt preparations follow the completion of the proximal gingival bevel and primary flares. Experienced operators often prepare the skirt extensions at the same time that the gingival bevel is placed, however, working from the lingual toward the facial, or vice versa. Maintaining the long axis of the instrument parallel to the line of draw, the operator translates the rotating instrument into the tooth to create a definite vertical margin, just beyond the line angle of the tooth, providing at the same time a 140-degree cavosurface enamel angle (40-degree metal angle) (see Fig. 17-30, *D* through *F*). The occlusogingival length of this entrance cut varies, depending on the length of the clinical crown and the amount of extracoronal retention and resistance forms desired. Extending into the gingival third of the anatomic crown is usually necessary for an effective

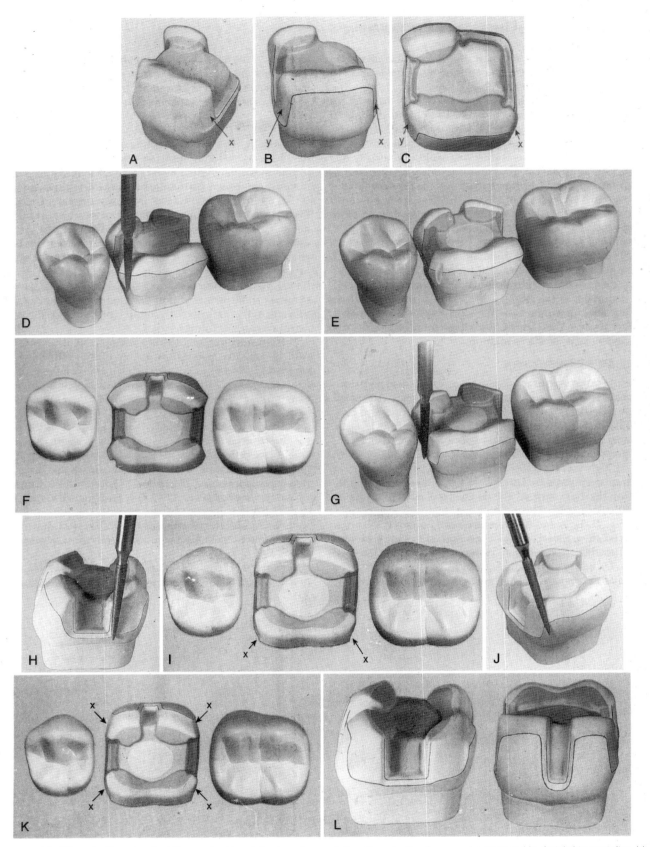

Fig. 17-30 A, When the lingual wall of the proximal box is inadequate or missing, the retention form can be improved by facial skirt extension (*x*). **B,** Facio-occlusal view of *A*. Maximal resistance form is developed by skirting the distofacial (*y*) and mesiofacial (*x*) transitional line angles. **C,** Occlusal view of *B*. **D–F,** The initial cut for the skirt is placed just past the transitional line angle of the tooth. **G** and **H,** Blending the skirt into the primary flare. **G** and **H,** Blending the skirt into the primary flare. **I,** Occlusal view showing the mesiolingual and distolingual skirts. Caution is exercised to prevent the over-reduction of transitional line angles (*x*). Facial surface groove extension also improves the retention and resistance forms. **J,** The junction of the skirt and the counterbevel is slightly rounded. **K,** Skirting all four transitional line angles of the tooth further enhances the retention and resistance forms. Caution is exercised to prevent the over-reduction of transitional line angles (*x*). **L,** Mesial and facial views of the preparation shown in *K*.

resistance form. In most instances, the gingival margin of the skirt extension is occlusal to the position of the gingival bevel of the proximal box (see Fig. 17-30, *H* and *L*).

The operator should use less than half the tip diameter of the flame-shaped diamond instrument to avoid creating a ledge at the gingival margin of the skirt extension. Using high speed and maintaining the long axis of the diamond instrument parallel with the line of draw, the operator translates the instrument from the entrance cut toward the proximal box to blend the skirt into the primary flare and the proximal gingival margin (see Fig. 17-30, *G* and *H*). The operator must ensure that the line angle of the tooth is not over-reduced when preparing skirt extensions (see *x* in Fig. 17-30, *I* and *K*). If the line angle of the tooth is over-reduced, the bracing effect of the skirt is diminished. Holding the diamond instrument at the same angle that was used for preparing the counterbevel, the operator rounds the junction between the skirt and the counterbevel (see Fig. 17-30, *J*). Any sharp angles that remain after preparation of the skirt need to be rounded slightly because these angles often lead to difficulties in the subsequent steps of the restoration.

COLLAR PREPARATION

To increase the retention and resistance forms when preparing a weakened tooth for a mesio-occluso-distal onlay to cap all cusps, a facial or lingual "collar" or both may be provided (Fig. 17-31). To reduce the display of metal, however, the facial surfaces of maxillary premolars and first molars usually are not prepared for a collar. The operator uses a No. 271 carbide bur at high speed parallel to the line of draw to prepare a 0.8 mm–deep shoulder (equivalent to the diameter of the tip end of the bur) around the lingual (or facial) surface to provide for a collar about 2 to 3 mm high occlusogingivally (see Fig. 17-31, *A* and *B*). To provide for a uniform thickness of metal, the occlusal 1 mm of this reduction should be prepared to follow the original contour of the tooth (see Fig. 17-31, *C*), and any undesirable sharp line angle formed by the union of the prepared lingual and occlusal surfaces should be

rounded. This aspect of the preparation is completed by lightly beveling the gingival margin of the shoulder with the flame-shaped, fine-grit diamond instrument to achieve a 30-degree metal angle at the margin (see Fig. 17-31, *D*).

SLOT PREPARATION

Occasionally, the use of a slot in dentin is helpful in creating the necessary retention form. An example is the mandibular second molar that has no molar posterior to it and requires a mesio-occlusal onlay restoration that caps all of the cusps (Fig. 17-32, *A* through *C*). The distal, facial, and lingual surfaces are free of caries or other injury, and these surfaces also are judged not to be prone to caries. After cusp reduction, the vertical walls of the occlusal step portion of the preparation have been reduced so as to provide very little retention form. The necessary retention can be achieved by cutting a distal slot. Such a slot is preferred over preparing a box in the distal surface because (1) the former is more conserving of the tooth structure and of the strength of the tooth crown, and (2) the linear extent of marginal outline is less.

To form this slot, the dentist uses a No. 169L carbide bur with its long axis parallel to the line of draw (this must be reasonably close to a line parallel with the long axis of the tooth) (see Fig. 17-32, *A*). The slot is cut in dentin so that it would pass midway between the pulp and the DEJ if it were to be extended gingivally (see Fig. 17-32, *C*). The position and direction of the slot thus avert (1) the exposure of the pulp, (2) the removal of the dentin supporting the distal enamel, and (3) the perforation of the distal surface of the tooth at the gingival termination of the slot. The slot should have the following approximate dimensions: (1) the width (diameter) of the bur mesiodistally; (2) 2 mm faciolingually; and (3) a depth of 2 mm gingival of the normally positioned pulpal wall. To be effective, the mesial wall of the slot must be in sound dentin; otherwise, the retention form obtained is insufficient.

A comparable situation occurs occasionally: The maxillary first premolar requires a disto-occlusal onlay restoration to

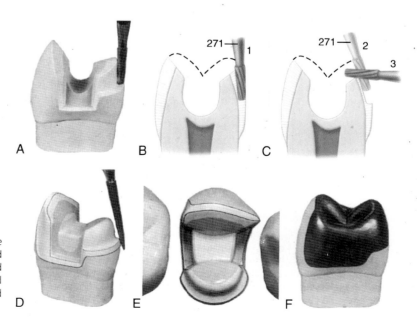

Fig. 17-31 **A,** First position of the bur in preparing for the lingual collar on a weakened maxillary premolar. **B** and **C,** Section drawings of the first position of the bur (*B*) and the second and third positions (*C*). **D,** Beveling the lingual margin. Note the distofacial skirt extension. **E,** Completed preparation. **F,** Completed onlay.

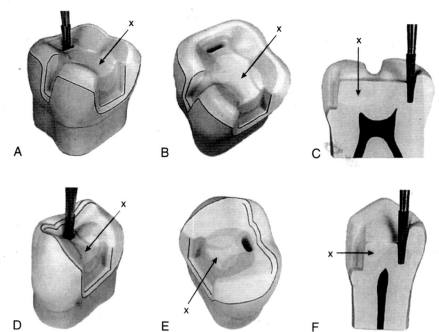

Fig. 17-32 **A** and **B,** Cutting a distal slot for the retention for the mesio-occlusal onlay to treat the terminal molar having a large cement base (*x*) resulting from extensive occlusal and mesial caries. **C,** Section of *A.* **D** and **E,** Preparing a mesial slot for the retention for the disto-occlusal onlay to treat the maxillary first premolar that has a large cement base (*x*). **F,** Section of *D.*

cap the cusps, and the mesial surface is non-carious and deemed not prone to caries (see Fig. 17-32, *D* through *F*). To reduce the display of metal and to conserve the tooth structure, a slot similar to that described in the preceding paragraph (except that it is mesially positioned and 1.5 mm wide faciolingually) may be used for the production of adequate retention. The mesio-occlusal marginal outline in this preparation should be distal of the height of the mesial marginal ridge.

MODIFICATIONS FOR ESTHETICS ON MAXILLARY PREMOLARS AND FIRST MOLARS

To minimize the display of metal on maxillary premolars and first molars, several modifications for esthetics are made to the basic onlay preparation. On the facial cusps of maxillary premolars and on the mesiofacial cusp of the maxillary first molar, the occlusal reduction should be only 0.75 to 1 mm on the facial cusp ridge to minimize the display of metal. This thickness should increase progressively to 1.5 mm toward the center of the tooth to provide rigidity to the capping metal. These cusps do not receive a counterbevel but are "stubbed" or blunted by the application of a sandpaper disk or the fine-grit diamond instrument held at a right angle to the facial surface (see Fig. 17-23, *C*). The surface created by this blunting should be approximately 0.5 mm in width.

To further decrease the display of metal on maxillary premolars and first molars, the mesiofacial margin is minimally extended facially of the contact to such a position that the margin is barely visible from a facial viewing position. To accomplish this, the secondary flare is omitted, and the wall and margin are developed with a chisel or enamel hatchet. Final smoothing with the fine-grit paper disk is recommended when access permits. The cavosurface margin should result in a gold angle of 40 to 50 degrees, if possible.

When more than ideal extension of the mesiofacial margin is necessary because of caries or previous restorations, and as dictated by the esthetic desires of the patient, the operator may choose to place a composite insert at this margin. This is a more conservative option than preparing the tooth to receive a porcelain-veneered metal crown. When preparing the mesiofacial margin, no attempt is made to develop a straight mesiofacial wall past the point of ideal extension. After caries excavation, a glass ionomer cement base is inserted to temporarily form the missing portion of the wall. The cement is contoured to the ideal form, and the preparation can continue, terminating the mesiofacial onlay margin in the ideal position in the cement. After cementation, the operator removes (with small round burs) the glass ionomer cement to a depth of 1 mm for a composite insert. Small undercuts should be prepared in the wall formed by the cast metal onlay (see Fig. 17-57, *A*). (It is best to carve the undercut in the wall formed by the onlay during the wax pattern stage.) After beveling the enamel cavosurface margin and preparing a gingival retention groove where, and if, enamel is thin or missing, the composite veneer is inserted (see Fig. 17-62, *A*).

ENDODONTICALLY TREATED TEETH

Routinely, teeth that have had endodontic treatment are weak and subject to fracture from occlusal forces. These teeth require restorations designed to provide protection from this injury (see Fig. 17-30, *K* and *L*). This particularly applies to posterior teeth, which are subjected to greater stress. The need for such protection is accentuated when much of the strength of the tooth has been lost because of extensive caries or previous restorations. When the facial and lingual surfaces of an endodontically treated tooth are sound, it is more conservative, for the health of the facial and lingual gingival tissue, to prepare the tooth not for a full crown, but for a full occlusal coverage onlay that has been designed with adequate resistance form to prevent future tooth fracture. Such features include skirt extensions and collar preparations. These features make the onlay more of an extracoronal restoration that encompasses the tooth such that the tooth is better

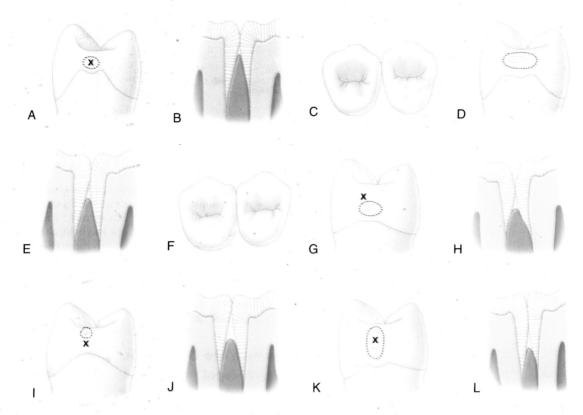

Fig. 17-50 **A–C,** Correct contact. Note the position and form of the contact and the form of the embrasures around the contact. The mesial and distal pits are below (gingival of) the proximal marginal ridges. **D–F,** Contact too broad faciolingually. **G** and **H,** Contact positioned too far gingivally. **I** and **J,** Contact too close to the occlusal surface. **K** and **L,** Contact too broad occlusogingivally. *(Modified from Black GV: Operative dentistry, vol 2, ed 8, Woodstock, IL, 1947, Medico-Dental.)*

To complete the occlusal wax-up, wax is added (where appropriate) to the fossae until they contact the opposing centric-holding cusps (see Fig. 17-51, *I*). Spillways for the movement of food are established by carving appropriately placed grooves. Flat-plane occlusal relationships are not desired.

This technique is a systematic and practical method of waxing the occlusal aspect of the pattern into proper occlusion. Forming one small portion at a time results in waxing each portion into proper occlusion before adding another, which simplifies the procedure. Building the occlusal aspect by such small increments should help develop a pattern with minimal stress and distortion. Whenever a large portion of wax is added, it creates a potential for pattern distortion caused by the large shrinkage of such an addition.

For establishing stable occlusal relationships, the operator should take care to place the cusp tips against flat plateaus or into fossae on the stone cast of the opposing teeth. In other areas, the wax is shaped to simulate normal tooth contours, using adjacent teeth as references. Some relief between the opposing cusp inclines should be provided because these incline contacts often interfere during mandibular movements. The maximum intercuspation record provides only information regarding the position of the opposing teeth in maximum intercuspation. Some adjustment to the casting may be necessary in the mouth to eliminate interferences during mandibular movements. See Chapter 1 for the

principles of cusp and fossa placement when using full-arch casts mounted on a semi-adjustable articulator.

Finishing the Wax Pattern

Careful attention to good technique is required for waxing the margins of the wax pattern. There must be a continuous adaptation of wax to the margins, with no voids, folds, or faults. If adaptation is questionable, the marginal wax should be re-melted to a distance into the pattern of approximately 2 mm. Finger pressure is applied immediately after surface solidification and before subsequent cooling of the wax, with pressure maintained for at least 4 seconds. This finger pressure helps develop close adaptation to the die by offsetting the cooling shrinkage of the wax. Additional wax should be added during the re-melting procedure to ensure a slight excess of contour and extension beyond the margin.

Wax that is along the margins is now carved back to the cavosurface outline with a warmed No. 7 wax spatula (Fig. 17-52, *A* through *E*). This warming of the spatula permits carving of the marginal wax with light pressure so that the stone margins are not damaged. A little practice helps the operator determine how much to heat the instrument for easy and effective carving. The No. 7 spatula should not have sharp edges; when it touches the die lightly, it should not abrade or injure the die surface. The operator uses the die surface just beyond the cavosurface margin to guide the position and

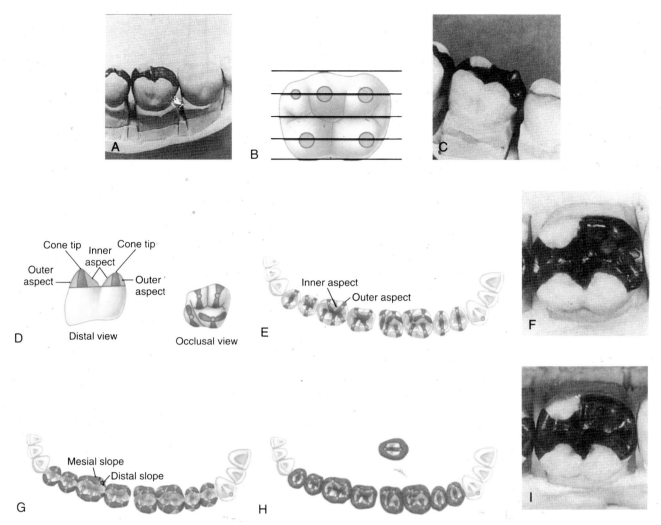

Fig. 17-51 A, The pattern base is completed and ready for waxing two reduced cusps (distolingual and distal) into occlusion by using Payne's waxing technique. **B,** The facial cusps are located on the first facial quarter line, and the lingual cusps fall on the first lingual quarter line. **C,** The distolingual and distal cusp tips are waxed into occlusion in the form of small cones. **D,** Cone tips and inner and outer aspects. **E,** Cone tips and inner and outer aspects of the cusps of teeth. **F,** The inner and outer aspects of the distolingual and distal cusps have been added to the pattern base. **G,** The mesial and distal slopes of the cusps of teeth. **H,** Marginal ridges of teeth. **I,** After the marginal ridge is added to the pattern base, fossae are waxed in, and grooves are carved to complete the wax pattern. *(Modified from Payne E: Reproduction of tooth form,* Ney Tech Bull *1, 1961.)*

direction of the carving instrument. The direction of the instrument movement is not dictated by the margin but by the contour of the unprepared tooth (die) surface just beyond the margin. The instrument blade is held parallel to this surface and used as a guide for the contour of the pattern near the margin; this should result in a continuity of contour across the margin. This principle of carving is too often neglected, resulting in the contour errors (see *x* in Fig. 17-52, *B* through *D*); correct application of the carving instrument results in correct contours (exemplified by *y*). The completed patterns are shown in Figure 17-52, *F* through *I*.

On accessible surfaces of the carved pattern, satisfactory smoothness can be imparted by a few strokes with the end of a finger if surfaces have been carefully carved with the No. 7 spatula. Rubbing with cotton that has been twisted onto a round toothpick may smooth less accessible surfaces such as grooves.

Initial Withdrawal and Reseating of the Wax Pattern

Care must be exercised when initially withdrawing the wax pattern from the die. The wax can be dislodged by holding the die and pattern as shown in Figure 17-53. When the pattern has been dislodged, it should be removed gently from the preparation. The operator should inspect the preparation side of the pattern to see if any wrinkles or holes are present. Such voids indicate poor wax adaptation and should be corrected if they are (1) in critical regions of the preparation designed to provide the retention form, (2) numerous, or (3) closer than 1 mm to the margin. To eliminate these voids, the operator first re-lubricates the die and reseats the pattern on the die. Then, a hot instrument is passed through the wax to the unadapted area. This usually results in the air (void) rising through the liquid wax to the pattern's surface as the wax takes

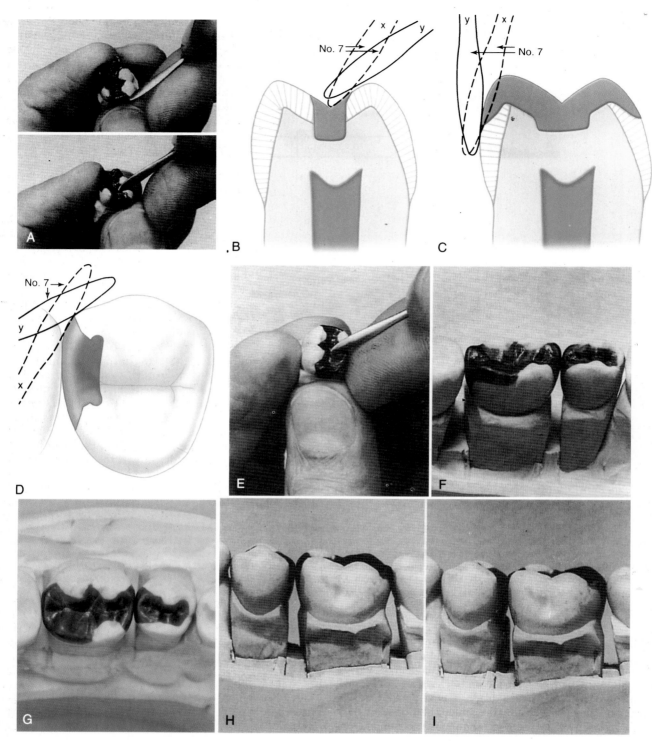

Fig. 17-52 **A,** Wax is carved to margins with a warm No. 7 spatula. **B–D,** Incorrect application of No. 7 spatula to carve the contour of the marginal wax is shown by *x*; the correct manner is labeled *y*. **E,** Carving the occlusal groove and pit anatomy. **F,** The adjacent marginal ridges should be on the same level as much as possible. **G,** Occlusal view of completed patterns. Note the shape of the facial and lingual embrasures and the position of the contact. **H** and **I,** Facial view of the completed patterns. Note the gingival and occlusal embrasures and the position of the contact.

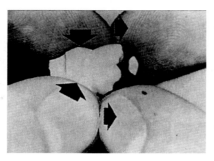

Fig. 17-53 Removing the wax pattern by using indirect finger pressure. Arrows indicate the direction of the pressure. Care must be exercised not to squeeze and distort the wax pattern as it is initially withdrawn.

the place of the air. A consequence of this correcting procedure on the occlusal surface is the obliteration of the occlusal carving in the affected region, requiring the addition of wax, re-carving, and rechecking the occlusion.

Spruing, Investing, and Casting

If a delay of several hours or more occurs between the forming of the wax pattern and the investing procedure, the pattern should remain on the die, and the margins should be inspected carefully again before spruing and investing. When such a delay is contemplated, it is suggested that the sprue be added to the pattern before the delay period. If the addition of the sprue caused the induction of enough stress to produce pattern distortion, such a condition is more evident after the rest period, and corrective waxing can be instituted before investing. The reader is referred to textbooks on dental materials for the principles and techniques of spruing, investing, casting, and cleaning the casting. All investment must be removed from the casting, and it should be properly pickled.

Seating, Adjusting, and Polishing the Casting

It is crucial to examine the casting closely, preferably under magnification, before testing the fit on the die. The internal and external surfaces should be examined with good lighting to identify any traces of investment, positive defects (blebs), or negative defects (voids). Voids in critical areas indicate rejection of the casting, unless they can be corrected by soldering. Any small positive defects on the internal surface should be carefully removed with an appropriately sized round bur in the high-speed handpiece.

The casting is then trial-fitted on the die before removing the sprue and sprue button, which serve as a handle to remove the casting, if removal is necessary. The casting should seat with little or no pressure (Fig. 17-54, *A*). Ideally, when being placed on the die, it should have the same feel as the feel of the wax pattern when it was seated on the die. If the casting fails to seat completely, it should be removed, and the die surface should be inspected for small scratches to see where it is binding. Usually, failure to seat is caused by small positive defects not seen on the first inspection. Attempts at forcing the casting into place cause irreparable damage to the die and difficulties when trial-seating the casting in the mouth.

After the accuracy of the casting is found to be satisfactory, the casting is separated from the sprue, as close to the inlay as possible, using a carborundum separating disk. The cut should be made twice as wide as the thickness of the disk to prevent binding and should not cut completely through the sprue (a small uncut portion should be left) (see Fig. 17-54, *B*). If the cut is made completely through, control of the disk is sometimes lost, often resulting in damage to the casting or to the operator's fingers. The uncut portion should be so small that bending with the fingers breaks it with very little effort (see Fig. 17-54, *C*).

Having seated the casting on the die, the technician hand burnishes the marginal metal using a ball or beaver-tail burnisher (see Fig. 17-54, *D*). An area approximately 1 mm in width is burnished, using strokes that increasingly approach the marginal metal and are directed parallel to the margin. Burnishing improves marginal adaptation and begins the smoothing process, almost imparting a polish to this rubbed surface. While burnishing, the adaptation of the casting along the margin is continually assessed by using magnification, as needed, to see any marginal opening 0.05 mm in size. Moderate pressure during burnishing is indicated during closure of small marginal gaps. When the casting is well adapted, pressure is reduced to a gentle rubbing for continued smoothing of the metal surface. At this stage, marginal openings and irregularities should not be detectable even under (×1.5 or ×2) magnification (see Fig. 17-54, *E* and *F*). Care must be taken not to over-burnish the metal because this can crush and destroy the underlying die surface. Over-burnished metal prevents complete seating of the casting on the prepared tooth. Proper burnishing usually improves the retention of the casting on the die so that the casting does not come loose during subsequent polishing steps. A casting must not be loose on the die if the inlay is to be polished properly.

The remaining sprue metal is carefully removed with a heatless stone or a carborundum disk (see Fig. 17-54, *G* and *H*). The grooves are accentuated by lightly applying a dull No. 1 round bur (see Fig. 17-54, *I*) or other appropriate rotary instrument. Next, a knife-edge rubber polishing wheel is used on accessible surfaces (see Fig. 17-54, *J*) (Flexie rubber disk, Dedico International Inc., Long Eddy, NY). The operator should guard against the polishing wheel touching the margins and the die because both can be unknowingly and quickly polished away, resulting in "short" margins on the tooth. Also, at this time, the proximal contacts are adjusted one at a time. If the distal surface of a mesio-occluso-distal casting on the first molar is being adjusted, only the first and second molar dies are on the cast. Proximal contacts are deemed correct when they are the correct size, correctly positioned, and passive. If a temporary restoration was made properly, these contact relationships would be the same in the mouth as on the cast. Chairtime can be reduced by carefully finishing the contacts on the cast.

The occlusion of the castings is checked by marking the occlusal contacts with articulating paper. Any premature contacts are corrected, and their locations are refined by selective grinding. Often, prematurities occur where the sprue was attached and insufficient sprue metal was removed. The operator applies a smaller, rubber, knife-edge wheel, which should reach some of the remaining areas not accessible to the larger disk (Fig. 17-55, *A* and *B*). The grooves, pits, and other most

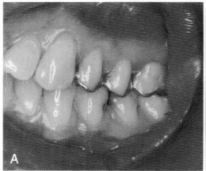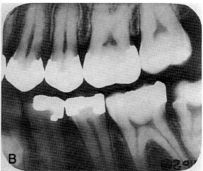

Fig. 17-62 A, Cemented castings on teeth first shown in Figure 17-41, *E.* This photo was taken immediately after cementation and insertion of the composite insert on the molar. **B,** Bitewing radiograph of the restored quadrant shown in *A.* Note the fit of inlays at the gingival margins and the contour of the proximal surfaces.

Cementation
Cement Selection

The selection of cement for permanent cementation is crucial to the success of the final restoration. The advantages and disadvantages of each cement are discussed in the chapter on dental materials. No cement is without shortcomings. Each product has specific requirements with regard to tooth surface conditioning, casting surface conditioning, and manipulation techniques. To obtain optimal performance from the cement, the dentist should carefully follow the manufacturer's instructions for dispensing, mixing, and application.

Cementation Technique

Before cementing the casting, the tooth is isolated from saliva with the aid of cotton rolls (and saliva ejector, if necessary) (Fig. 17-61, *A*). With the air syringe, the dentist dries the preparation walls but does not desiccate them. This air should eliminate visible moisture from the walls except possibly on the gingival bevel. The cement is mixed according to the manufacturer's instructions. With the cement mix applied generously to the preparation side of the casting (see Fig. 17-61, *B*), the dentist starts to place the casting with the fingers or with operative pliers. Next, the dentist places the ball burnisher in the pit areas (first one and then another), exerting firm pressure to seat the casting (see Fig. 17-61, *C*). The dentist places a small flexible rubber polishing disk over the casting, removes the saliva ejector, and requests the patient to close and exert biting force (see Fig. 17-61, *D* and *E*). The patient also is asked to move the mandible slightly from side to side, while continuing to exert pressure. A few seconds of this pressure is sufficient. When the disk is removed, much of the occlusal area should be clean of the cement mix and easier to inspect and to verify complete seating of the casting. When the cusps are capped, complete seating of the casting is verified by inspection of the facial and lingual margins after wiping the excess cement away (see Fig. 17-61, *F*). While the cement is still soft, all accessible margins are burnished. The saliva ejector is replaced in the mouth and the region kept dry during the setting of the cement. Excess moisture during this setting reaction can weaken many types of cement.

After the cement has hardened, any excess is cleaned off with an explorer and air-water spray. Dental floss should be passed through the contact, carried into the interproximal gingival embrasures and sulci, and pulled facially and lingually to help in the removal of cement in this region (see Fig. 17-61, *G*). Tying a small knot in the floss helps dislodge small bits of interproximal cement. Finally, directing a stream of air into the gingival sulcus opens it and reveals any remaining small pieces of cement, which should be removed. When cementing has been properly accomplished, a cement line should not be visible at the margins (see Fig. 17-61, *H*). A quadrant of inlays after cementation is illustrated in Figure 17-62.

Repair

The weak link of most cast metal inlays and onlays is the cement seal. At times, the operator may find discrepancies at margins that require replacement or repair. If the restoration is intact and retentive and if the defective margin area is small and accessible, small repairs can be attempted with amalgam or composite. If cement loss is found in one area of the restoration, however, other areas are usually suspect. When defects are found, the most common procedure is to remove the defective restoration and replace it.

Summary

Cast metal inlays and onlays offer excellent restorations that may be under-used in dentistry. The technique requires multiple patient visits and excellent laboratory support, but the resulting restorations are durable and long lasting. High noble alloys are desirable for patients concerned with allergy or sensitivity to other restorative materials. Cast metal onlays, in particular, can be designed to strengthen the restored tooth while conserving more tooth structure than does a full crown. Disadvantages such as high cost and esthetics limit their use, but when indicated, cast metal inlays and onlays provide a restorative option that is less damaging to pulpal and periodontal tissues compared with a full crown.

References

1. Donovan T, Simonsen RJ, Guertin G, et al: Retrospective clinical evaluation of 1,314 cast gold restorations in service from 1 to 52 years. *J Esthet Restor Dent* 16(3):194–204, 2004.
2. Wataha JC: Biocompatibility of dental casting alloys: A review. *J Prosthet Dent* 83:223–234, 2000.
3. Stanley HR: Effects of dental restorative materials: local and systemic responses reviewed. *J Am Dent Assoc* 124:76–80, 1993.

4. Hood JA: Biomechanics of the intact, prepared and restored tooth: Some clinical implications. *Int Dent J* 41:25–32, 1991.

5. Carson J, Rider T, Nash D: A thermographic study of heat distribution during ultra-speed cavity preparation. *J Dent Res* 58(7):1681–1684, 1979.

6. Fisher DW, Caputo AA, Shillingburg H, et al: Photoelastic analysis of inlay and onlay preparations. *J Prosthet Dent* 33:47–53, 1975.

7. Payne E: Reproduction of tooth form. *Ney Tech Bull* 1, 1961.

8. Grajower R, Shaharbani S, Kaufman E: Temperature rise in pulp chamber during fabrication of temporary self-curing resin crowns. *J Prosthet Dent* 41:535–540, 1979.

9. Hume WR: A new technique for screening chemical toxicity to the pulp from dental restorative materials and procedures. *J Dent Res* 64:1322–1325, 1985.

10. Moulding MB, Loney RW: The effect of cooling techniques on intrapulpal temperature during direct fabrication of provisional restorations. *Int J Prosthodont* 4:332–336, 1991.

11. Crispin BL, Watson JF, Caputo AA: The marginal accuracy of treatment restorations: A comparative analysis. *J Prosthet Dent* 44:283–290, 1980.

12. Malamed SF: *Handbook of local anesthesia*, ed 5, St. Louis, 2005, Mosby.

13. Dawson PE: A classification system for occlusions that relates maximal intercuspation to the position and condition of the temporomandibular joints. *J Prosthet Dent* 75:60–66, 1996.

Index

Page numbers followed by "f" indicate figures, "t" indicate tables, and "b" indicate boxes.